Lecture Notes in Computer Science　　　7766

Commenced Publication in 1973
Founding and Former Series Editors:
Gerhard Goos, Juris Hartmanis, and Jan van Leeuwen

T0074257

Bjoern H. Menze   Georg Langs
Le Lu   Albert Montillo   Zhuowen Tu
Antonio Criminisi (Eds.)

Medical Computer Vision

Recognition Techniques and Applications
in Medical Imaging

Second International MICCAI Workshop, MCV 2012
Nice, France, October 5, 2012
Revised Selected Papers

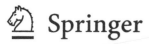 Springer

Volume Editors

Bjoern H. Menze
ETH Zurich, Sternwartstrasse 7, 8092 Zürich, Switzerland
E-mail: bjoern@ethz.ch

Georg Langs
Medical University of Vienna, Währinger Gürtel 18-20, 1090 Wien, Austria
E-mail: georg.langs@meduniwien.ac.at

Le Lu
Siemens Corporate Research, 755 College Road East, Princeton, NJ 08540, USA
E-mail: le-lu@siemens.com

Albert Montillo
GE Global Research, 1 Research Circle, Niskayuna, NY 12309, USA
E-mail: montillo@ge.com

Zhuowen Tu
University of California, 635 Charles E. Young Drive South
Los Angeles, CA 90095-7334, USA
E-mail: zhuowen.tu@loni.ucla.edu

Antonio Criminisi
Microsoft Research, 7 JJ Thomson Avenue, Cambridge, CB3 0FB, UK
E-mail: antcrim@microsoft.com

ISSN 0302-9743   ISSN 1611-3349
ISBN 978-3-642-36619-2   ISBN 978-3-642-36620-8 (eBook)
DOI 10.1007/978-3-642-36620-8
Springer Heidelberg Dordrecht London New York

Library of Congress Control Number: 2013931266

CR Subject Classification (1998): I.4.6-7, I.4.9, I.4.3, I.2.10, I.5.2-4, J.3

LNCS Sublibrary: SL 6 – Image Processing, Computer Vision, Pattern Recognition,
and Graphics

Typesetting: Camera-ready by author, data conversion by Scientific Publishing Services, Chennai, India

Printed on acid-free paper

Springer is part of Springer Science+Business Media (www.springer.com)

Preface

The Second MICCAI Workshop on Medical Computer Vision (MICCAI-MCV 2012) was held in conjunction with the 15th International Conference on Medical Image Computing and Computer-Assisted Intervention (MICCAI) on October 5, 2012 in Nice, France. It succeeded the First Workshop on Medical Computer Vision that was held in September 2010 in conjunction with MICCAI 2010 in Beijing.

The workshop aimed at exploring the use of modern computer vision technology in tasks such as automatic segmentation and registration, localization of anatomical features and detection of anomalies, as well as 3D reconstruction and biophysical model personalization. In this it focuses on principled approaches that go beyond the limits of current model-driven image analysis, which are provably efficient and scalable, and which generalize well to previously unseen images.

The goal of the workshop was to foster discussions among researchers working on novel computational approaches at the interface of computer vision, machine learning, and medical image analysis, and who are interested in pushing the boundaries of what current medical software applications can deliver in both clinical and medical research settings. To this end we invited Nikos Paragios from INRIA and Ecole Centrale Paris and Nassir Navab from TU Munich to discuss challenges and opportunities lying at the interface of medical computer vision and "classic" computer vision. The following panel discussion with the invited speakers – in which Nicholas Ayache, INRIA Sophia-Antipolis, and Simon Mercer, Microsoft Research, joined in – dealt with the following questions:

- How do we turn research into clinical use? How do we turn research into products?
- How do we make data available to the broader research community?
- What makes medical imaging data special compared to classic computer vision data and problems?
- How would we set up large data sets for training efficient computer vision like algorithms? And is this a good idea at all?
- How do we solve the annotation problem? What are perspectives in times of mechanical turk? What are effective incentives for clinical collaborators to share knowledge and to annotate data image?

Central to the workshop were the contributions of the participants. Our call for papers resulted in 42 submissions of up to 12 pages. Each paper received at least three reviews. Based on these peer reviews, we selected 24 submissions for presentation out of which 12 were presented as a poster and 12 as a poster together with a plenary talk. Three talks were awarded the "MCV Best Paper Award" based on the popular vote of the workshop attendees: Herve Lombaert et al. "Groupwise Spectral Log-Demons Framework for Atlas Construction," Tobias Gass et al. "Semi-supervised Segmentation Using Multiple Segmentation Hypotheses from a Single Atlas," and Rene Donner et al. "Fast Anatomical Structure Localization Using Top-down Image Patch Regression."

The present volume contains the reworked papers of the MICCAI-MCV 2012 workshop. It also features four selected papers by Zhong et al., Li et al., Song et al., and Wu et al. that were presented at the previous CVPR Medical Computer Vision Workshop, which was co-organized by L. Lu, B. Menze, G. Langs, Y. Zhan, and Z. Tu and was held in conjunction with the International Conference on Computer Vision and Pattern Recognition on June 21, 2012, in Providence, Rhode Island, USA.

December 2012

Bjoern H. Menze
Georg Langs
Le Lu
Albert Montillo
Zhuowen Tu
Antonio Criminisi

Organization

Workshop Chairs

Bjoern Menze	ETH Zurich, INRIA, Switzerland/France
Georg Langs	MU Vienna, MIT, Austria/USA
Albert Montillo	GE, USA
Zhuowen Tu	UCLA, USA
Antonio Criminisi	Microsoft Research, UK

Invited Speakers

Nassir Navab	TU Munich, Germany
Nikos Paragios	Ecole Centrale Paris, France

Program Committee

Alison Noble	Oxford, UK
Ben Glocker	Microsoft Research, UK
Cagatay Demiralp	Brown University, USA
Christian Barillot	IRISA Rennes, France
Christos Davatzikos	University of Pennsylvania, USA
Daniel Rueckert	Imperial College London, UK
Darko Zikic	Microsoft Research, UK
Ender Konukoglu	Microsoft Research, UK
Hayit Greenspan	Tel Aviv University, Israel
Helmut Grabner	ETH Zurich, Switzerland
Horst Bischof	TU Graz, Austria
Jan Margeta	INRIA, France
Juan Eugenio Iglesias	Harvard MGH, USA
Juergen Gall	Max-Planck Gesellschaft Tübingen, Germany
Kayhan Batmanghelich	MIT, USA
Kilian Pohl	University of Pennsylvania, USA
Koen Van Leemput	Harvard MGH, DTU, USA
Leo Grady	Siemens Corporate Research, USA
Lin Yang	University of Kentucky, USA
Marleen de Bruijne	EMC Rotterdam, University of Copenhagen, The Netherlands/Denmark
Matthew Blaschko	Ecole Centrale Paris, France

Michael Kelm   Siemens Corporate Research, Germany
Michael Wels   Siemens Corporate Research, Germany
Milan Sonka   University of Iowa, USA
Paul Suetens   KU Leuven, Belgium
Rachid Deriche   INRIA, France
Ron Kikinis   Harvard BWH, USA
Sebastian Ourselin   University College London, UK
Tammy Riklin Raviv   Harvard BWH, USA
Tom Vercauteren   Mauna Kea Technology, France
Victor Lempitsky   Yandex, Russia
Yefeng Zheng   Siemens Corporate Research, USA

Table of Contents

Detection, Localization, Tracking

3D Reconstruction

Biophysical Model Personalization

Real-Time 2D/3D Deformable Registration
Using Metric Learning

Chen-Rui Chou[1] and Stephen Pizer[1,2]

[1] Department of Computer Science, University of North Carolina at Chapel Hill,
Chapel Hill, NC 27599, USA
cchou@cs.unc.edu
[2] Department of Radiation Oncology, University of North Carolina at Chapel Hill,
Chapel Hill, NC 27599, USA

Abstract. We present a novel 2D/3D deformable registration method,
called Registration Efficiency and Accuracy through Learning Metric
on Shape (*REALMS*), that can support real-time Image-Guided Radiation Therapy (*IGRT*). The method consists of two stages: planning-time
learning and registration. In the planning-time learning, it firstly models
the patient's 3D deformation space from the patient's time-varying 3D
planning images using a low-dimensional parametrization. Secondly, it
samples deformation parameters within the deformation space and generates corresponding simulated projection images from the deformed 3D
image. Finally, it learns a Riemannian metric in the projection space
for each deformation parameter. The learned distance metric forms a
Gaussian kernel of a kernel regression that minimizes the leave-one-out
regression residual of the corresponding deformation parameter. In the
registration, REALMS interpolates the patient's 3D deformation parameters using the kernel regression with the learned distance metrics. Our
test results showed that REALMS can localize the tumor in 10.89 ms
(91.82 fps) with 2.56 ± 1.11 mm errors using a single projection image.
These promising results show REALMS's high potential to support real-
time, accurate, and low-dose IGRT.

1   Introduction

Tumor localization in 3D is the main goal of Image-guided Radiation Therapy (*IGRT*). It is usually accomplished by computing the patient's treatment-
time 3D deformations based on an on-board imaging system, usually x-ray. The
treatment-time 3D deformations can be computed by doing image registration
between the treatment-time reconstructed 3D image and the treatment-planning
3D image (3D/3D registration) or between the treatment-time on-board projection images and the treatment-planning 3D image (2D/3D registration). Recent
advances of the IGRT registration methods emphasize real-time computation
and low-dose image acquisition. Russakoff et al. [1,2], Khamene et al. [3], Munbodh et al. [4], Li et al. [5,6] rejected the time-consuming 3D/3D registration
and performed 2D/3D registration by optimizing similarity functions defined in

H. Menze et al. (Eds.): MCV 2012, LNCS 7766, pp. 1–10, 2013.
Springer-Verlag Berlin Heidelberg 2013

the projection domain. Other than the optimization-based methods, Chou et al. [7,8] recently introduced a faster and low-dose 2D/3D image registration by using a linear operator that approximates the deformation parameters. However, all of the above registration methods involve computationally demanding production of Digitally-Reconstructed Radiographs ($DRRs$) in each registration iteration (e.g., 15ms on a modern GPU to produce a 256×256 DRR from a $256 \times 256 \times 256$ volume [9]), which makes them difficult to be extended to support real-time (> 30 fps) image registration.

We present a novel real-time 2D/3D registration method, called Registration Efficiency and Accuracy through Learning Metric on Shape ($REALMS$), that does not require DRR production in the registration. It calculates the patient's treatment-time 3D deformations by kernel regression. Specifically, each of the patient's deformation parameters is interpolated using a weighting Gaussian kernel on that parameter's training case values. In each training case, its parameter value is associated with a corresponding training projection image. The Gaussian kernel is formed from distances between training projection images. This distance for the parameter in question involves a Riemannian metric on projection image differences. At planning time, REALMS learns the parameter-specific metrics from the set of training projection images using a Leave-One-Out (LOO) training.

To the best of our knowledge, REALMS is the first 2D/3D deformable registration method that achieves real-time (> 30 fps) performance. REALMS uses the metric learning idea firstly introduced in Weinberger and Tesauro [10] to tackle the 2D/3D image registration problem. Particularly, in order to make the metric learning work for the high dimensional ($D \gg 10^3$) projection space, REALMS uses a specially-designed initialization approximated by linear regression. The results have led to substantial error reduction when the special initialization is applied.

The rest of the paper is organized as follows: In section 2, we describe REALMS's novel registration scheme that uses kernel regression. In section 3, we describe its deformation space modeling approach for generating training samples in the deformation space. In section 4, we describe the metric learning scheme and the specialized initialization in REALMS. We show our synthetic and real results in section 5. Finally, we discuss the results and conclude in section 6.

2   2D/3D Registration Framework

In this section, we describe REALMS's 2D/3D registration framework. REALMS uses kernel regression (eq. 1) to interpolate the patient's n 3D deformation parameters $\mathbf{c} = (c^1, c^2, \cdots, c^n)$ separately from the on-board projection image $\mathbf{\Psi}(\theta)$ where θ is the projection angle. It uses a Gaussian kernel $K_{\mathbf{M}^i, \sigma^i}$ with the width σ^i and a metric tensor $\mathbf{M}^i$ on projection intensity differences to interpolate the patient's i^{th} deformation parameter c^i from a set of N training projection images $\{\mathbf{P}(I \circ T(\mathbf{c}_\kappa); \theta) \mid \kappa = 1, 2, \cdots, N\}$ simulated at planning time. Specifically, the training projection image, $\mathbf{P}(I \circ T(\mathbf{c}_\kappa); \theta)$, is the DRR of a 3D image deformed from the patient's planning-time 3D mean image I with sampled deformation parameters $\mathbf{c}_\kappa = (c_\kappa^1, c_\kappa^2, \cdots, c_\kappa^n)$. T and $\mathbf{P}$ are the warping and the DRR operators, respectively. $\mathbf{P}$ simulates the DRRs according to the treatment-time imaging geometry, e.g., the projection angle θ.

In the treatment-time registration, each deformation parameter c^i in $\mathbf{c}$ can be estimated with the following kernel regression:

$$c^i = \frac{\sum\limits_{\kappa=1}^{N} c_\kappa^i \cdot K_{\mathbf{M}^i, \sigma^i}(\boldsymbol{\Psi}(\theta), \mathbf{P}(I \circ T(\mathbf{c}_\kappa); \theta))}{\sum\limits_{\kappa=1}^{N} K_{\mathbf{M}^i, \sigma^i}(\boldsymbol{\Psi}(\theta), \mathbf{P}(I \circ T(\mathbf{c}_\kappa); \theta))}, \tag{1}$$

$$K_{\mathbf{M}^i, \sigma^i}(\boldsymbol{\Psi}(\theta), \mathbf{P}(I \circ T(\mathbf{c}_\kappa); \theta)) = \frac{1}{\sqrt{2\pi}\sigma^i} e^{-\frac{d^2_{\mathbf{M}^i}(\boldsymbol{\Psi}(\theta), \mathbf{P}(I \circ T(\mathbf{c}_\kappa); \theta))}{2(\sigma^i)^2}}, \tag{2}$$

$$d^2_{\mathbf{M}^i}(\boldsymbol{\Psi}(\theta), \mathbf{P}(I \circ T(\mathbf{c}_\kappa); \theta)) = (\boldsymbol{\Psi}(\theta) - \mathbf{P}(I \circ T(\mathbf{c}_\kappa); \theta))^\mathsf{T} \mathbf{M}^i (\boldsymbol{\Psi}(\theta) - \mathbf{P}(I \circ T(\mathbf{c}_\kappa); \theta)), \tag{3}$$

where $K_{\mathbf{M}^i, \sigma^i}$ is a Gaussian kernel (kernel width= σ^i) that uses a Riemannian metric $\mathbf{M}^i$ in the squared distance $d^2_{\mathbf{M}^i}$ and gives the weights for the parameter interpolation in the regression. The minus signs in eq. 3 denote pixel-by-pixel intensity subtraction.

We describe in section 3 how REALMS, at planning time, parameterizes the deformation space and describe in section 4 how it learns the metric tensor $\mathbf{M}^i$ and decides the kernel width σ^i.

3   Deformation Modeling at Planning Time

REALMS limits the deformation to a shape space. It models deformations as a linear combination of a set of basis deformations calculated through PCA analysis. In our target problem – lung IGRT, a set of Respiratory-Correlated CTs ($RCCTs$, dimension: $512 \times 512 \times 120$) $\{J_\tau \mid \tau = 1, 2, \cdots, 10\}$ are available at planning time. From these a mean image $I = \bar{J}$ and a set of deformations ϕ_τ between J_τ and $\bar{J}$ can be computed. The basis deformations can then be chosen to be the primary eigenmodes of a PCA analysis on the ϕ_τ.

3.1   Deformation Shape Space and Mean Image Generation

REALMS computes a respiratory Fréchet mean image $\bar{J}$ from the RCCT dataset via an $LDDMM$ (Large Deformation Diffeomorphic Metric Mapping) framework described in Lorenzen et al. [11]. The Fréchet mean $\bar{J}$, as well as the diffeomorphic deformations ϕ from the mean $\bar{J}$ to each image J_τ, are computed using a fluid-flow distance metric:

$$\bar{J} = \underset{J}{argmin} \sum_{\tau=1}^{10} \int_0^1 \int_\Omega ||v_{\tau,\gamma}(x)||^2 dx d\gamma + \frac{1}{s^2} \int_\Omega ||J(\phi_\tau^{-1}(x)) - J_\tau(x)||^2 dx, \tag{4}$$

where $J_\tau(x)$ is the intensity of the pixel at position x in the image J_τ, $v_{\tau,\gamma}$ is the fluid-flow velocity field for the image J_τ in flow time γ, s is the weighting variable on the image dissimilarity, and $\phi_\tau(x)$ describes the deformation at the pixel location x: $\phi_\tau(x) = x + \int_0^1 v_{\tau,\gamma}(x)d\gamma$.

3.2 Statistical Analysis

With the diffeomorphic deformation set $\{\phi_\tau \mid \tau = 1, 2, \cdots, 10\}$ calculated, our method finds a set of linear deformation basis vectors ϕ_{pc}^i by PCA analysis. The scores λ_τ^i on each ϕ_{pc}^i yield ϕ_τ in terms of these basis vectors.

$$\phi_\tau = \overline{\phi} + \sum_{i=1}^{10} \lambda_\tau^i \cdot \phi_{pc}^i \tag{5}$$

We choose a subset of n eigenmodes that captures more than 95% of the total variation. Then we let the n scores form the the the n-dimensional parametrization $\mathbf{c}$.

$$\mathbf{c} = (c^1, c^2, \cdots, c^n) = (\lambda^1, \lambda^2, \cdots, \lambda^n) \tag{6}$$

For most of our target problems, $n = 3$ satisfies the requirement.

4 Metric Learning at Planning Time

4.1 Metric Learning and Kernel Width Selection

REALMS learns a metric tensor $\mathbf{M}^i$ with a corresponding kernel width σ^i for the patient's i^{th} deformation parameter c^i using a Leave-One-Out (LOO) training strategy. At planning time, it samples a set of N deformation parameter tuples $\{\mathbf{c}_\kappa = (c_\kappa^1, c_\kappa^2, \cdots, c_\kappa^n) \mid \kappa = 1, 2, \cdots N\}$ to generate training projection images $\{\mathbf{P}(I \circ T(\mathbf{c}_\kappa); \theta) \mid \kappa = 1, 2, \cdots, N\}$ where their associated deformation parameters are sampled uniformly within three standard deviations of the scores λ observed in the RCCTs. For each deformation parameter c^i in $\mathbf{c}$, REALMS finds the best pair of the metric tensor $\mathbf{M}^{i\dagger}$ and the kernel width $\sigma^{i\dagger}$ that minimizes the sum of squared LOO regression residuals $\mathcal{L}_{c^i}$ among the set of N training projection images:

$$\mathbf{M}^{i\dagger}, \sigma^{i\dagger} = \underset{\mathbf{M}^i, \sigma^i}{arg\ min} \mathcal{L}_{c^i}(\mathbf{M}^i, \sigma^i), \tag{7}$$

$$\mathcal{L}_{c^i}(\mathbf{M}^i, \sigma^i) = \sum_{\kappa=1}^N \left(c_\kappa^i - \hat{c}_\kappa^i(\mathbf{M}^i, \sigma^i) \right)^2, \tag{8}$$

$$\hat{c}_\kappa^i(\mathbf{M}^i, \sigma^i) = \frac{\sum_{\chi \neq \kappa} c_\chi^i \cdot K_{\mathbf{M}^i, \sigma^i}(\mathbf{P}(I \circ T(\mathbf{c}_\kappa); \theta), \mathbf{P}(I \circ T(\mathbf{c}_\chi); \theta))}{\sum_{\chi \neq \kappa} K_{\mathbf{M}^i, \sigma^i}(\mathbf{P}(I \circ T(\mathbf{c}_\kappa); \theta), \mathbf{P}(I \circ T(\mathbf{c}_\chi); \theta))}, \tag{9}$$

where $\hat{c}^i_\kappa(\mathbf{M}^i, \sigma^i)$ is the estimated value for parameter c^i_κ interpolated by the metric tensor $\mathbf{M}^i$ and the kernel width σ^i from the training projection images χ other than κ; $\mathbf{M}^i$ needs to be a positive semi-definite $(p.s.d)$ matrix to fulfill the pseudo-metric constraint; and the kernel width σ^i needs to be a positive real number.

To avoid high-dimensional optimization over the constrained matrix $\mathbf{M}^i$, we structure the metric tensor $\mathbf{M}^i$ as a rank-1 matrix formed by a basis vector $\mathbf{a}^i$: $\mathbf{M}^i = \mathbf{a}^i \mathbf{a}^{i\mathsf{T}}$. Therefore, we can transform eq. 7 into a optimization over the unit vector $\mathbf{a}^i$ where $\left\lVert \mathbf{a}^i \right\rVert_2 = 1$:

$$\mathbf{a}^{i\dagger}, \sigma^{i\dagger} = \underset{\mathbf{a}^i, \sigma^i}{arg\,min} \mathcal{L}_{c^i}(\mathbf{a}^i \mathbf{a}^{i\mathsf{T}}, \sigma^i) \tag{10}$$

Then we can rewrite the squared distance $d^2_{\mathbf{M}^i} = d^2_{\mathbf{a}^i \mathbf{a}^{i\mathsf{T}}}$ used in the Gaussian kernel $K_{\mathbf{M}^i, \sigma^i}$ as follows:

$$d^2_{\mathbf{a}^i \mathbf{a}^{i\mathsf{T}}}(\mathbf{P}(I \circ T(\mathbf{c}_\kappa); \theta), \mathbf{P}(I \circ T(\mathbf{c}_\chi); \theta)) = (\mathbf{a}^{i\mathsf{T}} \cdot \mathbf{r}_{\kappa,\chi})^\mathsf{T}(\mathbf{a}^{i\mathsf{T}} \cdot \mathbf{r}_{\kappa,\chi}), \tag{11}$$

$$\mathbf{r}_{\kappa,\chi} = \mathbf{P}(I \circ T(\mathbf{c}_\kappa); \theta) - \mathbf{P}(I \circ T(\mathbf{c}_\chi); \theta), \tag{12}$$

where $\mathbf{r}_{\kappa,\chi}$ is a vector of intensity differences between projection images generated by parameters $\mathbf{c}_\kappa$ and $\mathbf{c}_\chi$; and $\mathbf{a}^i$ is a metric basis vector where the magnitude of the inner product of $\mathbf{a}^i$ and the intensity difference vector $\mathbf{r}_{\kappa,\chi}$, $\mathbf{a}^{i\mathsf{T}} \cdot \mathbf{r}_{\kappa,\chi}$ gives the Riemannian distance for the parameter c^i (eq. 11).

The learned metric basis vector $\mathbf{a}^{i\dagger}$ and the selected kernel width $\sigma^{i\dagger}$ form a weighting kernel $K_{\mathbf{a}^{i\dagger}\mathbf{a}^{i\dagger\mathsf{T}}, \sigma^{i\dagger}}$ to interpolate the parameter c^i in the registration (see eq. 1).

4.2   Linear-Regression Implied Initial Metric

Since the residual functional $\mathcal{L}$ (see eq. 7) that we want to minimize is non-convex, a good initial guess of the metric basis vector $\mathbf{a}$ is essential. Therefore, REALMS uses a vector $\mathbf{w}^i$ as an initial guess of the metric basis vector $\mathbf{a}^i$ for the parameter c^i. Let $\mathbf{W} = \begin{pmatrix} \mathbf{w}^1 & \mathbf{w}^2 & \cdots & \mathbf{w}^n \end{pmatrix}$ list these initial guesses. The matrix $\mathbf{W}$ is approximated by a multivariate linear regression (eq. 13 and eq. 14) between the projection difference matrix $\mathbf{R} = (\mathbf{r}_1 \mathbf{r}_2 \cdots \mathbf{r}_N)^\mathsf{T}$ and the parameter differences matrix $\Delta\mathbf{C}$. In particular, the projection difference vector $\mathbf{r}_\kappa = \mathbf{P}(I \circ T(\mathbf{c}_\kappa); \theta) - \mathbf{P}(I; \theta)$ is the intensity differences between the DRRs calculated from the deformed image $I \circ T(\mathbf{c}_\kappa)$ and the DRRs calculated from the mean image I (where $\mathbf{c} = \mathbf{0}$).

$$\Delta\mathbf{C} = \begin{pmatrix} c^1_1 & c^2_1 & \cdots & c^n_1 \\ c^1_2 & c^2_2 & \cdots & c^n_2 \\ \vdots & \vdots & \ddots & \vdots \\ c^1_N & c^2_N & \cdots & c^n_N \end{pmatrix} - \mathbf{0} \approx \begin{pmatrix} \mathbf{r}^\mathsf{T}_1 \\ \mathbf{r}^\mathsf{T}_2 \\ \vdots \\ \mathbf{r}^\mathsf{T}_N \end{pmatrix} \cdot \begin{pmatrix} \mathbf{w}^1 & \mathbf{w}^2 & \cdots & \mathbf{w}^n \end{pmatrix} \tag{13}$$

$$\mathbf{W} = (\mathbf{R}^\mathsf{T}\mathbf{R})^{-1}\mathbf{R}^\mathsf{T}\Delta\mathbf{C} \tag{14}$$

The inner product of the matrix $\mathbf{W}$, calculated by the pseudo-inverse in eq. 14, and the projection intensity difference matrix $\mathbf{R}$, $\mathbf{W}^\mathsf{T}\mathbf{R}$, gives the best linear approximation of the parameter differences $\Delta\mathbf{C}$. Therefore, we use $\mathbf{w}^i$ as the initial guess of the metric basis vector $\mathbf{a}^i$ for the parameter c^i.

4.3   Optimization Scheme

REALMS uses a two-step scheme to optimize the metric basis vector $\mathbf{a}^i$ and the kernel width σ^i in eq. 10.

First, for each candidate kernel width σ^i, it optimizes the metric basis vector $\mathbf{a}^i$ using the quasi-Newton method (specifically, the BFGS method) with the vector $\mathbf{w}^i$ as the initialization. The gradient of the function $\mathcal{L}_{c^i}$ with respect to $\mathbf{a}^i$ can be stated as

$$\frac{\partial \mathcal{L}_{c^i}}{\partial \mathbf{a}^i} = \frac{2\sqrt{2}}{\sigma^i}\mathbf{a}^i\sum_{\kappa=1}^{N}(\hat{c_\kappa^i}-c_\kappa^i)\sum_{\chi=1}^{N}(\hat{c_\chi^i}-c_\chi^i)K_{\mathbf{a}^i\mathbf{a}^{i\mathsf{T}},\sigma^i}(\mathbf{P}(I{\circ}T(\mathbf{c}_\kappa);\theta),\mathbf{P}(I{\circ}T(\mathbf{c}_\chi);\theta))\mathbf{r}_{\kappa,\chi}\mathbf{r}_{\kappa,\chi}^\mathsf{T}$$

$$(15)$$

Second, REALMS selects a kernel width $\sigma^{i\dagger}$ among the candidate kernel widths where its learned metric basis vector $\mathbf{a}^{i\dagger}$ yields minimum LOO regression residuals $\mathcal{L}_{c^i}$ for parameter c^i.

4.4   Projection Normalization

To account for variations caused by x-ray scatter that produces inconsistent projection intensities, REALMS normalizes both the training projection images $\mathbf{P}(I \circ T(\mathbf{c}_\kappa);\theta)$ and the on-board projection image $\mathbf{\Psi}(\theta)$. In particular, it uses the localized Gaussian normalization introduced in Chou et al. [8], which has shown promise in removing the undesired scattering artifacts.

5   Results

5.1   Synthetic Tests

We used coronal DRRs (dimension: 64 × 48) of the target CTs as synthetic on-board cone-beam projection images. The target CTs were deformed from the patient's Fréchet mean CT by normally distributed random samples of the first three deformation parameters.[1] We generated 600 synthetic test cases from 6 lung datasets and measured the registration quality by the average $mTRE$ (mean Target Registration Error) over all cases and all voxels at tumor sites.

---

[1] In our lung datasets, the first three deformation parameters captured more than 95% lung variation observed in their RCCTs.

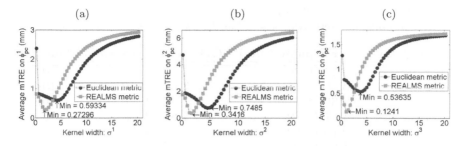

Fig. 1. Average mTREs over 600 test cases projected onto the (a) first, (b) second, and (c) third deformation basis vector versus the candidate kernel widths using $N = 125$ training projection images

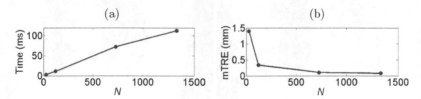

Fig. 2. (a) Time and (b) accuracy v.s. the number of training projection images N

With REALMS's registrations, the average mTRE and its standard deviation are down from 6.89 ± 3.53 mm to 0.34 ± 0.24 mm using $N = 125$ training projection images. The computation time for each registration is 11.39 ± 0.73 ms (87.79 fps) on Intel Core2 Quad CPU Q6700. As shown in figure 1, REALMS reduces the minimum errors produced by kernel regressions that use the Euclidean metric $(\mathbf{M}^i = \mathbf{I})$.

Figure 2 shows the computation time and registration accuracy tradeoff in REALMS.

5.2 Real Tests

We tested REALMS on 6 lung datasets with an on-board CBCT system where a *single* coronal on-board CB projection (dimension downsampled to 64×48 for efficient computation) at both *EE* (End-Expiration) and *EI* (End-Inspiration) phases were used for the testing. See the top image of figure 4(b) for illustration. For each dataset, we generated $N = 125$ training DRRs to learn the metrics and select optimal interpolation kernel widths. The learned metrics and the selected kernel widths were used to estimate deformation parameters for the testing EE and EI on-board projections. The estimated CTs were deformed from the Fréchet mean CT with the estimated deformation parameters. The results were validated with reconstructed CBCTs at target phases.[2] Table 1 shows the

---

[2] The CBCTs were reconstructed by the retrospectively-sorted CB projections at target breathing phases.

Table 1. Tumor Centroid Differences (*TCD*) after REALMS's registration at EE and EI phases of 6 lung datasets. Numbers inside the parentheses are the initial TCDs.

dataset#	TCD at EE phase (mm)	TCD at EI phase (mm)	Time (ms)
1	2.42 (9.70)	4.06 (7.45)	10.40
2	3.60 (4.85)	3.60 (4.89)	10.92
3	2.30 (8.71)	3.60 (4.03)	10.91
4	1.27 (2.69)	2.80 (2.29)	10.91
5	0.70 (9.89)	3.28 (8.71)	11.15
6	1.98 (2.03)	1.12 (1.72)	11.08

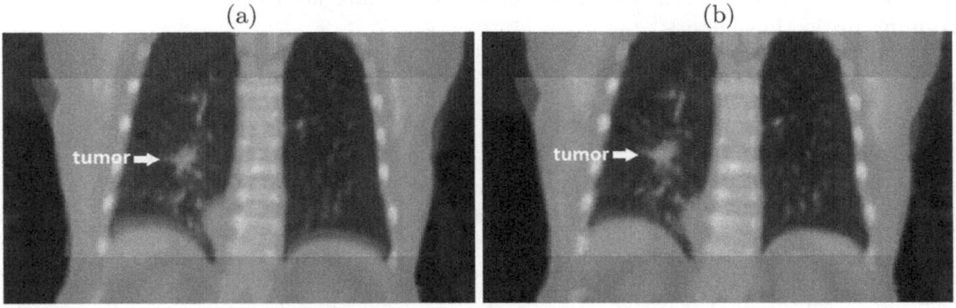

(a)   (b)

Fig. 3. (a) Image overlay of the reconstructed CBCT at EE phase (red) and the Fréchet mean CT (green) (b) Image overlay of the reconstructed CBCT at EE phase (red) and the REALMS-estimated CT (green) calculated from an on-board cone-beam projection image at EE phase. The yellow areas are the overlapped region.

3D Tumor Centroid Differences (*TCD*s) between REALMS-estimated CTs and the reconstructed CBCTs at the same respiratory phases. Tumor centroids were computed via Snake active segmentations. As shown in table 1, REALMS reduces the TCD from 5.58 ± 3.14 mm to 2.56 ± 1.11 mm in 10.89 ± 0.26 ms (91.82 fps).

Figure 3 illustrates an example REALMS registration on a lung dataset where the tumor, the diaphragm, and most of the soft tissues are correctly aligned.

5.3   The Learned Metric Basis Vector

The learned metric basis vector $\mathbf{a}^{i\dagger}$ will emphasize projection pixels that are significant for the distance calculation of the deformation parameter c^i (e.g. give high positive or high negative values). As shown in figure 4(a), the learned metric basis vector $\mathbf{a}^{1\dagger}$ emphasized the diaphragm locations and the lung boundaries as its corresponding deformation basis vector ϕ^1_{pc} covers the expansion and contraction motion of the lung. See the bottom image of figure 4(b) for illustration.

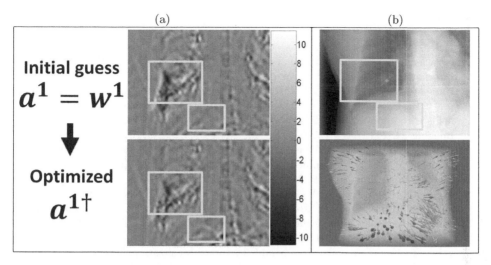

Fig. 4. (a) Initial guess of the metric basis vector $\mathbf{a}^1 = \mathbf{w}^1$ (top) and the optimized metric basis vector $\mathbf{a}^{1\dagger}$ (bottom) of a lung dataset. They are re-shaped into projection image domain for visualization. As shown in the figure, the diaphragm locations and the lung boundaries (yellow boxes) were emphasized after metric learning. (b) Top: a coronal on-board CB projection at EE phase of the lung dataset used in (a). The yellow boxes in (a) and (b) correspond to the same 2D locations. Bottom: the first deformation basis vector ϕ_{pc}^1 (the color arrows indicate heat maps of the deformation magnitudes) overlaid with the volume rendering of the Fréchet mean CT of the lung dataset used in (a). For this dataset, ϕ_{pc}^1 covers the expansion and contraction motion of of the lung.

6   Conclusion and Discussion

This paper presents an accurate and real-time 2D/3D registration method, REALMS, that estimates 3D deformation parameters from a single projection image using kernel regressions with learned rank-1 projection distance metrics. The learned distance metrics are optimized with an initialization approximated by linear regression that we found, is essential to the success of this high dimensional metric learning. Without this special initialization, the optimization would have easily converged to local minimum and thus produce wrong distance metrics. With this special initialization, the regression estimation on both synthetic and real test cases showed its good promise in supporting real-time and low-dose IGRT by using a single projection image. In this paper, we use highly down-sampled projection images for efficient learning at planning time. To support efficient learning for projection images of higher dimensions, the future work of REALMS will incorporate neighborhood approximation methods in the leave-one-out training such that the computation complexity will be reduced from $O(N^2)$ to $O(kN)$ if only k nearest training neighbors are considered for the regression estimation.

References

1. Russakoff, D.B., Rohlfing, T., Maurer, C.: Fast intensity-based 2D-3D image registration of clinical data using light fields. In: Proceedings of the Ninth IEEE International Conference on Computer Vision, vol. 1, pp. 416–422 (2003)
2. Russakoff, D.B., Rohlfing, T., Mori, K., Rueckert, D., Ho, A., Adler, J.R., Maurer, C.R.: Fast generation of digitally reconstructed radiographs using attenuation fields with application to 2d-3d image registration. IEEE Transactions on Medical Imaging 24, 1441–1454 (2005)
3. Khamene, A., Bloch, P., Wein, W., Svatos, M., Sauer, F.: Automatic registration of portal images and volumetric ct for patient positioning in radiation therapy. Medical Image Analysis 10, 96–112 (2006)
4. Munbodh, R., Jaffray, D.A., Moseley, D.J., Chen, Z., Knisely, J.P.S., Cathier, P., Duncan, J.S.: Automated 2d-3d registration of a radiograph and a cone beam ct using line-segment enhancement. Medical Physics 33, 1398–1411 (2006)
5. Li, R., Jia, X., Lewis, J.H., Gu, X., Folkerts, M., Men, C., Jiang, S.B.: Real-time volumetric image reconstruction and 3d tumor localization based on a single x-ray projection image for lung cancer radiotherapy. Medical Physics 37, 2822–2826 (2010)
6. Li, R., Lewis, J.H., Jia, X., Gu, X., Folkerts, M., Men, C., Song, W.Y., Jiang, S.B.: 3d tumor localization through real-time volumetric x-ray imaging for lung cancer radiotherapy. Medical Physics 38, 2783–2794 (2011)
7. Chou, C.R., Frederick, B., Chang, S., Pizer, S.: A Learning-Based patient repositioning method from Limited-Angle projections. In: Angeles, J., Boulet, B., Clark, J.J., Kövecses, J., Siddiqi, K. (eds.) Brain, Body and Machine. AISC, vol. 83, pp. 83–94. Springer, Heidelberg (2010)
8. Chou, C.R., Frederick, B., Liu, X., Mageras, G., Chang, S., Pizer, S.: Claret: A fast deformable registration method applied to lung radiation therapy. In: Fourth International (MICCAI) Workshop on Pulmonary Image Analysis, pp. 113–124 (2011)
9. Miao, S., Liao, R., Zheng, Y.: A hybrid method for 2-d/3-d registration between 3-d volumes and 2-d angiography for trans-catheter aortic valve implantation (tavi). In: ISBI, pp. 1215–1218 (2011)
10. Weinberger, K., Tesauro, G.: Metric learning for kernel regression. In: Eleventh International Conference on Artificial Intelligence and Statistics, pp. 608–615 (2007)
11. Lorenzen, P., Prastawa, M., Davis, B., Gerig, G., Bullitt, E., Joshi, S.: Multi-modal image set registration and atlas formation. Medical Image Analysis 10(3), 440–451 (2006)

Groupwise Spectral Log-Demons Framework for Atlas Construction

Herve Lombaert[1,2], Leo Grady[3], Xavier Pennec[2], Jean-Marc Peyrat[4],
Nicholas Ayache[2], and Farida Cheriet[1]

[1] Ecole Polytechnique de Montreal, Canada
[2] INRIA Sophia Antipolis, France
[3] Siemens Corporate Research, Princeton, NJ
[4] Siemens Molecular Imaging, Oxford, UK

Abstract. We introduce a new framework to construct atlases from images with very large and complex deformations. The atlas is build in parallel with groupwise registrations by extending the symmetric Log-Demons algorithm. We describe and evaluate two forms of our framework: the *Groupwise Log-Demons* (GL-Demons) is faster but is limited to local nonrigid deformations, and the *Groupwise Spectral Log-Demons* (GSL-Demons) is slower but, due to isometry-invariant representations of images, can construct atlases of organs with high shape variability. We demonstrate our framework by constructing atlases from hearts with high shape variability.

1   Introduction

Statistics on complex characteristics with high anatomical and functional variability require the normalization of measurements across subjects to establish a population average and deviations from that average. The process of shape averaging [22,5,27] becomes particularly complex, and still remains unsolved, with organs undergoing large shape disparities. In the present state-of-the-art, the concept of geodesic shape averaging allows unbiased constructions of atlases through diffeomorphic methods [12,2,17], i.e., the transformation of a reference shape toward an average (the geometry of the atlas) follows a geodesic path on a Riemannian manifold (the space of diffeomorphic transformations). While the LDDMM [4,3,6] or forward scheme approaches [1,8] provide elegant mathematical frameworks for averaging shapes, these methods could be slow and find their limitations with high shape variability. Guimond *et al.* [10] proposed a fast and efficient algorithm [19,16,26] with sequential (pairwise) registrations to a reference image. A new simultaneous (groupwise) registration approach would enable the construction of an atlas in parallel, during the registration process (rather than with a series of pairwise registrations). To do so, *firstly*, we extend the symmetric Demons algorithm [25] to perform a groupwise registration of a set of images in order to construct their atlas. However, as in most registration methods, transformation updates based on the image gradients are inherently limited by their local scope. *Secondly*, we introduce a new update scheme for groupwise

B.H. Menze et al. (Eds.): MCV 2012, LNCS 7766, pp. 11–19, 2013.

registration based on the spectral decomposition of graph Laplacians [7,23,13], that is invariant to shape isometry and is capable of capturing large deformations during the construction of the atlas. We provide *two forms* of our groupwise registration framework that we name the *Groupwise Log-Demons* (**GL-Demons**, faster and suited for local nonrigid deformations), and the *Groupwise Spectral Log-Demons* (**GSL-Demons**, slower but capable of capturing very large deformations). We evaluate the two forms of our new framework by constructing atlases of images with very large deformations.

2   Method

The atlas is defined as the set of N images $\{I_i\}_{i=1..N}$ nonrigidly aligned to their average shape $\tilde{I}$. Our new shape averaging framework extends the symmetric Log-Demons algorithm [25] and can use classical gradient-based updates (*GL-Demons*) or an improved spectral matching for groupwise registration (*GSL-Demons*). We begin by briefly reviewing each component.

2.1   Diffeomorphic Registration

A diffeomorphic transformation ϕ between two images (such that $F(\cdot) \mapsto M(\phi(\cdot))$ or simply $F \mapsto M \circ \phi$) guarantees a smooth one-to-one mapping (i.e., differentiable and invertible, without creating foldings in space). From the theory of Lie groups, the exponential map of a stationary velocity field v generates a diffeomorphic transformation $\phi = \exp(v)$ (approximated with the scaling-and-squaring method [24]). The Log-Demons algorithm alternates the optimization of a similarity term and a regularization term by decoupling them with a hidden variable (the correspondence c). The algorithm is slightly modified from [25] to converge toward an average shape by minimizing the following energy (controlled with $\alpha_i, \alpha_x, \alpha_T$):

$$E(F, M, c, v) = \alpha_i^2 \mathrm{Sim}(F', M') + \alpha_x^2 \mathrm{dist}(c, v)^2 + \alpha_T^2 \mathrm{Reg}(v), \text{ where} \quad (1)$$
$$\mathrm{Sim}(F', M') = (F' - M')^2, \ \mathrm{dist}(c, v) = \|c - v\||, \text{ and } \mathrm{Reg}(v) = \|\nabla v\|^2$$

The similarity term incorporates diffeomorphism and symmetry with $F' = F \circ \exp(-c)$ and $M' = M \circ \exp(+c)$. Both images F' and M' effectively converge toward an average shape $\tilde{I} = F \circ \phi^{-1} + M \circ \phi$ (similar to the approaches in [2,6]).

2.2   Spectral Correspondence

The computation of the velocity field updates in the Log-Demons is inherently limited by the local scope of the update forces derived from the image gradient, i.e., it requires texture data which is generally local information. We now describe a new update scheme based on spectral correspondence [21,11,18,14,13] that will enable the construction of atlases with large deformations. Let us first consider I_Ω, the portion of an image I bounded by a contour Ω. We build a connected graph $\mathcal{G} = (\mathcal{V}, \mathcal{E})$ where the vertices $\mathcal{V}$ represent the pixels of I_Ω and the edges $\mathcal{E}$ define the neighborhood structure within I_Ω. The corresponding adjacency matrix W [9] represents the edge weights ($W_{ij} = w_{ij}$ if pixels (i, j) are neighbors, 0 otherwise), such that pixels with similar intensity and close in space would have strong links in $\mathcal{G}$ (e.g., $w_{ij} = \exp(-\beta(I(i) - I(j))^2) / \|\mathbf{x}(i) - \mathbf{x}(j)\|^2$ where $\mathbf{x}$ are Euclidean coordinates and β a parameter). The Laplacian operator on a graph [9] is formulated as a $|\mathcal{V}| \times |\mathcal{V}|$ matrix with the form $\mathcal{L} = D^{-1}(D - W)$, where D is the (diagonal) degree matrix containing the node degrees $D_{ii} = \sum_j W_{ij}$.

Spectral Coordinates. The decomposition of the Laplacian matrix $\mathcal{L} = \mathscr{X}^T \Lambda \mathscr{X}$ reveals the graph spectrum [7] which comprises the eigenvalues $\Lambda = \mathrm{diag}$ $(\lambda_0, \lambda_1, ..., \lambda_{|\mathcal{V}|})$ (in increasing order) and their associated eigenmodes $\mathscr{X} = (\mathscr{x}^{(0)}, \mathscr{x}^{(1)}, ..., \mathscr{x}^{(|\mathcal{V}|)})$ (a $|\mathcal{V}| \times |\mathcal{V}|$ matrix where columns $\mathscr{x}^{(\cdot)}$ are eigenmodes). The first eigenmode is trivial ($\lambda_0 = 0$) and the following non-trivial eigenmodes are the fundamental modes of vibrations of a shape depicted by I_Ω. The eigenmodes associated with the first k smallest non-zero eigenvalues (the lower frequencies) represent the k-dimensional *spectral coordinates* (each point $i \in I_\Omega$ has the coordinates $\mathscr{x}(i) = (\mathscr{x}^{(1)}(i), \mathscr{x}^{(2)}(i), ..., \mathscr{x}^{(k)}(i))$ defined in a spectral domain). These lowest modes of vibration have the strong property of being smooth and invariant to shape isometry (i.e., shapes in different poses would share the same spectral coordinates at each point, see *below*).

However, the eigenmodes need to be rearranged as a result of sign ambiguity ($\mathscr{x}^{(\cdot)}$ and $-\mathscr{x}^{(\cdot)}$ are both valid eigenmodes), algebraic multiplicity (many eigenmodes can share the same eigenvalue), and imperfection in isometry (changing the multiplicity and ordering of the eigenvalues). Firstly, their values are scaled to fit the range $[-1; +1]$, i.e., for negative values:

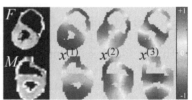

Three lowest frequency eigenmodes of two images

$\mathscr{x}^{(\cdot)-} \leftarrow \mathscr{x}^{(\cdot)-} / \min\{\mathscr{x}^{(\cdot)-}\}$ and for positive values: $\mathscr{x}^{(\cdot)+} \leftarrow \mathscr{x}^{(\cdot)+} / \max\{\mathscr{x}^{(\cdot)+}\}$. Secondly, the eigenmodes of two images, $\mathscr{X}_F$ and $\mathscr{X}_M$, are reordered with the optimal permutation π (where $\mathscr{x}_F^{(\cdot)} \mapsto \mathscr{x}_M^{\pi \circ (\cdot)}$) which may be found with the Hungarian algorithm that minimizes the following dissimilarity matrix:

$$C(u, v) = \sqrt{\frac{1}{|I_\Omega|} \sum_{i \in I_\Omega} \left(\mathscr{x}_F^{(u)}(i) - \mathscr{x}_M^{(v)}(i) \right)^2} + \sqrt{\sum_{i,j} \left(h_F^{\mathscr{x}_F^{(u)}}(i,j) - h_M^{\mathscr{x}_M^{(v)}}(i,j) \right)^2} \tag{2}$$

The first term is the difference in spectral coordinates between the images. The second term measures the dissimilarities between the joint histograms $h(i, j)$ (a 2D matrix where the element (i, j) is the joint probability of having at the same time the intensity i and the eigenmodal value $\mathscr{x}^{(\cdot)} = j$). The sign ambiguity can be removed by optimizing, instead, the dissimilarity matrix $Q(u, v) = \min\{C(u, v), C(u, -v)\}$. To keep the notation simple in the next sec-

Algorithm 1. Spectral Correspondence

Input: Images F, M.
Output: Correspondence c mapping F to M
- Compute general Laplacians $\mathcal{L}_F$, $\mathcal{L}_M$.
  $\mathcal{L} = D^{-1}(D - W)$, where
  $W_{ij} = \exp(-\beta(I(i) - I(j))^2)/\|\mathbf{x}(i) - \mathbf{x}(j)\|^2$
  $D_{ii} = \sum_j W_{ij}$,
- Compute first k eigenmodes of Laplacians
- Reorder $\mathscr{X}_M$ with respect to $\mathscr{X}_F$ (Eq. (2))
- Build embeddings:
  $\mathbf{F} = (I_F, \mathbf{x}_F, \mathscr{X}_F)$; $\mathbf{M} = (I_M, \mathbf{x}_M, \mathscr{X}_M)$
- Find c mapping nearest points $\mathbf{F} \mapsto \mathbf{M}$

Algorithm 2. Groupwise Demons Framework

Input: N images with initial reference (e.g., $\tilde{I} = I_1$)
Output: Transformations $\phi_i = \exp(v_i)$ mapping $\tilde{I}$ to I_i
Average shape is $\tilde{I} = \frac{1}{N} \sum_{i=1}^{N} I_i \circ \exp(v_i)$
repeat
for $i = 1 \to N$ **do**
- Find updates $u_i \leftarrow \text{mapping}(\tilde{I}, I_i \circ \exp(v_i))$.
  (mapping() differs in GL and GSL-Demons)
- Smooth updates: $u_i \leftarrow K_{\text{fluid}} \star u_i$.
  (convolution of a Gaussian kernel on u_i)
- Update velocity fields: $v_i \leftarrow \log(\exp(v_i) \circ \exp(u_i))$
  (approximated with $v_i \leftarrow v_i + u_i$).
- Smooth velocity fields: $v_i \leftarrow K_{\text{diff}} \star v_i$.
end for
- Get reference update: $u_{\text{ref}} = -\frac{1}{N} \sum_{i=1}^{N} v_i$
- Update velocity fields: $v_i \leftarrow v_i + u_{\text{ref}}$.
- Update reference: $\tilde{I} \leftarrow \frac{1}{N} \sum_{i=1}^{N} I_i \circ \exp(v_i)$.
until convergence

tions, we assume the spectral coordinates have been appropriately signed, scaled and reordered using this method.

Spectral Matching. The correspondence between two images F and M is established (Alg. (1)) by finding the nearest neighbors in the spectral domain (e.g., with fast k-d trees). Put differently, if $\mathscr{X}_F(i)$ is the closest point to $\mathscr{X}_M(j)$ then the pixel i corresponds with j. This simple nearest-neighbor scheme is extended to add similarity constraints on intensity and space by adding image intensities and Euclidean coordinates to the spectral embedding: $\mathbf{X} = (\alpha_i I, \alpha_s \mathbf{x}, \alpha_g \mathscr{X})$. Nearest points between $\mathbf{X}_F$ and $\mathbf{X}_M$ actually locate the best compromise among three strong properties: points with similar isometric (or geometric) properties, similar image intensities, and similar location (each weighted with $\alpha_{\text{g,i,s}}$). To be more precise, this corresponds to minimizing the energy $E(F, M, \phi) = \text{Sim}(F, M)$ where the regularization (similarly to [14]) is enforced with the smoothness of the spectral and spatial components:

$$\text{Sim}(F, M) = (F - M \circ \phi)^2 + \frac{\alpha_s^2}{\alpha_i^2}(\mathbf{x}_F - \mathbf{x}_{M \circ \phi})^2 + \frac{\alpha_g^2}{\alpha_i^2}(\mathscr{X}_F - \mathscr{X}_{M \circ \phi})^2, \quad (3)$$

where $\mathscr{X}_F$ and $\mathscr{X}_{M \circ \phi}$ are the spectral coordinates of corresponding points. This matching technique that is invariant to isometry will enable the capture of large deformations for our atlas construction.

2.3 Groupwise Demons Framework

Our framework is based on Guimond's *et al.* approach [10] where they construct the average image $\tilde{I}$ *sequentially* by alternating between pairwise registrations

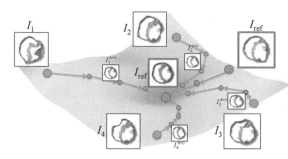

Fig. 1. Groupwise Demons: Simultaneous registration of 4 images (blue circles) toward a reference image that evolves in the space of diffeomorphisms (colored manifold). The reference image is computed in parallel and converges to the average shape (middle red circle).

(fixing a reference image) and updates of the average image (transforming the reference image). Our novelty is to directly compute $\tilde{I}$ *in parallel* with simultaneous (groupwise) registrations (illustrated in Fig. 1). To do so, Eq. (1) is extended to incorporate N velocity fields that warp all images $\{I_i \circ \exp(c_i)\}$ toward the average image $\tilde{I}$. The new groupwise framework is summarized in Alg. (2) and the underlying energy is:

$$E(\tilde{I}, \{I_i, c_i, v_i\}) = \frac{1}{N} \sum_{i=1}^{N} \left(\alpha_i^2 \mathrm{Sim}(\tilde{I}, I_i \circ \exp(c_i)) + \alpha_x^2 \mathrm{dist}(c_i, v_i)^2 + \alpha_T^2 \mathrm{Reg}(v_i) \right)$$

(4)

The reference image can be optionally generated with weighted contributions from all images (e.g., weights different than $1/N$ in order to remove outliers). The minimization of all similarity terms, $\{\mathrm{Sim}(\tilde{I}, I_i')\}$, causes all warped images to become similar to the reference image and the sum of all velocity fields is brought to a minimal value at convergence. Similar to the convergence of [10], the Groupwise Demons framework effectively brings the reference image toward the barycenter of all images. The average image is simply generated with $\tilde{I} = \frac{1}{N} \sum_{i=1}^{N} I_i \circ \exp(c_i)$.

Groupwise Spectral Log-Demons. The update schemes based on image gradients and on spectral correspondence can be used in the Groupwise Demons framework. The *Groupwise Log-Demons* (GL-Demons) algorithm uses update forces derived from the image gradient and is well suited for images with local nonrigid deformations, while the *Groupwise Spectral Log-Demons* (GSL-Demons) algorithm uses spectral correspondences as update forces (i.e., u is found with Alg. (1)) and is better suited for large and highly non-local deformations. GSL-Demons enables large jumps during the construction of the atlas where points move toward their isometric equivalents even if they are far away in space. The atlas construction can handle very large deformations and convergences in fewer iterations (typically 5 iterations are sufficient). The energy has the same form of Eq. (4) and uses the similarity term of Eq. (3).

Multilevel Scheme. Moreover, large and complex deformations can be captured in a low resolution level with *GSL-Demons*, improving thus the processing time, while the remaining small and local deformations can be recovered with

GL-Demons in higher resolutions. This multilevel approach keeps the computation of the eigenmodes tractable.

3   Results

GL-Demons and *GSL-Demons* are evaluated by constructing atlases of images with large deformations. In the synthetic experiment, we verify convergence toward an average shape, and the handling of highly complex deformations (parameters: $\sigma_{\text{fluid,diff}} = 1, \alpha_x = 1, k = 5, \alpha_g = 0.1, \alpha_s = 0.2, \alpha_i = 0.7$ in 2D). In a second experiment, we use both algorithms with real cardiac images that exhibit high shape variability (parameters: $\sigma_{\text{fluid,diff}} = 0.75, \alpha_x = 1, k = 5, \alpha_g = 0.25, \alpha_s = 0.35, \alpha_i = 0.4$ in 3D).

Synthetic Deformations. Convergence and capture of large deformations are now evaluated. $N/2$ velocity fields v are generated randomly using 15 control points with random locations in the image and random displacements of at most 15 pixels (20% of the image size) that are diffused over the image. Their forward and background transformations ($\exp(v)$ and $\exp(-v)$) are applied to an initial image I_0, holding thus the average shape to I_0 (establishing our ground truth). Since we compare the convergence and its rate, and not the final performance, the multi-level scheme (which should be used in real applications) is not applied. Fig. 2 shows the groupwise registrations of 10 random hearts (2D 75×75 images) through 100 trials (a total of 1000 hearts). The average Dice metric (measuring the overlap) between all computed average shapes and I_0 as well as the intensity errors (MSE) reveal that the reference shape (defined arbitrarily as one of the 10 images) evolves toward the ground truth (i.e., Dice increases and MSE decreases). Moveover, the N deformation fields become closer to the

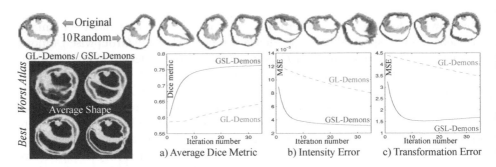

Fig. 2. Groupwise registration of 10 images deformed randomly (100 trials, 1 sample on top row, with known ground truth) using *GL-Demons* and *GSL-Demons, Left)* Best and worst atlases (based on Dice metric among 100 trials) demonstrating the capability of the *GSL-Demons* to handle large deformations, *a)* Average Dice metric with ground truth, *b)* Intensity difference between average shape and ground truth, *c)* transformation error with ground truth. *GSL-Demons* converges faster toward the average shape.

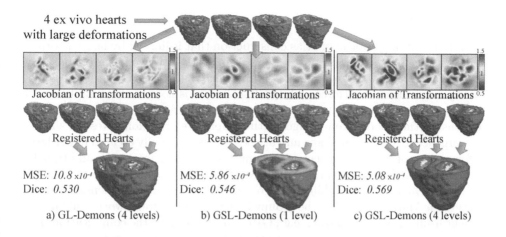

Fig. 3. Atlas of *ex vivo* hearts (isosurfaces are shown) using *a) GL-Demons* (4 levels, showing failure in the right ventricle), *b) GSL-Demons* (1 level), *c)* and *GSL-Demons* (4 levels, with correct right ventricle). *GSL-Demons* capture successfully large deformations. Jacobian determinants (axial planes) show that spectral matching capture smooth and large deformations while gradient-based updates capture local deformations.

ground truth during registration. The striking difference in the convergence rates shows the full power of GSL-Demons (less than 5 iterations are required) while *GL-Demons* might not converge with such large deformations (we stopped the algorithms after 200 iterations). Time-wise, 35 iterations takes 194 seconds with GSL-Demons, and 53 seconds with *GL-Demons* (using unoptimized Matlab code on a 2.53GHz Core 2 Duo). GSL-Demons shows a better performance with high deformations than *GL-Demons*.

Cardiac Atlases. We now evaluate the construction of atlases with organs of high shape variability. *Ex vivo* hearts are particularly challenging to register as they present a high variability in fixture poses due to flabby ventricular walls. The human *ex vivo* DTMRI dataset [20,16,15] provides good candidates to evaluate our algorithms. We use four hearts ($b = 0$ images of size 64^3) that were excluded in the construction of the human atlas [15] due to their hypertrophy and highly deformed shapes (see Fig. 3). GL-Demons (with 4 resolution levels) fail in recovering the shapes of the right ventricles, while GSL-Demons successfully constructs the atlas even with 1 level of resolution (downsampled images at size 28^3). As a comparison, 35 iterations takes 40 minutes in Matlab with *GSL-Demons* and 9 minutes with *GL-Demons*. Using *GSL-Demons* with 4 resolution levels reduce the intensity error (MSE) by half (from 10.8 to 5.08). Moreover, the Jacobian determinants of the transformation fields show that the large and highly non-local deformations are successfully captured with the spectral-based update scheme (high and smooth Jacobian in Fig. 3 b) while local deformations are captured with the gradient-based update scheme in the higher levels of *GSL-Demons* (Fig. 3 c).

4 Conclusion

We addressed the problem of atlas construction that is limited by large deformations between images. We proposed a new framework with two forms to construct an atlas in parallel with groupwise registrations: *GL-Demons* is faster but is limited by its gradient-based forces, while *GSL-Demons* is slower but can capture very large deformations due to its spectral components. We evaluated our framework by constructing atlases from images with complex deformations. Results showed convergence to an average shape and atlases were successfully created under large deformations of 20% of the image size using 1000 random hearts. We additionally showed that *GSL-Demons* can construct an atlas for a challenging dataset of *ex vivo* hearts with high shape variability. Future work will focus on implementation (converting the Matlab code, also, the groupwise nature of our framework could highly benefit from parallel computing, e.g., GPU) and improving the computation time of the spectral decomposition (e.g., reuse of pre-computations, approximations). Nevertheless, our current framework enables the construction of atlases from images with very large and complex deformations.

Acknowledgements. The authors wish to thank Pierre Croisille for *ex vivo* herts as well as Hervé Delingette for helpful comments. The project was supported financially by the National Science and Engineering Research Council of Canada (NSERC).

References

1. Allassonnière, S., Amit, Y., Trouvé, A.: Towards a coherent statistical framework for dense deformable template estimation. J. Royal Stat. Soc. 69, 3–29 (2007)
2. Avants, B., Gee, J.C.: Geodesic estimation for large deformation anatomical shape averaging and interpolation. NeuroImage 23, 139–150 (2004)
3. Beg, M.F., Khan, A.: Computing an average anatomical atlas using LDDMM and geodesic shooting. In: ISBI, pp. 1116–1119 (2006)
4. Beg, M.F., Miller, M.I., Trouvé, A., Younes, L.: Computing large deformation metric mappings via geodesic flows of diffeomorphisms. IJCV 61, 139–157 (2005)
5. Bhatia, K.K., Hajnal, J.V., Puri, B.K., Edwards, A.D., Rueckert, D.: Consistent groupwise non-rigid registration for atlas construction. In: ISBI, pp. 908–911 (2004)
6. Bossa, M., Hernandez, M., Olmos, S.: Contributions to 3D Diffeomorphic Atlas Estimation: Application to Brain Images. In: Ayache, N., Ourselin, S., Maeder, A. (eds.) MICCAI 2007, Part I. LNCS, vol. 4791, pp. 667–674. Springer, Heidelberg (2007)
7. Chung, F.: Spectral Graph Theory. AMS (1997)
8. Durrleman, S., Fillard, P., Pennec, X., Trouvé, A., Ayache, N.: Registration, atlas estimation and variability analysis of white matter fiber bundles modeled as currents. NeuroImage 55, 1073–1090 (2011)
9. Grady, L., Polimeni, J.R.: Discrete Calculus: Applied Analysis on Graphs for Computational Science. Springer (2010)
10. Guimond, A., Meunier, J., Thirion, J.P.: Average brain models: a convergence study. In: Computer Vision and Image Understanding, pp. 192–210 (2000)
11. Jain, V., Zhang, H.: Robust 3D shape correspondence in the spectral domain. In: Int. Conf. on Shape Modeling and App., p. 19 (2006)

12. Joshi, S., Davis, B., Jomier, M., Gerig, G.: Unbiased diffeomorphic atlas construction for computational anatomy. NeuroImage 23, 151–160 (2004)
13. Lombaert, H., Grady, L., Pennec, X., Ayache, N., Cheriet, F.: Spectral Demons – Image Registration via Global Spectral Correspondence. In: Fitzgibbon, A., Lazebnik, S., Perona, P., Sato, Y., Schmid, C. (eds.) ECCV 2012, Part II. LNCS, vol. 7573, pp. 30–44. Springer, Heidelberg (2012)
14. Lombaert, H., Grady, L., Polimeni, J.R., Cheriet, F.: Spectral correspondence for brain matching. In: IPMI, pp. 660–670 (2011)
15. Lombaert, H., Peyrat, J.-M., Croisille, P., Rapacchi, S., Fanton, L., Cheriet, F., Clarysse, P., Magnin, I., Delingette, H., Ayache, N.: Human atlas of the cardiac fiber architecture: Study on a healthy population. IEEE Trans. on Med. Imaging 31, 1436–1447 (2012)
16. Lombaert, H., Peyrat, J.-M., Croisille, P., Rapacchi, S., Fanton, L., Clarysse, P., Delingette, H., Ayache, N.: Statistical Analysis of the Human Cardiac Fiber Architecture from DT-MRI. In: Metaxas, D.N., Axel, L. (eds.) FIMH 2011. LNCS, vol. 6666, pp. 171–179. Springer, Heidelberg (2011)
17. Marsland, S., Twining, C.J., Taylor, C.J.: Groupwise Non-rigid Registration Using Polyharmonic Clamped-Plate Splines. In: Ellis, R.E., Peters, T.M. (eds.) MICCAI 2003. LNCS, vol. 2879, pp. 771–779. Springer, Heidelberg (2003)
18. Mateus, D., Horaud, R., Knossow, D., Cuzzolin, F., Boyer, E.: Articulated shape matching using Laplacian eigenfunctions and unsupervised point registration. In: CVPR, pp. 1–8 (2008)
19. Peyrat, J.-M., Sermesant, M., Pennec, X., Delingette, H., Xu, C., McVeigh, E.R., Ayache, N.: A computational framework for the statistical analysis of cardiac diffusion tensors: application to a small database of canine hearts. IEEE Trans. on Med. Imaging 26(11), 1500–1514 (2007)
20. Rapacchi, S., Croisille, P., Pai, V., Grenier, D., Viallon, M., Kellman, P., Mewton, N., Wen, H.: Reducing motion sensitivity in free breathing DWI of the heart with localized Principal Component Analysis. In: ISMRM (2010)
21. Shapiro, L.S., Brady, J.M.: Feature-based correspondence: an eigenvector approach. Image and Vision Computing 10, 283–288 (1992)
22. Studholme, C., Cardenas, V.: A template free approach to volumetric spatial normalization of brain anatomy. Pattern Recogn. Lett. 25, 1191–1202 (2004)
23. van Kaick, O., Zhang, H., Hamarneh, G., Cohen-Or, D.: A survey on shape correspondence. Eurographics 30(6), 1681–1707 (2011)
24. Vercauteren, T., Pennec, X., Perchant, A., Ayache, N.: Non-parametric Diffeomorphic Image Registration with the Demons Algorithm. In: Ayache, N., Ourselin, S., Maeder, A. (eds.) MICCAI 2007, Part II. LNCS, vol. 4792, pp. 319–326. Springer, Heidelberg (2007)
25. Vercauteren, T., Pennec, X., Perchant, A., Ayache, N.: Symmetric Log-Domain Diffeomorphic Registration: A Demons-Based Approach. In: Metaxas, D., Axel, L., Fichtinger, G., Székely, G. (eds.) MICCAI 2008, Part I. LNCS, vol. 5241, pp. 754–761. Springer, Heidelberg (2008)
26. Wu, G., Jia, H., Wang, Q., Shen, D.: SharpMean: groupwise registration guided by sharp mean image and tree-based registration. NeuroImage 56(4), 1968–1981 (2011)
27. Zollei, L., Miller, L.E., Grimson, W.E.L., Wells, W.M.: Efficient population registration of 3D data. In: ICCV 2005, Computer Vision for Biomedical Image Applications (2005)

Robust Anatomical Correspondence Detection by Graph Matching with Sparsity Constraint

Yanrong Guo[1,2], Guorong Wu[2], Yakang Dai[2], Jianguo Jiang[1], and Dinggang Shen[2,*]

[1] School of Computer and Information, Hefei University of Technology, Hefei, China
[2] IDEA Lab, Department of Radiology and BRIC, University of North Carolina at Chapel Hill
dgshen@med.unc.edu

Abstract. Graph matching is a robust correspondence detection approach which considers potential correspondences as graph nodes and uses graph links to measure the pairwise agreement between potential correspondences. In this paper, we propose a novel graph matching method to augment its power in establishing anatomical correspondences in medical images, especially for the cases with large inter-subject variations. Our contributions have twofold. First, we propose a robust measurement to characterize the pairwise agreement of appearance information on each graph link. In this way, our method is more robust to ambiguous matches than the conventional graph matching methods that generally consider only the simple geometric information. Second, although multiple correspondences are allowed for robust correspondence, we further introduce the sparsity constraint upon the possibilities of correspondences to suppress the distraction from misleading matches, which is very important for achieving accurate one-to-one correspondences in the end of the matching procedure. We finally incorporate these two improvements into a new objective function and solve it by quadratic programming. The proposed graph matching method has been evaluated in the public hand X-ray images with comparison to a conventional graph matching method. In all experiments, our method achieves the best matching performance in terms of matching accuracy and robustness.

1   Introduction

Robust anatomical correspondence detection is very important in many medical image applications, such as deformable image registration [1] and organ motion correction [2]. Although a lot of local image descriptors have been proposed with great success in computer vision area in the last decade, it remains a big challenge in establishing correspondences between subjects with large anatomical differences.

Recently, graph matching has emerged as a robust correspondence detection approach by modeling not only the point-to-point correspondence [3] but also the pair-to-pair matching consistency in a graph [4]. Specifically, each possible correspondence is considered as a node in the graph and the pairwise agreement between any two possible correspondences is described as a link in the graph. Then,

---

* Corresponding author.

B.H. Menze et al. (Eds.): MCV 2012, LNCS 7766, pp. 20–28, 2013.

the problem of correspondence matching becomes an optimization problem for finding a cluster of these nodes that can produce the maximal pairwise agreement.

In general, the advantages of graph matching over other pointwise correspondence detection methods lie in two aspects: (1) the matching coherence is explicitly modeled in the graph to leverage the problem of ambiguous matches; (2) multiple correspondences are allowed in correspondence detection while the final one-to-one correspondences are simultaneously solved on all correspondences by the spectral-based optimization method [5]. However, there are two major issues in the current graph matching methods: (1) only simple geometric information is generally used for constructing the graph links; (2) its solution is usually suboptimal due to the lack of effective mechanism to control the quality of each possible correspondence established.

To alleviate these two issues, we present a novel graph matching method to augment its power in establishing anatomical correspondences, especially for the cases with large inter-subject shape variations in the medical images. Our contributions have twofold. **First**, we propose a robust appearance measurement to characterize the pairwise agreement on each graph link. Specifically, for any two possible matches (with the two starting points in the template image and the two ending points in the subject image), a sequence of local intensity profiles (called *line patch*) along the line connecting two starting points in template image, or two ending points in the subject image, is constructed. Then the appearance discrepancy between these two line patches is computed to measure their pairwise agreement. Using this novel measurement, our method is more robust to ambiguous matches than the conventional graph matching methods that generally use only the simple geometric compatibility. **Second**, inspired by the discriminative power of sparse representation in machine learning and pattern recognition [6, 7], we apply a sparsity constraint on the possibilities of multiple correspondences, which requires to seek for only a small number of qualified correspondences for each feature point. Thus, the risk of ambiguous matches can be significantly avoided when determining one-to-one correspondences in the end of matching procedure. We finally construct a new objective function by integrating these two improvements. An efficient solution is further provided, via quadratic programming, to jointly estimate correspondences for all feature points. Our graph matching method has been evaluated in the public hand X-ray images and compared with the state-of-the-art graph matching method, namely Spectral Matching with Affine Constraint (SMAC) [4], which was reported with one of the best matching performances among the conventional graph matching methods. In all experiments, our method outperforms SMAC in terms of both matching accuracy and robustness.

2   Methods

Considering a feature point set $T = \{t_i | i = 1, \dots, n\}$ in the template image and another feature point set $S = \{s_{i'} | i' = 1, \dots, n'\}$ in the subject image, our goal is to find an assignment matrix $\boldsymbol{X} = [X_{i,i'}]_{n \times n'}, (X_{i,i'} \in \{0,1\})$ between these two point sets, where each assignment $X_{i,i'}$ indicates whether a feature point t_i in the template is matched to a feature point $s_{i'}$ in the subject with '1' denoting correspondence and '0' denoting non-correspondence. Fig. 1 schematically illustrates the main idea of our method by using the hand X-ray images as example. Given the template feature point set T (Fig. 1(a)) and the subject feature point set S (Fig. 1(b)), all possible correspondences between T and S are established as shown by the white lines in Fig. 1(c). Then, the $nn' \times nn'$ affinity matrix M (Fig. 1(d)) can be constructed to describe the confidence of all established correspondences as well as the pairwise agreement between any two possible matches. Specifically, each diagonal element (shown with boxes in Fig. 1(d)) in the affinity matrix M represents the pointwise similarity between two feature points $t_i \in T$ and $s_{i'} \in S$. Each off-diagonal element (shown with pink triangle in Fig. 1(d)) measures the pairwise agreement between two possible matches $((i, i')$ indicated by the red box and (j, j') indicated by the blue box in Fig. 1(d)), where we propose to use appearance-based line patch, combined with simple geometric relationship [4], to robustly characterize their coherence. The continuous relaxed assignment matrix $X = [X_{i,i'}]_{n \times n'} (X_{i,i'} \in [0,1])$ can be optimized by finding the cluster of correspondences among the diagonal elements of M while maximizing its pairwise agreements. To alleviate the potential ambiguity in determining one-to-one correspondences in Fig. 1(e) directly from the one-to-many assignment matrix X, the sparsity constraint is applied to X to suppress the distraction of ambiguous matches during the correspondence detection procedure.

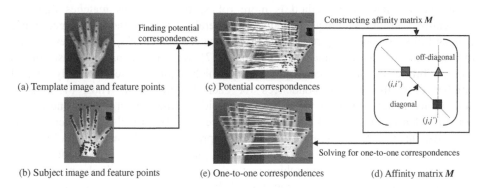

Fig. 1. The scheme of the proposed anatomical correspondence detection by graph matching

2.1   Limitation of Conventional Graph Matching Method

In the conventional graph matching method, such as the SMAC method, the coherence between possible matches (i, i') and (j, j') is usually measured by the geometric distance $\frac{|d(i,j)-d(i',j')|}{\min(d(i,j),d(i',j'))}$, and the angle between two matches/correspondences (i, i') and (j, j'). Here, $d(.,.)$ denotes the Euclidian distance of two points. Then, the energy function is defined to maximize the following quadratic score function of x:

$$J(x) = x^T M x \quad s.t. \; Ax = 1^T \text{ and } \{0 \le x_m \le 1 | m = 1, ..., nn'\} \quad (1)$$

where assignment vector x is a nn' column vector after concatenating each row of X. Thus, each element x_m $(m = 1, ..., nn')$ in the vector x is associated with a particular correspondence (i, i') in the assignment matrix X, i.e., $x_m = X_{i,i'}$. Since the optimization of $J(x)$ is NP-hard, each element in x is relaxed to be a continuous value between 0 and 1. Thus, the objective function $J(x)$ is subject to the affine constraint $Ax = 1^T$ (as in [3]) to enforce the one-to-one correspondences. A is a $(n + n') \times (nn')$ selection matrix applied to vector x (vectorization of X^T) to represent the summation of each column or each row of X equals to 1, i.e., $\sum_{i=1}^{n} X_{i,i'} = 1$ or $\sum_{i'=1}^{n'} X_{i,i'} = 1$. Spectral relaxation technique can be used to maximize the energy function in Eq. 1.

Fig. 2(a) shows the optimized assignment matrix X by the SMAC method. It can be observed that the distribution of assignment in most rows (or columns) of X is not sharp (with an example of $X_{i,i'}$ values along the pink line shown in the top of Fig. 2 (c)), indicating that it is still very difficult to determine the one-to-one correspondence for each feature point based on the one-to-many correspondences (each with similar likelihood). Thus, a good solution is to keep the large assignments only for the good matches while suppress the distractions from ambiguous matches. To achieve this, we propose to (1) utilize the appearance-based line patch to exclude the in-correct matches when constructing the affinity matrix M and (2) further apply sparsity to the assignment matrix X during the optimization procedure to suppress the influence from ambiguous matches, as will be presented below.

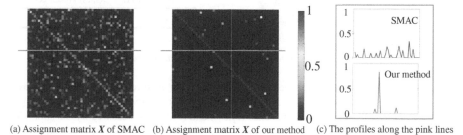

(a) Assignment matrix X of SMAC   (b) Assignment matrix X of our method   (c) The profiles along the pink lines

Fig. 2. The assignment matrix X optimized from the same affinity matrix by SMAC method (without sparsity constraint) and our method (with sparsity constraint)

2.2   Improved Graph Matching Method

Construction of Robust Affinity Matrix with Line Patch: It is clear that the matching performance is largely dependent on the established affinity matrix M, especially the off-diagonal elements which characterize the pairwise agreement between two possible correspondences (i, i') and (j, j'). However, the conventional graph matching methods only consider the geometric coherence between (i, j) and (i', j'). Although local image descriptor can be used to measure the appearance similarities between feature point t_i and $s_{i'}$, as well as between t_j and $s_{j'}$, it still fails to discriminate the unreasonable matches as shown in Fig. 3. In this example, there are two template feature points and three subject feature points. Subject feature points $s_{1'}$ and $s_{2'}$ (blue circles) are the correct matches of template feature points t_1 and t_2 (white circles) in the template image, while $s_{3'}$ (blue triangle) is the incorrect match to t_2. However, neither the geometric coherence nor local descriptor based measurement is able to distinguish the incorrect correspondence $(2, 3')$ from the correct one $(2, 2')$ in the affinity matrix M, which affects the optimization of assignment matrix X in Eq. 1.

To solve this problem, we define the *line patch* by utilizing a sequence of intensity profiles along the line connecting the two feature points in the template or subject image. In Fig. 3, the image intensity profiles along the lines $\overline{t_1 t_2}$, $\overline{s_{1'} s_{2'}}$ and $\overline{s_{1'} s_{3'}}$ are displayed as blue, green, and white stripes, respectively. Thus, a collection of intensity profiles along the underlying stripe can be captured, which is referred to as the *line patch* in our method, to measure the pairwise agreement of two possible matches. Specifically, normalized cross correlation is used to measure the similarity between line patches. As shown in the right part of Fig. 3, the pairwise agreement measured by the line patches is able to distinguish between the correct and incorrect matches. Here we note that the radius of intensity profile is set to 5 pixel and we uniformly sample 60 local intensity profiles for each line patch. Thus, the number of intensity values included in the line patch of our method is 11×60.

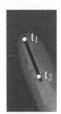 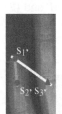

	Normalized cross correlation between line patches	
	$(s_{1'}, s_{2'})$ (correct)	$(s_{1'}, s_{3'})$ (incorrect)
(t_1, t_2)	0.7616	0.1750

(a) Line patch on template T (b) Line patches on subject S (c) Similarity between line patches

Fig. 3. Demonstration of using line patches in removing incorrect matches. Three possible correspondences are shown, i.e., $(t_1, s_{1'})$ (correct), $(t_2, s_{2'})$ (correct), $(t_2, s_{3'})$ (incorrect). The pairwise agreement between correct matches $(t_1, s_{1'})$ and $(t_2, s_{2'})$ is measured by the similarity of blue and green line patches, while another pairwise agreement is measured by blue and white line patches for incorrect match. Since each line patch utilizes the intensity profiles between two feature points, it is able to suppress the incorrect matches in the affinity matrix, as quantitatively measured by the normalized cross correlation listed in the right part of this figure.

Sparse Constraint on Assignment Vector: Although the one-to-many correspondence strategy ensures detection of all possible matches for each feature point, it also introduces many ambiguous matches, which could affect the final determination of one-to-one correspondences as shown in Fig. 2(a). Inspired by the discriminative power of sparse representation, we apply the l_1-norm on the assignment vector x to require the number of non-zero elements in x to be as small as possible. Since the affine constraint $Ax = \mathbf{1}^T$ in Eq. 1 specifies each feature point to have at least one correspondence, the l_1-norm regularization term on the entire vector x eventually leads to the sparsity on the possible matches for each feature point.

The advantage of using l_1-norm regularization $\|x\|_1$ is demonstrated in Fig. 2(b). Compared with the assignment matrix obtained by SMAC without l_1-norm constraint, the distribution of assignments along each row and each column of matrix X is much sharper by our method. Thus, it is easier to finally apply the Hungarian algorithm to binarize X and obtain the one-to-one correspondences. It is worth noting that both methods are performed on the same affinity matrix, in order to evaluate only the effectiveness of including l_1-norm regularization in correspondence detection.

New Energy Function for Graph Matching: Incorporating the two improvements described above, our energy function for graph matching is given as:

$$F(x) = x^T M x - \gamma \cdot \|x\|_1 \quad s.t. \ Ax = 1^T \ and \ \{0 \le x_m \le 1 | m = 1, ..., nn'\} \quad (2)$$

Apparently, the first term is similar to SMAC method, except that the affinity matrix M is constructed by adding our newly-defined line patch to measure the pairwise agreement (i.e., off-diagonal elements in M). The second term $\|x\|_1$ is called as sparsity constraint term, with its strength being controlled by the parameter γ.

2.3   Optimization for the Improved Graph Matching

We can incorporate the affine constraint $Ax = 1^T$ into the energy function in Eq. 2 as:

$$F'(x) = x^T M x - \gamma \cdot \|x\|_1 - \lambda \cdot \|Ax - 1^T\|_2^2 \quad s.t. \ \{0 \le x_m \le 1 | m = 1, ..., nn'\} \ (3)$$

Since each element x_m in x is non-negative, we can simplify $\|x\|_1$ as $\sum_{m=1}^{nn'} x_m = 1x$. Then the energy function $F'(x)$ becomes the quadratic function of x. Finally the maximization of $F'(x)$ falls into the constrained indefinite quadratic programming problem and can be efficiently solved by the trust region reflective algorithm [8].

3   Experiments

A publicly available USC hand atlas[1] is used for evaluation of our method. The resolution for each image is $0.1mm \times 0.1mm$ [9]. Thirty landmarks were manually placed for each of 43 left hand radiographs, randomly selected from the images of 11-year-old children, and these manual landmarks are used as ground-truth in this paper. Correspondence results are evaluated by the matching errors computed as the Euclidean distances between the automatically detected correspondences and the ground-truth.

In order to demonstrate the advantages of line patch and sparsity constraint separately, we compare the following four methods: (1) SMAC, (2) SMAC with line patch, (3) our method without line patch, and (4) our full method (equipped with both

---

[1] http://www.ipilab.org/BAAweb/

line patch and sparsity constraint). For the four methods, the normalized cross correlation between local intensity patches are used to measure the pointwise similarities in establishing possible correspondences (i.e., diagonal elements in affinity matrix M). The experiments are conducted by randomly selecting one image as the template image and the rest 42 images as the subject images. In each round of cross validation case, affine registration is performed for each subject image before detecting its correspondence with the selected template image. For the template image, 30 manually placed landmarks are used as its feature points, while, for each subject image, we follow the automatic landmark detection method in [10] to select around 450 feature points.

Typical correspondence matching results by SMAC and our full method are shown in Fig. 4, where correct matches are displayed by solid cyan lines and incorrect matches are displayed by dashed pink lines. By visual inspection, it can be concluded that our full method is able to correctly identify all 30 correspondences, while SMAC method failed at two landmarks (#3 and #30). For the better illustration, we also zoom in the regions enclosing the landmarks #3 and #30 (see black rectangle in the original images), and show them in the right of Fig. 4(a) and Fig. 4(b), respectively. For matching two images of size about 1500×2000, the average runtimes for SMAC and our full method are 451seconds and 537 seconds by a Matlab implementation.

Table 1 shows the mean and standard deviation of matching errors between the ground-truth and the estimated correspondences by the four methods, with respect to the two different templates. It can be seen that (1) our full method achieves the highest matching accuracy; and (2) each improvement strategy proposed in our method has significant effect in enhancing the performance of correspondence detection.

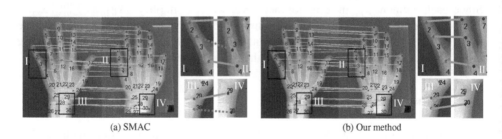

| (a) SMAC | (b) Our method |

Fig. 4. Matching results by (a) SMAC and (b) our full method, with solid cyan lines showing correct matches and dashed pink lines showing incorrect matches. In the right of (a) and (b), regions I and III represent the enlarged views at landmarks 3 and 30 of the template image, and regions II and IV represent the corresponding enlarged views of the subject image.

Table 1. Mean and standard deviation of matching errors between the manual ground-truth and the estimated correspondences by the four methods (mm)

	SMAC	SMAC + line patch	Our method (without line patch)	Our method (line patch + sparsity)
Template 1	1.78 ± 2.54	1.33 ± 1.79	1.20 ± 1.50	0.98 ± 1.08
Template 2	2.12 ± 4.57	1.78 ± 3.96	1.36 ± 1.89	1.07 ± 1.28

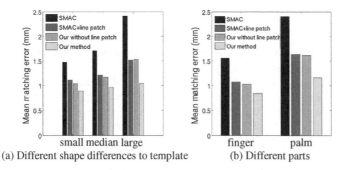

Fig. 5. Mean matching errors of four methods (a) under different amounts of shape difference from the selected template, and (b) at different parts of hand images

Furthermore, we demonstrate the robustness of the four methods under two different cases: (a) shape variation (such as difference between subject image and the template image), and (b) image contrast (such as in different parts of hand images). Specifically, for the first case, we classify all subject images into three groups (i.e., small, median, large) according to the total shape distance of their 30 manually labeled landmarks to the selected template image after affine alignment. Fig. 5(a) shows the mean distance errors by the four methods, which indicate that our full method achieves the lowest distance error. It is worth noting that, for the group with large shape difference, the matching error by our full method is almost 50% lower than that by SMAC method. This shows the great performance of our method in dealing with large inter-subject variations. For the second case, we separate landmarks into two different groups, i.e., located in the finger areas with high image contrast or in the palm areas with poor contrast. According to the results in Fig. 5(b), our method in difficult areas (i.e., palm areas) achieves even lower distance error than the SMAC method in the easy areas (i.e., finger areas).

4   Conclusion

In this paper, we have proposed a new graph matching method to improve the accuracy in establishing anatomical correspondences between two images. Our contributions have twofold: (1) a new concept of line patch is proposed to robustly characterize the pairwise agreement of two possible matches/correspondences; and (2) sparsity constraint is further introduced for the correspondence assignment, to suppress the influence from ambiguous matches. Promising results have been achieved by our method on the hand X-ray images, outperforming the state-of-the-art SMAC graph matching method. In the future, we will extend our method to other medical applications, e.g., deformable registration and motion correction for lung 4D-CT images by extending our method to deal with large number of feature points under the framework of hierarchical correspondence matching.

References

1. Chui, H., Rangarajan, A.: A New Point Matching Algorithm for Non-Rigid Registration. Comput. Vis. Image Underst. 89(2-3), 114–141 (2003)
2. Castillo, E., Castillo, R., Martinez, J., et al.: Four-Dimensional Deformable Image Registration Using Trajectory Modeling. Phys. Med. Biol. 55(1), 305–327 (2010)
3. Maciel, J., Costeira, J.P.: A Global Solution to Sparse Correspondence Problems. IEEE Trans. on Pattern Anal. Mach. Intell. 25(2), 187–199 (2003)
4. Cour, T., Srinivasan, P., Shi, J.: Balanced Graph Matching. In: Advances in Neural Information Processing Systems 19, pp. 313–320. MIT Press (2006)
5. Leordeanu, M., Hebert, M.: A Spectral Technique for Correspondence Problems Using Pairwise Constraints. In: International Conference of Computer Vision, vol. 2, pp. 1482–1489. IEEE Computer Society (2005)
6. Tibshirani, R.: Regression Shrinkage and Selection Via the Lasso. Journal of the Royal Statistical Society Series B 58(1), 267–288 (1996)
7. Wright, J., Yang, A.Y., Ganesh, A., et al.: Robust Face Recognition Via Sparse Representation. IEEE Trans. on Pattern Anal. Mach. Intell. 31(2), 210–227 (2009)
8. Nocedal, J., Wright, S.J.: Numerical Optimization, 2nd edn. Springer, New York (2006)
9. Cao, F., Huang, H.K., Pietka, E., et al.: An Image Database for Digital Hand Atlas. In: Proceedings of SPIE Medical Imaging: PACS and Integrated Medical Information Systems: Design and Evaluation, vol. 5033, pp. 461–470 (2003)
10. Zhang, P., Cootes, T.: Automatic Construction of Parts+Geometry Models for Initialising Groupwise Registration. IEEE Transactions on Medical Imaging 31(2), 341–358 (2012)

Semi-supervised Segmentation Using Multiple Segmentation Hypotheses from a Single Atlas

Tobias Gass, Gábor Székely, and Orcun Goksel

Computer Vision Lab, Dep. of Electrical Engineering, ETH Zurich, Switzerland
{gasst,gszekely,ogoeksel}@vision.ee.ethz.ch

Abstract. A semi-supervised segmentation method using a single atlas is presented in this paper. Traditional atlas-based segmentation suffers from either a strong bias towards the selected atlas or the need for manual effort to create multiple atlas images. Similar to semi-supervised learning in computer vision, we study a method which exploits information contained in a *set* of unlabelled images by mutually registering them non-rigidly and propagating the single atlas segmentation over multiple such registration paths to each target. These multiple segmentation hypotheses are then fused by local weighting based on registration similarity. Our results on two datasets of different anatomies and image modalities, corpus callosum MR and mandible CT images, show a significant improvement in segmentation accuracy compared to traditional single atlas based segmentation. We also show that the bias towards the selected atlas is minimized using our method. Additionally, we devise a method for the selection of intermediate targets used for propagation, in order to reduce the number of necessary inter-target registrations without loss of final segmentation accuracy.

1 Introduction

Image segmentation is an essential problem in medical image processing. Among automatic segmentation methods, the amount of prior information needed is a major distinguishing characteristic of different approaches. It is desirable to limit the constraints posed by prior knowledge both to retain generalizability and to reduce the effort required to acquire the information needed. Arguably, intensity-based approaches are among the methods that require the least amount of prior information. However, these methods are often susceptible to imaging artifacts, ambiguous intensities, and low contrast low signal-to-noise ratio imaging modalities, since no prior knowledge of shape or pose is assumed. Examples of such methods are active contours [1] and MRF-based segmentation [2, 3]. A straight-forward method for incorporating anatomical knowledge into automatic segmentation is the registration of an *atlas* image with known segmentation to a target image, namely *atlas based segmentation* [4, 5]. Then, the resulting transformation can be applied to the labelled atlas, yielding a segmentation of the target image. As the registration is ill-posed due to ambiguous and non-convex criteria [6], only approximate solutions can be achieved and these are influenced

B.H. Menze et al. (Eds.): MCV 2012, LNCS 7766, pp. 29–37, 2013.

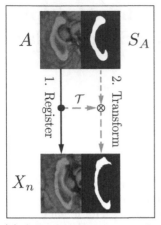 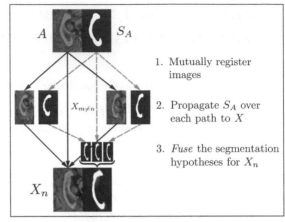

(a) Atlas based segmentation   (b) The proposed method

Fig. 1. Illustration of standard atlas based segmentation (left) and our proposed method (right). In the latter, additional segmentation hypotheses are created by deforming the atlas segmentation multiple times along each path to each target. In a last step, these hypotheses are then fused to create the final segmentations.

strongly by the choice of the atlas image [7]. To remedy this, the use of multiple atlases is a common approach [7–12]: The information contained in such set of atlases can be used to create an average atlas [11]; to train statistical models of shape [8] or deformations [12]; or to register them individually to the target and fuse these segmentations afterward [13]. While all these methods improve segmentation accuracy compared to single atlas based segmentation, several studies indicate that the latter fusion of multiple deformed atlas segmentations is superior to registering an average atlas [7, 9].

In contrast to increasing the amount of manual annotation, harnessing information from unlabelled data has been a major research focus in computer vision. To this end, semi-supervised learning [14] is an established framework which enables tasks like image classification in large and diverse databases [15, 16]. For medical image segmentation, the situation is similar: large amounts of raw data are readily available while annotated data (atlases) are scarce.

In this paper, we study a method that propagates atlas segmentation labels via a graph of inter-target registrations. This is inspired by label propagation in semi-supervised learning [17] and similar to a method presented in [13], which used *indirect propagation* of atlas labels to validate multi-atlas segmentation results. In our framework, the traditional single atlas segmentation can be seen as direct, or *zero-hop* propagation. Multiple segmentation hypotheses per target can be obtained by allowing more *hops* via other target images, generating a different segmentation hypothesis for each path from the atlas to the target (c.f. Fig. 1b), which are then fused. In this paper, different strategies are studied for fusing such propagated labels for the segmentation of each target. Experiments with different anatomies and image modalities show significant improvement over the traditional atlas-based segmentation. In order for the method to scale successfully to larger datasets, we also investigate methods to reduce the number of propagation connections in the graph, which in turn reduces the computational complexity by removing registrations that would otherwise be necessary.

2   Label Propagation

In this section, we present our method of generating and fusing multiple segmentation hypotheses for each target image X_n in a set of N unlabelled images using a single atlas A. An image is a function $\Omega \to \mathbb{R}$, where $\Omega \in \mathbb{N}^D$ is the discrete coordinate domain and D is the dimensionality of the image. We define a binary segmentation as $S_{(.)} = \Omega \to \{0, 1\}$. A transformation is denoted with $\mathcal{T}$, e.g. $\mathcal{T}(A)$ is the transformed atlas A. While $\mathcal{T}$ can be an arbitrary transformation, we will assume non-rigid deformations represented by dense displacement fields throughout this paper. Let $\mathcal{T}_{source,target}$ denote a registration from X_m to X_n. We first mutually register all images $\{A, X_1, \ldots, X_N\}$, finding all possible combinations of $\mathcal{T}$, which are also connections in the graph. The traditional atlas based segmentation for a target X_n is then given by a *zero-hop* segmentation $S_n^0 = \mathcal{T}_{A,n}(S_A)$. Such segmentations can then be *propagated* to a target X_n over other target images $X_{m \neq n}$ as secondary (*one-hop*) segmentation hypotheses:

$$S_{m,n}^1 = \mathcal{T}_{m,n}(S_m^0). \tag{1}$$

These hypotheses must then be *fused*: We use a function F to first generate a spatial segmentation probability map $\hat{S}_n = \Omega \to [0, 1]$ and subsequently binarize this using thresholding. The said probability map is generated as a weighted average of the zero- and one-hop segmentation hypotheses:

$$\hat{S}_n = F\left(S_n^0, \{S_{m,n}^1 | m \neq n\}\right) = \frac{1}{\sum \lambda}\left(\lambda_n^0 S_n^0 + \sum_{m \neq n} \lambda_{m,n}^1 S_{m,n}^1\right). \tag{2}$$

We propose and evaluate two different strategies for the choice of weights λ:

Global Similarity Weighting (GSW):   Assuming correlation between segmentation accuracy and a normalized post-registration similarity f_G, the latter can be used as a scalar weight. Using the zero-hop deformed atlas image $A_n^0 = \mathcal{T}_{A,n}(A)$, the zero-hop weight is then $\lambda_n^0 = f_G(X_n, A_n^0)$. The atlas image is propagated analogously to the atlas segmentation along each path, i.e. $A_{m,n}^1 = \mathcal{T}_{m,n}(A_m^0)$, which leads to one-hop weights as follows:

$$\lambda_{m,n}^1 = f_G\left(X_n, A_{m,n}^1\right). \tag{3}$$

Locally Adaptive Weighting (LAW): In contrast to the constant weights per hypothesis in GSW, a spatially-varying *local* weighting scheme is used:

$$\lambda_{m,n}^1(p) = f_L\left(X_n(p), A_{m,n}^1(p)\right), \forall p \in \Omega . \tag{4}$$

In contrast to GSW, such locally adaptive weighting is expected to leverage useful information even from partially mis-registered images.

3   Compact Graphs

To use all one-hop segmentation hypotheses, all graph connections should be computed requiring N^2 registrations. With large datasets this may easily become computationally challenging. Below, different methods are proposed for selecting a target image subset $\mathbb{X}$, called *support-samples*, that will act as intermediate nodes via which the atlas segmentation is propagated using (1). Reducing the size $K=|\mathbb{X}|$ then decrease the number of edges in $\mathcal{G}$ and hence the number of necessary inter-target registrations. A natural choice is to sort nodes by their GSW-based zero-hop weights λ_n^0, as this corresponds to image similarity to deformed atlas, and to use the highest ranked images as support samples. We call this GSW-based ranking. This scheme makes two assumptions: first, that it is utmost important to propagate 'good' zero-hop segmentations; and second, that the quality of these segmentations can be assessed reliably using the similarity function f. Using our label propagation framework, we propose the following two additional ranking criteria for selecting support samples.

In segmenting a target X_n, we wish to quantify how reliable a one-hop segmentation hypotesis $S_{m,n}^1$ via an intermediate node X_m is. As we only know the segmentation of the atlas, we define an *atlas reconstruction error* (ARE) for such quantification. Exploiting the fact that most non-rigid registration algorithms are not symmetric, we compute deformations $\mathcal{T}_{m,A}$ to obtain back-propagated one-hop atlas segmentation hypotheses $S_{m,A}^1 = \mathcal{T}_{m,A}(S_m^0)$ via each graph node. Then, ARE for each node is defined based on Dice's similarity coefficient:

$$\text{ARE}\,(m) = 1 - \text{Dice}\left(S_A, S_{m,A}^1\right), \tag{5}$$

and support samples are selected from the smallest error nodes. While such ranking is expected to perform superior to GSW-based ranking, it cannot ensure that complementary information is contained in the set. For example, a subset $\mathbb{X}$ might have individually low AREs, however, their one-hop hypotheses may all contain similar errors which are then amplified when they are fused to create a target segmentation. It is thus desirable to find a *complementary* basis, where each support sample is likely to contain information that other samples do not provide. We therefore propose a *groupwise* error criterion (ARE-G) to score a *set* of K graph nodes:

$$\text{ARE-G}(S_A, \{m_1, \ldots, m_K\}) = 1 - \text{Dice}\left(S_A, F\left(S_{m_1,A}^1, \ldots, S_{m_K,A}^1\right)\right), \tag{6}$$

where F is the fusion function in (2). As it is not feasible to evaluate all $\binom{N}{K}$ K-sized sets of support samples, we rely on a greedy scheme where we pick the first support sample based on its individual ARE, and iteratively add support samples that reduce ARE-G the most.

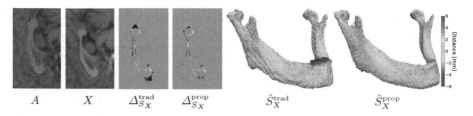

Fig. 2. Sample results for both datasets. For the MR dataset, the atlas, a target image and the difference of both the traditional single-atlas based segmentation $\Delta_{S_X}^{\text{trad}}$ and our proposed method $\Delta_{S_X}^{\text{prop}}$ from the ground-truth are shown. False positives and false negatives are shown in black and white, respectively. For the CT dataset, the traditional atlas based segmentation and our method are shown for the same atlas/target, and the surface is colored with the distance error to the ground-truth.

4   Results and Discussion

We evaluated our method using a set of 70 mid-saggital slices of MR brain scans containing the corpus callosum and a set of 15 3D CT scans of the head. Both datasets were rigidly pre-aligned. In the MR dataset a fixed region of interest containing the corpus callosum was cropped out in all images. The images are 120x200 pixels with 0.3 mm spacing in the MR dataset and 160x160x129 voxels with 1 mm spacing in the CT dataset. We used the Dice coefficient to measure volume overlap, the Hausdorff distance (HD) for estimating maximum surface-to-surface distance, and the mean surface distance (MSD) as an additional distance based metric. In both datasets we performed a leave-one-out (l1o) evaluation scheme, using each image as atlas in turn to segment all remaining images. We used our own implementation of the MRF-based registration in [4] as the registration method of choice in our experiments. We used normalized cross correlation (NCC) as the registration similarity criterion throughout our experiments, and accordingly defined GSW weights using $f_{\text{G}} = \frac{1-\text{NCC}}{2}$. Since NCC is not suitable as a point-wise metric for LAW, we used the following intensity difference based radial basis function $\lambda_{m,n}^{1}(p) = \exp\left(-\frac{|X_n(p) - A_{m,n}^1(p)|}{\sigma^2}\right)$ where σ^2 is the intensity variance over all images. Sample results are given in Fig. 2.

Quantitative results can be found in Tab. 1. For both datasets, the improvement over traditional atlas based segmentation is significant, especially considering the distance based metrics which are outperformed by $\approx 35\%$(HD) and $\approx 60\%$(MSD). The CT images also show a strong improvement in Dice similarity metric, and LAW expectedly performed superior to GSW. GSW only slightly outperforms an uniform weighting, which results in a simple max-voting scheme. We also compared our method to a recent group-wise registration approach (ABSORB [11]) a 3D implementation of which is publicly available. This method uses the atlas as a reference image, on which all test images are aligned iteratively to improve a mean image. Similarly to ours, this method also utilizes

Table 1. Mean segmentation accuracy from leave-one-out evaluation on the MR(2D) and CT(3D) datasets

	Corpus Callosum in MR			Mandibles in CT		
	DICE	HD	MSD	DICE	HD	MSD
single-atlas [4]	0.926	2.45	0.088	0.828	12.37	0.50
Propagation-maxvote	0.944	1.50	0.027	0.852	9.24	0.32
Propagation-GSW	0.944	1.49	0.027	0.859	9.32	0.27
Propagation-LAW	**0.946**	**1.46**	**0.025**	**0.886**	**8.42**	**0.18**
ABSORB [11]	-	-	-	0.698	14.74	0.86
multi-atlas-LAW	0.965	1.06	0.014	0.917	5.77	0.13

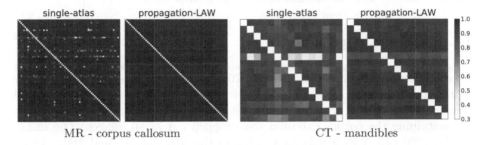

MR - corpus callosum   CT - mandibles

Fig. 3. Segmentation accuracy (Dice) of traditional single atlas based segmentation and our proposed method with LAW fusion for each atlas (x-axis) and target (y-axis) image combination. (The diagonal values were not computed.)

image information contained in the entire dataset. However, unlike the probabilistic map in our method, ABSORB generates a single binary segmentation per target and thus suffers from a bias towards the atlas similarly to the traditional atlas based segmentation. This is seen in the results as it is outperformed by our proposed method. In order to estimate an upper bound for the expected performance of our method, we also computed multi-atlas segmentation of each target by using all remaining images and their ground-truth segmentations as multiple atlases. We used the same registration method and LAW weighting to achieve comparable results. As seen in Tab. 1, even though our method did not reach the performance of such multi-atlas segmentation, it performed remarkably close to it while using orders of magnitude less prior knowledge.

In Fig. 3, the Dice measure is plotted for each atlas/target pair of our l1o-experiments. For both datasets, it is seen that using traditional atlas based segmentation some atlases lead to sub-optimal segmentations. Using our method, however, these sub-optimal pairs seen as 'speckles' disappear, indicating an improved performance for arbitrary atlas selection.

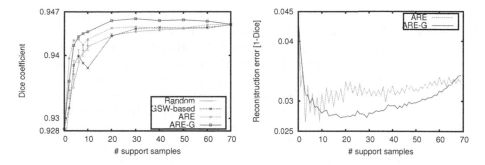

Fig. 4. Dice metric for support sample selection for a single atlas using random selection, GSW-based, individual ARE, and ARE-G ranking criteria (left). The progression of error as more support samples are added.

Support Sample Reduction: We first evaluated a random selection of K support samples for each target and repeated this 10 times each. As shown in Fig. 4(left), Dice metric improves rapidly until reaching 20 support samples, which is also the point at which the standard deviation becomes negligible. We then used the GSW-based ranking, which did not provide any improvement over random draws. Individual ARE based ranking expectedly outperformed random draws, and the group-wise ARE ranking was superior to all other support sample selection methods. Interestingly, the results indicate the presense of support sample subsets that can perform *better* in comparison to using all the samples (the full graph). We also analyzed the progression of error during the expansion of the support-sample subset. As seen in Fig. 4(right), error using ARE-G based ranking starts deteriorating beyond a certain number of subset size. This number is also near the optimal Dice metric shown in Fig. 4(left) as the posterior target segmentation accuracy. Based on this observation, we propose to use the deflecting point (minimum value) of ARE-G to determine optimal graph size. Note that individual ARE does not exhibit such a behaviour. Accordingly, we have repeated the 11o-experiments on the MR dataset using only 20 support samples selected by ARE-G ranking. This yielded mean Dice of 94 % and mean HD of 1.56 mm, which are nearly identical to the results using all target images while requiring less than three times the number of intermediate target images and their registrations.

Discussion: Our method was shown to increase segmentation accuracy substantially compared to the standard atlas based segmentation. This can be attributed to the boosting nature of the approach, which can be seen as creating and fusing multiple weak classifiers in a semi-supervised manner. Our results being close to that of multi-atlas segmentation, we conclude that a substantial amount of the information contained in a set of *atlas* images is indeed available in the support (*target*) images, and that is the information leveraged by our method. Note that this contradicts partially with the findings of [13], which concludes that the major benefit of multi-atlas segmentation is due to the increase in anatomical variation in the available ground-truth. We believe that this difference in findings might be due to different registration algorithms and datasets, which will be important to explore in the future work. Additionally, it will be interesting to explore whether a principled, probabilistic approach can be employed to also take into account the improved segmentations in an iterative manner. A similar method was proposed in [18] for images aligned to a single template, whereas we aim to include information from inter-target registrations as well. For the CT images, we used the probabilistic segmentation output as shape prior in an MRF-based segmentation [2]. This led to a considerable improvement in results with a mean Dice of 93 %. As this relies on strong edges to find bone boundaries, it does not yield a significant improvement in the MR images.

5 Conclusions

We presented a novel method that augments single-atlas based segmentation using multiple segmentation hypotheses for each target obtained by propagating atlas segmentation along different paths. This outperforms both the traditional single-atlas based registration and group-wise registration. We also demonstrated that a smaller set of support samples providing complementary information can be found automatically. Using such reduced set of support samples both decreases the computational complexity of the method and improves the results as redundant and possibly detrimental information is then discarded.

Acknowledgements. This work has been funded by the Swiss National Center of Competence in Research on Computer Aided and Image Guided Medical Interventions (NCCR Co-Me) supported by the Swiss National Science Foundation.

References

1. Kass, M., Witkin, A.: Snakes: Active contour models. International Journal of Computer Vision 331, 321–331 (1988)
2. Furnstahl, P., Fuchs, T., Schweizer, A., Nagy, L., Székely, G., Harders, M.: Automatic and robust forearm segmentation using graph cuts. In: ISBI, pp. 77–80 (2008)
3. Boykov, Y., Funke-Lea, G.: Graph Cuts and Efficient N-D Image Segmentation. International Journal of Computer Vision 70(2), 109–131 (2006)
4. Glocker, B., Komodakis, N., Tziritas, G., Navab, N., Paragios, N.: Dense image registration through MRFs and efficient linear programming. Medical Image Analysis 12(6), 731–741 (2008)
5. Rueckert, D., Aljabar, P., Heckemann, R.A., Hajnal, J.V., Hammers, A.: Diffeomorphic Registration Using B-Splines. In: Larsen, R., Nielsen, M., Sporring, J. (eds.) MICCAI 2006. LNCS, vol. 4191, pp. 702–709. Springer, Heidelberg (2006)
6. Fischer, B., Modersitzki, J.: Ill-posed medicine - an introduction to image registration. Inverse Problems 24(3), 1–19 (2008)
7. Rohlfing, T., Brandt, R., Menzel, R., Russakoff, D., Maurer, C.: Quo vadis, atlas-based segmentation? In: Handbook of Biomedical Image Analysis, pp. 435–486 (2005)

8. Heimann, T., Meinzer, H.P.: Statistical shape models for 3D medical image segmentation: A review. Medical Image Analysis 13(4), 543–563 (2009)
9. Isgum, I., Staring, M., Rutten, A., Prokop, M., Viergever, M.A., van Ginneken, B.: Multi-atlas-based segmentation with local decision fusion–application to cardiac and aortic segmentation in CT scans. IEEE T. Med. Imaging 28(7), 1000–1010 (2009)
10. van Rikxoort, E.M., Isgum, I., Arzhaeva, Y., Staring, M., Klein, S., Viergever, M.A., Pluim, J.P.W., van Ginneken, B.: Adaptive local multi-atlas segmentation: application to the heart and the caudate nucleus. Medical Image Analysis 14(1), 39–49 (2010)
11. Jia, H., Wu, G., Wang, Q., Shen, D.: NeuroImage ABSORB: Atlas building by self-organized registration and bundling. NeuroImage 51(3), 1057–1070 (2010)
12. Rueckert, D., Frangi, A.F., Schnabel, J.A.: Automatic Construction of 3D Statistical Deformation Models Using Non-rigid Registration. In: Niessen, W.J., Viergever, M.A. (eds.) MICCAI 2001. LNCS, vol. 2208, pp. 77–84. Springer, Heidelberg (2001)
13. Heckemann, R.A., Hajnal, J.V., Aljabar, P., Rueckert, D., Hammers, A.: Automatic anatomical brain MRI segmentation combining label propagation and decision fusion. NeuroImage 33(1), 115–126 (2006)
14. Chapelle, O., Schölkopf, B., Zien, A. (eds.): Semi-supervised learning, vol. 2. MIT Press, Cambridge (2006)
15. Wang, F., Wang, J., Zhang, C., Shen, H.C., Bay, C.W., Kong, H.: Semi-Supervised Classification Using Linear Neighborhood Propagation. Sci. & Tech. (2006)
16. Guillaumin, M., Verbeek, J., Schmid, C.: Multimodal semi-supervised learning for image classification. In: IEEE CVPR, pp. 902–909 (June 2010)
17. Zhu, X., Ghahramani, Z.: Learning from labeled and unlabeled data with label propagation. Technical report, School Comput. Sci. Carnegie Mellon Univ. (2002)
18. Riklin-Raviv, T., Van Leemput, K., Menze, B.H., Wells, W.M., Golland, P.: Segmentation of image ensembles via latent atlases. Medical Image Analysis 14(5), 654–665 (2010)

Carotid Artery Wall Segmentation by Coupled Surface Graph Cuts

Andres Arias[1], Jens Petersen[2], Arna van Engelen[1], Hui Tang[1,3],
Mariana Selwaness[4,5,6], Jacqueline C.M. Witteman[5], Aad van der Lugt[4],
Wiro Niessen[1,3], and Marleen de Bruijne[1,2]

[1] Biomedical Imaging Group Rotterdam, Departments of Radiology and Medical
Informatics, Erasmus MC, Rotterdam, The Netherlands
[2] Image Group, Department of Computer Science, University of Copenhagen,
Denmark
[3] Faculty of Applied Sciences, Department of Imaging Science and Technology, Delft
University of Technology, The Netherlands
[4] Department of Radiology, Erasmus MC, Rotterdam, The Netherlands
[5] Department of Epidemiology, Erasmus MC, Rotterdam, The Netherlands
[6] Department of Biomedical Engineering, Erasmus MC, Rotterdam, The Netherlands

Abstract. We present a three-dimensional coupled surface graph cut algorithm for carotid wall segmentation from Magnetic Resonance Imaging
(MRI). Using cost functions that highlight both inner and outer vessel
wall borders, the method combines the search for both borders into a single graph cut optimization. Our approach requires little user interaction
and can robustly segment the carotid artery bifurcation. Experiments on
32 carotid arteries from 16 patients show good agreement between manual segmentation performed by an expert and our method. The mean
relative area of overlap is more than 85% for both lumen and outer vessel wall. In addition, differences in measured wall thickness with respect
to the manual annotations were smaller than the in-plane pixel size.

Keywords: Carotid artery, flow lines, graph, segmentation.

1 Introduction

Atherosclerosis is one of the primary causes of death in the world [11]. Atherosclerotic plaques in the carotid arteries cause lumen narrowing. This may lead to
plaque rupture, which can cause a stroke or Transient Ischemic Attack (TIA).
Therefore, the early detection of plaque and accurate quantification of lumen
narrowing and plaque volume are important. In order to determine these parameters, segmentation of both the vessel lumen and the outer vessel wall are
required. As manual segmentation is highly time consuming and subject to
observer variability, automated techniques are needed.

Although most work on automated segmentation of blood vessels has focused
on segmenting the vessel lumen only, several automatic and semi-automatic
methods have been proposed in the past for segmenting the outer vessel wall.

B.H. Menze et al. (Eds.): MCV 2012, LNCS 7766, pp. 38–47, 2013.
© Springer-Verlag Berlin Heidelberg 2013

Active Shape Models (ASMs) have been used for detecting the outer vessel wall of the abdominal aorta in CTA scans [3]. These ASMs utilize a statistical model of shape and boundary grey level appearance to restrict the search space to anatomically reasonable solutions. To segment the carotid arteries in MRI, gradient-based ellipse fitting combined with fuzzy clustering [1] and Closed Contour Snakes (CCS) [14] have been proposed. A drawback of both these methods is that user interaction is required for each image slice. More recently, van 't Klooster et al. [8] proposed a three-dimensional (3D) deformable vessel model, in which a vessel is modeled using a 3D cylindrical surface that can be modified by moving control points located on the model surface. Good results were achieved on Black-Blood MRI images of the carotids. This method can however segment only a single, non-bifurcating vessel and will therefore not give reliable results in the bifurcation region. Furthermore, it uses a local optimization procedure with the lumen segmentation as initialization, which may get stuck in a local optimum in diseased vessels where the distance between the inner and outer wall can be large. Better segmentation results may be achieved if both walls are estimated jointly across the bifurcation and if local image information is combined with a globally optimal solution.

Global optimality can be guaranteed with graph based methods, and recently these have been used for vessel segmentation with promising results [9,5,13]. Surface based graph methods such as [9,10,13] as opposed to voxel based [5] make it possible to enforce topology constraints as well to encourage smoothness without biasing the solution towards smaller surfaces. To use these methods the problem has to be transformed from image space to a discretized graph space defined by a set of columns. Each column is associated with a point on the sought surface and represents the set of possible positions it can take. The suitability of the graph space depends on how well the graph columns cross the sought surface [10]. Xu et al. [13] oriented the graph columns in the normal direction of the centerline of the vessels, but this leads to long columns and thus in-efficiency if the sought surface is far from the centerline. Moreover, straight columns intersect in regions with curvature leading to possibly self-intersecting surfaces [10].

We propose to use a 3D coupled surface graph cut algorithm for carotid artery wall segmentation from MRI images. Similar to Petersen et al. [10] who applied such a technique for segmenting airway trees, we define the graph columns based on flow lines traced from a coarse initial segmentation. As such flow lines are non-intersecting this enables accurate segmentation across high curvature areas such as the carotid bifurcation. Moreover, as the inner and outer surfaces are estimated jointly, the proposed method can use information from both surfaces locally and globally to reach an optimal solution.

2   Method

2.1   Initial Segmentation

An initial segmentation of the lumen was obtained using the method proposed by Tang et al. [12]. In this method first the lumen centerlines are determined by finding a minimum cost path between three user-defined seed points in the common, internal, and external carotid arteries. To improve accuracy in high curvature regions, this path is refined iteratively by computing a new minimum cost path in a curved multi-planar reformatting based on the current center line estimate. Subsequently, the lumen is segmented using a levelset method, which is initialized by the extracted centerlines and steered by the MR intensities.

2.2   Graph Construction

First, to obtain the graph columns the initial segmentation is converted to a mesh. We located graph vertices at the center of each surface face. This set of vertices is denoted by V_B.

Flow Lines. The graph columns are traced from V_B, and follow the direction of flow lines of the gradient vector field of the smoothed segmentation. An example of columns traced along flow lines is depicted in figure 1. If this gradient vector field is defined in terms of a scalar potential field ϕ, the flow lines will follow the direction of largest change of this potential. We define the scalar field ϕ by the convolution of the initial segmentation with a Gaussian kernel G_σ as:

$$\phi(\boldsymbol{x}) = \int Q\left(\hat{\boldsymbol{x}}\right) G_\sigma\left(\hat{\boldsymbol{x}} - \boldsymbol{x}\right) d\hat{\boldsymbol{x}}, \tag{1}$$

where $Q\colon \mathbb{R}^3 \to \mathbb{Z}$ is the initial lumen segmentation represented by a binary scalar field. Flow lines traced along the gradient of ϕ are smooth and non-intersecting and the surfaces are thus non-self-intersecting [10], see figure 1.

The parametric flow lines $\boldsymbol{f}\colon \mathbb{R} \to \mathbb{R}^3$ that cross each vertex of the initial surface mesh $\boldsymbol{i}_0 \in V_B$ can be computed by solving the following differential equation:

$$\frac{\partial \boldsymbol{f}}{\partial t}(t) = \nabla\phi(\boldsymbol{f}(t)), \tag{2}$$

with initial value given by $\boldsymbol{f}(0) = \boldsymbol{i}_0$. Solving equation (2) for all vertices on the initial surface mesh V_B leads to all graph columns, where inner and outer graph columns are represented by the same flow lines. We use the Runge-Kutta-Fehlberg method to approximate the solution of these differential equations [4]. The solution of $\boldsymbol{f}(t)$ is approximated at regular intervals δ along the flow line. This defines the positions of the other graph vertices. The columns vary in length depending on the point where the gradient of the scalar field ϕ flattens.

Graph Construction and Optimization. To construct the coupled surface graph $G = (V, E)$ with vertices V and edges E, we define the set of vertices in a column by V_i with $i \in V_B$. Therefore, the complete set of vertices V is defined by:

$$V = \bigcup_{i \in V_B, m \in M} V_i^m \cup \{s, t\}. \tag{3}$$

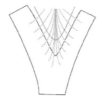

Fig. 1. Graph columns based on flow lines (green) traced from an initial segmentation (black), which are crossing the sought surface (blue)

Here M represents the surfaces to find and s and t denote the source and sink vertices respectively. In our case there are two surfaces, lumen and outer vessel wall surface. Moreover, given that the inner and outer columns are the same, we have $\forall_{m \in M} V_i^m = V_i$.

The edge set E of the coupled surface graph G consists of intra-column edges E_{intra} and edges between columns E_{inter}. For the intra-column edges E_{intra}, we define directed edges connecting each vertex to the next vertex in outward direction in the same column. We assign edges from the source vertex s to all innermost vertices in the graph, and from the outermost vertices to the sink vertex t. Topology preserving edges in the opposite direction with infinite capacity ensure that a minimum cut can cut each column only once. In addition, we assign a cost function $w^m (i_k^m) > 0$ to these edges, mapping a vertex with index k in column V_i to the inverse likelihood representation that it is part of surface m. An example of the intra-column edges and their respective costs is shown in figure 2(a) (for simplicity we do not show the infinity capacity edges).

Selecting a vertex for each column indicates a possible solution for all M surfaces. Therefore, a cut that separates the graph in two parts: sink and source, represents a solution to the segmentation problem. The main aim is then to find a cut that minimizes the cost of the edges that are being cut as depicted in figure 2(b). There are several approaches to solve this optimization problem. We used a min-cut/max-flow algorithm described in [2] to find the minimum cut.

Computing the minimum cut without considering any interaction between columns may lead to irregular surfaces and/or un-realistic relations between surfaces such as borders that are too far from each other, or an outer surface that is inside the inner surface. In order to deal with these problems, we include smoothing penalty edges connecting vertices in columns belonging to the same surface, separation penalty edges and separation constraint edges that connect vertices from columns of different surfaces. These represent the edges between columns E_{inter}.

To ensure smooth surfaces, we linearly penalize the distance in a cut between consecutive columns of the same surface. To do this, we assign edges with the same capacity p between vertices at the same column level. When the length of two consecutive columns are different, the remaining vertices at the inner most part of the column are connected to the source vertex, and the remaining vertices at the outer most part of the column are connected to the sink. If these edges

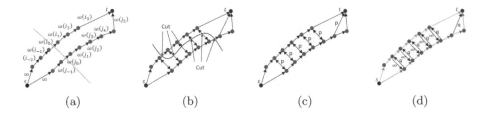

Fig. 2. Examples of intra and inter column edges and a graph cut. In figure 2(a) the intra-column edges, the initial segmentation (green), and the associated cost to each edge are depicted. An example of a graph cut is depicted in figure 2(b), indicating which edges are part of the cut. Figure 2(c) shows the smooth penalty edges which connect vertices from neighbor columns of the same surface. Finally, the separation penalty edges and separation constraint edges are depicted in figure 2(d). These edges connect vertices from columns of different surfaces lying at the same flow line (green: inner column, blue: outer column).

coincide with the intra-column edges, only one edge is assigned and the capacities are added. An example of these smoothing penalty edges is shown in figure 2(c). Using these edges we obtain a linear penalty function of the form $\psi(x) = px$, where x represents the vertex index difference. In a similar way, the separation between surfaces is penalized by assigning capacity q to edges between vertices of columns lying at the same flow line but belonging to different surfaces. In addition, to avoid solutions where parts of the outer surfaces are inside the inner surface, we assign constraint edges with infinite capacity at the same location of the separation edges but pointing from the inner column to the outer column. An example of these separation penalty edges and separation constraint edges is shown in figure 2(d).

2.3   Cost Functions

For the intra-column edges, we define a cost function $w^m(i_k^m) > 0$, which represents the inverse likelihood that the vertex i_k^m is associated to the edge $i_k^m \rightarrow i_{k+1}^m$ is part of surface m. In the case of the carotid walls in our MR images, the graph columns will start inside the lumen area, which looks dark in the image, move through the carotid wall where the voxels are normally brighter, and finally end up out of the carotid wall where the image is darker compared to the wall intensity. We therefore define a cost function for the inner wall w^i which is low for strong dark-to-bright edges, and a cost function for the outer wall w^o which is low for strong bright-to-dark edges. We use a similar approach to Petersen et al. [10] to define the cost functions. First, we define the functions $C^i : \mathbb{R} \rightarrow \mathbb{R}$ and $C^o : \mathbb{R} \rightarrow \mathbb{R}$ that highlight the inner and outer walls. These use a linear combination of the first and second order derivatives of the intensity along the columns:

$$C^i(t) = \gamma^i \frac{\partial P}{\partial t}(t) + \left(1 - |\gamma^i|\right) P(t), \tag{4}$$

$$C^o(t) = \gamma^o \frac{\partial N}{\partial t}(t) + \left(1 - |\gamma^o|\right) \left(-N(t)\right), \tag{5}$$

where $\gamma^i, \gamma^o \in [-1, 1]$ are weighting parameters that can be tuned to adjust the position of the edge slightly inwards or outwards, and P and N the positive and negative parts of the first order derivative respectively. These derivatives are computed using central differences from cubic interpolated values. Subsequently, we invert and normalize C^i and C^o in order to get a representation of the wall inverse likelihood given by w^i and w^o.

3 Experiments and Results

3.1 Data

Proton Density Weighted Black-Blood MRI (BBMRI) and Proton Density Weighted Echo Planar MRI (EPIMRI) images were obtained from 26 subjects that were randomly selected from the Rotterdam study [6]. BBMRI images were acquired using an in-plane pixel size of 1.105mm × 0.8125mm, and 0.9 mm slice thickness. The EPIMRI images have an in-plane pixel size of 0.43mm × 0.8125mm, and a slice thickness of 1.2 mm. BBMRI and EPIMRI images were interpolated on the scanner to a pixel size of 0.507mm × 0.507mm. B-spline registration from EPIMRI to BBMRI using mutual information was performed using with Elastix [7]. To train and evaluate our method, we used manually annotated cross-sectional images with a resolution of 0.05mm×0.05mm extracted at random positions perpendicular to center-lines of both carotid arteries. The manual annotations of the inner and outer carotid walls were drawn by an expert on the BBMRI images. Six manually annotated cross sections were extracted from each carotid artery.

3.2 Graph Parameters Tuning

The proposed method has several parameters: inner and outer smoothness penalties p^i and p^o, separation penalties q, inner and outer cost function derivative weightings γ^i and γ^o, the intervals for sampling the flow lines to define the positions of the vertices δ, and the standard deviation of the Gaussian kernel σ. We used the carotid arteries of ten patients randomly selected to search for the optimal values for these parameters on each image sequence (BBMRI and EPIMRI). The optimal values were obtained by searching the parameter space on the training data-set using an iterative binary search algorithm [10]. In this algorithm, manually annotated cross-sections and automatically segmented cross-sections are compared based on the relative area of overlap. The set of parameters that generated the highest overlap was selected. To reduce the searching time of the parameter optimization algorithm, we fixed the column sampling interval δ to 0.35 mm.

Table 1. Relative area of overlap, WTD, LAD, and OVAD for both sequences (mean absolute and P-values in parentheses)

	BBMRI	EPIMRI
φ^i	$85.2\% \pm 1.6\%$	$83.9\% \pm 5\%$
φ^o	$85.6\% \pm 2.7\%$	$84.1\% \pm 6\%$
WTD(mm)	$-0.25 \pm 0.24(0.28 \pm 0.19; p < 0.001)$	$0.04 \pm 0.23(0.17 \pm 0.15; p = 0.5)$
LAD(mm^2)	$2.7 \pm 2.1(3.0 \pm 1.7; p < 0.001)$	$-0.07 \pm 3.29(2.3 \pm 2.21; p = 0.9)$
OVAD(mm^2)	$-0.3 \pm 1.1(0.92 \pm 0.8; p = 0.3)$	$-0.3 \pm 1.05(0.76 \pm 0.75; p = 0.25)$

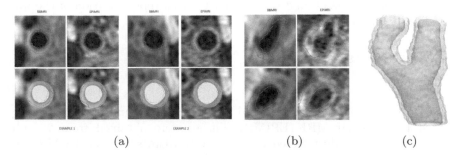

(a)   (b)   (c)

Fig. 3. Automatic segmentation results using the proposed method. In figure 3(a), two example of automated segmented cross-section in BBMRI and EPIMRI are depicted (top). The automatic segmentation is represented by green (inner wall) and blue (outer wall) lines. The overlay of the automatic segmentation to the manual annotations (yellow: lumen, red: vessel wall) is also depicted in figure 3(a) (bottom). Figure 3(b) shows two examples of automatic segmentations obtained in the bifurcation section. Finally, figure 3(c) shows a 3D representation of the automatic segmentation of the complete carotid artery in an image (darker gray: lumen, bright gray: outer wall).

3.3   Segmentation Results

Thirty two carotid arteries of 16 patients not included in the training set were used for the evaluation. Table 1 gives the average relative area of overlap (Dice coefficient) for inner φ^i and outer vessel surface φ^o on this testing data set. In addition, table 1 describes the mean signed and mean absolute difference between wall thickness (WTD) measured by the manual annotation and by the automatic segmentations in BBMRI and EPIMRI. Notice that these values are smaller than the image in-plane pixel size (0.51 mm). We observed good segmentation overlap for both sequences with a slightly higher overlap for BBMRI images. Using EPIMRI images we obtained lower WTD. The table shows also the mean cross-sectional lumen area difference (LAD), and mean cross-sectional outer vessel area difference (OVAD). P-values of the paired t-test including 95% of confidence intervals are also given in the table. Figure 3(a) shows examples of the automatic segmentation results using BBMRI and EPIMRI images together with the overlay to the manual annotations. Results in the bifurcation section, for which no manual annotations were available, are depicted in figure 3(b). Figure 3(c) shows a 3D representation of the automatic segmentation.

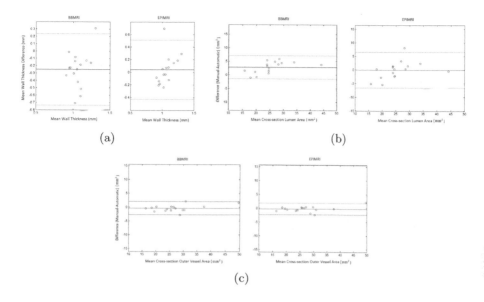

(a)   (b)

(c)

Fig. 4. Bland-Altman plots comparing manual annotations and automatic segmentation for both sequences BBMRI and EPIMRI. Figure 4(a) depicts the comparison of the mean wall thickness. Figure 4(b) and figure 4(c) show a comparison of the mean lumen area and outer vessel area respectively.

Bland-Altman analyses for the mean wall thickness, mean cross-section lumen area, and mean cross-section outer vessel area for the 16 patient data sets are shown in figure 4. From the figure a good agreement between automatic and manual area measurements for lumen and outer vessel wall is observed. Pearson correlation coefficients were 0.95 and 0.98 respectively for BBMRI, and 0.87 and 0.99 for EPIMRI.

4   Discussion and Conclusion

In this paper, we presented a new 3D method for carotid wall segmentation in MRI. Results show a good agreement between manual segmentation performed by an expert and our method. The mean relative area of overlap was about 84% and 85% for EPIMRI and BBMRI respectively. Our results are comparable to or slightly better than those reported in the literature. Van 't Klooster et al. [8] reported a WTD of 0.12mm$\pm$0.21mm. Their method only analyzes the common carotid artery and not the bifurcation. This section may represent the most difficult section to segment. In contrast, we analyze the complete carotid artery. We found a somewhat lower mean WTD with a similar variance (0.04mm $\pm$ 0.23mm) using the EPIMRI sequence.

Adame et al. [1] use similar in-plane resolution images of 17 patients. They reported a LAD of -2.19mm$^2 \pm 5.21$mm^2 and an OVAD of -5.56mm$^2 \pm 19.55$mm^2

with correlation coefficients of 0.92 and 0.91 respectively. Yuan et al. [14] reported a LAD of $1.05mm^2 \pm 2.26mm^2$ and an OVAD of $1.36mm^2 \pm 3.46mm^2$ on five patients, and focus on the internal carotid artery. We reported in general better results on our data compared to these two methods (see table 1). Furthermore, these two methods require a large amount of user interaction. In contrast, our method only requires the location of three seed points for obtaining the initial segmentation.

A potential drawback of our approach is that it relies on an initial lumen segmentation. Although this segmentation does not need to be very accurate, the smoothness constraints are most effective if the shape of the initial segmentation is similar to shape of the true vessel surfaces. Another potential source of errors in our method is related to registration errors of the EPIMRI images. Overall, segmentation results were best for the sequence in which the manual annotations were performed, the BBMRI. However, the EPIMRI images have better wall contrast, which generates better results in some images compared to the results obtained by BBMRI. Therefore, we expect that combining information from both image types in the cost function can still improve upon the results presented here.

To conclude, we propose a graph-based method for segmenting the carotid artery wall that shows good agreement with manual segmentations. In contrast to previous approaches, our method jointly optimizes both surfaces, finds a globally optimal solution, and can reliably segment the bifurcation section which may represent the most clinically relevant area to assess.

References

1. Adame, I.M., van der Geest, R.J., Wasserman, B.A., Mohamed, M.A., Reiber, J.H.C., Lelieveldt, B.P.F.: Automatic segmentation and plaque characterization in atherosclerotic carotid artery MR images. Magnetic Resonance Materials in Physics, Biology and Medicine 16, 227–234 (2004)
2. Boykov, Y., Kolmogorov, V.: An experimental comparison of min-cut/max-flow algorithms for energy minimization in vision. IEEE Transactions on Pattern Analysis and Machine Intelligence 26(9), 1124–1137 (2004)
3. de Bruijne, M., van Ginneken, B., Viergever, M.A., Niessen, W.J.: Adapting Active Shape Models for 3D Segmentation of Tubular Structures in Medical Images. In: Taylor, C.J., Noble, J.A. (eds.) IPMI 2003. LNCS, vol. 2732, pp. 136–147. Springer, Heidelberg (2003)
4. Butcher, J.: Numerical Methods for Ordinary Differential Equations. Wiley (2008)
5. Freiman, M., Frank, J., Weizman, L., Nammer, E., Shilon, O., Joskowicz, L., Sosna, J.: Nearly automatic vessels segmentation using graph-based energy minimization. The MIDAS Journal (2009)
6. Hofman, A., van Duijn, C., Franco, O., Ikram, M., Janssen, H., Klaver, C., Kuipers, E., Nijsten, T., Stricker, B., Tiemeier, H., Uiterlinden, A., Vernooij, M., Witteman, J.: The rotterdam study: 2012 objectives and design update. European Journal of Epidemiology, 1–30 (August 2011)
7. Klein, S., Staring, M., Murphy, K., Viergever, M., Pluim, J.: Elastix: a toolbox for intensity-based medical image registration. IEEE Transactions on Medical Imaging 29(1), 196–205 (2010)

8. van't Klooster, R., de Koning, P.J., Dehnavi, R.A., Tamsma, J.T., de Roos, A., Reiber, J.H., van der Geest, R.J.: Automatic lumen and outer wall segmentation of the carotid artery using deformable three-dimensional models in MR angiography and vessel wall images. Journal of Magnetic Resonance Imaging 35(1), 156–165 (2012)

9. Li, K., Wu, X., Chen, D.Z., Sonka, M.: Optimal surface segmentation in volumetric images – a graph-theoretic approach. IEEE Transactions on Pattern Analysis and Machine Intelligence 28(1), 119–134 (2006)

10. Petersen, J., Nielsen, M., Lo, P., Saghir, Z., Dirksen, A., de Bruijne, M.: Optimal Graph Based Segmentation Using Flow Lines with Application to Airway Wall Segmentation. In: Székely, G., Hahn, H.K. (eds.) IPMI 2011. LNCS, vol. 6801, pp. 49–60. Springer, Heidelberg (2011)

11. Ross, R.: Atherosclerosis — an inflammatory disease. New England Journal of Medicine 340(2), 115–126 (1999)

12. Tang, H., van Walsum, T., van Onkelen, R.S., Hameeteman, K., Klein, S., Schaap, M., Bouwhuijsen, Q.J.B., Witteman, J., van der Lugt, A., van Vliet, L.J., Niessen, W.: Semiautomatic carotid lumen segmentation for quantification of lumen geometry in multispectral MRI. Medical Image Analysis (May 2012)

13. Xu, X., Niemeijer, M., Song, Q., Garvin, M., Reinhardt, J., Abramoff, M.: Retinal vessel width measurements based on a graph-theoretic method. In: 2011 IEEE International Symposium on Biomedical Imaging: From Nano to Macro, pp. 641–644 (April 2011)

14. Yuan, C., Lin, E., Millard, J., Hwang, J.: Closed contour edge detection of blood vessel lumen and outer wall boundaries in black-blood MR images. Magnetic Resonance Imaging 17(2), 257–266 (1999)

Graph Cut Segmentation
Using a Constrained Statistical Model
with Non-linear and Sparse Shape Optimization

Tahir Majeed, Ketut Fundana, Silja Kiriyanthan,
Jörg Beinemann, and Philippe Cattin

Medical Image Analysis Center (MIAC), University of Basel, Switzerland
{tahir.majeed,ketut.fundana,philippe.cattin}@unibas.ch

Abstract. This paper proposes a novel segmentation method combining shape knowledge obtained from a constrained Statistical Model (SM) into the well known Markov Random Field (MRF) segmentation framework. The employed SM based on Probabilistic Principal Component Analysis (PPCA) allows to compute local information about the remaining variance *i.e.* uncertainty about the correct segmentation boundary. This knowledge about the local segmentation uncertainty is then used to construct a prior with a non-linear shape update mechanism, where a high cost is incurred in locations with little uncertainty and a low cost for shifting the segmentation boundary in locations with high uncertainty.

Experimental results for segmenting the masseter muscle from CT data are presented showing the advantage of including the knowledge about local segmentation uncertainties into the segmentation framework.

Keywords: Graph-Cut, MRF, Statistical Model, Shape Prior, PCA, Segmentaion, Facial, Muscles, Medical Image.

1 Introduction

Most of human's sense organs are located in the head and face area, which makes it one of the most important parts of the human body. The shape and the unique features of a face are largely determined by the musculoskeletal system underneath the facial skin. The importance of the face for socio-ecological interaction increases the demand on any surgical intervention on the facial musculoskeletal system. This explains the widespread need for pre-operative planning and simulations based on segmented patient specific data.

The goal of image segmentation is to partition the imaging data into multiple segments that will then be used for example patient specific simulations. At a lower level, the objective is to assign a label to each pixel in an image in a way that pixels with the same label share certain visual characteristics. Image segmentation is, however, an ill-posed problem that has been often casted in the Markov Random Field (MRF) framework in the literature. The recent advances in Graph-cut theory [2,3], that guarantee to globally optimize the MRF for a certain class of energy functions, made this approach even more attractive.

B.H. Menze et al. (Eds.): MCV 2012, LNCS 7766, pp. 48–58, 2013.

Graph-cuts are very successful at segmenting objects that can be distinguished from their background producing globally optimal results, but they fail when the object is similar in appearance to its adjacent structures [8]. To alleviate the problem, people suggested incorporating prior shape knowledge into the graph-cuts. Since shape knowledge is used as a prior, this knowledge is incorporated in the smoothness term of the energy function by Veksler [15], Freedman and Zhang [8] and Das et al. [5]. Others do not consider the shape knowledge as a prior but more as likelihood information, therefore, they proposed to incorporate it in the data term of the energy function such as El-Zehiry and Elmaghraby [7], Freiman et al. [9], Ali et al. [1], Slabaugh and Unal [14] and Malcolm et al. [13]. Slabaugh and Unal [14] describe a class of representable shapes and add a constant factor to the data term, while El-Zehiry and Elmaghraby [7], Freiman et al. [9] and Ali et al. [1] proposed a more elaborated factor in the data term. Common to all solutions is the creation of a probability map by registering the shapes in the training datasets. They all propose an iterative scheme to refine their initial estimates and shape probabilities. These methods are prone to generating invalid shapes as there is no statistical dependence between the shapes. Malcolm et al. [13] use non-linear shape priors learned through Kernel PCA which does not suffer from statistical non-dependence. They then iteratively refine the shape prior and the segmentation by fitting the shape prior in the high dimensional space to the segmentation. The pre-image of the fitted shape prior in the input space is computed and then the updated shape prior is used to obtain better segmentation in the next iteration.

This paper bases on the earlier work of Majeed et al. [12] but extends it in several ways. In particular we introduce a non-linear cost function together with L^1 regularization [17] to provide bolder and more accurate shape update than that of [12] which uses a linear cost function. The shape knowledge is provided by the variability constrained SM as explained in the earlier work [12]. The main advantages of the proposed method is that non-linear cost function and L^1 regularization provides better shape update and guard against the SM from degenerating and collapsing onto itself.

The paper is organized as follows: Sec. 2 lays out the segmentation framework and how shape knowledge is extracted from the variability constrained SM. The creation of the non-linear cost function over which the SM is optimized to get a better shape fitting to the segmentation is detailed in Sec. 3. The complete algorithm is given in Sec. 4. Sec. 5 provides the results of applying the proposed method to segment masseter muscle and finally Sec. 6 provides the conclusion.

2   Segmentation Framework

The segmentation problem is cast as a binary labeling problem in the MRF framework. Let $\mathcal{L} = \{0, 1\}$ be the set of binary labels, "1" for object and "0" for background, $\mathcal{P}$ be the set of voxels of the volume dataset and $\mathbf{z} = \{z_p : p \in \mathcal{P}, z_p \in \mathcal{L}\}$ be the set of labeling which defines the segmentation. The goal of our segmentation is to find a labeling z, which is a mapping from $\mathcal{P} \longmapsto \mathcal{L}$ by minimizing the energy functional

$$E(\mathbf{z}|\mathbf{I}, \mathbf{x}^*) = \sum_{p \in \mathcal{P}} \left\{ V_p(z_p|\mathbf{I}) + \mu V_p(z_p|\mathbf{x}^*) \right\} + \lambda \sum_{p \in \mathcal{P}} \sum_{q \in \mathcal{N}_p} V_{p,q}(z_p, z_q|\mathbf{I}), \qquad (1)$$

where $\mathbb{N} = \{N_p | \forall p \in \mathcal{P}\}$ is an unordered 26 neighborhood system over $\mathcal{P}$, $\mathbf{I}$ is the observed intensity data, $\mathbf{x}^*$ is the shape prior, λ is the smoothness parameter and μ is the shape parameter. $V_p(z_p|\mathbf{I})$ and $V_{p,q}(z_p, z_q|\mathbf{I})$ are the data and the smoothness terms respectively, based on the image intensity information. The data term encodes how likely a voxel is to belong to object and background given its intensity while the smoothness term encodes our prior assumption about the target object that it consists of a homogeneous region, therefore, the smoothness term assigns a penalty whenever adjacent voxels p, q are assigned different labels z_p and z_q. The data and the smoothness terms are based on the traditional graph-cut intensity based energy functional of Boykov and Jolly [2].

$V_p(z_p|\mathbf{x}^*)$ is the shape data term which encodes how likely a particular voxel p is to belong to the object "1" and the background "0", given the shape prior $\mathbf{x}^*$ obtained from a SM explained below. Shape knowledge is encoded by creating a probability map both for the object and the background from the unsigned distance map of the shape prior's contour and it is similar to that of Majeed et al. [12]. Based on the closeness to the shape's contour; the object probability map is created for the voxels enclosed by the contour while the background probability map is created for the voxels not enclosed by the contour.

2.1   Statistical Model

This section summarizes the method of Lüthi et al. [11]. The same anatomical structures show considerable shape variability among the population which cannot be represented by a fixed shape template. Statistical shape models have been extensively used as a mathematical framework to capture this shape variability [4,10,16]. A set of shapes in the training dataset are used to capture the shape variability of the particular structure. The shapes in the training dataset are assumed to be Independent and Identically Distributed (i.i.d) having an underlying unknown multivariate Gaussian distribution with probability density function $p \sim \mathcal{N}(\bar{\mathbf{x}}, \mathbf{\Sigma})$ with mean $\bar{\mathbf{x}}$ and covariance $\mathbf{\Sigma}$. The shapes in the training dataset $\{\mathbf{x}^i \in \mathbb{R}^{3m} | i = 1, \dots, n\}$, where n represents the number of training shapes each having m number of vertices, are brought into correspondence using the method of Dedner et al. [6], which results in all shapes having the same number of vertices. Singular Value Decomposition (SVD) is then applied to decompose $\mathbf{\Sigma} = \mathbf{U}\mathbf{D}^2\mathbf{U}^T$, where $\mathbf{U}$ are the eigenvectors while $\mathbf{D}^2$ represents the eigenvalues of $\mathbf{\Sigma}$.

Reconstruction from Partial Information. The shape is represented by a surface mesh $\mathbf{x}$ which can be partitioned into $\mathbf{x} := (\mathbf{x}_a, \mathbf{x}_b)^T$, based on the available l-landmark information $\mathbf{x}_b \in \mathbb{R}^{3l}$ and unknown $\mathbf{x}_a \in \mathbb{R}^{3m-3l}$. The landmarks ($l = 6$), which are manually labelled, provide the location of the muscle attachments at the facial bones. $\mathbf{x}_b$ is then used to estimate $\mathbf{x}_a$. Using the PPCA based approach of Lüthi *et al.* [11] a probability distribution over the shape $\mathbf{x}$ can be defined as

$$p(\mathbf{x}) = p(\mathbf{x}_a, \mathbf{x}_b) = \mathcal{N}\left(\begin{bmatrix} \bar{\mathbf{x}}_a \\ \bar{\mathbf{x}}_b \end{bmatrix}, \begin{bmatrix} \mathbf{W}_a\mathbf{W}_a^T & \mathbf{W}_a\mathbf{W}_b^T \\ \mathbf{W}_b\mathbf{W}_a^T & \mathbf{W}_b\mathbf{W}_b^T \end{bmatrix} + \sigma_m^2 \mathcal{I}_{3l} \right), \qquad (2)$$

where $\mathcal{I}_{3l}$ is a $3l \times 3l$ identity matrix, $\mathbf{W} = \mathbf{UD} = [\mathbf{W}_a\mathbf{W}_b]^T \in \mathbb{R}^{3m \times d}$ is the d-largest scaled eigenvectors and σ_m^2 is a parameter that controls the remaining variance of the SM. If $\sigma_m > 0$ then $\mathbf{x}_b$ is allowed to move. Since $\mathbf{x}$ has a multivariate normal distribution, the conditional distribution $p(\mathbf{x}_a|\mathbf{x}_b) \sim \mathcal{N}(\bar{\mathbf{x}}_{\mathbf{x}_a|\mathbf{x}_b}, \boldsymbol{\Sigma}_{\mathbf{x}_a|\mathbf{x}_b})$ is also a multivariate normal distribution with mean $\bar{\mathbf{x}}_{\mathbf{x}_a|\mathbf{x}_b}$ and covariance $\boldsymbol{\Sigma}_{\mathbf{x}_a|\mathbf{x}_b}$. $p(\mathbf{x}_a|\mathbf{x}_b)$ needs to be computed to reconstruct the shape $\bar{\mathbf{x}}_{\mathbf{x}_a|\mathbf{x}_b}$ from partial information $\mathbf{x}_b$. Since coefficients of the modes of variation $\boldsymbol{\alpha} = \mathcal{N}(0, I_n)$ of the SM defines a shape $\mathbf{x} = \mathbf{W}\boldsymbol{\alpha} + \bar{\mathbf{x}}$, therefore, first the coefficients are determined from the partial information $\mathbf{x}_b$ as $p(\boldsymbol{\alpha}|\mathbf{x}_b)$ and then $\bar{\mathbf{x}}_{\mathbf{x}_a|\mathbf{x}_b}$ can be reconstructed using

$$\bar{\mathbf{x}}_{\mathbf{x}_a|\mathbf{x}_b} = \arg \max_{x} p(\mathbf{x}|\boldsymbol{\alpha}) = \mathbf{W}\boldsymbol{\alpha} + \bar{\mathbf{x}}. \qquad (3)$$

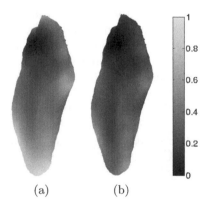

(a)   (b)

Fig. 1. Normalized variance of the SM. (a) Original variance, (b) Remaining variance (color online)

Remaining Variance. The known l-landmark information can be further utilized to constrain the variability of the SM. Since $\mathbf{x}_b$ provides additional information, therefore, in a probabilistic setting it is natural to assume that the uncertainty of the SM will reduce as further evidence is obtained. The covariance matrix $\boldsymbol{\Sigma}_{\mathbf{x}_a|\mathbf{x}_b}$ can be decomposed by applying SVD into its eigenvectors $\mathbf{U}_{\mathbf{x}_a|\mathbf{x}_b}$ and eigenvalues $\mathbf{D}_{\mathbf{x}_a|\mathbf{x}_b}^2$. $\mathbf{U}_{\mathbf{x}_a|\mathbf{x}_b}$, $\mathbf{D}_{\mathbf{x}_a|\mathbf{x}_b}^2$ and $\bar{\mathbf{x}}_{\mathbf{x}_a|\mathbf{x}_b}$ can now be used to generate an optimal shape $\mathbf{x}^*$ with the remaining flexibility of the model using

$$\mathbf{x}^* = \mathbf{U}_{\mathbf{x}_a|\mathbf{x}_b}\mathbf{D}_{\mathbf{x}_a|\mathbf{x}_b}\boldsymbol{\alpha} + \bar{\mathbf{x}}_{\mathbf{x}_a|\mathbf{x}_b}. \qquad (4)$$

As an illustration of the concept of remaining variability, we show in Fig. 1 the original variance of the model (a) and the remaining variance of the model after being fit to the muscle attachments (b). It is however, not possible to compute $\Sigma_{\mathbf{x}_a|\mathbf{x}_b}$ directly since it is potentially huge. For an in-depth analysis of the reconstruction of the shape given partial information and calculating the remaining variance see Lüthi *et al.* [11].

3   Adaptive Shape Optimization

For updating the shape prior with respect to the segmentation, we propose to use a shape optimization based on adaptive weights with respect to the remaining variances of the SM and sparse shape optimization.

3.1   Shape Cost Function

Creating the cost function for shape optimization is the second major step of our algorithm after the segmentation corresponding to the energy function E Eq. 1. Since the surface mesh is very dense consisting of 39156 vertices, therefore, adjacent vertices are close enough to occupy adjacent voxels. We have used the morphable model of Blanz and Vetter [16] which is very dense (around 76000 vertices) as compared to the active shape model of Cootes *et al.* [4] which are not dense (only 72 vertices). On average for all datasets there are 1.75 vertices per voxel with a density of 7.66 vertices per mm^2. Once a vertex is in a voxel, the cost of the vertex can be directly read out of the voxel, defined by

$$C(v) = \beta C_{obj}(v) + \eta C_{edge}(v) + C_{seg}(v), \qquad (5)$$

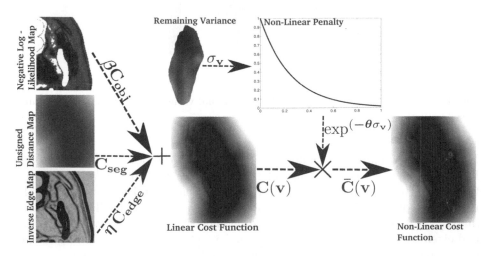

Fig. 2. Generating non-linear cost function $\bar{C}(v)$

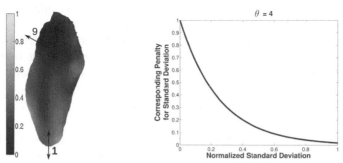

(a) Illustration of the adaptive cost. (b) Penalty $\exp^{(-\theta\sigma_v)}$ for the normalized standard deviation.

Fig. 3. Normalized standard deviations and their corresponding penalty

where η and β are weighting parameters, $v = (v_x, v_y, v_z)$ represents the x, y, z coordinates of a vertex of $\mathbf{x}$. The object intensity negative log-likelihood map (C_{obj}) is calculated using the parzen window estimation that has already been estimated during the graph-cut segmentation. An inverse edge map C_{edge} provides low values where there is an edge. The third term in Eq. 5 is the unsigned distance map (C_{seg}) which is calculated from the segmentation boundary. All the maps are then linearly combined as in Eq. 5 and shown in Fig. 2 to generate the linear cost function $C(v)$ which is then weighted with non-linear variance penalties $\exp^{(-\theta\sigma_v)}$ to generate non-linear cost function $\bar{C}(v)$ as shown in Fig. 2 over which the SM is optimized.

3.2   Shape Optimization

Once the non-linear cost function has been created, the next step is to optimize the SM over the generated cost function. We propose to use an adaptive cost instead of linear cost employed by Majeed *et al.* [12] in order to make the SM robust to local minima encountered during the shape update. The cost is adapted with respect to the remaining variance of the vertex σ_v. The sum of the cost of all the vertices for a particular setting of shape coefficients $\boldsymbol{\alpha}$ gives the cost of the shape as follows

$$\bar{C}(\mathbf{x}) = C(\mathbf{UD}\boldsymbol{\alpha} + \bar{\mathbf{x}})\exp^{(-\theta\sigma_v)} = \sum_v C(v)\exp^{(-\theta\sigma_v)}, \qquad (6)$$

where σ_v is the remaining variance of vertex v and θ is a weight parameter.

Here vertices with higher variance incur lower cost in comparison to vertices with lower variance. As a consequence, a vertex with higher remaining variance (color coded in light golden in Fig. 3(a)) as given by the SM is allowed to move further with less cost (cost 1) while a vertex with lower remaining variance (color coded in black) incurs higher cost (cost 9) when it moves the same distance. With linear cost, vertices irrespective of their remaining variance in the SM would incur

equal cost when they move equal distances. The adaptive weights with respect
to the variances are shown by the graph in Fig. 3(b).

The SM is optimized by minimizing the sum of the cost of vertices over the
non-linear cost function $\bar{C}(v)$. The coefficients $\boldsymbol{\alpha}$ corresponding to the main
modes of variation are obtained by solving the minimization problem

$$\min_{\boldsymbol{\alpha}} \left\{ \bar{C}(\mathbf{x}) + \xi |\boldsymbol{\alpha}|_{L^1} \right\}, \tag{7}$$

where ξ is a weight parameter. Since the adaptive cost is used, the SM has more
flexibility, therefore, it is required that the model be regularized to constrain
the solutions space and generate smoother shape priors. Note that we use L^1
regularization [17] to constrain the solution space and generate sparse and more
accurate solutions. Once the optimal $\boldsymbol{\alpha}$ are found, the optimized shape is then
constructed using Eq. 4 and used as a shape prior for the next iteration.

4   Algorithm

Figure 4 outlines the algorithm. The algorithm starts with the initial shape prior
obtained from the shape reconstruction from partial information (see Sec. 2.1),
therefore, $\bar{\mathbf{x}}_{\mathbf{x}_a|\mathbf{x}_b}$ which is the mean shape of the constrained variability SM is the
initial shape prior used for the first iteration. The shape prior is used to generate
the probability maps for the object and the background which is similar to the
one used by Majeed *et al.* [12] and encodes the shape knowledge. These maps

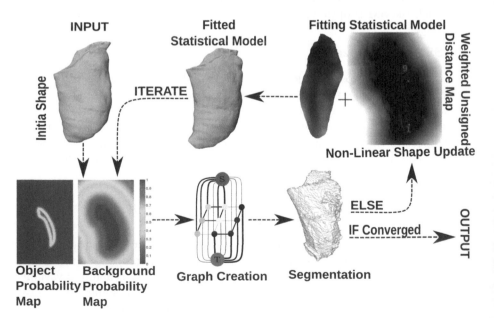

Fig. 4. Segmentation Process (color online)

are then used to create graph corresponding to the energy function E given by Eq. 1 and then the graph-cut algorithm of Boykov and Kolmogorov [3] is used to obtain the muscle segmentation. If the segmentation has not converged then a non-linear cost function $\bar{C}(\mathbf{x})$ outlined in Sec. 3.1 is created over which the shape prior is updated. Once the SM has been fitted to the current segmentation (see Sec. 3.2), the fitted SM provides better and more accurate shape knowledge for the next iteration. This process is repeated until segmentation converges.

The update of the shape prior is required as the initial estimate of the shape is not perfect, therefore, previous segmentation is used to update shape knowledge and get a better fitting of the SM to the specific patients muscle anatomy.

5   Experimental Results

The proposed segmentation method was tested on 20 CT datasets - the ground truth was provided by a medical expert - using a Leave-One-Out approach. The dataset dimensions were 79-156×148-214×125-384 voxels and spacing 0.3-0.5×0.3-0.5×0.3-1 mm^3. All datasets possessed high-density artifacts caused by dental fillings and dental implants. The parameters $\sigma_m = 10$, $\lambda = 0.016$ and $\mu = 0.0037$ were optimized on three different datasets and used throughout the entire segmentation experiments. The parameters $\beta = 0.01$, $\eta = 0.07$, $\theta = 4$ were used to generate the non-linear cost function while $\xi = 600000$ was used for sparse shape optimization. The dice coefficient, sensitivity and specificity of the segmentation were calculated as similarity measures to ascertain the accuracy of the proposed method.

Shape convergence was achieved within $5 - 11$ iterations. The algorithm is computationally quite fast; it takes on average 4.1 ± 1.5 minutes. 4 min. is not real time but on the other hand it takes around an hour and a medical expert to segment the muscle. It should be noted that although the mesh employed is very dense, the algorithm itself is independent of the density of the mesh.

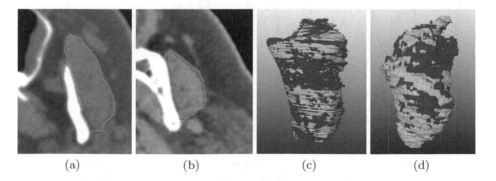

(a)   (b)   (c)   (d)

Fig. 5. (a,b) Qualitative segmentation result in 2D where red is the ground truth and green is the segmentation boundary. (c,d) Qualitative segmentation result in 3D where ground truth is in gray and segmentation is in blue (color online).

The cost function is evaluated where the vertices end up and that gives the total cost of the shape. The algorithm will work equally well with a less dense mesh.

Figure 5(a+b) shows qualitative results of our technique in 2D, while the qualitative results in 3D are shown in Fig. 5(c+d). The experimental results obtained using the proposed method is clinically acceptable as validated by the medical expert.

The graphs in Fig. 6 show the results of the method of [12] using a linear cost function (black curve) and the proposed method with non-linear cost function (red curve). The gray curve shows the results of using the method of Freedman *et al.* [8]. The proposed method is statistically significantly better than both the methods [8] with p-value $p < 0.01$ and [12] with p-value $p < 0.01$. The improvemnt over [12] is mainly due to the use of the non-linear cost function using L^1 regularization. The dice coefficient (see Fig. 6(a)) and specificity (see Fig. 6(c)) for the proposed method is better for all datasets except for a few. Table 1 lists the mean, median, standard deviation and the smallest and the largest dice coefficient values for the methods.

We show that our novel approach shows a further improvement in the segmentation accuracy. In this paper we showed that SM models can not only be used to restrict the shape variability during segmentation but also how to make use of the remaining shape variability in the SMs to even further improve the segmentation.

Table 1. The table list the mean, median and the standard deviation of the dice coefficient of the proposed method, method with linear cost [12] and Freedman [8]

	DC (Mean ± Std)	DC (Median)	DC (Smallest - Largest)
Proposed	0.895 ± 0.022	0.900	(0.857 - 0.930)
Linear [12]	0.884 ± 0.029	0.890	(0.822 - 0.922)
Freedman [8]	0.861 ± 0.054	0.877	(0.751 - 0.923)

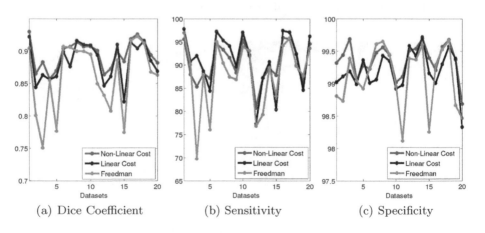

(a) Dice Coefficient   (b) Sensitivity   (c) Specificity

Fig. 6. Quantitative segmentation result: (a) Dice coefficient. (b) Sensitivity. (c) Specificity; for all the methods (color online).

6 Conclusion

In this paper we have proposed an improved segmentation approach that combines a constrained SM with an MRF-based segmentation approach. As compared to the state-of-the-art methods we employ a non-linear cost function when fitting the SM. This new cost function has shown to be superior as it generates more consistent shape updates. The method's performance has been evaluated on 20 masseter CT dataset and quantitatively compared to state-of-the-art segmentation approaches. Although the method has been shown and evaluated on the masseter muscle it is of general use and can be applied whenever SM is available.

Acknowledgment. We would like to thank Marcel Lüthi for providing the registered PCA based statistical model of the masseter muscle. This work has been supported by the NCCR/CO-ME research network of the Swiss National Science Foundation.

References

1. Ali, A.M., Farag, A.A., El-Baz, A.S.: Graph Cuts Framework for Kidney Segmentation with Prior Shape Constraints. In: Ayache, N., Ourselin, S., Maeder, A. (eds.) MICCAI 2007, Part I. LNCS, vol. 4791, pp. 384–392. Springer, Heidelberg (2007)
2. Boykov, Y., Jolly, M.P.: Interactive Graph Cuts for Optimal Boundary and Region Segmentation of Objects in N-D Images. In: ICCV, vol. 1, pp. 105–112 (2001)
3. Boykov, Y., Kolmogorov, V.: An Experimental Comparison of Min-Cut/Max-Flow Algorithms for Energy Minimization in Vision. PAMI 26(9), 1124–1137 (2004)
4. Cootes, T., Taylor, C., Cooper, D., Graham, J.: Active Shape Models; Their Training and Application. Computer Vision and Image Understanding 61(1), 38–59 (1995)
5. Das, P., Veksler, O., Zavadsky, V., Boykov, Y.: Semi-Automatic Segmentation with Compact Shape Prior. Image and Vision Computing 27(1), 206–219 (2009)
6. Dedner, A., Lüthi, M., Albrecht, T., Vetter, T.: Curvature Guided Level Set Registration using Adaptive Finite Elements. In: Pattern Recognition, pp. 527–536 (2007)
7. El-Zehiry, N., Elmaghraby, A.: Graph Cut Based Deformable Model with Statistical Shape Priors. In: ICPR, pp. 1–4 (2008)
8. Freedman, D., Zhang, T.: Interactive Graph Cut Based Segmentation with Shape Priors. In: CVPR, pp. 755–762 (2005)
9. Freiman, M., Kronman, A., Esses, S.J., Joskowicz, L., Sosna, J.: Non-parametric Iterative Model Constraint Graph min-cut for Automatic Kidney Segmentation. In: Jiang, T., Navab, N., Pluim, J.P.W., Viergever, M.A. (eds.) MICCAI 2010, Part III. LNCS, vol. 6363, pp. 73–80. Springer, Heidelberg (2010)
10. Leventon, M.E., Grimson, W.E.L., Faugeras, O.: Statistical Shape Influence in Geodesic Active Contours. In: CVPR, p. 1316 (2000)
11. Lüthi, M., Albrecht, T., Vetter, T.: Probabilistic Modeling and Visualization of the Flexibility in Morphable Models. In: Mathematics of Surfaces, pp. 251–264 (2009)

12. Majeed, T., Fundana, K., Lüthi, M., Kiriyanthan, S., Beinemann, J., Cattin, P.C.: Using a Flexibility Constrained 3D Statistical Shape Model for Robust MRF-Based Segmentation. In: MMBIA, pp. 57–64 (2012)
13. Malcolm, J., Rathi, Y., Tannenbaum, A.: Graph Cut Segmentation with Nonlinear Shape Priors. In: ICIP, vol. 4, pp. 365–368 (2007)
14. Slabaugh, G.G., Unal, G.: Graph Cuts Segmentation Using an Elliptical Shape Prior. In: ICIP, pp. 1222–1225 (2005)
15. Veksler, O.: Star Shape Prior for Graph-Cut Image Segmentation. In: Forsyth, D., Torr, P., Zisserman, A. (eds.) ECCV 2008, Part III. LNCS, vol. 5304, pp. 454–467. Springer, Heidelberg (2008)
16. Blanz, V., Vetter, T.: A Morphable Model for the Synthesis of 3D Faces. In: Computer Graphics and Interactive Techniques, pp. 187–194 (1999)
17. Zhang, S., Zhan, Y., Dewan, M., Huang, J., Metaxas, D.N., Zhou, X.S.: Sparse Shape Composition: A New Framework for Shape Prior Modeling. In: CVPR, pp. 1025–1032 (2011)

Novel Context Rich *LoCo* and *GloCo* Features with Local and Global Shape Constraints for Segmentation of 3D Echocardiograms with Random Forests

Kiryl Chykeyuk, Mohammad Yaqub, and J. Alison Noble

Institute of Biomedical Engineering, Department of Engineering Science,
University of Oxford, Oxford, UK

Abstract. This work addresses the challenging problem of segmenting the myocardium in 3D LV echocardiograms by Random Forests (RF). While the RF framework has proven to be a good discriminative classifier for segmentation of 3D echocardiography [1], our hypothesis is that richer features than those traditionally used (Haar etc) need to be employed for accurate segmentation to tackle artifacts in ultrasound images such as missing anatomical boundaries. To address this, we propose two new context rich and shape invariant features, called *LoCo* and *GloCo*. The new features impose a local and global constraint on the coupled endocardial and epicardial shape of the left ventricle and use barycentric coordinates to uniquely identify the position of a voxel with respect to a number of landmarks on the epicardial and endocardial border. The landmarks are found using a new measure (COFA) to separate the two boundaries. Experimental results show that the new features provide a smoother segmentation and improve the accuracy compared with a classic RF implementation.

Keywords: Random forests, 3D echocardiographic segmentation, the monogenic signal, feature asymmetry, barycentric coordinates.

1   Introduction

Accurate automatic segmentation of the myocardium of the left ventricle (LV) provides quantitative data from 3D echocardiographic images that helps in the assessment of heart abnormalities and diseases. However, automatic segmentation of 3D echocardiography is challenging due to ultrasound artifacts such as shadowing, attenuation, signal drop-out, speckle, missing boundaries and similarity in appearance of different tissues, for instance of the left and right ventricles.

The accuracy of image-based classification techniques reported in the literature to segment and/or detect structures in medical images varies depending on, for example, the classification model, chosen feature set or the complexity of the structure of interest. Segmentation of the LV is challenging. Therefore, the classification model and features need to be chosen and developed carefully. Random Forests (RF) have

B.H. Menze et al. (Eds.): MCV 2012, LNCS 7766, pp. 59–69, 2013.

proven to show good performance in recent publications [1-6] and was adopted in this work on 3D echocardiography segmentation. In the RF framework, segmentation is formalized as a voxel classification problem. Although the choice of the classifier is important, the accuracy of the model is pre-dominantly determined by the features used within the classifier. In our approach, first a novel image alignment method is proposed to make the widely used position features stronger. Second, a novel set of context rich features is introduced to improve automated segmentation of 3D echocardiography.

The contributions of this work are twofold. Firstly, as a pre-segmentation step, we propose a new method for left ventricular long axis detection in 3D echocardiography. The robust detection of the mid line is an important step in alignment of echocardiography volumes which is done prior to segmentation. Our method is based on a Feature Asymmetry measure (FA), Local Orientation (LO) and a modified Hough transform. Secondly, we introduce a set of new context rich features that utilize the relevant position of a voxel with respect to a specific landmark or landmarks at the epicardial and/or endocardial boundaries of the left ventricle. The landmarks are detected using the new Centrally Oriented Feature Asymmetry measure (COFA) to highlight and separate the epicardial and endocardial boundaries in an image.

1.1   Random Forests

Random Forests [2] is a learning-based technique gaining popularity in medical imaging, in which training using a gold standard segmentation is done by building multiple decision trees. Each node in the tree, except the leaves, is a decision node and contains a feature and a threshold. Each leaf node contains a class distribution for the voxels that reached the node. Testing is performed by traversing voxels over the trees starting from the root of each tree to a leaf node. The voxels are split at a given node based on the learned feature and the threshold value at that node. The mean class distribution from all trees is considered the final probabilistic class distribution of the test case. For more information see [1-6].

1.2   The Monogenic Signal and Feature Asymmetry Images

In echocardiography, low-level feature extraction is an important step before the segmentation of the LV is performed. For LV segmentation, the goal is to detect endocardial and epicardial boundaries. It is usually assumed that they have step-like edge characteristics. It has been shown that intensity based methods do not perform well due to the low-contrast nature of echocardiographic images, whereas local-phase based techniques have been shown to be intensity-invariant and less sensitive to speckle [7]. In [7], the original Phase Congruency measure [8] was adapted to the Feature Asymmetry (FA) measure, and outperformed the intensity based methods for detecting step-like edges in echocardiographic images. It has since been modified in [9] using the monogenic signal [10].

The monogenic signal is a high dimensional generalization of the analytic signal. It is based on the Riesz transform, which is used instead of the Hilbert transform. The monogenic signal is formed by combining the original band-pass image with its Riesz components:

$$I_M(x,y,z) = [I(x,y,z)*g(x,y,z), I(x,y,z)*g(x,y,z)*h_x(x,y,z), I(x,y,z)*g(x,y,z)*$$
$$h_y(x,y,z), I(x,y,z)*g(x,y,z)*h_z(x,y,z)], \tag{1}$$

where $g(x,y,z)$ is the spatial domain representation of a bandpass filter and $h_i(x,y,z)$ are the Riesz filter components.

The odd and even filter responses are then defined as follows:

$$even(x,y,z) = I_{M,1}(x,y,z) \tag{2}$$
$$odd(x,y,z) = \sqrt{I_{M,x}(x,y,z)^2 + I_{M,y}(x,y,z)^2 + I_{M,z}(x,y,z)^2}$$

In computing the monogenic signal, aside from choosing how to combine the results from different scales, the selection of a bandpass filter has to be made. In our case we used the log-Gabor filter though other filters could have been used.

The feature asymmetry (FA) measure is defined as:

$$FA_{3D}(x,y,z) = \sum_s \frac{\lfloor \|odd_s(x,y,z)\| - \|even_s(x,y,z)\| - T_s \rfloor}{\sqrt{(even_s(x,y,z))^2 + (odd_s(x,y,z))^2 + \varepsilon}} \tag{3}$$

where ε is a small constant to avoid division by zero and T_s is a scale specific threshold that suppresses any response due to noise or symmetric points of the image:

$$T_s = \exp\left[mean\left(\log(\sqrt{(even_s(x,y,z))^2 + (odd_s(x,y,z))^2})\right)\right] \tag{4}$$

2   Method

In this section, we describe the procedure for myocardium segmentation using the RF with the new *LoCo* and *GloCo* features, see Fig. 1. We first describe the pre-segmentation steps for the *LoCo* and *GloCo* features extraction.

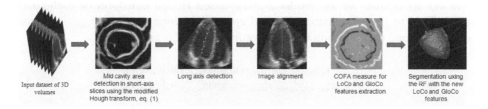

Input dataset of 3D volumes — Mid cavity area detection in short-axis slices using the modified Hough transform, eq. (1) — Long axis detection — Image alignment — COFA measure for LoCo and GloCo features extraction — Segmentation uxing the RF with the new LoCo and GloCo features

Fig. 1. Algorithm flowchart

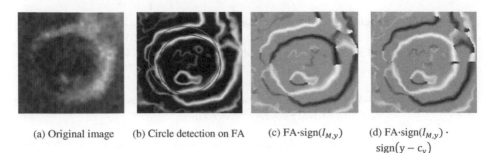

(a) Original image   (b) Circle detection on FA   (c) FA·sign($I_{M,y}$)   (d) FA·sign($I_{M,y}$) · sign($y - c_y$)

Fig. 2. Circle detection on a short-axis slice from the 3D echocardiogram. (a) The original image. (b) The FA image and the detected circles by the original Hough transform for circles (in red, failed) and by the proposed modified Hough transform for circles (in blue) defined by (5). (c) and (d) The intermediate measures used by the modified Hough transform (5). In (d) the clear separation of epicardial and endocardial borders makes it feasible for the modified Hough transform not to confuse between the two borders.

2.1 Detection of the Long Axis

We propose a novel method for long axis detection from 3D echocardiographic images utilizing a modified Hough transform for circles, the 3D monogenic signal and the FA images as edge maps.

Specifically, a local-phased based version of the Hough transform for circle detection can be defined as follow:

$$H_z(c_x, c_y, r) = \sum_s \sum_\theta \text{sign}(x - c_x) \cdot \text{sign}(I_{M,x}^s) \cdot FA_z^s(x, y) + \text{sign}(y - c_y) \cdot \text{sign}(I_{M,y}^s) \cdot FA_z^s(x, y); \quad (5)$$

$$\text{where} \quad \begin{cases} x = c_x + r\cos\theta \\ y = c_y + r\sin\theta \end{cases} \quad (6)$$

c_x, c_y, r parameterize the circle, and $I_{M,x}^s$ and $I_{M,y}^s$ are the x and y monogenic signal components respectively, as defined in (1). See also Fig. 2.

In our implementation the summation is performed over multiple scales s of the band-pass filter. Notice that the Hough transform can be fairly accurately computed using only one of the summands in (5). However, we have found in our application that employing both terms leads to better accuracy and robustness.

In our application we use the local-phase based Hough transform on each short-axis slice z, to give the endocardial and epicardial center points, $(x_{c,endc}^z, y_{c,endc}^z)$ and $(x_{c,epic}^z, y_{c,epic}^z)$, and the endocardial and epicardial radii, r_{endc}^z and r_{epic}^z, as:

$$\begin{aligned} x_{c,epic}^z, y_{c,epic}^z, r_{epic}^z &= \text{argmax}_{c_x, c_y, r} \, H_z(c_x, c_y, r); \\ x_{c,endc}^z, y_{c,endc}^z, r_{endc}^z &= \text{argmin}_{c_x, c_y, r} \, H_z(c_x, c_y, r); \end{aligned} \quad (7)$$

Having detected the center points, the long axis is then fitted as the first principal component of the detected endocardial centers. The long axis is utilized to align the 3D LV images, to facilitate the extraction of a new set of features as described next.

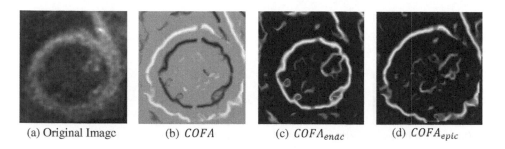

(a) Original Image   (b) $COFA$ (c) $COFA_{endc}$ (d) $COFA_{epic}$

Fig. 3. Visualisation of the COFA measure. (a-b) The original image and COFA measure defined in (9). (c-d) The COFA measures for the endocardial and epicardial borders defined in (10) and (11).

2.2 Centrally Oriented Feature Asymmetry (COFA) Measure for Separating and Highlighting the Epicardial and Endocardial Boundary

The Centrally Oriented Feature Asymmetry (COFA) measure is defined in terms of the detected epicardial and endocardial points for each of the short-axis slices z, as follows:

$$COFA_z(x,y) = \sum_s \sum_{i=epic,endc} sign(x - x_{c,i}^z) \cdot sign(I_{M,x}^s) \cdot FA_z^s(x,y) + sign(y - y_{c,i}^z) \cdot sign(I_{M,y}^s) \cdot FA_z^s(x,y) \tag{8}$$

See also Fig. 3 (b). The epicardial and endocardial boundaries can be separated in the following way:

$$COFA_{z,epic}(x,y) = \sum_s \sum_{i=epic,endc} \lfloor sign(x - x_{c,i}^z) \cdot sign(I_{M,x}^s) \cdot FA_z^s(x,y) \rfloor + \lfloor sign(y - y_{c,i}^z) \cdot sign(I_{M,y}^s) \cdot FA_z^s(x,y) \rfloor \tag{9}$$

$$COFA_{z,endc}(x,y) = \sum_s \sum_{i=epic,endc} \lfloor sign(x - x_{c,i}^z) \cdot sign(I_{M,y}^s) \cdot FA_z^s(x,y) \rfloor + \lceil sign(y - y_{c,i}^z) \cdot sign(I_{M,x}^s) \cdot FA_z^s(x,y) \rceil \tag{10}$$

where $(x_{c,i}, y_{c,i})$ is either epicardial or endocardial center point in the slice z, determined by (7), $\lfloor\rfloor$ and $\lceil\rceil$ are the operators that zero the negative and positive values correspondingly. See also Fig. 3 (c) and (d).

2.3 Feature Sets

Having estimated the center lines, each volume is rotated to a common co-ordinate system so that the long axis is positioned vertically and centered in the aligned image. This corresponds to two translations and two rotations. The remaining five parameters (1 translation, 1 rotation and 3 scaling) are found using a standard rigid registration technique (in our work we used the FLIRT registration tool, http://www.fmrib.ox.ac.uk/fsl/flirt/), fixing the determined four parameters. The process of long axis detection and image alignment is repeated in an iterative manner until no further improvement is achieved. By aligning the images, features extracted from different images correspond, which improves the testing accuracy.

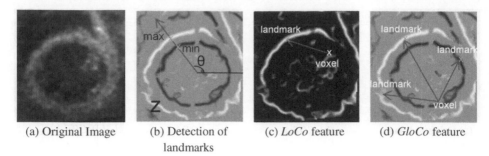

| (a) Original Image | (b) Detection of landmarks | (c) *LoCo* feature | (d) *GloCo* feature |

Fig. 4. Visualisation of the *LoCo* and *GloCo* features. The landmark detection is illustrated in (b): randomly chosen z and θ define the slice and the direction of the search (red line) for the endocardial landmark (minimum along the line) or the epicardial landmark (maximum along the line). (c) An example of the *LoCo* feature using the epicardial landmark. (d) An example of the *GloCo* feature (shown in 2D for illustration purposes). Four randomly selected landmarks form a simplex in 3D, the *GloCo* features are Barycentric coordinates of this voxel with respect to the simplex.

Conventional Local Appearance Features. In this work we adopted several classic low level features. We used rectangle3D, Haar3D and Difference3D features [4-6]. These features capture local appearance information, but in practice can be sub-optimal for analysis of low quality images.

Absolute Voxel Position Features. Following the work of [1], we employ a position3D feature to capture the absolute position of the voxels in the image. The alignment procedure boosts the strength of such features. However, due to the global and local geometric variability of the myocardium, position features only provide a weak geometric constraint.

Local Shape Constraint Contextual Features (LoCo). Here, we introduce a novel set of context rich features $\mathbf{F}(z,\theta)$ that capture geometric variability of the myocardium and can be regarded as a shape constraint. This type of feature is determined by the relative position of a considered voxel $\mathbf{v}^k = (v_x^k, v_y^k, v_z^k)$ to a pre-chosen landmark $\mathbf{p}^k = (p_x^k, p_y^k, p_z^k)$ on the endocardial or epicardial boundary shape in image k. The *LoCo* feature set is thus defined as:

$$f_{LoCo}^x(\mathbf{v}^k;\mathbf{p}^k) = v_x^k - p_x^k \quad f_{LoCo}^y(\mathbf{v}^k;\mathbf{p}^k) = v_y^k - p_y^k \qquad f_{LoCo}^z(\mathbf{v}^k;\mathbf{p}^k) = v_z^k - p_z^k \quad (11)$$

$$f_{LoCo}^{xy}(\mathbf{v}^k;\mathbf{p}^k) = \sqrt{(v_x^k - p_x^k)^2 + (v_y^k - p_y^k)^2} \qquad f_{LoCo}^{dist}(\mathbf{v}^k;\mathbf{p}^k) = |\mathbf{v}^k - \mathbf{p}^k|$$

Landmark selection and detection. With all the images globally aligned endo- and epicardial points can be corresponded in different images. Two randomly chosen parameters, the short-axis slice z and the polar angle θ, define in which slice and in what direction from the center of the cavity area the (aligned) epicardial or endocardial landmark will be detected, Fig. 4 (b). To find the epicardial and endocardial landmarks along the chosen direction, COFA images, described in sect. 3.2, are utilized. The maximum COFA detected feature along the θ direction defines the epicardial landmark, whereas the minimum defines the endocardial landmark, Fig. 4 (b).

Thus, a detected landmark is defined by the two parameters z and θ, and is detected in each image independently as follows:

$$\begin{cases} p_x^{k,q}, p_y^{k,q} = \text{argmax}_{x,y} \left| COFA_{z,q}(x,y) \right| \\ \qquad\qquad p_z^{k,q} = z \end{cases} \text{ subject to } \begin{cases} x^q = x_{c,q}^z + r\cos\theta \\ y^q = y_{c,q}^z + r\sin\theta \end{cases} \qquad (12)$$

$$\text{where } r_q^z - \text{shift} < r < r_q^z + \text{shift}$$

Here the endocardial/epicardial centers $(x_{c,q}^z, y_{c,q}^z)$ and radii r_q^z in the slice z are found by (7).

Global Shape Constraint Contextual Features (GloCo). Unlike *LoCo* features, *GloCo* features use the relative position of a voxel to a number of structures on the epicardial and endocardial boundary shapes. Barycentric coordinates are utilized to uniquely specify the location of the voxel with respect to the specified structures on the boundary shapes. To calculate the barycentric coordinates in 3D space, the 3D simplex, a tetrahedron, is constructed by randomly selecting four structure points on endo- and epicardial boundaries. Mathematically, the scalars u_1, u_2, u_3, u_4 are the barycentric coordinates of an arbitrary voxel $\mathbf{v} = (v_1 \ v_2 \ v_3)$ with respect to the four nonplanar structure points $\mathbf{p_1}, \mathbf{p_2}, \mathbf{p_3}, \mathbf{p_4}$ if

$$\mathbf{v} = u_1\mathbf{p_1} + u_2\mathbf{p_2} + u_3\mathbf{p_3} + u_4\mathbf{p_4} \qquad (13)$$

$$\text{subject to } \quad u_1 + u_2 + u_3 + u_4 = 1 \qquad (14)$$

where $\mathbf{v}$ and $\mathbf{p_i}$ denote the Euclidean coordinates. The four structure points are defined by randomly selecting a short-axis slice z and a directional angle θ for each of the points. The four landmarks are further detected separately in each image using (12). To ensure invariance to arbitrary pose of the epicardial and endocardial shape the coefficients are constrained to sum to one (14).

The proposed *GloCo* features are barycentric coordinates and computed as follows:

$$f_{GloCo}^1(\mathbf{v}^k; \mathbf{p}_1^k, \mathbf{p}_2^k, \mathbf{p}_3^k, \mathbf{p}_4^k) = u_1 \qquad\qquad f_{GloCo}^2(\mathbf{v}^k; \mathbf{p}_1^k, \mathbf{p}_2^k, \mathbf{p}_3^k, \mathbf{p}_4^k) = u_2$$
$$\qquad\qquad\qquad\qquad\qquad\qquad\qquad\qquad\qquad\qquad\qquad\qquad\qquad (15)$$
$$f_{GloCo}^3(\mathbf{v}^k; \mathbf{p}_1^k, \mathbf{p}_2^k, \mathbf{p}_3^k, \mathbf{p}_4^k) = u_3 \qquad\qquad f_{GloCo}^4(\mathbf{v}^k; \mathbf{p}_1^k, \mathbf{p}_2^k, \mathbf{p}_3^k, \mathbf{p}_4^k) = u_4$$

where

$$(u_1 \ u_2 \ u_3)^{\mathrm{T}} = \mathbf{T}^{-1}(\mathbf{v} - \mathbf{p_4}), \quad u_4 = 1 - u_1 - u_2 - u_3 \qquad (16)$$

$$\mathbf{T} = \begin{pmatrix} x_1-x_4 & x_2-x_4 & x_3-x_4 \\ y_1-y_4 & y_2-y_4 & y_3-y_4 \\ z_1-z_4 & z_2-z_4 & z_3-z_4 \end{pmatrix}, \ x_i, y_i, z_i \text{ are the coordinates of landmark } \mathbf{p_i}$$

Comparison of position and LoCo and GloCo features. A position feature does not exploit image intensity information and considers only the absolute position of the voxel in the image. Thus, it provides a weak constraint on geometric variability of the myocardium. On the contrary, the *GloCo* feature quantifies the relative position of the voxel with respect to four landmarks detected using intensity information from the COFA images. The detected landmarks are the tetrahedron vertices used in calculation of the barycentric coordinates and have different spatial locations across the images. Thus, the tetrahedron captures the coupled endo- and epicardial shape variability enforcing a strong constraint on the geometry of the myocardium.

3   Experimental Results

3.1   Dataset

25 3D end-diastolic echocardiograms from health subjects were used in this study. A Philips iE33 ultrasound system was used to acquire the images. Volume dimensions are (224×208×208) with an average of 0.88mm^3 spatial resolution. The myocardium and the blood pool of all volumes were manually segmented by an expert.

3.2   Validation Methodology

20 volumes were chosen randomly to train the RFs and the remaining 5 volumes were used in testing to report the results. To understand the impact of the new *LoCo* and *GloCo* features, two RF classifiers were trained: 1) using the previously reported local appearance and position features on the original images and 2) using the conventional local appearance, position features and also the new *LoCo* and *GloCo* features on the aligned images. The two RF were trained with 15 trees. The stopping criteria for growing the tree were the maximum depth - 16, no information gain of splitting and the minimum number of points at a node - 50. For the classic RF, 100 conventional features were randomly chosen at a node and further investigated to find the one that gives the highest information gain. For the RF with the new *LoCo* and *GloCo* features, 100 randomly chosen conventional features and 150 randomly chosen *LoCo* and *GloCo* features were used.

The RF was implemented in C++. Testing volumes were segmented in 20 seconds per volume using Intel Xeon 2.8GHz computer with 12 cores and 48GB RAM running Win7. With a parallel tree implementation, training required about 3 hours and only needed to be done once.

Fig. 5 shows a visual comparison of the segmentation from the classic RF and from the RF using the new features.

For quantitative analysis, the mean and standard deviation of the Dice and Jaccard similarity coefficients for both the myocardium and the blood pool are reported in Table 1. The Dice similarity coefficient is defined as Dice $= \frac{2 \times |GT \cap Auto|}{|GT| + |Auto|}$, while the Jaccard is defined as Jaccard $= \frac{|GT \cap Auto|}{|GT \cup Auto|}$, where GT is the ground truth represented as manual segmentation and Auto is the automatic segmentation, |.| is the cardinality of a set.

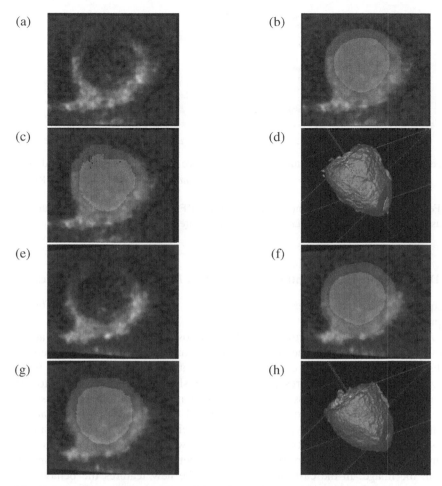

Fig. 5. (a) and (e) Short-axis slice of the original images ((e) is vertically aligned). (b) and (f) Manual segmentations of (a) and (e). (c) Automatic segmentation by the RF with the classic features (g) Automatic segmentation by the RF with the new LoCo and GloCo features. (d) and (h) 3D mesh of the automatically segmented volumes (a) and (e).

Table 1. Mean (μ) ± standard deviation (σ) of the dice and Jaccard coefficients for the myocardium and the blood pool

		Classic RF	RF with *LoCo* and *GloCo*
Myocardium	Dice	0.77 ± 0.06	0.77 ± 0.05
	Jaccard	0.63 ± 0.08	0.63 ± 0.06
Blood pool	Dice	0.88 ± 0.04	0.90 ± 0.02
	Jaccard	0.79 ± 0.06	0.82 ± 0.04

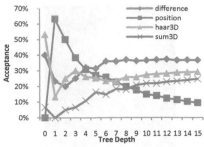
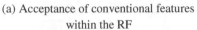
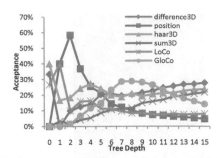

(a) Acceptance of conventional features   (b) Acceptance of conventional features and the
within the RF   new *LoCo and GloCo* features within the RF

Fig. 6. Feature acceptance at different depth with (a) the RF using the classic features and (b) the RF using the classic and the new *LoCo and GloCo* features

3.3   Discussion on the Conventional and the New *LoCo* and *GloCo* Features

The frequency of each type of feature selected during the training stage for different tree depths is shown in Fig. 6.

Position and appearance features. Recall that a position feature looks only at the absolute position of a voxel. The position features are pre-dominantly selected by both RFs at depths 1-4 when the complexity of the data is the highest, see Fig. 6. At this stage, the appearance features poorly distinguish the classes well due to the similar appearance of different tissues or the different appearance of the same tissue.

LoCo and GloCo features. Both the position and the *LoCo* and *GloCo* features divide the image domain spatially. In the case of the classic RF, the position features tend to split the data spatially until the depth 4, after which, as seen in Fig. 6 (a), the appearance features prove to separate the classes better within each of the spatial regions in the image. In the case of the RF with the new features the behavior is different. After depth 4, the *GloCo* features are shown to dominate. They continue splitting the image spatially into regions until the depth 11. This suggests that the *GloCo* features carry more detailed contextual information than the position or the *LoCo* features. Fig. 6 (b) suggests that after the depth 11, the separation is mainly done using the appearance information within each of the regions in the image. Note that by splitting the image spatially, the *LoCo* and *GloCo* features also encode a constraint on local and global shape variability.

We caveat our findings with two comments related to the dataset we used. The current training set consists of 20 3D volumes which is relatively small to capture the complexity of coupled variability of the epicardial and endocardial shapes. Thus firstly one would hypothesise an improvement of the Jaccard/Dice measures for the myocardial segmentation with an increase of training dataset size. Secondly one cannot guarantee that the small testing dataset used fairly captures the variability seen in the training dataset. Having said this, the results are encouraging and convincingly demonstrate the usefulness of the new proposed features for 3D echocardiography segmentation.

4   Conclusions

This paper proposes new context rich *LoCo* and *GloCo* features for medical imaging machine learning based segmentation that embed local and global shape constraints respectively. Our first contribution is the detection of the ventricular long axis based on image intensity information. This enables a) accurate alignment of all the volumes, which decreases the variability of LV position and thus, improves the quality of classic features; and b) detection of corresponding landmarks throughout the images, which are needed for the proposed features. Our second contribution is the new *LoCo* and *GloCo* features that encode local and global variability of coupled endo- and epicardial shapes.

We demonstrated improvement of 3D echocardiography segmentation over classic RF segmentation. The proposed features need to be tested on a larger training set to draw strong conclusions on the accuracy for myocardial segmentation which will be the subject of future work.

Acknowledgement. This research was funded by the UK EPSRC on grant EP/G030693/1.

References

1. Lempitsky, V., Verhoek, M., Noble, J.A., Blake, A.: Random Forest Classification for Automatic Delineation of Myocardium in Real-Time 3D Echocardiography. In: Ayache, N., Delingette, H., Sermesant, M. (eds.) FIMH 2009. LNCS, vol. 5528, pp. 447–456. Springer, Heidelberg (2009)
2. Breiman, L.: Random Forests. Machine Learning 45(1), 5–32 (2001)
3. Schroff, F., Criminisi, A., Zisserman, A.: Object Class Segmentation using Random Forests. In: BMVC (2008)
4. Shotton, J., Johnson, M., Cipolla, R.: Semantic Texton Forests for Image Categorization and Segmentation. In: CVPR (2008)
5. Yaqub, M., et al.: Efficient Volumetric Segmentation using 3D Fast-Weighted Random Forests. In: MICCAI-MLMI, Toronto, Canada (2011)
6. Geremia, E., Menze, B.H., Clatz, O., Konukoglu, E., Criminisi, A., Ayache, N.: Spatial Decision Forests for MS Lesion Segmentation in Multi-Channel MR Images. In: Jiang, T., Navab, N., Pluim, J.P.W., Viergever, M.A. (eds.) MICCAI 2010, Part I. LNCS, vol. 6361, pp. 111–118. Springer, Heidelberg (2010)
7. Mulet-Parada, M., Noble, J.A.: 2D+T Acoustic Boundary Detection in Echocardiography. Medical Image Analysis 4, 21–33 (2000)
8. Kovesi, P.: Image Features from Phase Congruency. Journal of Computer Vision Research 1 (1999)
9. Rajpoot, K., Grau, V., Noble, J.A.: Local-phase based 3D boundary detection using monogenic signal and its application to real-time 3-D echocardio images. In: ISBI (2009)
10. Felsberg, M., Sommer, G.: The Monogenic Signal. IEEE Transactions on Signal Processing 49, 3136–3144 (2001)

Novel Vector-Valued Approach
to Automatic Brain Tissue Classification

Nataliya Portman and Alan Evans

McConnell Brain Imaging Centre, Montreal Neurological Institute
3801 University H3A 2B4, Montreal, Quebec, Canada
{nataliya,alan}@bic.mni.mcgill.ca
http://www.bic.mni.mcgill.ca

Abstract. In this work we propose a novel SSIM (Structural Similarity
Index Measure)-guided brain tissue classification approach, implement-
ing Kernel Fisher Discriminant Analysis (KFDA). In Computer Vision,
KFDA has been shown to be competitive with other state-of-the-art techniques. In the KFDA-based framework, we exploit the complex structure
of grey matter, white matter and cerebro-spinal fluid intensity clusters
to find an optimal classification. We illustrate our novel technique using
a dataset of early normal brain development in the age range from 10
days to 4.5 years. The SSIM metric, an objective measure of an image
quality as perceived by the Human Visual System, is used to evaluate the
quality of brain segmentation. SSIM comparison of the quality of classification obtained by the KFDA-based and the Expectation-Maximization
algorithms shows the superior performance of the proposed technique.

Keywords: Kernel Fisher Discriminant Analysis, classification, testing
set, partial volume effect, feature space, brain tissue classes.

1   Introduction

Motivation. This paper addresses the problem of automatic classification of
brain tissue into white matter (WM), grey matter (GM) and cerebrospinal fluid
(CSF) for an MR pediatric dataset of early brain development from birth through
4.5 years of age [1].
This dataset exhibits dramatic qualitative changes in GM/WM contrast during
early brain maturation. The MRI signal is affected by myelinated axons of the
major pathways (white matter and the corpus callosum). As a result of poor
and highly variable GM/WM contrast and tight sulcal packing, automatic classification via INSECT [2] was difficult to implement.
We set out to achieve high quality classification of this dataset as this is fundamental for the accuracy of cortical surface extraction and the following assessment of normal surface variability in children before 4.5 years of age.

Classification Techniques in NeuroImaging. Many brain tissue classification techniques have been proposed, e.g. a k Nearest Neighbour classifier [3], an

B.H. Menze et al. (Eds.): MCV 2012, LNCS 7766, pp. 70–81, 2013.
© Springer-Verlag Berlin Heidelberg 2013

Artificial Neural Network classifier [4], an Expectation-Maximization (EM) algorithm [5], a modified EM-based algorithm using a Markov Random Field model [6] and a watershed-based segmentation [7], being among the most popular.

Different methods for the evaluation of classifier performance show that existing automatic classification algorithms do not fully capture expert tracings [8]. The major drawback is incorrect classification of the CSF into either background or GM.

The MR brain tissue labeling process is complicated by the presence of a partial volume (PV) effect due to the limited spatial resolution of the scanner, which leads to the presence of multiple tissue types within a single voxel. PV estimation (PVE) or computation of the mixing proportions of tissue classes per voxel is essential for an accurate quantification of tissue volumes and cortical surface extraction [9]. Among the proposed PVE techniques, a Trimmed Minimum Covariance Determinant (TMCD) approach [9] provides a generalized segmentation framework since it uses Gaussian distributions with different covariance matrices for modeling tissue intensity histograms and it can be applied to multi-channel data.

The disadvantage of the TMCD method is its computational complexity. We seek a simpler approach that would classify brain image data with high accuracy.

Why KFDA? We introduce *the first of its kind* KFDA-based brain tissue classification algorithm to the NeuroImaging field that explores the structure of GM, WM and CSF clusters, reveals their non-linearity in the original space and exploits this non-linearity for improved classification [10]. KFDA [11] is particularly useful for the separation of input data into classes when their histogram distributions overlap as is the case with the MR pediatric dataset. KFDA attempts to make the image data more separable by non-linearly mapping them from the original space to an abstract feature space and classify them via optimal discriminant hyperplanes.

The KFDA-based approach is natural for the identification of PV voxels that lie near the boundaries between tissue types. Since KFDA finds complex decision surfaces that best separate the data into GM, WM and CSF in the original space then overlapping subsets (e.g., WM voxels trapped in the intensity range of GM) and class cluster outliers located near these separating surfaces identify the voxels with significant PV effect. KFDA is related to kernel-based classifiers such as the Support Vector Machine (SVM) approach [13]. The superior performance of KFDA over SVM as shown in [11] can be explained by the fact that KFDA uses all training samples to compute the discriminant function, not only the ones that lie closest to the decision surface, i.e. the Support Vectors. The appealing features of KFDA include:

- KFDA is vector-valued, i.e. applied to multi-channel data
- Non-linear generalization of LDA (Linear Discriminant Analysis) that implies a higher prediction accuracy.
- Precision; algebraic formulation of the maximization of the discriminant criterion provides an exact solution.

- Minimal dependency on parameters (unlike SVM whose performance depends also on the number of support vectors and training samples). The
parameters that are used in KFDA define kernel functions.

Dataset. The pediatric dataset (NIHPD) collected by the National Institutes
of Health (NIH) [15] consists of 72 healthy subjects aged 10 days to 4.5 years
scanned repeatedly at quarterly intervals. Imaging data includes structural MRI
(T1w, T2w, PDw). Data were acquired on a 1.5 T Siemens Sonata scanner with
a $1 \times 1 \times 3$ mm spatial resolution. MR brain scans were corrected for image
intensity non-uniformity [16] and registered to the MNI stereotaxic space using
spatial normalization [17]. The data were resampled to 1 mm^3 grid using tri-
cubic interpolation. T1w, T2w and PDw average atlases have been created for
important developmental age ranges for the NIHPD data[1] [12].

2   KFDA-Based Algorithm

1. *Initialization.* We started with a template for the oldest age range (44-60
months) and transferred GM, WM and CSF probability maps known for the age
range 4.5 to 8.5 years [12] [2] onto the oldest pediatric template via registration
mni_autoreg [17] of the T1w template (4.5 to 8.5 years) (see Fig. 1.a) with
the T1w template (44-60 months) (see Fig. 1.b). The *mni_autoreg* procedure
estimates a 3D non-linear deformation field iteratively in a multiscale hierarchy,
i.e. by matching blurred template volumes and subsequent refining of a resulting
displacement field. Hard labeling of the template for the age range of 44 to 60
months is then used as the best guess for initialization (see Fig. 1.c).

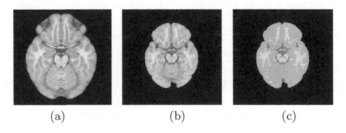

(a)   (b)   (c)

Fig. 1. (a) T1w pediatric template (4.5-8.5 years), (b) T1w pediatric template (44-60
months), (c) Hard labels of the template (b) obtained from tissue probability maps of
older brains registered with (b).

2. *Preliminary Quantile Analysis.* In the posterior brain, the MRI signal in
WM tends to weaken towards the occipital lobe introducing more uncertainty to

---

[1] The   age-dependent   pediatric   atlas   is   available   for   download   at
http://www.bic.mni.mcgill.ca/ServicesAtlases/NIHPD-obj2
[2] This probabilistic brain atlas was obtained from 82 normal subjects within the age
range 4.5 to 8.5 years using an unsupervised genetic tissue classification algorithm.

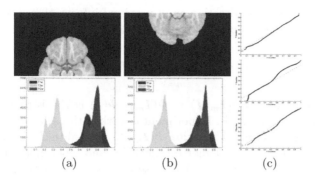

(a)   (b)   (c)

Fig. 2. T1w, T2w and PDw intensity histograms in (a) the anterior and (b) posterior parts of the 3D template (44-60 months), (c) quantile-quantile plots of the anterior (X-axis) versus posterior (Y-axis) intensity samples in 3D (from top to bottom) T1w, T2w and PDw templates

GM/WM boundary location. This results in a greater overlap of GM and WM intensity histograms as shown in Fig. 2.a-b. Scatter plots of quantiles computed from samples of grey levels in the anterior and posterior parts of the 3D template brain suggest that they come from different probability distributions (see Fig. 2.c). Therefore, we explore tissue cluster structures in each of the brain halves.

3. 3D Brain partitioning. To proceed with KFDA implementation in MAT-LAB, namely, to solve an eigen-value problem in a high-dimensional feature space the brain partitioning into subvolumes is needed. Due to MATLAB limitations on the maximum matrix size and available system memory it is not possible to carry out computations for each interior brain half (containing $\approx 300,000$ voxels). Therefore, given a vector-valued image function

$$\boldsymbol{I}(i,j,k) = (T1w(i,j,k), T2w(i,j,k), PDw(i,j,k)),$$

where $1 \leqslant i \leqslant M,\ 1 \leqslant j \leqslant N,\ 1 \leqslant k \leqslant L$ are voxel coordinates of the interior brain, we partition each brain half into subsets of K slices in the axial direction. Due to insufficient system memory we have chosen $K = 3$. That is, we have $\left[\frac{L}{2}\right]$ subvolumes

$$\{\boldsymbol{I}\}_k = \{(T1w(i,j,k+l-1), T2w(i,j,k+l-1), PDw(i,j,k+l-1))\}_{l=1}^3,$$

where $k = 1, 3, 5, ..., L - 2$.

4. Kernel transformation of the data and optimal projection in the feature space. We partition the non-binary brain tissue classification problem into two two-class problems, namely, separation of the image data into G+W matter and CSF and then separation of G+W matter into GM and WM. We consider each vector-valued intensity at the interior brain voxel as a training sample. Given the brain subvolume $\{\boldsymbol{I}\}_k$ with M_1 labeled training samples we implicitly transform them to the M_1-dimensional feature space $\mathcal{F}$ with a non-linear map

Φ. We then calculate the direction w of maximal information discrimination in $\mathcal{F}$ [11] and project the mapped data $\Phi(I)$ onto the vector w

$$w \cdot \Phi(I) = \sum_{m=1}^{M_1} \alpha_m k(I_m, I) + \beta, \qquad (1)$$

where β is an offset and $k(I_m, I) = \Phi(I_m) \cdot \Phi(I)$ is the kernel function that computes a dot product in $\mathcal{F}$. Experimental work with various kernel functions shows that a sigmoid kernel function $k(I_m, I) = \tanh(a(I_m^T \cdot I) + b)$ yields the best separation into G+W matter and CSF, and a polynomial of a degree 3 $k(I_m, I) = (I_m^T \cdot I + b)^3$ or higher best separates GM and WM.

Figures 3.b and 4.b show optimal projections of G+W matter (in red) and CSF (in blue) classes and GM (in blue) and WM (in red) classes correspondingly (according to their initial classifications). In both Figures, X-axis represents column-wise enumeration of the interior brain voxels from 1 to M_1 and Y-axis represents the projected values $w \cdot \Phi(I_i)$, $1 \leqslant i \leqslant M_1$. When calculated with the offset β they are positive for one class and negative for another.

Classification into G+W Matter and CSF. For the anterior subvolume displayed in Fig. 3 KFDA identified 22 CSF and 384 G+W matter outliers shown in cyan and green, respectively in Fig. 3.c. Their spatial positions in stereotaxic space (see Fig. 3.a) suggest that they are likely to be PV voxels. To determine the dominant tissue type for each of these outliers we split the projected data into testing and training sets. Namely, the outliers form the testing set and the rest of the projected data forms the training set.

Using Mahalanobis distance, KFDA predicted CSF membership for all 384 G+W matter outliers from the classified training set (see Fig. 3.c). As a result, a new classification detects more CSF (see Fig. 3.d).

A separating surface corresponding to this new classification is shown in Fig. 4.e with G+W matter and CSF intensities depicted in red and blue, respectively. The template decision surface is used for the subject classification into G+W matter and CSF shown in cyan and magenta, respectively in Fig. 4.e. Notice the complexity of the separating surfaces displayed in Fig. 4.e-f due to the fact that all training samples are used to compute them.

Classification into GM and WM. Unlike the case with G+W matter and CSF clusters, both GM and WM distributions of the projected data contain only a few if any outliers. There is a significant number of GM voxels trapped in the negative range of WM distribution as seen from Fig. 4.b. More precisely, KFDA has identified 1647 overlapping GM voxels and 74 overlapping WM voxels shown in cyan and green correspondingly in Fig. 4.b. Fig. 4.a suggests that these voxels are likely to contain a significant PV effect. Treating them as testing samples we predict their labels via a kNN classifier ($k = 8$ neighbours) from a training set comprised of the rest of the projected subvolume in $\mathcal{F}$ (see Fig. 4.c).

The separating polynomial surface corresponding to the KFDA classification of the posterior subject subvolume into GM (in magenta) and WM (in cyan) is shown in Fig. 4.g.

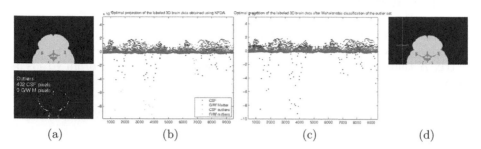

(a)   (b)   (c)   (d)

Fig. 3. (a) top: Labeled input data (one of the three anterior slices is shown) from the template (44-60 months), bottom: spatial location of outliers in stereotaxic space, (b) data projection onto w in $\mathcal{F}$: G+W (in red) and CSF (in blue), (c) Mahalanobis classification of the outliers, (d) KFDA classification into G+W matter and CSF

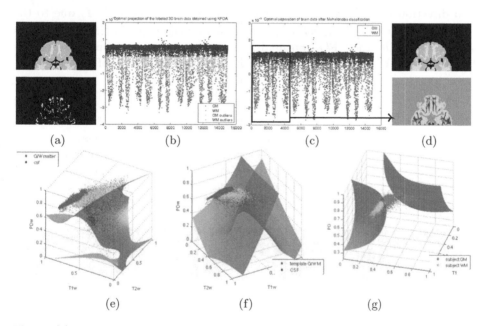

(a)   (b)   (c)   (d)

(e)   (f)   (g)

Fig. 4. (a) top: Initial GM and WM labels of G+W matter (one of the three anterior slices is shown) in the template subvolume (44-60 months), bottom: overlapping voxels in the stereotaxic space, (b) optimal projection in the feature space, (c) kNN classification of GM and WM overlapping voxels, WM (in red), GM (in blue), (d) top: KFDA classification into GM and WM, bottom: An image display of projected anterior subvolume (one slice out of $K = 3$ is shown) in $\mathcal{F}$ contained in a rectangular area (c). Red peaks in (c) correspond to interior WM voxels. Optimal decision surfaces for the CSF and G+W matter (e) in the anterior part, (f) in the posterior part, (g) optimal separation of the posterior subject data into GM and WM.

3   Spatial Regularization

To increase robustness to misclassification, we introduce a spatial regularization term that penalizes local kernel projected intensity differences in $\mathcal{F}$. We define matrix H that describes local relationships between the interior brain voxels as follows

$$H_{ij} = \begin{cases} 1, & \text{if voxels } i \text{ and } j \text{ are neighbours } ((i,j) \text{ is an edge)}; \\ -d_{ij}, & \text{if } i = j, \text{ the degree of vertex (voxel) } i; \\ 0, & \text{otherwise.} \end{cases}$$

$$\text{Then for } \forall \boldsymbol{V} \in R^{M_1} \quad \boldsymbol{V}^T H \boldsymbol{V} = - \sum_{(i,j) \in E} (V_i - V_j)^2, \tag{2}$$

where E is an edge set comprised of edges $\{V_i, V_j\}$.

Let $\boldsymbol{V} = \boldsymbol{w} \cdot \Phi(\boldsymbol{I})$ be the kernel projection of the input data $\boldsymbol{I}$ onto the optimal direction $\boldsymbol{w}$ in $\mathcal{F}$. $\boldsymbol{V}$ can be rewritten as $\boldsymbol{V} = \sum_{i=1}^{M_1} \alpha_i k(\boldsymbol{I_i}, \boldsymbol{I})$ due to the expansion of $\boldsymbol{w} = \sum_{i=1}^{M_1} \alpha_i \Phi(\boldsymbol{I_i})$ in $\mathcal{F}$ spanned by the mapped training samples $\Phi(\boldsymbol{I_i})$. We modify the KFDA optimality criterion by adding the penalty term of the form $V^T HV = \alpha^T K H K^T \alpha$, where K is the kernel matrix of size $M_1 \times M_1$

$$\hat{\alpha} = \arg \max_{\alpha} \left(\frac{\alpha^T M \alpha + \lambda \alpha^T K H K^T \alpha}{\alpha^T N \alpha} \right). \tag{3}$$

Here, M is a between-class covariance matrix and N is a within-class covariance matrix in $\mathcal{F}$ (see [11], [14] for details). In this setup the penalty function forces misclassified voxels closer to another class cluster centroid. The problem (3) can be solved by computing a leading eigen-vector of $N^{-1}(M + \lambda K H K^T)$.

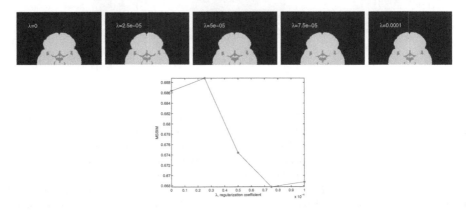

Fig. 5. Upper panel: anterior template brain classified into G+W M and CSF for $\lambda_i = 0.000025 \cdot i$, $i = 0, ..., 4$; Lower panel: MSSIM between T1w template and each of the classified anterior brains shown in the upper panel

A modified version of the KFDA criterion (3) depends on the value of the regularization coefficient λ. The upper panel in Fig. 5 shows the influence of λ-coefficient on the quality of segmentation into G+W M and CSF as it increases by an increment of 0.000025 from 0 to 0.0001. By a visual inspection, the classification corresponding to $\lambda = 0.000025$ is most plausible as the CSF pattern appears to be most connected compared to that with other λ-values. This choice was operationalized with the SSIM metric described below.

4 Objective Quality Evaluation via SSIM

For the automatic control of λ-parameter we need a quantitative assessment of segmentation quality. Such measures to MR brain segmentation as the Jaccard coefficient and the Dice coefficient are commonly used, however, they rely on knowledge of a reference segmentation. We seek a similarity measure to evaluate λ-dependent classifications in the absence of a ground truth and use the Structural Similarity Index Measure (SSIM) [18], [19]. The SSIM is an objective similarity metric that quantifies the degree of structural similarity between ideal and distorted images. It is based on the assumption that the Human Visual System (HVS) is an optimal extractor of structural information from images.

We evaluated the performance of our classification algorithm relying on the Computer Vision hypothesis that the HVS focuses on image components with high information content [20]. In our case, these image components are WM/GM and G+W matter and CSF boundaries. We evaluated how well these boundaries are captured by our algorithm versus the boundaries that we can visually extract from T1w data (we use one imaging modality for simplicity).

We created classified brain subvolumes in the form of mean T1w intensity values for the two tissue types. We computed the SSIM between each classified and T1w brain slices and the mean SSIM (MSSIM) defined by

$$MSSIM = \frac{1}{M_1} \sum_{i=1}^{M_1} SSIM(x_i, y_i), \ \ SSIM(x_i, y_i) = l(x_i, y_i) \cdot c(x_i, y_i) \cdot s(x_i, y_i),$$

x_i and y_i are local image patches[3] and $l(x_i, y_i)$, $c(x_i, y_i)$, $s(x_i, y_i)$ are the luminance, contrast and structure comparison measures defined by

$$l(x, y) = \frac{2\mu_x\mu_y + C_1}{\mu_x^2 + \mu_y^2 + C_1}; \ c(x, y) = \frac{2\sigma_x\sigma_y + C_2}{\sigma_x^2 + \sigma_y^2 + C_2}; s(x, y) = \frac{\sigma_{xy} + C_3}{\sigma_x\sigma_y + C_3}.$$

Here, $\mu_x(\mu_y)$, $\sigma_x(\sigma_y)$ and σ_{xy} represent the local mean, standard deviation and cross-correlation estimates, respectively, and C_1, C_2, C_3 are small constants [18].

Shown in the lower panel of Fig. 5 is the MSSIM computed between the T1w and classified anterior template subvolumes and plotted against the values of λ. It achieves its maximum at $\lambda = 0.000025$ as expected. Thus, by choosing λ-value corresponding to the largest MSSIM we are able to automatically guide the classification procedure.

---

[3] a sliding window that moves across the entire brain slice pixel by pixel. For the MSSIM the background patches have been excluded.

5   Results

We compared classification results obtained by prior hard labeling, KFDA-based and EM approaches using MSSIM. Figures 7 and 8 show single slices from the classified template (44-60 months) and subject brain subvolumes obtained by joining overlapping anterior and posterior parts. Namely, if $I_1(i,j,k)$, $i \in \{1,2,3,...,\left[\frac{N}{2}\right]+2\}$ is an anterior brain, and $I_2(i,j,k)$, $i \in \{\left[\frac{N}{2}\right]-1,...,N\}$ is a posterior brain, where $y = \left[\frac{N}{2}\right]$ is the middle plane, then the whole brain image function $I(i,j,k)$ is defined as follows

$$I(i,j,k) = \begin{cases} I_1(i,j,k), & \text{for } i \in \{1,2,3,...,\left[\frac{N}{2}\right]\}, \\ I_2(i,j,k), & \text{for } i \in \{\left[\frac{N}{2}\right]+1,...,N\}. \end{cases}$$

Note that in order to preserve neighbourhood relations of the middle plane voxels in anterior and posterior parts, we defined I_1 and I_2 as subsets with an overlapping region $R(i,j,k)$, $i \in \{\left[\frac{N}{2}\right]-1,..,\left[\frac{N}{2}\right]+2\}$.

Remark. In order to better accommodate grey level intensity inhomogeneities present in brain tissues, we intend to optimally partition the brain into regions that differ significantly in average intensity values. Shown in Fig. 6 are transverse and coronal slices of the template brain subdivided into parallelepipeds using a binary space partition. Having created and classified overlapping parallelepipeds, 3D image stitching can then be performed via simulated annealing.

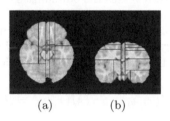

(a)   (b)

Fig. 6. 3D template brain partitioning based on mutual information maximization between the intensity histogram bins and the regions of the subdivided image: (a) transverse slice 37 (out of 105), (b) coronal slice 110 (out of 235). The total number of the brain regions is 32.

Fig. 7.a-c show that the CSF structure captured by KFDA is more similar to the one seen in T1w. The comparison of MSSIMs given in Fig. 7.b-c suggests that our proposed algorithm improves CSF detection.

The comparison of the classified WM patterns (see Fig. 7.d-e) with the one seen in T1w (see Fig. 7.a) and of their respective MSSIMs for the template shows that the proposed algorithm also improves classification into GM and WM. EM algorithm with a prior seen in Fig. 7.f yields a reasonable estimate of CSF and a significant underestimate of WM. MSSIM comparison of the GM/WM classified results demonstrates a superior performance of KFDA over EM algorithm. Seen

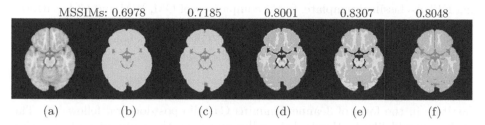

(a)   (b)   (c)   (d)   (e)   (f)

Fig. 7. (a) T1w template (44-60 months) and its classification into G+W matter and CSF: (b) prior, (c) KFDA; into GM and WM: (d) prior, (e) KFDA, (f) EM classification into GM, WM and CSF with a prior

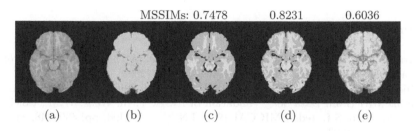

(a)   (b)   (c)   (d)   (e)

Fig. 8. (a) T1w image of a 4.5 year old subject and its classification into G+W matter and CSF: (b) KFDA; into GM and WM: (c) prior, (d) KFDA, (e) EM with a prior.

in Fig. 8.a is a T1w scan of a 4.5 year old subject. We generated classification into G+W matter and CSF by treating the entire subject data as a testing set and by its kernel projection onto w in $\mathcal{F}$ spanned by the template samples $\Phi(I_i)$. The resulting classification is displayed in Fig. 8.b.

The comparison of a WM pattern seen in Fig. 8.a with the classified WM seen in Fig. 8.c-e demonstrates the remarkable capability of KFDA to reveal a complex WM structure given a poor GM/WM contrast. The EM algorithm with a prior applied to the vector-valued subject subvolume tends to overestimate WM and CSF (see Fig. 8.e). The comparison of MSSIMs given in Fig. 8.c-e shows that KFDA yields the most similar WM pattern to the one extracted by our visual system.

6 Conclusion

We have developed a novel and elegant KFDA-based algorithm for automatic brain tissue classification. It is a vector-valued non-parametric approach that relies on prior hard labels of tissue types for initialization. The proposed algorithm takes into account spatial correlations between interior brain intensities, identifies voxels with PV effect, predicts the dominating tissue types in the PV set and constructs complex optimal decision surfaces precisely.

In this work, we classified the oldest template (44-60 months) of this dataset and showed how a subject chosen from the same age range can be labeled using KFDA-classified template. SSIM comparison of GM, WM and CSF patterns detected by KFDA and EM approaches showed a superior performance of the latter. Our next incentive is to apply the KFDA-based technique for the classification of age-dependent templates for earlier age ranges.

Acknowledgement. This research was supported by the Montreal Neurological Institute in the form of Jeanne Timmins Costello postdoctoral fellowship. The authors would like to thank their colleagues from the University of Waterloo (Canada), Dr. Zhou Wang, a Prof. in the ECE Department, and Dr. Edward Vrscay, a Prof. in the Department of Applied Mathematics, for the discussion and insightful comments on the proposed KFDA-based methodology.

References

1. Evans, A.C., Brain Development Cooperative Group: The NIH MRI study of normal brain development. NeuroImage 30, 184–202 (2006)
2. Zijdenbos, A.P., Forghani, R., Evans, A.: Automatic Quantification of MS Lesions in 3D MRI Brain Data Sets: Validation of INSECT. In: Wells, W.M., Colchester, A.C.F., Delp, S.L. (eds.) MICCAI 1998. LNCS, vol. 1496, pp. 439–448. Springer, Heidelberg (1998)
3. Warfield, S.: Fast kNN classification for multichannel image data. Pattern Recogn. Lett. 17(7), 713–721 (1996)
4. Zijdenbos, A.P., Dawant, B.M., et al.: Morphometric Analysis of White Matter Lesions in MR Images: Method and Validation. IEEE Trans. Med. Imag 21(10), 1280–1291 (1994)
5. Wells, W.M., Kikinis, R., Grimson, W.E.L., Jolesz, F.: Adaptive Segmentation of MRI Data. IEEE Trans. Med. Imag. 23, 429–442 (1996)
6. Pohl, K.M., Bouix, S., Kikinis, R., Grimson, W.E.L.: Anatomical Guided Segmentation with non-Stationary Tissue Class Distributions in an Expectation-Maximization Framework. In: IEEE Int. Symposium on Biomed. Imag., Arlington, VA, pp. 81–84 (2004)
7. Grau, V., Mewes, A.U.J., et al.: Improved Watershed Transform for Medical Image Segmentation Using Prior Information. IEEE Trans. Med. Imag. 23(4), 447–458 (2004)
8. Bouix, S., Martin-Fernandez, M., Ungar, L., et al.: On Evaluating Brain Tissue Classifiers without a Ground Truth. NeuroImage 36, 1207–1224 (2007)
9. Tohka, J., Zijdenbos, A., Evans, A.: Fast and Robust Estimation for Statistical Partial Volume Models in Brain MRI. NeuroImage 23, 84–97 (2004)
10. Portman, N., Evans, A.: Novel Vector-Valued Approach to Automatic Brain Tissue Classification. Poster 6488, 18th Annual Meeting of the OHBM, Beijing (2012)
11. Mika, S., Ratsch, G., Weston, J., et al.: Fisher Discriminant Analysis with Kernels. In: Neural Networks for Signal Processing IX: Proc. of the 1999 IEEE Signal Proc. Soc. Workshop, pp. 41–48 (1999)
12. Fonov, V., Evans, A.C., Botteron, K., et al.: Unbiased Average Age-Appropriate Atlases for Pediatric Studies. Neuroimage 54(1), 313–327 (2011)
13. Vapnik, V.N.: Statistical learning theory. John Wiley & Sons (1998) (manuscript)
14. Baudat, G., Anouar, F.: Generalized Discriminant Analysis Using a Kernel Approach. Neural Computation 12(10), 2385–2404 (2000)

15. Almli, C.R., Rivkin, M.J., McKinstry, R.C., Brain Development Cooperative Group: The NIH MRI study of normal brain development (Objective-2): Newborns, infants, toddlers, and preschoolers. NeuroImage 35(1), 308–325 (2007)
16. Sled, J.G., Zijdenbos, A.P., Evans, A.C.: A Non-Parametric Method for Automatic Correction of Intensity Non-Uniformity in MRI Data. IEEE Trans. Med. Imag. 17, 87–97 (1998)
17. Collins, D.L., Neelin, P., Peters, P.M., Evans, A.C.: Automatic 3D Intersubject Registration of MR Volumetric Data in Standardized Talairach Space. J. Comput. Assist. Tomogr. 18(2), 192–205 (1994)
18. Wang, Z., Bovik, A.C.: A Universal Image Quality Index. IEEE Signal Processing Letters 9, 81–84 (2002)
19. Wang, Z., Simoncelli, E.P., Bovik, A.C.: Multi-scale Structural Similarity for Image Quality Assessment. In: IEEE Proc. Asilomar Conf. Signals, Syst.,Comput., pp. 1398–1402 (2003)
20. Wang, Z., Bovik, A.C., Sheikh, H.R.: Image Quality Asessment: From Error Visibility to Structural Similarity. IEEE Trans. Image Proc. 13(4), 600–612 (2004)

Atlas-Based Whole-Body PET-CT Segmentation Using a Passive Contour Distance

Fabian Gigengack[1,2], Lars Ruthotto[3], Xiaoyi Jiang[2], Jan Modersitzki[3], Martin Burger[4], Sven Hermann[1], and Klaus P. Schäfers[1]

[1] European Institute for Molecular Imaging (EIMI), University of Münster, Germany
[2] Department of Mathematics and Computer Science, University of Münster, Germany
[3] Institute of Mathematics and Image Computing, University of Lübeck, Germany
[4] Institute for Computational and Applied Mathematics, University of Münster, Germany

Abstract. In positron emission tomography (PET) imaging, the segmentation of organs is necessary for many quantitative image analysis tasks, e.g., estimation of individual organ concentration or partial volume correction. To this end we present a fully automated approach for whole-body segmentation which enables large-scale and reproducible studies. The approach is based on joint segmentation and atlas registration. The classical active contour approach by Chan and Vese is modified to a novel *passive contour* energy term with implicitly incorporated information about shape and location of the organs. This new energy is added to a registration functional which is based on both functional (PET) and morphological (CT) data. The proposed method is applied to medical data, given by 13 PET-CT data sets of mice, and quantitatively compared to manually drawn VOIs. An average Dice coefficient of 0.73 ± 0.10 for the left ventricle, 0.88 ± 0.05 for the bladder, and 0.76 ± 0.07 for the kidneys shows the high accuracy of our method.

Keywords: Segmentation, Active Contour, Passive Contour, Registration, Atlas, PET-CT, Whole-Body.

1 Introduction

Positron emission tomography (PET) is widely used in medical imaging to assess functional information in the body. However, quantitative evaluation of PET images is challenging due to the rather limited spatial resolution and low signal-to-noise ratio which makes the segmentation of organs necessary for various applications. Estimating organ concentration in biodistribution studies [6], [9], or analyzing organ specific diseases such as myocardial infarction demands for an adequate whole-body segmentation. In addition, organ segmentation is mandatory for many partial volume correction techniques [15]. To this end we developed a general approach for whole-body segmentation based on joint segmentation and registration.

B.H. Menze et al. (Eds.): MCV 2012, LNCS 7766, pp. 82–92, 2013.

1.1   Related Work

Many approaches originating from computer vision are transferred to medical imaging as they are well understood and, at the same time, also efficiently applicable to volumetric (3D) medical images. A popular approach in computer vision for automatic segmentation is active contours as introduced by Chan and Vese [2]. The method was successfully applied to medical imaging based on brain MRI data [3]. The main idea of active contours is also exploited in our work, but in a reversed interpretation, cf. Sec. 2.

There is a large demand for automatic segmentation in medical imaging as the manual segmentation of organs is time-consuming for 3D data sets. Further, inter- and intra-observer variability can have a high impact. This is why manual segmentation is inapplicable for large-scale and reproducible studies. We restrict the following discussion to related literature on segmentation of PET and CT and joint registration and segmentation.

An automated method for whole-body segmentation in Micro-CT data of mice was introduced by Baiker et al. [1]. The approach consists of a model-based registration with a subsequent intensity-based registration. They achieved high accuracies for skin and skeleton. However, they did not report results for inner organs which are the focus of this work. This might be due to the low soft tissue contrast of the CT images which makes the localization of inner organs challenging. We overcome this limitation (inter alia) by using functional information in terms of PET images (and additional CT images).

Wang et al. presented a registration approach based on a statistical shape model for small-animal PET segmentation [13]. High uptake organs guide the registration using a conditional Gaussian model and allow good estimates for low uptake organs as well. However, for the labeling of organs the method requires user interaction.

Recently various techniques were published combining registration and segmentation. A taxonomy on this topic is given in [8]. A method, which is basically similar to our proceeding, was presented by Yezzi et al. [14]. They propose a variational framework that uses active contours for segmentation with a simultaneous registration of features. The level-set based segmentation separates only one object from the background which makes this method inapplicable for multiple organ segmentation tasks. Further, only rigid and affine transformations were practically explored.

2   Methods

In this paper we present a novel atlas-based segmentation approach. The general scheme is illustrated in Fig. 1. Given a pair of spatially aligned PET and CT images (real data on the left of Fig. 1) of the same subject, we follow a two-step strategy. After aligning the atlas (atlas data on the right of Fig. 1) and the real data with an affine transformation, a tailored registration functional with joint segmentation is minimized. Three distance terms drive the registration: 1. Distance of the atlas CT and real CT, 2. Distance of the atlas PET and real PET,

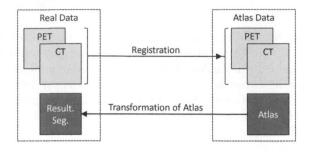

Fig. 1. General scheme: The inverse of the estimated transformation is applied to the atlas to segment the real data

3. Segmentation distance motivated by Chan and Vese [2]. Instead of matching a contour to the data, the novel segmentation distance is used to optimize for the transformation that aligns the data best to the (passive) contours. This turns around the interpretation of standard active contours models. Finally, the atlas organ definitions are transformed with the inverse transformation and yield the resulting segmentation of the real data, cf. bottom of Fig. 1.

In particular, we address the following points:

1. Transition of 2D active contours to 3D passive contours for medical image segmentation
2. Fully automation to make large-scale studies possible (user interaction is time-consuming)
3. Non-rigidity of atlas-based whole-body segmentation
4. Multimodality treatment (function and morphology)
5. Handling of multiple organs for joint registration and segmentation

2.1   Joint Passive Contour Segmentation and Registration

As a technical preprocessing step, a rough alignment of the atlas dataset and the real dataset is performed by matching the atlas CT to the real CT with an affine transformation to overcome differences in the orientation, scaling, and translation. As both images are of the same modality we choose the sum of squared differences (SSD) distance measure.

To overcome anatomical variations of organs, the information of the PET and the CT images is used simultaneously in a joint registration functional. Hence, anatomical and functional information is exploited at the same time. In addition, we include a novel segmentation distance term into the functional, inspired by Chan and Vese [2]. The Chan-Vese distance measures the in-class variance according to the atlas organ definitions. We derive the complete registration model by first looking at standard image registration for the CT images.

For the alignment of the CT images, the real data $\mathcal{T}_{CT} : \Omega \to \mathbb{R}$ (template image) is registered to the atlas CT image $\mathcal{R}_{CT} : \Omega \to \mathbb{R}$ (reference image), where

$\Omega \subset \mathbb{R}^3$ is the image domain. The output of the registration is a transformation $y : \mathbb{R}^3 \to \mathbb{R}^3$ representing point-to-point correspondences between $\mathcal{T}_{CT}$ and $\mathcal{R}_{CT}$. To find y, the following functional has to be minimized

$$\min_{y} \left\{ \mathcal{D}^{\mathrm{SSD}}(\mathcal{T}_{CT} \circ y, \ \mathcal{R}_{CT}) + \alpha_{\mathcal{S}} \cdot \mathcal{S}(y) \right\} . \tag{1}$$

$\mathcal{D}^{\mathrm{SSD}}$ is the SSD distance functional and $\alpha_{\mathcal{S}} \in \mathbb{R}^+$ is a weighting factor of the regularization functional $\mathcal{S}$. By using regularized spline image interpolation we reduce artifacts in the PET images which justifies the usage of the SSD measure.

We assume that the PET and corresponding CT measurement approximately share the same geometry and hence y can be used to align both modalities. In practice the images provide complementary information which motivates the exploration of both modalities in a joint registration functional. The CT images guide the registration whereas the PET images provide important information in soft tissue regions. As the scanned mice are anesthetized the spatial variations are kept to a minimum. However, changes due to, e.g., bladder filling, are possible.

Our joint registration functional is an extension of (1) by adding a term for the PET data and an additional passive contour term $\mathcal{D}_{PC}$

$$\min_{y} \left\{ \alpha_{CT} \cdot \mathcal{D}^{\mathrm{SSD}}(\mathcal{T}_{CT} \circ y, \ \mathcal{R}_{CT}) + \alpha_{PET} \cdot \mathcal{D}^{\mathrm{SSD}}(\mathcal{T}_{PET} \circ y, \ \mathcal{R}_{PET}) \right.$$

$$\left. + \alpha_{PET}^{PC} \cdot \mathcal{D}_{PC}(\mathcal{T}_{PET} \circ y, \ A) + \alpha_{\mathcal{S}} \cdot \mathcal{S}(y) \right\} , \tag{2}$$

where $\mathcal{T}_{PET}, \mathcal{R}_{PET} : \Omega \to \mathbb{R}$ are the real PET image and the atlas PET image. $\alpha_{CT}, \alpha_{PET}, \alpha_{PET}^{PC}, \alpha_S \in \mathbb{R}^+$ are weighting factors for the individual distance functionals and are discussed later. $\mathcal{D}_{PC}$ is the passive contour distance and A denotes the delineation of the atlas organs.

Passive Contour Distance. Let us now derive the passive contour term $\mathcal{D}_{PC}$. The classical Chan-Vese functional [2] is defined as follows

$$\mathcal{CV}(C) = \int_{C^{in}} (\mathcal{T}(x) - \mu(\mathcal{T}, C^{in}))^2 \ dx + \int_{C^{ex}} (\mathcal{T}(x) - \mu(\mathcal{T}, C^{ex}))^2 \ dx . \tag{3}$$

The function μ computes an average value of $\mathcal{T}$ (we omit the subscript for simplicity) according to the interior (C^{in}) respectively the exterior (C^{ex}) of the contour C. The aim is to find the (active) contour C that minimizes the energy $\mathcal{CV}(C)$. We can rewrite this formulation as a functional of the transformation y

$$\mathcal{CV}(y) = \int_{y(\Omega)} (\mathcal{T}(x) - \mu(\mathcal{T}, \ A \circ y; \ x))^2 \ dx . \tag{4}$$

$\mu(\mathcal{T}, \ A \circ y; \ \cdot)$ is constant inside each organ containing the average intensity of $\mathcal{T}$ over the respective segment. A simple 2D example to illustrate the function μ is given in Fig. 2.

The atlas definitions A in Fig. 2(b) exactly match the contours of the blurred and noisy input image (a). By applying the segmentation function μ we result in a recovered image without noise and blur (c).

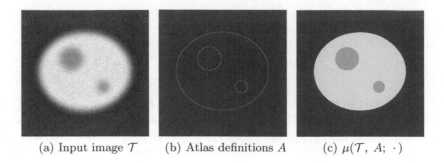

(a) Input image $\mathcal{T}$ (b) Atlas definitions A (c) $\mu(\mathcal{T}, A; \cdot)$

Fig. 2. Illustration of μ (2D). Given the image $\mathcal{T}$ (left) and the atlas definitions A (middle) we can apply the segmentation function $\mu(\mathcal{T}, A; \cdot)$ (right).

By substitution $x \rightarrow y(x)$ in (4) we receive

$$\mathcal{CV}(y) = \int_\Omega (\mathcal{T}(y(x)) - \mu(\mathcal{T} \circ y, A; x))^2 \cdot |\det(\nabla y(x))| \, dx . \qquad (5)$$

The term $\mathcal{D}_{PC}$ is then defined as:

$$\mathcal{D}_{PC}(\mathcal{T} \circ y, A) := \frac{1}{2} \int_\Omega (\mathcal{T}(y(x)) - \mu(\mathcal{T} \circ y, A; x))^2 \cdot \det(\nabla y(x)) dx . \qquad (6)$$

Thus, by finding an adequate transformation y the in-class variance of $\mathcal{T} \circ y$ according to the atlas A is minimized. Note that we can drop the absolute value bars for the Jacobian determinant, if the transformation is diffeomorphic, cf. Sec. 2.2.

Instead of adjusting the contour to the data (active contour, analogously deformable templates), the data is adjusted to the contour (passive contour) in our case. Hence we have an optimization problem in the transformation y and not in the contour. This allows us directly to treat multiple segments at once and not only to separate one foreground object from the background (note that there exist also active contour approaches for multiple segments [12]). A further advantage of passive contours compared to active contours is the implicitly incorporated information about shape and location of the organs. In contrast to active contours, contours can not split in multiple objects. Further, active contour approaches require proper initialization. In our case the initialization of the passive contours is directly given by the atlas definitions. Furthermore, the fixed integration domain for segmentation simplifies computations compared to exiting atlas-based segmentation methods.

2.2   Regularization

The non-rigid nature of whole-body segmentation poses challenges to the estimation of the transformation y. To guarantee diffeomorphic transformations and to be highly robust against noise, we utilize hyperelastic regularization [5]. The regularization functional $\mathcal{S}$ controls changes in length and volume of the transformation y. The weighting factor $\alpha_{\mathcal{S}}$ in (2) is thus a compact notation for the weighting of two regularization terms.

Local adaptive regularization prevents unphysiological contraction or expansion of organs. The organ definitions are given by our atlas organ delineations A. The areas inside organs get a higher volume regularization value ($2 \cdot 10^5$) compared to normal body tissue ($1 \cdot 10^5$) which keeps volumetric changes inside organs to a minimum.

2.3 Evaluation

The resulting segmentations are compared to manually drawn VOIs. The Dice coefficient is used to quantitatively compare our segmentation to the ground-truth. For two sets X and Y the Dice coefficient is defined as $D(X, Y) = \frac{2|X \cap Y|}{|X|+|Y|}$.

To assess whether the registration algorithm performs successful or not we analyze the Jacobian determinant. It specifies the volumetric change due to the transformation. A value of 1 represents no volumetric change and a value smaller (greater) than 1 indicates compression (expansion). For positive values the transformations are diffeomorphic. Fig. 4 shows a distribution of the Jacobian for all results.

2.4 Implementation

The implementation is based on the FAIR registration toolbox [10] in MATLAB®. In a first step the images are brought to the same resolution (voxel size of 0.35 mm). We use a multi-level strategy with a scaling of 0.5 between two adjacent levels, starting with a resolution of $16 \times 10 \times 40$ (voxel size of 2.77 mm) and going to a final resolution of $64 \times 40 \times 160$ (voxel size of 0.69 mm). Optimization is performed with a Gauss-Newton scheme in combination with a PCG solver for the linear system of equations, cf. [10]. Spline interpolation is used along with a regularization of the moments. The parameter controlling the amount of regularization is chosen to be 1 for the affine pre-registration and 0.5 for the joint registration. The regularization for the affine pre-registration is higher to reduce the amount of details in the images for the rough alignment.

3 Experimental Results

3.1 Data

This work is based on ^{18}F-FDG-PET/CT data of 13 healthy adult C57/Bl6 mice (without any intervention), representing the most widely used radiotracer and mouse strain in preclinical PET studies.

PET experiments were carried out using a high resolution (0.7 mm full width at half maximum) small animal scanner (32 module quadHIDAC, Oxford Positron Systems Ltd., Oxford, UK) with uniform spatial resolution over a large cylindrical field-of-view (165 mm diameter, 280 mm axial length). Mice were anesthetized with oxygen/isoflurane inhalation (2% isoflurane, 0.4 l/min oxygen) and body temperature was maintained at physiological values by a heating pad. One hour after intravenous injection of 10 MBq ^{18}F-FDG in 100 μl 0.9% saline list-mode data were acquired for 15 min. Subsequently, the scanning bed was transferred to the CT scanner (Inveon, Siemens Medical Solutions, USA) and a CT acquisition with a spatial resolution of ∼80 μm was performed for each mouse after intravenous injection of a contrast agent. The reconstructed image data sets were aligned with a rigid transformation based on extrinsic markers attached to the scanning bed and the image analysis software (Inveon Research Workplace 3.0, Siemens Medical Solutions, USA).

3.2 Atlas

The Digimouse software phantom [4] serves as an atlas. The organ delineations of the pixel atlas are filled with realistic values according to our scanning protocol to construct a pseudo-PET and pseudo-CT phantom image. This has to be done only once in advance. The resulting images are spatially aligned phantom images with a known ground-truth segmentation. No blurring or noise is added to the images.

For the heart, the used ^{18}F-FDG tracer accumulates mainly in the left ventricle. As Digimouse provides only a combined segment for the whole heart (including left and right ventricle and the blood pool) we apply some minor modifications, see Fig. 3. The heart region of the atlas is replaced by a manual threshold segmentation of the left ventricle using the accompanied Digimouse PET data. In addition, the bladder is slightly moved in posterior direction to better fit our real data (this stabilizes the transformation estimation by minimizing the local average deformation). The original image is shown in Fig. 3(a) and the modified version in (b).

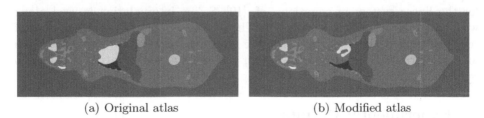

(a) Original atlas   (b) Modified atlas

Fig. 3. The heart's segmentation (green area) and the bladder (orange area) in the original version of the Digimouse phantom (a) is replaced in the modified atlas (b) to better match the real data

3.3 Results

For the non-parametric registration, the following approach is used to provide meaningful values for the various parameters in (2). An exhaustive parameter

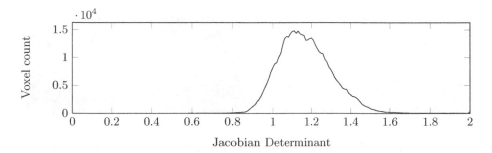

Fig. 4. Summed histograms of the Jacobian determinant of all data set

Table 1. Dice coefficients of the 13 mice for the heart (left ventricle), bladder and kidneys

Mouse	1	2	3	4	5	6	7	8	9	10	11	12	13	Avg.	Std.
Heart	0.85	0.84	0.84	0.85	0.79	0.62	0.77	0.72	0.60	0.60	0.68	0.60	0.75	0.73	0.10
Bladder	0.90	0.88	0.78	0.91	0.92	0.88	0.93	0.92	0.93	0.79	0.86	0.82	0.87	0.88	0.05
Kidneys	0.83	0.63	0.80	0.82	0.73	0.65	0.66	0.83	0.80	0.73	0.80	0.78	0.84	0.76	0.07
Avg.	0.86	0.78	0.81	0.86	0.81	0.72	0.79	0.82	0.77	0.71	0.78	0.74	0.82		
Std.	0.04	0.13	0.03	0.05	0.10	0.14	0.14	0.10	0.17	0.10	0.09	0.11	0.06		

search is performed for a randomly selected mouse. For each parameter combination the estimated segmentation is compared to the manual segmentation. The estimation giving the best fit is declared as the optimal parameter set for all experiments as they follow all the same protocol. We found the following optimal parameter set: $\alpha_{CT} = 10$, $\alpha_{PET} = 10$, $\alpha_{PET}^{PC} = 100$. For the hyperelastic regularization we found an optimal weighting for the length term of 1000 and for the volumetric regularization we refer to the regularization paragraph in Sec. 2.2.

For all transformations, the Jacobian determinant is everywhere positive and centered around 1, see Fig. 4. The global minimum is 0.26 and the global maximum is 2.66 which implicates diffeomorphisms. Note that the small shift of the maximum peak to a value greater than 1 in Fig. 4 is due to the affine component of the transformations indicating that the atlas is on average a little bit bigger than the real mice.

For all datasets an average Dice coefficient of 0.73 ± 0.10 could be achieved for the left ventricle, 0.88 ± 0.05 for the bladder, and 0.76 ± 0.07 for the kidneys. The estimated segmentation for one mouse is exemplified in Fig. 5. The Dice coefficients for all analyzed organs and mice can be found in Table 1.

The improvement due to our new passive contour distance can be assessed by setting $\alpha_{PET}^{PC} = 0$ and thus disabling the segmentation input. The objective is to analyze whether the additional passive contour distance can even improve the high accuracy of our multimodal PET-CT registration functional alone. For $\alpha_{PET}^{PC} = 0$, the Dice coefficient for the left ventricle was 0.61 ± 0.12, for the bladder 0.80 ± 0.07, and for the kidneys 0.76 ± 0.08. This means an improvement

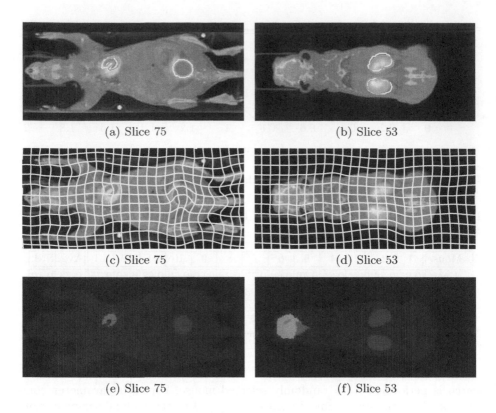

(a) Slice 75   (b) Slice 53

(c) Slice 75   (d) Slice 53

(e) Slice 75   (f) Slice 53

Fig. 5. Visualization of 3D registration results for whole-body segmentation. Overlay of 2D projections of PET, CT and contours ((a) heart and bladder, (b) kidneys) and transformation grid y_{opt} ((c), (d)). The estimated segmentations are plotted with white contours and the ground-truth segmentation is shown in green. The estimated contour of the body is plotted for additional visual assessment of the registration accuracy. Slices of the piecewise constant approximations $\mu(\mathcal{T}_{PET} \circ y_{opt}, A)$ are shown in (e) and (f).

of 16% for the left ventricle and 9% for the bladder. We found no improvement for organs with relatively low uptake like the kidneys.

4   Conclusion and Future Work

A novel fully automated approach for whole-body segmentation of PET data is presented in this work. The centerpiece of the proposed joint segmentation and registration method is the introduction of a novel segmentation distance for registration inspired by Chan and Vese [2]. As the interpretation is reversed to active contour models, we denote this as passive contours. Further, the registration is performed based on functional and morphological data simultaneously.

A validation based on the Dice coefficient and the Jacobian determinant demonstrates the high accuracy of our method. Further, the benefit of the additional Chan-Vese distance, in contrast to multimodal PET-CT registration alone, was shown.

Compared to existing atlas-based segmentation methods the novelty of our passive contours approach is given by implicitly incorporated information about shape and location of the organs. The general shape of the contour can not degrade (e.g. split in multiple objects) as we control the spatial regularity of the guaranteed diffeomorphic transformation by using hyperelastic regularization. Local adaptive volume regularization additionally prevents unnatural contraction or expansion of organs.

We overcome the limitation of low soft tissue contrast in CT by using additional PET images. Although the spatial resolution of PET is magnitudes lower compared to CT, the function information does not perturb the CT registration, but provides important complementary information in some soft tissue regions.

The primary goal is to apply our method to human data in future work. In addition, we will extend this work by analyzing a larger number of data sets with a larger number of VOIs. In this context it is also planned to analyze the applicability of the proposed method to subjects with tumors. It is planned to extend our method to dynamic PET data as activity over time carries important information for segmentation. An integration of our passive contour distance into the intensity-based registration of [1] is particularly promising. In future work we further plan to extend the data term to handle Poisson statistics and inhomogeneous areas as in [11].

Acknowledgments. The authors would like to thank Thomas Kösters for providing his reconstruction software EMRECON (http://emrecon.uni-muenster.de, [7]) used for the reconstruction of the PET datasets. This work was partly funded by the Deutsche Forschungsgemeinschaft, SFB 656 MoBil (projects B2 and B3).

References

1. Baiker, M., Staring, M., Löwik, C.W.G.M., Reiber, J.H.C., Lelieveldt, B.P.F.: Automated Registration of Whole-Body Follow-Up MicroCT Data of Mice. In: Fichtinger, G., Martel, A., Peters, T. (eds.) MICCAI 2011, Part II. LNCS, vol. 6892, pp. 516–523. Springer, Heidelberg (2011)
2. Chan, T., Vese, L.: Active contours without edges. IEEE Trans Image Process 10(2), 266–277 (2001)
3. Chan, T., Vese, L.: Active contour and segmentation models using geometric PDE's for medical imaging. In: Malladi, R. (ed.) Geometric Methods in Bio-Medical Image Processing: Mathematics and Visualization, pp. 63–75. Springer (2002)
4. Dogdas, B., Stout, D., Chatziioannou, A., Leahy, R.: Digimouse: a 3D whole body mouse atlas from CT and cryosection data. Physics Med. Biol. 52(3), 577 (2007)
5. Gigengack, F., Ruthotto, L., Burger, M., Wolters, C., Jiang, X., Schäfers, K.: Motion correction in dual gated cardiac PET using mass-preserving image registration. IEEE Trans. Med. Imag. 31(3), 698–712 (2012)

6. Hugenberg, V., Breyholz, H.J., Riemann, B., Hermann, S., Schober, O., Schäfers, M., Gangadharmath, U., Mocharla, V., Kolb, H., Walsh, J., Zhang, W., Kopka, K., Wagner, S.: A new class of highly potent matrix metalloproteinase inhibitors based on triazole-substituted hydroxamates (radio)synthesis, *in vitro* and first *in vivo* evaluation. J. Med. Chem. 55(10), 4714–4727 (2012)
7. Kösters, T., Schäfers, K., Wübbeling, F.: EMrecon: An expectation maximization based image reconstruction framework for emission tomography data. In: NSS/MIC Conference Record. IEEE (2011)
8. Erdt, M., Steger, S., Sakas, G.: Regmentation: A new view of image segmentation and registration. Journal of Radiation Oncology Informatics, 1–23 (2012)
9. Massoud, T., Gambhir, S.: Molecular imaging in living subjects: seeing fundamental biological processes in a new light. Genes Dev. 17(5), 545–580 (2003)
10. Modersitzki, J.: FAIR: Flexible Algorithms for Image Registration. SIAM, Philadelphia (2009)
11. Sawatzky, A., Tenbrinck, D., Jiang, X., Burger, M.: A variational framework for region-based segmentation incorporating physical noise models. CAM Report 11-81, UCLA (December 2011)
12. Vese, L., Chan, T.: A multiphase level set framework for image segmentation using the Mumford and Shah model. International Journal of Computer Vision 50, 271–293 (2002)
13. Wang, H., Olafsen, T., Stout, D., Chatziioannou, A.: Quantification of organ uptake from small animal PET images via registration with a statistical mouse atlas. In: MICCAI Workshop Proceedings (2011)
14. Yezzi, A., Zöllei, L., Kapur, T.: A variational framework for integrating segmentation and registration through active contours. Med. Image Anal. 7(2), 171–185 (2003)
15. Zaidi, H., Ruest, T., Schoenahl, F., Montandon, M.: Comparative assessment of statistical brain MR image segmentation algorithms and their impact on partial volume correction in PET. Neuroimage 32(4), 1591–1607 (2006)

Spatially Aware Patch-Based Segmentation (SAPS): An Alternative Patch-Based Segmentation Framework

Zehan Wang, Robin Wolz, Tong Tong, and Daniel Rueckert

Department of Computing, Imperial College London, UK
zehan.wang06@imperial.ac.uk

Abstract. Patch-based segmentation has been shown to be successful in a range of label propagation applications. Performing patch-based segmentation can be seen as a k-nearest neighbour problem as the labelling of each voxel is determined according to the distances to its most similar patches. However, the reliance on a good affine registration given the use of limited search windows is a potential weakness. This paper presents a novel alternative framework which combines the use of kNN search structures such as ball trees and a spatially weighted label fusion scheme to search patches in large regional areas to overcome the problem of limited search windows. Our proposed framework (SAPS) provides an improvement in the Dice metric of the results compared to that of existing patch-based segmentation frameworks.

Keywords: patch-based segmentation, label propagation, multi-atlas, nearest neighbour search, spatial.

1 Introduction

Accurate segmentations in medical imaging form a crucial role in many applications from patient diagnosis to clinical research. The amount of data generated from medical images can take a substantial amount of time for clinicians to manually segment, often becoming prohibitive as a regular task. Consequently, automatic methods for performing these tasks are becoming more important for image analysis. However, obtaining accurate results is highly important and still poses a challenge in many medical imaging applications.

Patch-based approaches for label propagation [1], [2] have been shown to be a robust and effective solution for applications in medical images. These methods label each voxel of a target image by comparing the image patch centred on the voxel with patches from an atlas library and choosing the most probable label according to the closest matches.

In this paper, we propose an alternative framework for patch-based segmentation which uses efficient k nearest neighbour structures, such as ball trees and a spatially weighted label fusion method which is loosely based on a non-local means approach [3] to allow segmentation of data with greater variability in alignment after affine registration. We validate this approach on 202 images from the ADNI database and compare the results with an existing method.

B.H. Menze et al. (Eds.): MCV 2012, LNCS 7766, pp. 93–103, 2013.
© Springer-Verlag Berlin Heidelberg 2013

2   Methods

2.1   Pre-processing

Atlases are all registered to a common template space using affine registration and intensities are normalised using the method proposed by Nyúl and Udupa [4]. A general mask is then created for each label of interest in the atlas by taking the union of the labels from all the training data and dilating the result. This mask is used to narrow the search space and restrict search to valid areas where a label might appear. The mask needs to be large enough to allow for possible variations in anatomical variability, but not too large as this would make the search process less efficient.

The training data is also denoised to improve robustness. We used Total Variation denoising as a quick and easy to apply method which is effective in regularizing images without smoothing boundaries and edges [5].

2.2 kNN Data Structure Construction

Performing patch-based segmentation can be seen as a k-nearest neighbour problem as the labelling of each voxel is determined according to the distances to its most similar patches. An exhaustive search would have a computational complexity that is linearly proportional to the size of the dataset and can be quite prohibitive in large datasets, especially given the number of voxels that require this process in an image. This is one reason why existing methods use a small search volume size, such as in the region of $11 \times 11 \times 11 = 1331$ voxels, and why a good alignment of images is required.

To increase the search volume size without a detrimental impact to the search speed, an efficient kNN search data structure is required. Any exact kNN data structure could be used in this framework, but in our implementation, a ball tree [6] was used. Ball trees provide much better search performance than kd trees or brute force searches for high dimensional data [7]. Ball trees are metric trees which use a given distance metric to partition the data so that only a small part of the data need to be queried. The distance metric used must obey the triangle inequality for metric trees to work correctly. Since Euclidean distances are used in both patch based comparisons and atlas selection, and this obeys the triangle inequality, ball trees can then be used to provide the results to kNN queries.

In principle all patches could be stored in a single tree, however, the memory requirements would grow prohibitively large as the number of atlases increases as well as giving decremental search performances. So instead, a ball tree is constructed offline for each label in each atlas region of every atlas in the training set. Each patch stored in the ball tree also has its spatial coordinates within the template space stored with it. This information is used in a soft-weighting scheme when performing patch selection as spatial correspondence can help distinguish between patches with homogeneous intensities which provide very little structural information. This is particularly the case in brain images where patches from different structures of the brain can be very similar when only voxel intensities are compared.

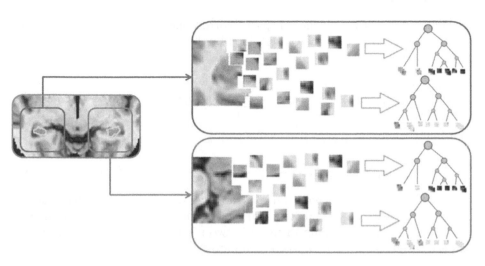

Fig. 1. Example: ball tree construction from patches. Split the brain into 2 regions centred around the left and right hippocampus and create a tree in each region for each label, including the background label.

2.3   Search Strategy

Target images undergo the same pre-processing steps as the training images prior to segmentation as some degree of spatial correspondence is required for an effective segmentation.

Atlas Selection by Region. For each of the regions of interest that requires labelling, the nearest N atlases are found for each region by comparing their Euclidean distance. Using a limited selection of the best subjects from the atlas library has been shown to provide more effective segmentation results [8]. Another kNN data structure such as the ball tree can be built offline to allow fast atlas selection in the case of a large atlas library. The corresponding kNN data structure for those atlas regions are then used for segmentation. By performing atlas selection on the regional level, more appropriate atlases can be chosen for each region rather than selecting a single set of atlases to use for the whole image. This can be improve the accuracy of segmentations in cases where images differ in their similarity from region to region. For example, for performing a hippocampus segmentations, the set of atlases selected for the left hippocampus can differ to those selected for the right hippocampus.

Patch Search and Label Fusion. The corresponding kNN data structures for the nearest N regions are then used for finding the nearest k patches for each voxel location i in target image x. The Euclidean distance between the patch, $P(x_i)$, in the target image and the nearest k patches, $\{P(y_j)\}$, from the atlas library are weighted with the Euclidean distance on their spatial location to provide an overall weighting for each label. An additional weighting, α, can be applied to control the influence of spatial correspondence. The resulting weighting for label l at voxel i is then determined by the sum of weights between patch $P(x_i)$ and the k nearest patches, $\{P(y_j)\}$ as follows:

$$w_{l_i}(x) = \sum_{j=1}^{k} w_l(x_i, y_j) \tag{1}$$

coordinate where

$$w_l(x_i, y_j) = e^{\dfrac{-\{||P(x_i) - P(y_j)||_2^2 + \alpha||x_i - y_j||_2^2\}}{h^2}} \tag{2}$$

h is a decay parameter which controls the level of influence of patches as the distance increases, an automatic estimation of this parameter is used for each voxel based on the minimum distance between patch $P(x_i)$ and the nearest k patches, weighted by their spatial coordinates:

$$h^2(x_i) = \min\{||P(x_i) - P(y_j)||_2^2 + \alpha||x_i - y_j||_2^2\} \tag{3}$$

An overall weight for each label at each voxel i is then calculated from the sum of the distances of these patches and the resulting label is decided based on majority voting of the labels according to these weights:

$$L(x_i) = \arg\max_{l} w_{l_i}(x) \tag{4}$$

3   Experiments and Results

3.1   Dataset

Images from the Alzheimers Disease Neuroimaging Initiative (ADNI) database (www.loni.ucla.edu/ADNI) were used for validation. These images consists of 202 subjects (68 normal, 93 with mild cognitive impairment, 41 with Alzheimer's disease) imaged using different scanners. Reference segmentations were obtained semi-automatically using a commercially available high dimensional brain mapping tool (Medtronic Surgical Navitgation Technologies, Louisville, CO) by propagating 60 manually labelled images. Images were pre-processed by the ADNI pipeline [9] and were linearly registered to the MNI152 template space using affine registration.

To test the proposed framework, a leave-one-out validation strategy was applied where each image was segmented in turn, using the remaining dataset as the atlas database. A patch size of $7 \times 7 \times 7$ was used whilst we experimented with the number of atlases used, N, the spatial weights, α, and the number of nearest neighbours for each patch, k. All image intensities were normalised and scaled to the same range and TV denoising [5] was applied to the training data.

3.2   Implementation

The main framework was implemented in Python using open source modules such as NumPy, SciPy and SciKit-learn. The computation time is around 10 minutes for each image using 8 cores clocked at 2.67GHz each when using 20 atlases and using the 100 nearst neighbours. Given that Python is an interpreted language, further speed ups can be achieved if the framework was implemented in C/C++.

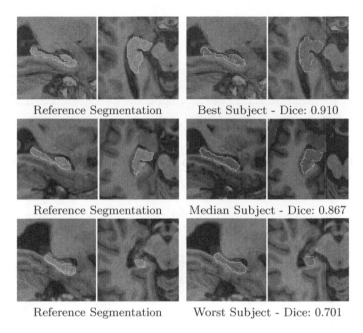

Fig. 2. Segmentations of the right hippocampus with parameters $N = 40$, $k = 79$, $\alpha = 13$

3.3   Effect of the Number of Nearest Patches and Atlases Used

With the spatial weight fixed at $\alpha = 13$, we experimented using a range of values for the number of patches, k, as well as the number of atlases, N. k is dependent on N as using more atlases would present a bigger selection of patches to choose from and we see in figure 3 that the optimal k value differs for the different N values.

Generally, we find that accuracy increases as k increases, but reaches a limit after $k > 60$. There is an increase in computational cost as k increases as more comparisons must be made in the kNN data structures, so it is most computationally optimal to select the lowest k value that provides the desired segmentation accuracy.

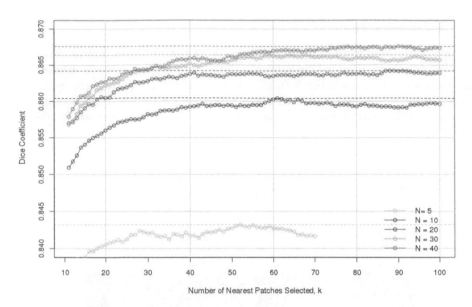

Fig. 3. Median Dice coefficients for the whole hippocampus whilst using a range of k values with different N values

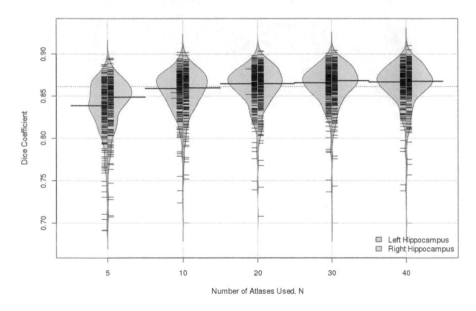

Fig. 4. Beanplot showing overall Dice coefficients distributions for a range of N values with $k = 64$. Large thick lines indicate medians, dotted line indicates median across all k values. The shape of the "bean" shows the distribution of the results and individual data points are shown as small lines on the bean.

Table 1. Dice Coefficients for the hippocampus (HC) when using different number of atlases, N, with $k = 64$. Highest values are show in bold.

N	Left HC			Right HC			Overall		
	Best	Worst	Median	Best	Worst	Median	Best	Worst	Median
5	0.887	0.691	0.839	0.895	0.707	0.849	0.886	0.719	0.842
10	**0.902**	0.724	0.860	0.902	0.700	0.859	0.898	0.719	0.860
20	0.898	**0.740**	0.864	0.904	**0.708**	0.865	0.899	**0.724**	0.864
30	0.901	0.737	0.866	0.904	0.700	**0.868**	0.899	0.719	0.866
40	0.900	0.738	**0.867**	**0.910**	0.700	0.868	**0.902**	0.719	**0.867**

An increase in the number of atlases used generally increases segmentation accuracy, but the gain accuracy after $N > 20$ is marginal. Given that the computational cost increases linearly with the number atlases used, this suggests that using more than 30 atlases would not provide a sufficient trade-off between the extra time spent and the accuracy gained. Our findings on here agree with those presented in [1] on the number of training subjects used, with proportional gains in accuracy as N increases.

3.4 Effect of the Spatial Weight, α

Experiments using several values for spatial weights, α, showed that using spatial information to provide a soft-weighting has significant impact on the

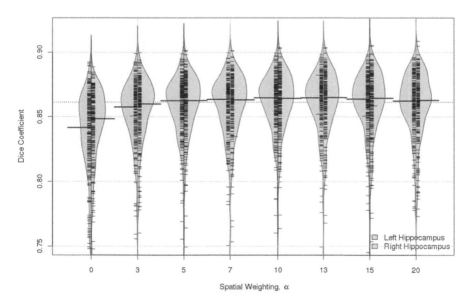

Fig. 5. Beanplot showing Dice coefficients distributions for a range of spatial weighting values, α with $N = 20$, $k = 64$. Large thick lines indicate medians, dotted line indicates median across all α values. The shape of the "bean" shows the distribution of the results and individual data points are shown as small lines on the bean.

Table 2. Dice Coefficients for the hippocampus (HC) when using different spatial weights, α, with $k = 64$ and $N = 20$. Highest values are show in bold.

α	Left HC			Right HC			Overall		
	Best	Worst	Median	Best	Worst	Median	Best	Worst	Median
0	0.892	0.669	0.842	0.889	0.674	0.848	0.884	0.702	0.844
5	0.899	0.736	0.862	0.902	0.700	0.862	0.897	0.718	0.862
10	**0.900**	**0.744**	**0.865**	0.906	0.692	0.864	0.899	0.723	0.863
13	0.898	0.740	0.864	0.904	0.708	**0.865**	0.899	**0.724**	**0.864**
15	0.898	0.736	0.864	0.905	0.704	0.864	**0.900**	0.720	0.863
20	0.860	0.729	0.862	**0.909**	**0.710**	0.863	**0.900**	**0.724**	0.862

segmentation accuracy (see figure 5 and table 2). The distribution of the results as seen in the beanplots shows that the consistency of the results increases significantly when we use spatial information. The values attempted suggests that segmentation accuracy peaks between $\alpha = 12$ and $\alpha = 13$. If the spatial weighting is too high, there is a detrimental effect on the segmentation accuracy as this soft-weighting becomes too restrictive when comparing patch intensities.

3.5   Effect of Denoising

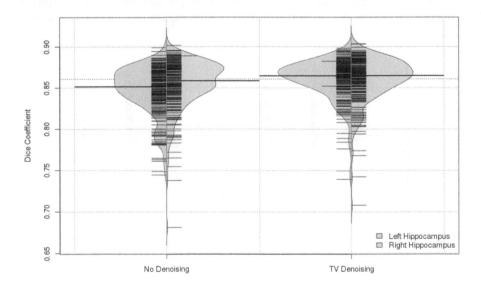

Fig. 6. Dice coefficients distributions for results using denoised and non-denoised training data with $N = 20$, $k = 64$, $\alpha = 13$. Large thick lines indicate medians, dotted line indicates median across both datasets. The shape of the "bean" shows the distribution of the results and individual data points are shown as small lines on the bean.

Comparing results from using non-denoised training data to those from using denoised training data, it can be seen that using denoised training data provides an improvement to the median segmentation accuracy (see figure 6). Further to this, the range of the results is significantly smaller with a more favourable distribution when using denoised training data, suggesting that this does indeed improve the generality and robustness of the framework.

3.6   Comparison of Results to an Existing Method

Finally, with the same dataset of ADNI images, we compared the results obtained by our proposed method to that using the method described in [1] (see figure 7 and table 3), with 10 training atlases in both cases. It can be seen that our

Table 3. Median Dice coefficients for the hippocampus (HC) comparing with the existing method in [1] with the number of atlases, $N = 10$ (*and* $N = 40$ *for reference*). Proposed method uses $k = 64$, $\alpha = 13$ as its other parameters.

Method	Left HC			Right HC			Overall		
	Best	Worst	Median	Best	Worst	Median	Best	Worst	Median
Existing[1]	0.894	0.696	0.842	**0.910**	0.644	0.848	**0.901**	0.709	0.844
Proposed, $N = 10$	**0.902**	**0.724**	**0.860**	0.902	**0.700**	**0.859**	0.898	**0.719**	**0.860**
Proposed, $N = 40$	*0.900*	*0.738*	*0.867*	*0.910*	*0.700*	*0.868*	*0.902*	*0.719*	*0.867*

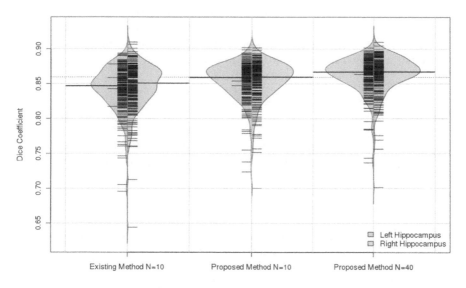

Fig. 7. Dice coefficients distributions for results comparing SAPS with an existing method [1]. Other parameters for SAPS are $k = 64$, $\alpha = 13$. Large thick lines indicate medians, dotted line indicates median across both datasets. The shape of the "bean" shows the distribution of the results and individual data points are shown as small lines on the bean.

method generally outperforms the existing method and is more robust. The two methods performs quite similarly when no spatial information is used (see table 2). This is because the label fusion would be equivalent to the non-local means method if the spatial weight, α, is 0.

Employing Welch's two sample t-test on these results gave p-values of 0.00003, 0.007 and 0.004 for the left, right and overall hippocampus respectively. Additionally, our proposed method has a 0.05 decrease in the standard deviation of the results.

4   Conclusion

We have presented a new generalized framework for applying patch based segmentation which is able to robustly segment data in conditions where images can have large variations in alignment by looking at a much larger search windows in addition to applying a spatial location weighting to each patch. We validated the proposed framework against 202 ADNI images of patients at various stages of Alzheimer's disease and achieved an overall median dice coefficient of 0.867 using patches from the 40 most similar atlases. The framework allows a trade-off between segmentation accuracy and speed. If we use patches from half as many atlases, we can complete the segmentation in half as much time and are still able to attain a median dice coefficient of 0.864. At the lowest limit tested, using 5 atlases is still able to yield a median Dice coefficient of 0.842 for the whole hippocampus whilst taking around 2-3 minutes on a machine with 8 cores.

In future work, we plan on further validating our proposed framework using a multi-scale extension against different anatomical structures and image types. We are currently working on a multi-scale extension to speed up segmentation of large structures such as bones in knee images or when performing brain extraction.

References

1. Coupé, P., Manjón, J.V., Fonov, V., Pruessner, J., Robles, M., Collins, D.L.: Patch-based segmentation using expert priors: application to hippocampus and ventricle segmentation. NeuroImage 54(2), 940–954 (2011)
2. Rousseau, F., Habas, P., Studholme, C.: A supervised patch-based approach for human brain labeling. IEEE Transactions on Medical Imaging 30(10), 1852–1862 (2011)
3. Coupe, P., Yger, P., Prima, S., Hellier, P., Kervrann, C., Barillot, C.: An optimized blockwise nonlocal means denoising filter for 3-D magnetic resonance images. IEEE Transactions on Medical Imaging 27(4), 425–41 (2008)
4. Nyúl, L.G., Udupa, J.K.: On standardizing the MR image intensity scale. Magnetic Resonance in Medicine 42(6), 1072–1081 (1999)
5. Chambolle, A.: An Algorithm for Total Variation Minimization and Applications. Journal of Mathematical Imaging and Vision 20(1), 89–97 (2004)
6. Omohundro, S.M.: Five Balltree Construction Algorithms. Technical Report 1, International Computer Science Institute (1989)

7. Kumar, N., Zhang, L., Nayar, S.K.: What Is a Good Nearest Neighbors Algorithm for Finding Similar Patches in Images? In: Forsyth, D., Torr, P., Zisserman, A. (eds.) ECCV 2008, Part II. LNCS, vol. 5303, pp. 364–378. Springer, Heidelberg (2008)

8. Aljabar, P., Heckemann, R.A., Hammers, A., Hajnal, J.V., Rueckert, D.: Multi-atlas based segmentation of brain images: atlas selection and its effect on accuracy. NeuroImage 46(3), 726–738 (2009)

9. Jack, C.R., Bernstein, M.A., Fox, N.C., Thompson, P., Alexander, G., Harvey, D., Borowski, B., Britson, P.J., Whitwell, J., Ward, C., Dale, A.M., Felmlee, J.P., Gunter, J.L., Hill, D.L.G., Killiany, R., Schuff, N., Fox-Bosetti, S., Lin, C., Studholme, C., DeCarli, C.S., Krueger, G., Ward, H.A., Metzger, G.J., Scott, K.T., Mallozzi, R., Blezek, D., Levy, J., Debbins, J.P., Fleisher, A.S., Albert, M., Green, R., Bartzokis, G., Glover, G., Mugler, J., Weiner, M.W.: The Alzheimer's disease neuroimaging initiative (ADNI): MRI methods. Journal of Magnetic Resonance Imaging 27(4), 685–691 (2008)

Efficient Geometrical Potential Force Computation for Deformable Model Segmentation

Igor Sazonov[1], Xianghua Xie[2], and Perumal Nithiarasu[1]

[1] College of Engineering, Swansea University, Singleton Park, Swansea, UK SA2 8PP
[2] Department of Computer Science, Swansea University, Singleton Park, Swansea,
UK SA2 8PP
{i.sazonov,x.xie,p.nithiarasu}@swansea.ac.uk

Abstract. Segmentation in high dimensional space, e.g. 4D, often requires decomposition of the space and sequential data process, for instance space followed by time. In [1], the authors presented a deformable model that can be generalized into arbitrary dimensions. However, its direct implementation is computationally prohibitive. The more efficient method proposed by the same authors has significant overhead on computer memory, which is not desirable for high dimensional data processing. In this work, we propose a novel approach to formulate the computation to achieve memory efficiency, as well as improving computational efficiency. Numerical studies on synthetic data and preliminary results on real world data suggest that the proposed method has a great potential in biomedical applications where data is often inherently high dimensional.

1 Introduction

Among many others, deformable modeling is a popular approach to image segmentation, e.g. [2–4]. Conventional techniques suffer from weak edge, image noise and convergence issues. For instance, in [2] a constant pressure force is necessary in order to improve its capture range, resulting in monotonic expanding or shrinking of the mode that is problematic. There have been numerous work reported in the literature to improve the performance of both image gradient based methods, such as [5–7], and region based approaches, e.g. [8]. In [1], Yeo *et al.* proposed a 3D deformable model that is based on a hypothesised geometrical interactions between image gradient vectors and embedding level set surface normal vectors. It is shown that the geometrical potential force (GPF) is robust towards noise interference, weak edges, and exhibits invariant convergence capabilities such that the model can be initialized across object boundary and converge to deep concavities and propagate through narrow passages to recover complex geometries, that are conventionally difficult for image gradient based deformable modeling techniques. The authors also showed its theoretical relationship to the 2D Magnetostatic Active Contour (MAC) model [7] , which

B.H. Menze et al. (Eds.): MCV 2012, LNCS 7766, pp. 104–113, 2013.
© Springer-Verlag Berlin Heidelberg 2013

is inspired by a physical analogy. The MAC model can be considered a special case of GPF in 2D, whereas GPF can be more conveniently extended to higher dimensional applications.

The computation of the GPF comprises two stages. At the first stage, the so-called geometrical potential (GP) $G(x, y, z)$ is computed through the convolution of the image gradient and the kernel $\mathbf{K}$:

$$G(\mathbf{x}) = \sum_{\mathbf{x}' \in \Omega} \nabla I(\mathbf{x}') \cdot \mathbf{K}(\mathbf{x} - \mathbf{x}'), \qquad \mathbf{K}(\mathbf{x}) = \begin{cases} \mathbf{x}/\left\|\mathbf{x}\right\|^{n+1}, & \mathbf{x} \neq \mathbf{0} \\ 0, & \mathbf{x} = \mathbf{0} \end{cases} \qquad (1)$$

where $\mathbf{x} = [x, y, z]^T$ is the vector of coordinates of the image grid-points (voxel centres), $I(\mathbf{x})$ is the greyscale image, ∇I is its gradient, Ω is the image domain, dot denotes the scalar product of two vector functions (∇I and kernel $\mathbf{K}(\mathbf{x})$), and n is the image dimension ($n = 3$ for 3D images).

At the second stage, the derived geometrical potential is then integrated into the deformable surface evolution under the level set framework. The active surface, $S(t)$, is embedded in the level set function, $\Phi(t, \mathbf{x})$: $S(t) = \{\mathbf{x}, \Phi(t, \mathbf{x}) = 0\}$, and its deformation is achieved by solving the following PDE proposed and developed in [9–11] and related to the energy minimization approach:

$$\partial \Phi / \partial t = \alpha \, g \kappa \|\nabla \Phi\| - (1 - \alpha) \, \mathbf{F} \nabla \Phi \qquad (2)$$

where α is a weighting parameter, $g(\mathbf{x}) = 1/(1 + \|\nabla I\|^2)$ is the stopping function, $\kappa(t, \mathbf{x}) = \nabla \hat{\mathbf{n}}$ denotes the curvature of isosurfaces of Φ, $\hat{\mathbf{n}}(t, \mathbf{x})$ is the unit vector normal to isosurfaces of Φ, and $\mathbf{F}(t, \mathbf{x}) = G \, \hat{\mathbf{n}}$ is the GPF that acts as the external force.

Direct calculation of the geometrical potential G is computationally expensive, particularly in 3D. However, Eq. (1) can be computed as a convolution of two functions. Hence a natural approach is to apply the fast Fourier transform (FFT) to compute the convolution, which is described in [1].

However, a significant drawback of using the FFT based computation as proposed in [1] is that it requires lots of computer memory for a large number of intermediate arrays of the same size as the initial image I. That is, it needs to compute and store 3 components of the image gradient $\nabla I = [I_x, I_y, I_z]^T$ and twice more for the real and imaginary part of their Fourier image, also 3 components of the kernel $\mathbf{K}$ and twice more for the Fourier image. Thus, it requires about 20 times more than the direct method, which can be problematic when dealing with volumetric data or extending this method to 4D, i.e. dynamic volumetric data. Dedicated memory management may become necessary and even crucial. Memory economic and computationally efficient method to evaluate the GP is thus desirable.

In this paper, we propose to compute spectrum of the kernel by an analytical formula so that there is no need to store components of the vector kernel and the real or imaginary part of its spectrum. We also change the vector form of the integrand into a scalar form to achieve further efficiency. The proposed methods are valuated on both numerical examples and real world 3D data.

2   Analytical Formula for Kernel's Spectrum

One of the possible approaches to reduce memory usage is to use an analytical formula for the kernel spatial spectrum rather than kernel's formula (1) in the x-space. To derive an analytical formula for the kernel Fourier image, it is useful to consider the computation of G in the continuous infinite 3D Euclidian space. In this case the kernel should be described by a generalized function (distribution) (see, e.g. [12]):

$$G(\mathbf{x}) = \int_{\mathbf{x}' \in \mathbb{R}^3} \nabla I(\mathbf{x}') \cdot \mathbf{K}(\mathbf{x} - \mathbf{x}') \, d^3\mathbf{x}, \qquad \mathbf{K}(\mathbf{x}) = P.V. \frac{\mathbf{x}}{\|\mathbf{x}\|^{n+1}} \tag{3}$$

where $P.V.$ denotes *principal value*, i.e. integral in (3) diverging when $\mathbf{x}' \to \mathbf{x}$, should be treated as the limit

$$G(\mathbf{x}) = \lim_{\varepsilon \to 0^+} \int_{\|\mathbf{x}' - \mathbf{x}\| > \varepsilon} \nabla I(\mathbf{x}') \cdot \frac{\mathbf{x} - \mathbf{x}'}{\|\mathbf{x} - \mathbf{x}'\|^{n+1}} \, d^3\mathbf{x}' \tag{4}$$

Performing the Fourier transform

$$\tilde{\mathbf{K}}(\mathbf{k}) = \mathcal{F}[\mathbf{K}](\mathbf{k}) = \int \mathbf{K}(\mathbf{x}) e^{i\mathbf{k}\mathbf{x}} \, d^3\mathbf{x}, \qquad i = \sqrt{-1} \tag{5}$$

we can show that that the spectrum depends only on direction of wavevector $\mathbf{k}$ and is independent of its magnitude

$$\tilde{\mathbf{K}}(\mathbf{k}) = -i\pi^2 \frac{\mathbf{k}}{\|\mathbf{k}\|}. \tag{6}$$

Comparing spectrum $\tilde{\mathbf{K}}(\mathbf{k})$ computed analytically via Eq. (6) and that computed by performing FFT for the kernel calculated in the x-space by (1) (see Figure 1(left)), we see that near the origin they have close values. However, the spectrum computed via the FFT decays when any component of the wavevector grows. Moreover, it vanishes when any component of the wavevector reaches its maximum value which is determined by the grid size in the correspondent direction: $k_{i,\max} = \pi/h_i$ where h_1, h_2, h_3 are voxel sizes in x,y,z direction, respectively. Therefore, to obtain the G-function close to that computed by FFT based method, spectrum (6) should be multiplied by a function $f(\mathbf{k})$ which equals 1 in the origin and smoothly decays when $k_i \to k_{i,\max}$. As numerical computation shown later, a good approximation of a 3D spectrum can be formulated as

$$\tilde{\mathbf{K}}(\mathbf{k}) = i\pi^2 \frac{\mathbf{k}}{\|\mathbf{k}\|} f(\mathbf{k}), \qquad f(\mathbf{k}) = (1 - \|\mathbf{k}'\| + V(\mathbf{k})) \tag{7}$$

where

$$V = \frac{(\xi \|\mathbf{k}'\| - 1)^2}{(\xi + \xi \|\mathbf{k}'\| - 2)\,\xi}, \qquad \mathbf{k}' = \left[\frac{k_1}{k_{1,\max}}, \frac{k_2}{k_{2,\max}}, \frac{k_3}{k_{3,\max}} \right]^T, \qquad \xi = \max_{i=1,2,3} |k_i'|.$$

This makes the computation much more memory economic; however, we still have to compute the FFT for components of ∇I and then multiply every element of the arrays of the kernel spectrum computed directly for every element.

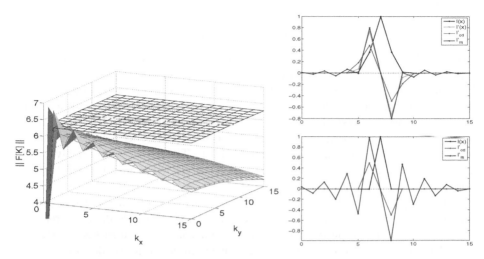

Fig. 1. Left: Absolute value of spectrum $\|\operatorname{Im}\tilde{\mathbf{K}}\|$ in the 128×128 2D domain (only first 16 positive wave components are shown) computed via Eq. (6) (black), computed by FFT from kernel evaluated in the x-space (blue) and approximated by Eq. (7) (red). Right: Function $I(x)$ (black), its exact derivative (green, on the top only), its derivative computed by central-difference (red), the same—through FFT (blue). Top: $I(x) = \exp\{-(x-7)^2\}$, bottom: $I(x) = \delta(x-7)$.

3   Use of a Scalar Kernel

Alternatively, we may rearrange the intergrand shown in Eqn. (3) as a product of scalar function and a scalar kernel, instead of a dot product between vectors. To derive the correspondent formula in x-space, we again temporally consider continuous infinite space in which initial integral takes the form given in (3). We then reforumate (3) as

$$G(\mathbf{x}) = \int_{\mathbf{x}' \in \mathbb{R}^3} I(\mathbf{x}') \cdot \nabla K(\mathbf{x} - \mathbf{x}')\, \mathrm{d}^3\mathbf{x} \qquad (8)$$

Thus, we only have to deal with the scalar kernel which is the divergence of the vector kernel $\mathbf{K}$. In the discretized finite domain Eqn. (8) can be approximated as

$$G(\mathbf{x}) = \sum_{\mathbf{x}' \in \Omega} I(\mathbf{x}') \cdot K(\mathbf{x} - \mathbf{x}'), \qquad K(\mathbf{x}) = \nabla K(\mathbf{x}) \qquad (9)$$

where the best way to calculate $\nabla \mathbf{K}$ is to compute vector kernel $\mathbf{K}$ and compute the spatial derivatives by central differences.

4   Combined Approach

However, we may combine the above two methods together to achieve even more efficient computation. In the k-space, the calculation of the geometrical potential spectrum, $\tilde{G}(\mathbf{k})$, is read as

$$\tilde{G} = (\mathrm{i}\mathbf{k}\tilde{I}) \cdot \tilde{\mathbf{K}} = \tilde{I}\,(\mathrm{i}\mathbf{k} \cdot \tilde{\mathbf{K}}) = \tilde{I}\tilde{K} \qquad (10)$$

where $\tilde{K}(\mathbf{k})$ is spectrum of the scalar kernel ($K = \nabla\mathbf{K}$), factor $\mathrm{i}\mathbf{k}$ in the k-space corresponds to the nabla (∇) operator in the infinite continuous x-space. Because we are dealing with discretized images with noise, the computation of the gradient through multiplication by $\mathrm{i}\mathbf{k}$ in the k-space can result in undesired sensitivity to noise. Derivative of a function on a finite uniform grid can be approximated by forward, backward or central differences, but also can be computed through the direct and inverse FFT. The latter method gives very high accuracy for smooth functions (periodic or decaying fast toward the grid borders).

For example, for a 1D function $I(x) = \exp\{-(x-7)^2\}$ set on $x = \{0, 1, \ldots, 15\}$ the error of derivative computed by the central differences is 0.24 whereas the error of derivative computed trough FFT is only 0.08 as seen in Figure 1(right-top). But if the function is not smooth (for example, contains delta-correlated noise) the situation is quite opposite. Consider, as an example, a discrete implementation of Dirac's delta $\delta(x - 7)$. Then the derivative computed by the central differences gives a reasonable approximation of $\delta'(x - 7)$ with a three point support, whereas the FFT method gives an oscillating result, as depicted in Figure 1(bottom right).

Thus, for image segmentation when noise is common in presence it is more appropriate to use central differences approximation than the FFT method. Fortunately though, the Fourier transform can be used to compute the central differences as well. Recall that in a continuous infinite space the derivative can be expressed as a convolution with $\delta'(x)$

$$\partial I / \partial x = I * (\delta'(x)) = \int_{-\infty}^{+\infty} I(x')\,\delta'(x - x')\,\mathrm{d}x', \qquad (11)$$

Computing this derivative by use of the Fourier transform, we should recall its spectrum $\mathcal{F}[\delta'(x)] = \mathrm{i}k$. The central differences can be computed analogously as a convolution with the function $\frac{1}{2h}\big(\delta(x+h) - \delta(x-h)\big)$ having spectrum

$$\mathcal{F}\big[\tfrac{1}{2h}\big(\delta(x+h) - \delta(x-h)\big)\big] = \frac{\mathrm{i}}{h}\sin(kh). \qquad (12)$$

which tends to $\mathrm{i}k$ when $h \to 0$.

In 3D case, spectrum of the gradient operator, $\mathrm{i}\mathbf{k}$, should be substituted by vector

$$\mathbf{g}(\mathbf{k}, \mathbf{h}) = \left[\frac{\mathrm{i}\sin k_1 h_1}{h_1}, \frac{\mathrm{i}\sin k_2 h_2}{h_2}, \frac{\mathrm{i}\sin k_3 h_3}{h_3}\right]^T \qquad (13)$$

Then Eqn. (10) should be transformed to

$$\tilde{G} = \tilde{I} \times \big(\mathbf{g}(\mathbf{k}, \mathbf{h}) \cdot \tilde{\mathbf{K}}\big). \qquad (14)$$

Thus, for this combined approach we perform FFT on the image $I(\mathbf{x})$; then for every element of the obtained arrays we calculate the scalar kernel spectrum by employing Eqn. (7) for the vector kernel and Eqn. (13) for the modified nabla operator in the k-space; finally we carry out the inverse Fourier transform. It requires memory space 4 times less than that for the initial image $I(\mathbf{x})$: I, Re $\tilde{I}$, Im $\tilde{I}$, G.

5   3D Numerical Examples

To compare different methods for computation of the geometrical potential, an artificial 3D star-like gray-scale image is created shown in Figure 2(right). Its dimension is $64 \times 64 \times 32$ pixel: this relatively small size image is chosen for the sake of convenience in visualizing the results. To understand the noise interference, the 3D data is then added with 5% Gaussian noise.

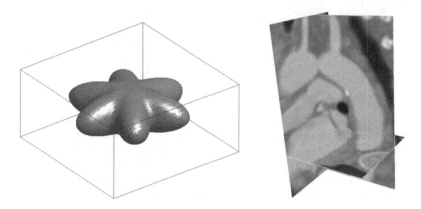

Fig. 2. Left: Isosurface of the 3D image (without added Gaussian noise). Right: an example of 3D scan of a human aorta.

Figure 3(left) shows the mid-slice along the z-axis. Note, the zero-crossings in the geometrical potential are in effect indicating the locations where the deformable model will converge, since on either side of the zero crossing the deformable model will converge towards zero-crossings. Hence, in the numerical studies, we examine the accuracy of the zero-crossings of different methods compared to the object boundary (groundtruth). The colored contours in Figure 3(left) indicate the results from different methods. Also the black curve shows the isoline for $I(x, y, z_m) = I_m$, i.e. result of segmentation performed by thresholding [13]: the middle value $I_m = \frac{1}{2}(I_{\max} + I_{\min})$ is used as the threshold.

All the lines are very close to each other, which suggests that the proposed methods are close approximation to the direct method. Plots of geometrical potential $G(x, y_m, z_m)$ along the x-coordinates is shown in Figure 3(right), where $y_m = \frac{1}{2}(y_{\min} + y_{\max})$. The curve $I_m - I(x, y_m)$ is plotted in black. It shows that the difference zero crossing is small. The rectangular region indicated by the dotted

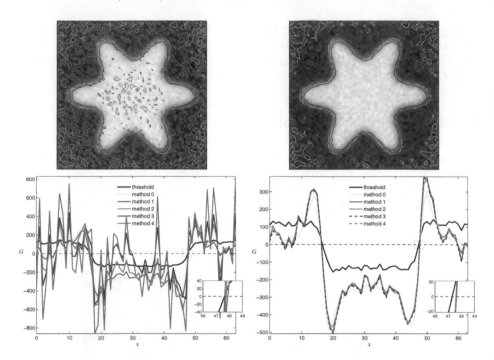

Fig. 3. Top: A slice of the 3D image; the colored curved indicate isolines of $G = 0$. Bottom: The G variation along the x direction through the center of the 3D image computed by the different methods explained in the legend. Method 0 is direct computation of the geometric potential; method 1 is the FFT based implementation of method 0; method 2 is using analytical formula for kernel's spectrum; method 3 using the scalar kernel alone; and method 4 is combining methods 2 and 3. Left: methods 2–4 without corrections, right: methods 2–4 with corrections (7) and (14).

line is zoomed and depicted at the right border of the plot. The difference is in sub-pixel level.

The direct computation is less susceptible to noise, but it is too slow to be practical. The proposed methods produce very similar result to that using FFT computation as proposed in [7, 1]. However, the proposed methods, particularly the combined approach, are far more memory efficient.

The CPU time of all the methods can be found in Table 1. Note, the combined approach (method 4) uses 4 times less memory than the FFT based computation used in [1]. The experiment was carried out on Linux, Intel(R) Xeon 3.00GHz, RAM 4G. A typical 3D scan of 512^3 voxels can only be pratically processed by method 4 and it requires 8 min of the CPU time and 3G of memory.

To demonstrate the effectiveness of the proposed combined approach, we show an example of segmenting a human aorta from a 3D CT dataset. The testing data and the results are shown in Figures 2(left) and 4. The initial surface is a sphere placed inside the lower part of the aorta and the model is able to propagate efficiently and converge accurately.

Table 1. CPU time and memory comparison for a 256^3 image. Method 0 is direct computation of the geometric potential; method 1 is the FFT based implementation of method 0; method 2 is using analytical formula for kernel's spectrum; method 3 using the scalar kernel alone; and method 4 is combining methods 2 and 3.

	method 0	method 1	method 2	method 3	method 4
CPU time	~ 7days	91s	55s	42s	30s
Memory required	0.6G	1.8G	1.0G	0.6G	0.4G

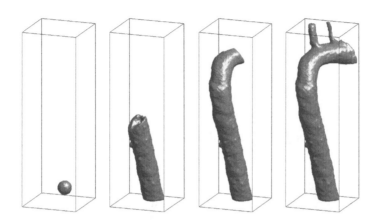

Fig. 4. An example of segmenting human aorta in 3D CT shown in Fig. 2(right) using the combined approach. From left: initial surface, intermediate stages, and final converged result.

6 4D Numerical Examples

Note that all the equations derived for the proposed methods can be readily generalised to 4D medical scans (dynamic volumetric data). We should treat the coordinate vector as $\mathbf{x} = \{x, y, z, t\}$, use the 4D wavenumber vector $\mathbf{k}$ with k_4-component treated as the frequency, and substitute $n = 4$ into the correspondent formulae for the kernel in Eqns. (1) and (3).

Here, we present a numerical study that is similar to that in the 3D case, but using a dynamic 3D shape. We vary the ray length shape parameters of the 3D star-like harmonic object periodically in time with the maximum near the middle of the cycle. The ray length parameter evolution is given as $[\frac{1}{2}(1 + \cos(2\pi(t - t_m - \frac{1}{3})/N_t))]^{1.5}$ where $N_t = 16, t_m = N_t/2$. The image dimension is $64 \times 64 \times 32 \times 16$. Thus the image contains 16 3D images, some of which are shown in Figure 5. Similarly, Gaussian noise is also added to the dynamic shape.

Figure 6(left) shows a slice of the image at instant $t = t_m = 7$ (the maximal length of the star-rays) and $z = z_m$. Here one can find colored contours $G(x, y, z_m, t_m) = 0$ with the geometrical potential computed by the different methods implemented in 4D. Spatial zero-crossings of geometrical potential:

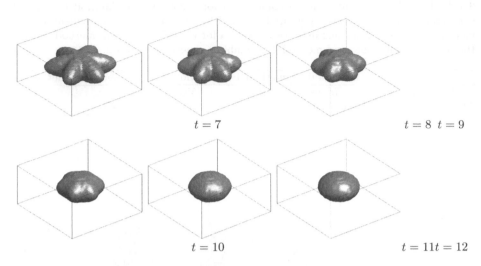

Fig. 5. Object shape at instances of 7 to12

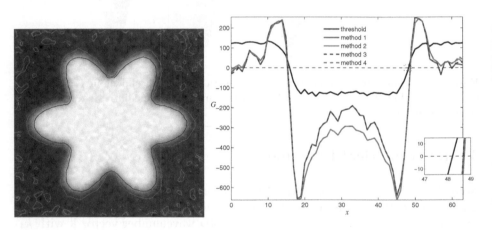

Fig. 6. Left: A slice of the 4D image; the colored curved indicate isolines of $G = 0$. Right: The G variation along the x direction through the center of the 3D image computed by the different methods explained in the legend. Method 1 is the FFT based implementation of direct computation; method 2 is using analytical formula for kernel's spectrum; method 3 using the scalar kernel alone; and method 4 is combining methods 2 and 3.

$G(x, y_m, z_m, t_m)$ where y_m, z_m, t_m are plotted in Figure 6(right). Note, the direct method is not shown as it takes prohibitive amount of time to compute the geometrical potential. There is no discernible difference among methods with improved computational efficiency. However, the proposed combined approach requires significantly less memory. This is particularly advantageous in dealing with 4D dataset.

7   Conclusion

We proposed several computationally efficient and memory economic methods to evaluate the geometrical potential in the GPF model [1]. The approach which combines analytical kernel spectrum and scalar kernel conversion provides most satisfactory results. The methods were evaluated on 3D and 4D synthetic datasets, as well as 3D real world data. This preliminary work provided promising results which suggest that the proposed method has a great potential in efficient deformable modelling in high dimensional space without decomposing the space into a sequential order.

References

1. Yeo, S.Y., Xie, X., Sazonov, I., Nithiarasu, P.: Geometrically induced force interaction for three-dimensional deformable models. IEEE T-IP 20(5), 1373–1387 (2011)
2. Malladi, R., Sethian, J.A., Vemuri, B.C.: Shape modelling with front propagation: A level set approach. IEEE T-PAMI 17(2), 158–175 (1995)
3. Whitaker, R.: Modeling deformable surfaces with level sets. IEEE Computer Graphics and App. 24(5), 6–9 (2004)
4. Xie, X.: Active contouring based on gradient vector interaction and constrained level set diffusion. IEEE T-IP 19(1), 154–164 (2010)
5. Xu, C., Prince, J.L.: Snakes, shapes, and gradient vector flow. IEEE T-IP 7(3), 359–369 (1998)
6. Xiang, Y., Chung, A., Ye, J.: A new active contour method based on elastic interaction. In: IEEE CVPR, pp. 452–457 (2005)
7. Xie, X., Mirmehdi, M.: MAC: Magnetostatic active contour model. IEEE T-PAMI 30(4), 632–647 (2008)
8. Chan, T., Vese, L.: Active contours without edges. IEEE T-IP 10(2), 266–277 (2001)
9. Caselles, V., Kimmel, R., Sapiro, G.: Geodesic active contour. IJCV 22(1), 61–79 (1997)
10. Paragios, N., Deriche, R.: Geodesic active regions and level set methods for supervised texture segmentation. IJCV 46(3), 223–247 (2002)
11. Parigios, N., Mellina-Gottardo, O., Ramesh, V.: Gradient vector flow geometric active contours. IEEE T-PAMI 26(3), 402–407 (2004)
12. Vladimirov, V.S.: Methods of the Theory of Generalized Functions. Taylor & Francis (2002)
13. Smith, C.M., Smith, J., Williams, S.K., Rodriguez, J.J., Hoying, J.B.: Automatic thresholding of three-dimensional microvascular structures from confocal microscopy images. J. Microscopy 225(3), 244–257 (2007)

Shape Prior Model for Media-Adventitia Border Segmentation in IVUS Using Graph Cut

Ehab Essa[1], Xianghua Xie[1], Igor Sazonov[2], Perumal Nithiarasu[2], and Dave Smith[3]

[1] Department of Computer Science, Swansea University, Singleton Park, Swansea, UK SA2 8PP
[2] College of Engineering, Swansea University, Singleton Park, Swansea, UK SA2 8PP
[3] ABM University NHS Trust, Swansea, UK
{csehab,x.xie,i.sazonov,p.nithiarasu}@swansea.ac.uk

Abstract. We present a shape prior based graph cut method which does not require user initialisation. The shape prior is generalised from multiple training shapes, rather than using singular templates as priors. Weighted directed graph construction is used to impose geometrical and smooth constraints learned from priors. The proposed cost function is built upon combining selective feature extractors. A SVM classifier is used to determine an optimal combination of features in presence of calcification, fibrotic tissues, soft plaques, and metallic stent, each of which has its own characteristics in ultrasound images. Comparative analysis on manually labelled ground-truth shows superior performance of the proposed method compared to conventional graph cut methods.

Keywords: IVUS, graph cut, image segmentation, shape prior.

1 Introduction

Intra-vascular Ultrasound (IVUS) imaging is a catheter-based technology, which shows 2D cross-sectional images of the coronary artery. A typical IVUS image consists of lumen, vessel that includes intima and media layers, and adventitia that surrounds the vessel wall. The media-adventitia border represents the outer coronary arterial wall located between the media and adventitia. The media layer exhibits as a thin dark layer in ultrasound and has no distinctive feature. It is surrounded by fibrous connective tissues called adventitia. The appearance of the media-adventitia border in IVUS is affected by various forms of artifact, such as acoustic shadow which can be caused by catheter guide wire, dense fibrous tissue or calcification. Fig. 1 gives an example of IVUS image.

Segmentation in IVUS images has shown to be an intricate process and often requires user initialisation to achieve meaningful results. Among many others, graph based segmentation has shown to be a promising approach to IVUS segmentation. In [1], dynamic programming is used to search a minimum path in a cost function, which incorporates edge information with a simplistic prior based on echo pattern and border thickness. Manual initialisation is necessary. In [2],

B.H. Menze et al. (Eds.): MCV 2012, LNCS 7766, pp. 114–123, 2013.

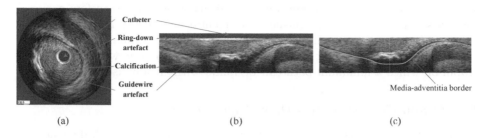

Fig. 1. Pre-Processing steps. (a) Original IVUS image. (b) Polar transformed image. (c) After removing the catheter region.

the authors applied spatio-temporal filters to enhance the lumen region based on the assumption that the blood speckles have higher spatial and temporal variations than arterial wall. However, image features introduced by acoustic shadow or metallic stent would seriously undermine this assumption when searching for media-adventitia border. The s-t cut method [3] is employed in [4] to segment 3D IVUS data. Intensity distribution in the radial directions from catheter origin and regional features based on piecewise constant assumption are used to design the cost function. However, intensity based features are susceptible to artifacts.

Learning *a priori* using a set of representative shapes is an effective approach to impose a general constraint in searching global minimum using graph cut. Freedman and Zhang [5] defined the shape template as a distance function and embedded the average distance between every pair of pixels into the neighbourhood edges in the graph. However, this method effectively requires the user to place landmarks to define the initial shape. In [6], the authors proposed an iterative graph cut method. Kernel PCA was used to build the shape model. The method ignores the affine transformation, and needs a rectangle window initialisation of the location of the objects. Iterative graph cut framework was also adopted in [7]. The method penalises the terminal edges of the graph according to the similarity between the previous segmentation and the shape template.

In this paper, we propose an efficient graph cut algorithm to segment media-adventitia border in IVUS images without user initialisation. Its objective functional consists of boundary based cost and shape penalties that are generalised from multiple training shapes. The boundary based features are dynamically selected to optimise the cost function based on trained classifier. The generalised shape prior is incorporated in the cost function, as well as embedded in graph construction. The method is evaluated on a large set of real data with groundtruth.

2   Proposed Method

The images are first transformed from Cartesian coordinates to polar coordinates and the catheter regions are removed (see Fig. 1). This transformation not only facilitates our feature extraction and classification but also transfers a closed contour segmentation to a "height-field" segmentation (see Fig. 1(c)). The border to be extracted intersects once and once only with each column of pixels. This particular form of segmentation allows us to construct a node-weighted directed graph, on which a minimum path can be found without any user initialisation.

2.1   Graph Construction without Shape Prior

We first present our basic graph construction, following [8], which does not require user initialisation. Our extended version with incorporated shape prior will be discussed later in Section 2.5. Let $G = \langle V, E \rangle$ denote the graph, where each node $V(x, y)$ corresponds to a pixel in the transformed IVUS image $I(x, y)$ in polar coordinates. The graph G consists of two arc types: intra-column arcs and inter-column arcs. For intra-column, along each column every node $V(x, y)$, where $y > 0$, has a directed arc to the node $V(x, y-1)$ with $+\infty$ weight assigned to the arc to ensure that the desired interface intersects with each column exactly once. In the case of inter-column, for each node $V(x, y)$ a directed arc with $+\infty$ weight is established to link with node $V(x+1, y - \Delta_{p,q})$, where $\Delta_{p,q}$ is the maximum difference between two neighbouring columns p and q and acts as a smoothness constraint. Similarly, node $V(x+1, y)$ is connected to $V(x, y - \Delta_{p,q})$. For IVUS segmentation, the first and the last columns are connected by inter-column arcs to enforce connectivity. Finally, the nodes in the last row of the graph are connected to each other with $+\infty$ weight to maintain a closed graph. Inter-columns and intra-columns arcs are illustrated in Figure 2 (a).

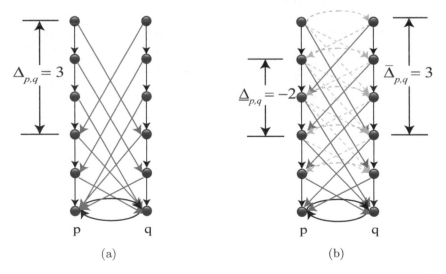

(a)   (b)

Fig. 2. Graph construction. (a) without shape prior where shape constraint is a global constant. (b) shape prior model (refer to Section 2.5 for details).

2.2   Feature Extraction and Classification

The media layer is usually thin and generally dark, and the adventitia layer tends to be brighter, see Fig. 1 as an example. Hence, edge based features are appropriate to extract the media-adventitia border. However, calcification and other interfering image features commonly exist above the media-adventitia border and cast acoustic shadows over the border, disrupting its continuity. Those imaging artifacts generally have large responses to image gradient based feature extraction. In this work, we propose to detect those artifacts and treat them differently when incorporating into the cost function.

To highlight the media-adventitia border, we use a combination of derivative of Gaussian (DoG) features and local phase features. A set of first and second order DoG filters are applied to capture the intensity difference between media and adventitia.

Local phase [9] has shown to be effective in suppressing speckles in ultrasound images. We use the dark symmetry feature [9] to highlight bar-like image patterns, which are useful to detect the thin media layer. This feature extraction operates at a coarser scale and complements to the edge features extracted using DoG filters.

For those parts of media-adventitia border that are beneath various forms of image artifacts, such as calcification, their image features are suppressed by those artifacts. Hence, it is desirable to detect those artifacts and treat those columns of pixels differently to others. However, instead of a usual attempt of localising those image artifacts based on intensity profile, e.g. [10,11], which is problematic, we classify entire columns of pixels that contain those image artifacts. The detection result will then have an influence on the formulation of the cost function. To this end, we train a SVM classifier to classify individual columns of pixels in the polar coordinates into one of the following five categories: calcification, fibrous plaque, stent, guide-wire artifact, and normal tissue or soft plaque. Each of those has their characteristics; however, the difference between some categories may be small, e.g. calcification and fibrous plaque. To achieve efficient classification, the matching pursuit algorithm is used to reduce the number of support vectors.

2.3   Boundary Based Cost Function

The boundary based energy term can be expressed as $E_B = \sum_{V \in S} \hat{c}_B(x, y)$, where $\hat{c}_B$ denotes the normalised cost function ($\hat{c}_B(x, y) \in [0, 1]$) and S is a path in the directed graph. The formulation of the pre-normalisation cost function, c_B, is determined by the SVM classification result as presented below.

For normal tissue (or soft plaque), the media layer has a good contrast to adventitia. Hence, c_B is defined as $c_B(x, y) = D_1(x, y) - D_2(x, y)$ where D_1 is a summation of raw filtering response of the first order DoG at four different orientations and D_2 denotes maximum response of second order DoG filtering from different orientations across three scales. That is D_1 measures total edge strength and D_2 is rotational invariant measurement of bar-like feature. Note, the media layer is generally darker than the lower layer, adventitia. The first order DoG filters are designed so that the stronger the media-adventitia border the lower the raw filtering response, i.e. negative values.

Calcified plaque exhibits strong edge features and casts varying degree of acoustic shadow on the media-adventitia border.

Thus, we use the second order DoG responses to suppress calcification and enhance possible media layer. Fibrous tissue behaves similarly to calcification, except in majority cases media-adventitia border is still discernible. Hence, bar feature detection is more appropriate and to enhance the effect we combine it with phase symmetry feature, i.e. $c_B(x, y) = -D_2(x, y) - FS(x, y)$ where FS is the local phase feature.

The presence of stent causes scattering of ultrasound signals, leading to very bright pixels. Once stent is detected by SVM, it is straight forward to localise the stent region which should not be part of media or adventitia. The cost for stent region is assigned a positive constant. Second order DoG responses are used to assign cost value for non-stent region. As for guide-wire artifact, there are also very bright pixels but it casts complete shadow over entire column. Hence, we do not extract any feature and a positive constant is used as their cost value.

2.4   Shape Prior Based Cost Function

The shape prior is defined as a likelihood term of each node in the graph, which is based on the similarity between the initial shape (obtained through finding the minimum closed set of our basic graph) and a set of templates from the training set. The graph construction is then modified so that inter-column arcs change dynamically according to the prior. The energy term for shape prior can be expressed as:

$$E_S = \sum_{x,y \in S} c_P(x, y) + \sum_{(p,q) \in \mathcal{N}} f_{p,q}(S(p) - S(q)), \tag{1}$$

where c_P denotes the cost function associated to prior and f is a convex function penalising abrupt changes in S between neighbouring columns p and q in the set $\mathcal{N}$ of neighbouring columns in the graph. The second term is realised through graph construction, detailed in the following Section 2.5. Notably in [7] the authors also used multiple templates in the graph cut. The terminal edge connection is determined by comparing the initial labelling with the template, e.g. if the node is in the template but not in the initial labelling, it connects to the source.

Each shape in the training set is treated as a binary template, ψ where the area inside shape is one and the outside area is zero. The distance between two templates ψ^a and ψ^b is defined using a discrete version of Zhu and Chan distance [12]:

$$d^2(\psi^a, \psi^b) = \sum_P (\psi^a - \psi^b)^2. \tag{2}$$

where P denotes the image domain. This distance measure is a true metric and is not influenced by image size. Let $\Psi = \psi^1, ..., \psi^N$ denote the N number of aligned shapes from the training set. Given a possible cut in the graph which produces an aligned binary shape f, its similarity to a shape template ψ^n in the training set is computed as $\alpha(f, \psi^n) = exp(-\frac{1}{2\sigma^2}d^2(f, \psi^n))$. Thus, the likelihood of this particular cut can be evaluated by taking into account of all training shapes:

$$c_{R_0} = \frac{\sum_{n=1}^{N} \alpha(f, \psi^n)\psi^n}{\sum_{n=1}^{N} \alpha(f, \psi^n)}. \tag{3}$$

In our case, an initial cut can be conveniently obtained by minimising the boundary based cost function alone. Note, it is fully automatic and there is no need for user initialisation. The labelling of the shape likelihood and initial cut needs to be compared in order to assign appropriate terminal arcs. The shape prior cost is defined as:

$$c_P(x, y) = \lambda_1 |c_{R_0}(x, y) - c_{R_1}(x, y)|, \tag{4}$$

where c_{R_0} and c_{R_1} denote the cost associated to prior for the inferior region (the region under the border) and superior region (the region above the border) respectively, and λ_1 is the weight for the shape prior cost. The normalised weighted templates c_{R_0} is in effect the inferior-region cost and is inversely proportional to the likelihood of a pixel belong to the region underneath the media-adventitia border. To define the superior-region prior cost c_{R_1}, we simply compute the complement of c_{R_0}, i.e. $c_{R_1} = \max_{x,y} c_{R_0}(x, y) - c_{R_0}(x, y)$. As shown in Section 2.6, the shape prior cost $c_P(x, y)$ is used to assign weights for each pixel according to its position from the border. By assigning the shape prior cost in this way, we eliminate the need to identify the terminal connection type.

2.5   Graph Construction Using Shape Prior

In non-prior graph construction the inter-column maximum distance Δ is set as a constant. For our prior model, inter-column change should be influenced by the derived shape prior. In calculating the shape prior cost function, the training shapes are aligned to our initial graph cut. The inter-column changes are then generalised using mean $m_{p,q}$ and standard deviation $\sigma_{p,q}$ at individual column. These statistics are then used in determining maximum and minimum distances when connecting neighbouring columns in graph construction, i.e. $\bar{\Delta}_{p,q} = m_{p,q} + c \cdot \sigma_{p,q}$, $\underline{\Delta}_{p,q} = m_{p,q} - c \cdot \sigma_{p,q}$, and c is a real constant. Note, these inter-column arcs alone will impose a hard constraint on shape regularisation.

Hence, additional inter-column arcs are necessary in order to allow smooth transition (see dashed arcs in Fig. 2 (b)), that is intermediate values, $h \in [\underline{\Delta}_{p,q}, \bar{\Delta}_{p,q}]$, are used to construct inter-column arcs. The direction of these arcs is based on the first order derivative of the function $f_{p,q}(h)$ as in (1). Here, we employ a quadratic function, $f_{p,q} = \lambda_2 (x - m_{p,q})^2$ where λ_2 is a weighting factor for smoothness constraint. If $f'_{p,q}(h) \geq 0$ an arc from $V(x, y)$ to $V(x + 1, y - h)$ is established; otherwise, the arc is connected from $V(x + 1, y)$ to $V(x, y + h)$. The weight for these arcs is assigned as the second order derivative of $f_{p,q}$. Note, when $f'_{p,q}(h) = 0$, only single arc is defined to reduce the shape prior influence in presence of strong boundary features, instead of using bi-directional arcs on the mean difference $m_{p,q}$.

2.6   Compute the Minimum Closed Set

The cost function $C(x, y) = c_B(x, y) + c_P(x, y)$ is inversely correlated to the likelihood that the border of interest passes through pixel (x, y). The weight for each node on the directed graph can be assigned as:

$$w(x, y) = \begin{cases} C(x, y) & \text{if } y = 0, \\ C(x, y) - C(x, y - 1) & \text{otherwise.} \end{cases} \tag{5}$$

For a feasible path $\mathcal{P}$ in the graph, the subset of nodes on or below $\mathcal{P}$ form a closed set and it can be shown that the cost of $\mathcal{P}$ is equivalent to the cost of nodes in the corresponding subset (differ by a constant) [8]. Hence, segmenting the media-adventitia is equivalent to finding the minimum closed set in the directed graph. The s-t cut algorithm [3] can then be used to find the minimum closed set, based on the fact that the weight can be used as the base for dividing the nodes into nonnegative and negative sets. The source s is connected to each negative node and every nonnegative node is connected to the sink t, both through a directed arc that carries the absolute value of the cost node itself.

The smoothing parameter in graph construction prevents sudden drastic changes in the extracted interfaces. However, the segmented media-adventitia may still contain local oscillations. Here, efficient 1D RBF interpolation using thin plate base function is used to obtain the final interface.

3   Experimental Results

A total of 1197 IVUS images of 240×1507 pixels in the polar coordinates from 4 sequences are used to evaluate the proposed method. These images contain various forms of fibrous plaque, calcification, stent, and acoustic shadow. Manual labelling was carried out on every 10 frames, i.e. 1197 frames in total, to establish groundtruth for quantitative analysis. The training set contains 278 images.

First, we compared our method against the $s - t$ cut algorithm [13]. The boundary cost function was kept the same, and careful manual initialisations were carried out for $s - t$ cut. The proposed method does not need user intervention. The first column in Fig. 3 shows typical results achieved using $s - t$ cut. Manual initialisations are shown in blue and green, and segmentation results are shown in red. Despite reasonable care in initialisation, the $s - t$ cut result was not satisfactory. The corresponding results of the proposed method are shown in the second column. The bottom of the each image shows the classification result of detecting different types of tissue. The proposed method achieved better accuracy and consistency. The quantitative comparison was carried out on a randomly selected subset of 50 images, since manual initialisation of 1197 images is too labour intensive. Table 1 shows that the proposed method clearly outperformed $s - t$ cut in both area difference measure (AD) and absolute mean difference measure (AMD) based on groundtruth.

Next, the proposed method was tested on the full dataset (1197 images) and its performance based on 1197 labelled groundtruth can be summarised as: 9.00 % mean AD with standard deviation of 6.35 and 9.16 pixel mean AMD with standard deviation of 6.20. This is marginally better than the first subset. Fig. 4 shows example comparisons to groundtruth. It is evident that the proposed method can handle various forms of ultrasound artifacts. Overall, the quantitative results suggest that the proposed method is an effective method in segmentation media-adventitia border in IVUS.

Table 1. Quantitative comparison to $s - t$ cut. AD: area difference in percentage; AMD: absolute mean difference in pixel in comparison to groundtruth.

	$s - t$ cut		proposed method	
	AD	AMD	AD	AMD
Mean	22.54	23.91	9.286	10.05
Std.	8.87	7.49	5.03	5.41

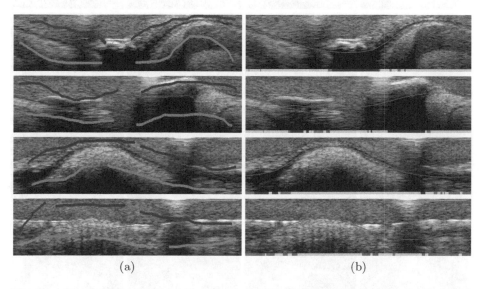

(a)   (b)

Fig. 3. (a) $s - t$ cut result (red) with user initialization (object: blue, background: green). (b) proposed method result; the bottom of each image also shows the classification result: calcified plaque (blue), fibrotic plaque (dark green), stent (dark red), guide-wire shadowing (cyan), and soft plaque/normal tissue (light green).

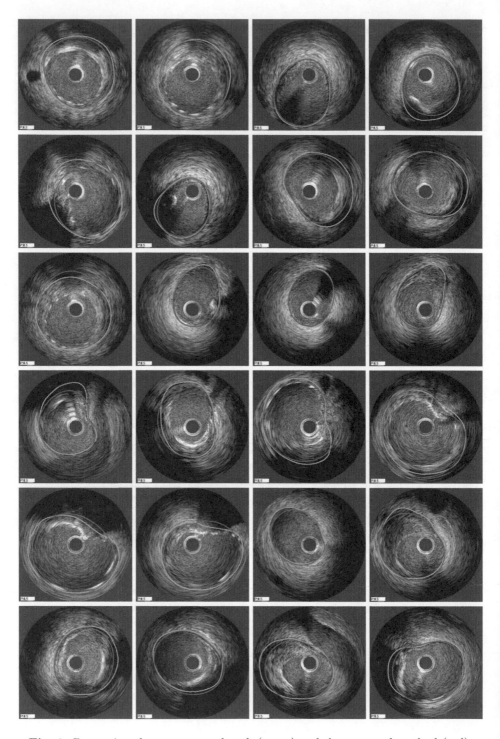

Fig. 4. Comparison between groundtruth (green) and the proposed method (red)

4   Conclusions

We presented an automatic graph based segmentation method for delineating the media-adventitia border in IVUS images. Boundary based features were dynamically selected to optimise the cost function. The use of multiple training shapes proved to be beneficial. The generalised shape prior was used in both incorporating the cost function but also graph construction. Smoothness constraint was intrinsically imposed in graph construction. Qualitative and quantitative results on a large number of IVUS images showed superior performance of the method.

Acknowledgement. We would like to thank Welsh Government NISCHR for funding this research work (Grant ID: HA09/035).

References

1. Sonka, M., et al.: Segmentation of intravascular ultrasound images: A knowledge-based approach. T-MI 14, 719–732 (1995)
2. Takagi, A., et al.: Automated contour detection for high frequency intravascular ultrasound imaging: A technique with blood noise reduction for edge enhancement. Ultrasound in Medicine and Biology 26(6), 1033–1041 (2000)
3. Boykov, Y., Kolmogorov, V.: An experimental comparison of min-cut/max-flow algorithms for energy minimization in vision. T-PAMI 26(9), 1124–1137 (2004)
4. Wahle, A., et al.: Plaque development, vessel curvature, and wall shear stress in coronary arteries assessed by x-ray angiography and intravascular ultrasound. MIA 10(1), 615–631 (2006)
5. Freedman, D., Zhang, T.: Interactive graph cut based segmentation with shape priors. In: CVPR, pp. 755–762 (2005)
6. Malcolm, J., Rathi, Y., Tannenbaum, A.: Graph cut segmentation with nonlinear shape priors. In: ICIP, pp. 365–368 (2007)
7. Vu, N., Manjunath, B.S.: Shape prior segmentation of multiple objects with graph cuts. In: CVPR, pp. 1–8 (2008)
8. Li, K., Wu, X., Chen, D.Z., Sonka, M.: Optimal surface segmentation in volumetric images-a graph-theoretic approach. T-PAMI 28(1), 119–134 (2006)
9. Mulet-Parada, M., Noble, J.: 2D + T acoustic boundary detection in echocardiography. MIA 4(1), 21–30 (2000)
10. Filho, E., et al.: Detection & quantification of calcifications in ivus by automatic thresholding. Ultrasound in Medicine and Biology 34(1), 160–165 (2008)
11. Unal, G., et al.: Shape-driven segmentation of the arterial wall in intravascular ultrasound images. IEEE Trans. Info. Tech. Biomed. 12(3), 335–347 (2008)
12. Chan, T., Zhu, W.: Level set based shape prior segmentation. In: CVPR (2005)
13. Boykov, Y., Funka-Lea, G.: Interactive graph cuts for optimal boundary and region segmentation of objects in n-d images. IJCV 70(2), 109–131 (2006)

Multiple Atlases-Based Joint Labeling of Human Cortical Sulcal Curves

Ilwoo Lyu[1], Gang Li[2], Minjeong Kim[2], and Dinggang Shen[2]

[1] Department of Computer Science, University of North Carolina,
Chapel Hill, NC 27599, USA
ilwoolyu@cs.unc.edu
[2] Department of Radiology and BRIC, University of North Carolina,
Chapel Hill, NC 27599, USA
{gang_li,mjkim,dgshen}@med.unc.edu

Abstract. We present a spectral-based sulcal curve labeling method by considering geometrical information of neighboring curves in a multiple atlases-based framework. Compared to the conventional method, we propose to use neighboring curves for avoiding ambiguity in curve-by-curve labeling and to integrate the labeling results obtained from multiple atlases for consistent labeling. In particular, we compute a histogram of points on the neighboring curves as a new feature descriptor for each point on a sulcal curve under consideration. To better resolve ambiguity in the curve labeling, we also employ the neighboring curves that are parallel to major sulcal curves. Moreover, we further integrate all the results from multiple atlases into a linear system, by solving which our method ultimately gives accurate labels to the major curves in the subjects. Experimental results on evaluation of 12 major sulcal curves of 12 human cortical surfaces indicate that our method achieves higher labeling accuracy 7.87% compared to the conventional method, while reducing 4.41% of false positive labeling errors on average.

Keywords: sulcal curve labeling, multiple atlases, spectral matching.

1 Introduction

The sulcal folding patterns of human cortical fundic regions are used as key features for analyzing brain function, monitoring brain growth, and discovering diseases. Since sulcal curves can be defined along fundic regions, automatic labeling of sulcal curves is important for these studies. There have been recent studies on automatic extraction of sulcal curves on human cortical surfaces [1,2]. However, these methods extract not only major curves but also many extraneous minor curves, which should be further removed for sulcal curve labeling. Due to the extremely complicated and variable sulcal folding patterns and extraneous minor sulcal branches, even if sulcal curves can be perfectly extracted, it is still challenging to identify major curves among the automatically extracted ones.

Atlas(es)-based sulcal curve labeling methods have been proposed for automatic labeling of major curves [3,4,5]. Compared to the single atlas-based methods [3,4], the multiple atlases-based labeling method is thought to be able to

B.H. Menze et al. (Eds.): MCV 2012, LNCS 7766, pp. 124–132, 2013.

give more accurate labels by considering individual sulcal variability. Recently, a spectral-based sulcal curve labeling method using multiple atlases has been reported [5]. In their method, they just picked the most matched sulcal curve from the multiple atlases to label the corresponding curve in the subject. The correspondence is established by solving an affinity matrix that stores all possible assignments based on the geometric features between two curves under consideration. However, there are two main drawbacks in their method. First, since only the best matched curve is considered as the candidate to label the subject, large false positive errors can be introduced if there is no similar curve in the atlases or the number of atlases is too small. Second, the labeling process is done independently for each major curve without considering its neighboring curves. This could reduce a chance for the major curves to be accurately labeled due to the ambiguity in the curve matching.

In this paper, we present a sulcal curve labeling method for cortical surfaces, which jointly exploits the geometric information of multiple atlases and neighboring curves in the subject space. We focus on "finding correct assignments", which can be formulated as a linear system similarly as in [6]. Specifically, for the feature description, each curve stores its neighboring curves' information (i.e., a histogram of position information of points on the neighboring curves), and in the curve matching, a major curve finds the most similar curves in the subject, guided by its neighboring curves. In addition, we incorporate all labeling results obtained from multiple atlases since it is likely that major curves in the atlases are only partially similar to those in the subject. To this end, we extend the affinity matrix in [6] to integrate labeling results into a linear system. Experimental results indicate that our method achieves 7.87% improvement of labeling accuracy as well as 4.41% reduction of false positive labeling errors on average for 12 major curves on 12 cortical surfaces, compared to the conventional method [5].

2   Method

Given a set of sulcal curves P in atlases and that of unlabeled sulcal curves Q in the subject, our goal is to label major curves in Q while discarding minor ones in Q. Note that the curves in P are pre-labeled major curves by following neuroanatomical conventions while Q contains (possibly disconnected) major curves and many minor ones. For curve labeling, we first automatically extract sulcal curves from the triangulated cortical surface using [1] and deform all curves in each atlas to the subject space using a diffeomporphic surface registration method [7]. It is worth noting that landmark-free surface registration methods can only roughly align the sulcal folding patterns [8], thus still leaving a certain amount of ambiguity in the curve labeling (see Fig. 1a). To better resolve ambiguity in the labeling, unlike the "hard" matching strategy in the conventional method, we use the geometric features of the major curve and its nearby curves for measuring curve similarity. Moreover, the final label is jointly determined by all atlases, which differs from the conventional method that directly retrieves the label from the most similar curve in a selected atlas.

2.1   Spectral-Based Curve Matching Using Neighboring Curves

To measure similarity for every possible pair of curves $p \subseteq P$ and $q \subseteq Q$, we basically measure the individual and pairwise affinities of an assignment $a = (p_i, q_j)$, where $p_i \in p$ and $q_j \in q$. For an assignment a, we denote $D(a)$ as the displacement vector between geometric features of p_i and q_j, each element of which is normalized with respect to its maximum value. Let w be a nonnegative weight vector that gives the importance of every element in $D(a)$. The individual affinity is then defined as follows:

$$A(a) = \exp(-\frac{\|D(a)\|_w^2}{2\sigma^2}) \,, \tag{1}$$

where $\|D\|_w$ denotes the weighted L_2-norm of D with respect to the weight vector w and σ is a user-provided regularization parameter. Similarly, for two distinct assignments a and b, the pairwise affinity is given by

$$A(a, b) = \exp(-\frac{\|D(a, b)\|_w^2}{2\sigma^2}) \,, \tag{2}$$

where $D(a, b) = D(a) - D(b)$.

Geometric Features Considering Neighboring Curves. Several geometric features are defined for each sulcal point, i.e., positions, curvatures, and unit tangent vectors from the major curve under consideration. Besides, we further incorporate the features from its neighboring curves. Basically, we calculate a histogram based on the position information of the neighboring curves in the Euclidean space. Given a major curve $p = \{p_1, \cdots, p_i, \cdots, p_N\}$ with N sulcal points for $p \subseteq P$, let S_p be a set of its neighboring curves. To compute a histogram of the neighboring sulcal points around a point $p_i \in p$, we first build a spherical kernel K centered at p_i with radius r. The size of r is automatically determined by the maximum Hausdorff distance between p and s for $\forall s \subseteq S_p$.

$$r = \max_{s \subseteq S_p} d_H(p, s) \,, \tag{3}$$

where $d_H(\cdot, \cdot)$ denotes the Hausdorff distance between two curves. The size of K is identical for any point on p. Let $F(\cdot)$ be the position-information vector of a sulcal point in the atlases, which stands for location information in the Euclidean space. Once the size of spherical kernel K is determined, an initial set of neighboring points L_{p_i} within K is obtained as follows:

$$L_{p_i} = \left\{ x \mid x \in s \subseteq S_p, \frac{\|F(x) - F(p_i)\|^2}{r^2} \leq 1 \right\} \,. \tag{4}$$

Our interest is to find sulcal points on the neighboring curves that are "parallel" to curve p, referring to those with similar global shapes and orientations to p. To emphasize such neighboring points in L_{p_i}, we apply the principal component analysis (PCA) on L_{p_i} since the principal direction u_1 of L_{p_i} stands for the direction of the parallel curves. We then discard as many sulcal points on the neighboring curves as possible that are not parallel to curve p within K, by reducing spherical kernel K to an ellipsoid with its three axes aligned to the three eigenvectors of PCA, $u_n, n = 1, 2, 3$. The eigenvalue λ_1 is given along the first major axis. We then have the following final set of neighboring points L'_{p_i} by letting $l_1 = \sqrt{\lambda_1}$ and $l_2 = l_3 = r$:

$$L'_{p_i} = \left\{ x \mid x \in L_{p_i}, \sum_{n=1}^{3} \frac{((F(x) - F(p_i)) \cdot u_n)^2}{l_n^2} \leq 1 \right\} . \tag{5}$$

Now, we build a bounding cube centered at p_i that fully contains the neighboring sulcal points in L'_{p_i}. Then, we uniformly divide the cube into m subvolumes. Let h_k be a ratio of points in L'_{p_i} that belong to a subvolume b_k, $1 \leq k \leq m$. We finally have a histogram $H_{p_i} = [h_1, h_2, \cdots, h_m]^T$ by the following equation.

$$h_k = \frac{\sum_{x \in L'_{p_i}} I(x, b_k)}{|L'_{p_i}|} , \tag{6}$$

$$I(x, b_k) = \begin{cases} 1 & \text{if } \{x\} \cap b_k \not\subseteq \emptyset, \\ 0 & \text{otherwise.} \end{cases} \tag{7}$$

For a sulcal point q_j in the subject, it is difficult to compute its actual spherical kernel because its neighboring major curves are unknown. Therefore, for an assignment $a = (p_i, q_j)$, we use the same kernel as p_i in the atlas for computing the histogram of q_j.

Synchronized Curve Matching. To account for sulcal shape variability, we generate the mean curve for each major curve [5]. We denote $\phi(\cdot)$ as the corresponding point on the mean curve to a given sulcal point in the atlas. For an assignment $a = (p_i, q_j)$, we now set a threshold of the distance between p_i and q_j with respect to the covariance of $\phi(p_i)$. Thus, the assignment a is rejected if

$$\sum_{n=1}^{3} \frac{((F(q_j) - F(p_i)) \cdot v_n)^2}{(3\tau_n)^2} > 1 , \tag{8}$$

where $\tau_n^2 (n = 1, 2, 3)$ are the covariances along the corresponding principal axes of the covariance matrix of $\phi(p_i)$. This constrains assignments statistically valid in terms of the sulcal shape variability.

Let s be a neighboring curve for a given major curve p as we defined above. We first measure affinities for p and s, respectively. To incorporate affinities of the neighboring curves into the affinity matrix M, we also measure all possible pairwise affinities between p and s. For $p_i \in p$ and $s_{i'} \in s$, suppose that assignments are given by $a = (p_i, q_j)$ and $b = (s_{i'}, q_{j'})$, where $q_j, q_{j'} \in q \subseteq Q$. Since a major curve is unable to share an identical label with its neighboring curves, in such a undesirable case of the coexistence of a and b, the pairwise affinity between a and b is set to zero. Once M is built, we compute the principal eigenvector of M to find the highly confident assignments. Since s only helps find the correspondences between p and q, the possibly remaining assignments in s will be left out.

2.2   Joint Labeling Using Multiple Atlases

It is worth noting that major curves in the atlases could be only partially similar to those in the subject. For all major sulcal curves in P, once the highly confident assignments with the corresponding curves in Q are selected, we incorporate the assignments to determine final labels based on their correspondences. Let p^α and p^β be the distinct major sulcal curves in P with an identical label. For two distinct assignments $a = (p_i^\alpha, q_j)$ and $b = (p_{i'}^\beta, q_{j'})$, it is highly desirable that $q_j = q_{j'}$ if $\phi(p_i^\alpha) = \phi(p_{i'}^\beta)$. To implement that idea, we construct a new affinity matrix M that describes relationships of all possible assignments between p^α and p^β. The diagonal entries of M are filled with confidence values that are obtained from the principal eigenvector of the affinity matrix in Sect. 2.1. For two distinct assignments $a = (p_i^\alpha, q_j)$ and $b = (p_{i'}^\beta, q_{j'})$, $M(a, b)$ is set to $A(a, b)$ as defined in Eq. 2. Then, $M(a, b)$ is updated as follows by letting $c = (q_j, q_{j'})$ if $\phi(p_i^\alpha) = \phi(p_{i'}^\beta)$:

$$M(a, b) = A(a, b) \cdot A(c) . \tag{9}$$

Finally, we compute the principal eigenvector of M to select the highly confident assignments for the joint labeling.

3   Experimental Results

Since the dataset in [5] is not publicly available, we used the MRIs Surfaces Curves dataset [8] for validation (total 12 subjects). However, in this dataset, several major curves delineated by experts were still crossed gyral regions, which slightly differ from the automatically extracted curves we used in the experiment. Thus, we generated ground-truth curves by combining the manual delineation results with the automatically extracted sulcal curves.

Given an automatically labeled curve q and its corresponding ground-truth curve q_g, the labeling accuracy $acc(q, q_g)$ and false positive labeling error $err(q, q_g)$ were measured by the following equations:

$$acc(q, q_g) = \frac{l(q \cap q_g)}{l(q_g)} \text{ and } err(q, q_g) = \frac{l(q - q_g)}{l(q_g)} , \tag{10}$$

where $l(\cdot)$ denotes the length of a curve.

In our experiment, we adapted a jackknife technique to validate the accuracy and false positive errors: For each validation set, one subject was left out from the subject set to be labeled, and other subjects were regarded as the atlases.

Table 1. 12 Major curves and their neighboring curves

Curve	Neighbors	Curve	Neighbors	Curve	Neighbors	Curve	Neighbors
STS	ITS	ITS	STS, OTS	CS	preCS, postCS	preCS	CS
postCS	CS	SFS	IFS	IFS	SFS	CingS	-
CalcS	colS	OcPS	-	OTS	ITS, colS	colS	OTS, CalcS

12 out of major curves for both left and right hemispheres were used for validation: the superior temporal sulcus (STS), inferior temporal sulcus (ITS), central
sulcus (CS), precentral sulcus (preCS), postcentral sulcus (postCS), superior
frontal sulcus (SFS), inferior frontal sulcus (IFS), cingulate sulcus (CingS), cal-
carine sulcus (CalcS), occipito parietal sulcus (OcPS), occipito temporal sulcus
(OTS), and collateral sulcus (colS). We selected the neighboring curves for each
major sulcal curve based on neuroanatomical prior knowledge as summarized in
Table 1. For fair comparison of different methods in all experiments, we used the
same set of the deformed atlases obtained by the same registration method [7],
even for the conventional method.

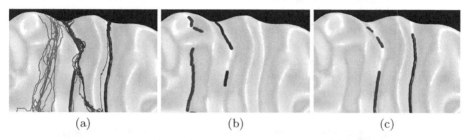

(a)   (b)   (c)

Fig. 1. Poorly deformed atlases and labeling results for the central sulcus (blue) and
postcentral sulcus (red): (a) deformed atlases (thin curves) and the ground-truth curves
(bold curves), (b) the labeling results by the conventional method, and (c) the labeling
results with neighboring curves

3.1   Neighboring Curves

We employed neighboring curves and chose the most similar curve among multiple atlases for the final result. For the histogram computation, we subdivided
the bounding cube into $4 \times 4 \times 4$ subvolumes, i.e., $m = 64$. For the affinity
matrix computation, we set the weight vector $w = [0.75, 0.15, 0.05, 0.05]^T$ and
the regularization parameter $\sigma = 0.3$. Each of the elements in w corresponds
to weight of the position, curvature, tangent vector, and histogram of neighboring sulcal points, respectively. We rejected an assignment if the norm of the
difference between the two histograms is greater than 0.1. Note that the parameters were empirically set according to [5] and by our experiment. In Fig. 1, the
labeling results with neighboring curves are consistent although the atlases are
poorly deformed. The results with neighboring curves exhibited better agreement

Table 2. Average labeling accuracy and false positive errors in the left (lh) and right hemispheres (rh) (unit: %):

	Conventional method		Neighboring curves (a)		Joint labeling (b)		Our method (a+b)	
	lh	rh	lh	rh	lh	rh	lh	rh
Accuracy	68.65	69.19	71.22	72.27	74.53	74.87	77.12	76.47
False positives	20.22	19.85	25.06	23.41	16.82	15.53	15.79	15.46

with the ground-truth than the conventional spectral-based method as summarized in Table 2. Interestingly, the average false positive errors also increased because several false positive assignments that had a low confidence value in the conventional method can gain a higher confidence, resulting from guidance of neighboring curves.

3.2 Joint Labeling Using Multiple Atlases

We applied the joint labeling without guidance of neighboring curves. The results obtained from 12 atlases were incorporated to determine the final label to each major sulcal curve. The same parameter setting as in Sect. 3.1 was used here. Figure 2 shows that the the joint labeling also gives labels to a part of major sulcal curves that is missed in the conventional spectral-based method. Compared to the conventional method, the labeling accuracy increased while the false positive errors decreased as summarized in Table 2.

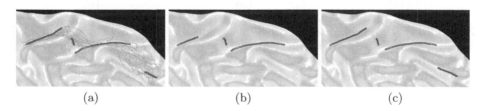

(a)   (b)   (c)

Fig. 2. Comparison of results by the conventional spectral-based method and joint labeling for the superior frontal sulcus: (a) deformed atlases (thin curves) and the ground-truth curves (bold curves), (b) the labeling results by the conventional spectral-based method, and (c) the labeling results by the joint labeling

3.3 Overall Performance

By incorporating two aspects, i.e., synchronized matching with neighboring curves and joint labeling using multiple atlases, into the our framework, we obtained the overall labeling accuracy and false positive errors as summarized in Table 2.

The labeling performance by our method was highly achieved after incorporating the two aspects. Also, our labeling results were comparable to the corresponding ground-truth curves (see an example in Fig. 3). Figure 4 demonstrates the statistical comparison of the labeling results for 12 major sulcal curves. The results show the average accuracy and false positive errors across subjects. This indicates that our labeling results were consistent on most of the curves, compared to the conventional method.

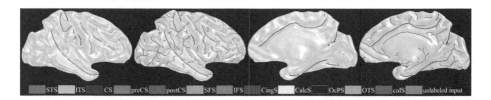

Fig. 3. A visual comparison of our automatic labeling results with the ground-truth for the right hemisphere: the lateral and medial views of ground-truth labeled curves (1st and 3rd columns) and the respective views of automatically labeled curves by our method (2nd and 4th columns). Note that there are many extraneous minor curves in the input (gray). For better visualization, a partially inflated surface model is used.

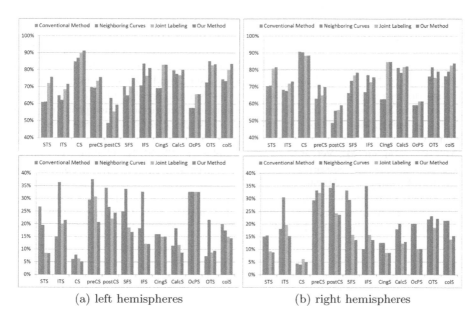

(a) left hemispheres   (b) right hemispheres

Fig. 4. Performance comparisons: average labeling accuracy (top row) and false positive errors (bottom row) for major sulcal curves in the left and right hemispheres

4   Conclusion

We presented a method for multiple atlases-based labeling of major sulcal curves on the cortical surface. Specifically, to resolve ambiguity in the labeling, we proposed a histogram feature for each sulcal point and incorporated the geometric information of neighboring curves into the affinity matrix for the curve matching. Since major curves in the atlases are likely to be partially similar to those in the subject, we incorporated the results obtained from all atlases into the linear system for accurate labeling. We have shown in experiment that compared to the conventional method, the performances were improved for 7.87% labeling accuracy and reduced for 4.41% of false positive errors. In our future work, we will employ a learning technique for optimizing parameters used in the curve matching.

References

1. Li, G., Guo, L., Nie, J., Liu, T.: An automated pipeline for cortical sulcal fundi extraction. Medical Image Analysis 14, 343–359 (2010)
2. Seong, J., Im, K., Yoo, S., Seo, S., Na, D., Lee, J.: Automatic extraction of sulcal lines on cortical surfaces based on anisotropic geodesic distance. Neuroimage 49, 293–302 (2010)
3. Lohmann, G., Von Cramon, D.: Automatic labelling of the human cortical surface using sulcal basins. Medical Image Analysis 4, 179–188 (2000)
4. Tao, X., Prince, J., Davatzikos, C.: Using a statistical shape model to extract sulcal curves on the outer cortex of the human brain. IEEE Trans. on Medical Imaging 21, 513–524 (2002)
5. Lyu, I., Seong, J., Shin, S., Im, K., Roh, J., Kim, M., Kim, G., Kim, J., Evans, A., Na, D., et al.: Spectral-based automatic labeling and refining of human cortical sulcal curves using expert-provided examples. Neuroimage 52, 142–157 (2010)
6. Leordeanu, M., Hebert, M.: A spectral technique for correspondence problems using pairwise constraints. In: Computer Vision, ICCV 2005, vol. 2, pp. 1482–1489. IEEE (2005)
7. Yeo, B., Sabuncu, M., Vercauteren, T., Ayache, N., Fischl, B., Golland, P.: Spherical demons: Fast diffeomorphic landmark-free surface registration. IEEE Trans. on Medical Imaging 29, 650–668 (2010)
8. Pantazis, D., Joshi, A., Jiang, J., Shattuck, D., Bernstein, L., Damasio, H., Leahy, R.: Comparison of landmark-based and automatic methods for cortical surface registration. Neuroimage 49, 2479–2493 (2010)

Fast Anatomical Structure Localization Using Top-Down Image Patch Regression

René Donner[1,2,*], Bjoern H. Menze[3,4,5], Horst Bischof[2], and Georg Langs[1,3]

[1] Computational Image Analysis and Radiology Lab, Department of Radiology,
Medical University Vienna, Austria
[2] Institute for Computer Graphics and Vision,
Graz University of Technology, Austria
[3] CSAIL, MIT, Cambridge MA, USA
[4] Asclepios Project, INRIA Sophia-Antipolis, France
[5] Computer Vision Laboratory, ETH Zurich, Switzerland
rene.donner@meduniwien.ac.at

Abstract. Fully automatic localization of anatomical structures in 2D and 3D radiological data sets is important in both computer aided diagnosis, and the rapid automatic processing of large amounts of data. We present a simple, accurate and fast approach with low computational complexity to find anatomical landmarks, based on a multi-scale regression codebook of informative image patches and encoded landmark contexts.

From a set of annotated training volumes the method captures the appearance of landmarks over several scales together with relative positions of neighboring landmarks and a spatial distribution model. During multi-scale search in a target volume, starting from the coarsest level, each landmark model predicts all landmark positions it has encoded, with the median of all predictions yielding the final prediction for each scale.

We present results on two challenging data sets (hand radiographs and hand CTs), where our method achieves comparable accuracy to the state of the art with substantially improved run-time.

Keywords: Anatomical structure localization, nearest neighbor regression, image patch codebooks.

1 Introduction

The accurate localization of anatomical landmarks in medical imaging data is a challenging problem, due to rich variability and frequent ambiguity of their appearance. Among the reasons for the difficulties are noise (including local

* This work was partly supported by the European Union FP7 Project KHRESMOI (FP7-257528), by the Austrian National Bank grants BIOBONE (13468) and AOR-TAMOTION (13497) and the Austrian Sciences Fund grant PULMARCH (P 22578-B19).

B.H. Menze et al. (Eds.): MCV 2012, LNCS 7766, pp. 133–141, 2013.

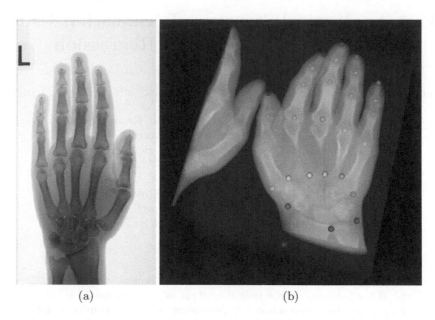

(a)   (b)

Fig. 1. Examples from the two data sets employed in this paper. a) Hand radiographs and b) high resolution hand CTs. The objective of the proposed method is to localize the depicted anatomical landmarks in an unseen target image or volume.

and global intensity changes), cluttered image data (overlapping structures in 2D projections, highly structured background in 3D organ segmentation), and anatomical structures that exhibit a high degree of similarity (e.g., fingers or vertebrae). We propose an algorithm that copes with these challenges and offers a general approach to accurately localize landmarks without initialization or subsequent refinement. The method constructs a multi-level regression codebook which associates image patches with the corresponding positions of anatomical landmarks depicted in the patch. During search the scale-pyramid is traversed, finding the most similar patch for each landmark using k-nearest neighbor search.

The localization of anatomical structures is crucial for several areas of medical imaging analysis: Segmentation approaches such as Level-Sets [4] and Appearance Models [3], typically require at least a coarse initial localization, while registration approaches can exploit spatial initialization to avoid local minima. The automatic localization of anatomical structures is fundamental for the field of Computer Aided Diagnosis [7] and for structuring image information in image retrieval, since it allows the algorithms to focus on target regions in the data and subsequently invoke more specialized analysis stages. Landmark localization can also be regarded as a form of semantic parsing [13] when point-wise rather than regional information is required.

State of the art. Several approaches to anatomical structure localization exist in recent literature. They mainly differ in the type of semantic representation that is obtained to describe the image data. We thus distinguish between approaches that either 1) indicate the *positions* of individual landmarks, 2) provide *bounding boxes* for entire organs, 3) result in *model parameters* which describe the position and shape of the object or 4) provide *voxel-wise labels* for different organs.

Localizing anatomical landmarks using the *positions* of selected interest points has been the objective of [8,1]. The methods learn interest point detectors on training data, estimate positions of landmark candidates in the target volume and finally disambiguate these candidates through a model matching step. Both methods rely on the classification of the entire volume. [9] reduces this computational burden by performing a low-resolution step and a refinement step using Hough regressors. Reducing the complexity by working on axial slices, [13] parse whole body CT data in a hierarchical fashion, but are concerned with finding larger organs. While substantially speeding up the localization this only works for objects which are rather large in respect to the overall volume size, since the objects have to be visible in at least one of the three central orthogonal slices. Using Random Forests for the localization of organs in thorax CTs through *bounding boxes* has been been proposed in [5]. An extension using Hough ferns was presented in [12] to predict the bounding boxes of multiple organs at once in full-body MR data. Relying on stochastic optimization instead of ensemble classification or regression, Marginal Space Learning [15] tries to find the parameters of a bounding box or a parametric and data-driven *shape model* [2] to localize and segment anatomical structures. This allows for fast localization, but instead of representing a global search algorithm, iterative approaches have to be used to cope with repetitive structures [10]. The task of assigning *voxel-wise labels* to segment entire organs or organ structures has been approached by [6] and [11] using Random Forest classification.

Contribution. We present a simple, fast method for the global, accurate localization of anatomical structures in 2D/3D data based on an appearance codebook, and location predictors that capture sub-configurations of a landmark set. It demonstrates that a top-down nearest neighbor matching strategy of image patches drastically reduces the number of required feature computations and yields localization results comparable to the state of the art.

Paper structure. The paper is structured as follows: Sec. 2.1 details the construction of the codebook, with the localization on a target volume described in Sec. 2.2. Sec. 3 introduces the experiments, with the results presented in Sec. 3.3. A discussion and an outlook can be found in Sec. 3.4 and Sec. 4.

2   Methods

The approach is divided into a training phase and a localization phase as shown in Fig. 2 and Fig. 3. During localization a multi-scale codebook of image patches and landmark positions is constructed, which is traversed during the localization phase to obtain increasingly accurate landmark estimates at each scale.

136   R. Donner et al.

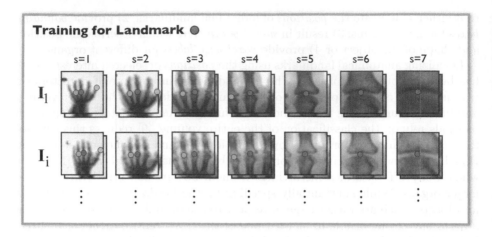

Fig. 2. Construction of the regression codebooks during training. For each landmark and scale patches at various offsets and the corresponding relative landmark positions are recorded, using all training images/volumes.

2.1   Training – Constructing the Landmark Regression Codebook

The training phase requires a set of N training images or volumes $\mathbf{I}_i$ with corresponding annotations. The annotations represent the coordinates $\mathbf{x}_x^i$ of the $x \in \{1, \ldots, L\}$ landmarks of the anatomical structure in question. Each landmark is present in each of the training volumes.

Codebook Construction to Connect Local Appearance and Landmark Information. Our aim is to build multi-scale regression codebooks $\mathcal{C}$ of image patches and corresponding relative landmark positions – one codebook per scale $s \in 1, \ldots, S$ and landmark x. The patches stored in the codebook are extracted around the landmarks with varying offsets and scaling, capturing the typical visual appearance around each landmark. For each patch the positions of all landmarks visible in the patch are recorded, relative to the patch's center. Each of the PN entries in the codebook $\mathcal{C}_{s,x}$ consists of the tuple $\langle \mathbf{P}^p, \mathbf{L}^p \rangle$ of the patch $\mathbf{P}^p$ and the corresponding relative $D \times L$ landmark coordinates $\mathbf{L}^p$ which are visible in the patch. $\mathbf{L}^p$ specifies the coordinates of the landmarks $x \in 1 \ldots L$ relative to the center of the given patch[1]. Landmarks which are outside of the patch are denoted as not visible.

The construction of the codebook proceeds as follows: At the top-most scale $s = 1$ each image or volume is represented by an an-isotropically downscaled miniature of size $m \times m \times m$ (similarly $m \times m$ for images). At each scale s the volume is considered to possess an edge length of $\sqrt{2}(s-1)m$. This re-sampling of the entire image is never actually computed, it simply forms the reference frame for each scale of the codebook generation.

---

[1] The necessary transformations between image coordinates and patch coordinates are omitted for clarity throughout the text.

At each scale s, patches $\mathbf{P}$ are extracted from the image or volume data using linear interpolation for each landmark x from all training volumes N. The patches are of size $m \times m \times m$, i.e. at scale $s = 1$ they correspond to the entire image, and for scales $s > 1$ the patches *zoom in* on the landmark, as illustrated in Fig. 2. Parts of patches which would be sampled from outside of the volume are set equal to the closest voxel on the volume's border. The gray values of each patch is normalized to zero mean and unit variance.

To explore the image information in the vicinity of a landmark the entries in the codebook $\mathcal{C}_{s,x}$ at a certain scale s and landmark x, are constructed by extracting several patches around the landmark with, empirically chosen, 7 off-sets in the range of $[-6, 6]$ voxels for each dimension, along with scaling factors of $\{0.9, 1, 1.1\}$, resulting in $P = 1029$ patches for one landmark in one training volume at one scale ($P = 147$ for images). To considerably reduce the memory requirements and computational complexity for the codebook lookup, dimensionality reduction of each codebook is performed using PCA, retaining 90% of variance, resulting in PCA coefficients $\mathbf{P}_{PCA}$ and final codebook tuples $\langle \mathbf{P}_{PCA}^p, \mathbf{L}^p \rangle$. This training scheme results in the $S \times L$ regression codebooks $\mathcal{C}_{s,x}$.

Shape model to regularize the localization. To be able to regularize the interme-diate solutions during the prediction phase, a model of the spatial distribution of the landmarks $\mathbf{s} = \langle \mathbf{x}_1^i, \ldots, \mathbf{x}_L^i \rangle$ in the training data is learned. We compute a point distribution model $\mathcal{S} = \langle \bar{\mathbf{s}}, \mathbf{S} \rangle$ using an eigen-decomposition of the co-variance matrix of the training landmarks $\mathbf{x}_x$ as proposed in [2], retaining all eigenvectors and thus the entire shape variance observable in the training set, where the shapes $\mathbf{s}$ in the model can be constructed through a parameter vector $\mathbf{b}$ such that:

$$\mathbf{s} = \bar{\mathbf{s}} + \mathbf{S}\mathbf{b}$$

2.2   Localization – Regularized Top-Down Matching

Similar to the training phase the localization is performed in a multi-scale fash-ion, shown in Fig. 3. The $D \times L$ landmark localization matrix $\mathbf{L}_{s=1}^*$ is initialized with all landmarks starting at the center of the test volume $\mathbf{I}_{target}$. Starting with scale $s = 1$, a patch $\mathbf{P}^x$ for each landmark x is extracted (without additional offsets or scaling variations). The patch is normalized and projected onto the patch PCA model of $\mathcal{C}_{s,x}$, resulting in $\mathbf{P}_{PCA}^x$. The most similar patch p^{x*} in the codebook is found using euclidean nearest neighbor search – leading to the tuple $\langle \mathbf{P}_{PCA}^{x*}, \mathbf{L}_p^{x*} \rangle$ and thus the landmark coordinate predictions $\mathbf{L}_p^{x*}$ as esti-mated by landmark x. Repeating this codebook lookup for all landmarks yields the $D \times L \times L$ prediction tensor $\mathbf{M}_{\mathbf{d,i,j}}$ with position estimates from each land-mark i to all landmarks that are visible in the same patch. The median over all predictions j which are not marked as not-visible yields the updated landmark localization matrix $\mathbf{L}_s^*$. This procedure is repeated through all scales, resulting in the final localization result $\mathbf{L}_S^*$.

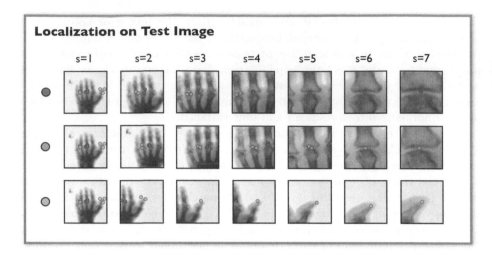

Fig. 3. The localization of three landmarks on a test image/volume descends the scale pyramid. At each level regression based on the image patch generates not only a position estimate for the primary landmak, but also for other landmarks visible in the patch. When progressing to a finer scale, for each landmark these estimates vote for the next estimate and center of the finer patch.

Shape regularization. The position estimates $\mathbf{L}_s^*$ are regularized by projecting them onto the shape PCA model $\mathcal{S}$ and reconstructing them again thereafter. This enforces landmark positions which can be modeled by a linear combination of the shapes observed in the training data. This regularization is performed for scales $s \leq S - 3$, to allow for landmark positions which can not be modeled though the shape model at scales $s > S - 3$.

3   Experiments

3.1   Data Sets

We evaluated the proposed approach on the two separate data sets shown in Fig. 1: 20 hand radiographs and 12 high resolution hand CTs.

Data set 1: Hand Radiographs $N = 20$ hand radiographs with an average size of 460×260 pixels with a resolution of 0.423mm/pixel were annotated with $L = 24$ landmarks. The landmarks include the five finger tips, as well as the distal interphalangeal (DIP), proximal interphalangeal (PIP), metacarpophalangeal (MCP) and carpometacarpal (CMC) joints for each finger.

Data set 2: Hand CTs The 3D hand CTs have a voxel size of $0.5mm \times 0.5mm \times 0.66mm$ resulting in an average size of $256 \times 384 \times 330$ voxels. They are annotated with the same 24 landmarks as the hand radiographs, with three additional landmarks placed around the carpus at the radiocarpal, radioulnar, and ulnocarpal joints, totaling in $L = 27$.

Table 1. Experimental results, localization accuracy in mm: Residual distances of the localization result to the ground truth annotation for the proposed method, in comparison with a state of the art approach

Residual in mm	MRF-based graph-matching			Proposed Patch-Regression Method		
	Median	Mean	Std	Median	Mean	Std
Hand Radiographs	0.80	0.99	0.82	0.63	0.77	0.64
Hand CTs	1.19	1.45	1.13	1.43	1.96	1.80

3.2 Setup

The experiments were run using four-fold cross validation, learning the landmark regression codebook on 75% of the N images / volumes and performing the localization on the remaining images / volumes. The main measure of interest for each landmark is the residual distance between the position of the predicted landmark position and the corresponding ground truth. The parameter settings are identical for the experiments on the two data sets, except for the size of the patches: 32×32 in the 2D case and $32 \times 32 \times 32$ for the 3D data. The results are compared with the recently proposed pre-filtered Hough regression Random forests [9], which in turn showed to outperform alternative approaches such as classification-based landmark candidate estimation with graph-based optimization [1] and classification + mean-shift based approaches [14].

3.3 Results

The results of the evaluation of the landmark localization are presented in Tab. 1, which shows the aggregated localization performance for the two data sets. The accuracy on the 2D radiograph data set is very high with a median residual of 0.63 mm and a mean/std of 0.77/0.64 mm. This result compares favorably with the results reported and methods tested on the same data in [9]. The result on the 3D hand CT data set show a median residual of 1.43 mm and a mean/std of 1.96/1.80 mm. It can be seen that despite a similar median residual, the proportion of localizations with higher error is slighty larger in this case. The run-times of the proposed approach were in the order of 0.6sec for the 2D data set and 4.5sec for the 3D data set on a single core of a 2009 Xeon MacPro. The method was entirely implemented in Matlab - we expect a potential speed-up by a factor of 10 to 100 through a more optimized implementation.

3.4 Discussion - Feature Computation Complexity

The main contribution of this work is the demonstration of a feature computation scheme which requires significantly less memory accesses then existing methods.

Voxel-wise classification / prediction approaches such as those proposed in [1,11] scale with the number of voxels, while pre-filtered Hough regression [9] reduces

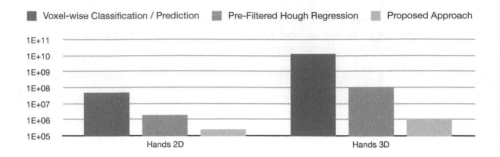

Fig. 4. Number of image/volume accesses necessary to compute the features required during the localization phase. Voxel-wise classification / prediction approaches [1,11] scale with the number of voxels, while pre-filtered Hough regression [9] works on strongly downsampled volumes. In constrast to this, the proposed approach is indepedent of the number of voxels and scales with the number of landmarks.

computational complexity by working on strongly down-sampled volumes. A typical number of 400 memory accesses to compute the classification for a single voxel was assumed in the calculation, corresponding to e. g. 20 individual features in an ensemble of 20 individual classifiers.

In contrast to this, the proposed approach is independent of the number of voxels and only depends on the number of landmarks, with $m \times m \times m$ voxels sampled for the patch at each landmark and scale. The proposed approach thus requires one to four orders of magnitude less image/volume accesses, allowing for fast localization even in unoptimized implementations or cheap commodity hardware.

4   Conclusion and Outlook

We present an approach for localizing complex, partly repetitive anatomical structures in 2D and 3D data. We demonstrate that a top-down nearest neighbor matching strategy of image patches drastically reduces the number of required feature computations and that the prediction of relative landmark positions using codebook regression is feasible.

The results on the two data sets clearly demonstrate the ability of the proposed approach to find the landmark positions in the target volume with accuracy comparable to the state of the art, with the consistent localization of detailed anatomical structures with a median residual of 1.7 to 2.7 pixels/voxels.

We consider the results to be very promising for such a simple method, and will focus on several topics in upcoming work: A detailed analysis of the parameters involved, namely the patch size and the perturbation strategy during codebook generation, as well as approximations of the nearest neighbor search through random subspaces.

References

1. Bergtholdt, M., Kappes, J., Schmidt, S., Schnörr, C.: A Study of Parts-Based Object Class Detection Using Complete Graphs. IJCV 87(1-2), 93–117 (2010)
2. Cootes, T.F., Taylor, C.J., Cooper, D.H., Graha, J.: Active Shape Models - Their Training and Application. CVIU 61(1), 38–59 (1995)
3. Cootes, T.F., Edwards, G.J., Taylor, C.J.: Active Appearance Models. TPAMI 23(6), 681–685 (2001)
4. Cremers, D., Rousson, M., Deriche, R.: A Review of Statistical Approaches to Level Set Segmentation: Integrating Color, Texture, Motion and Shape. IJCV 72(2), 195–215 (2007)
5. Criminisi, A., Shotton, J., Robertson, D., Konukoglu, E.: Regression forests for efficient anatomy detection and localization in ct studies. In: Medical Computer Vision 2010: Recognition Techniques and Applications in Medical Imaging, MICCAI Workshop (2010)
6. Criminisi, A., Shotton, J., Bucciarelli, S.: Decision Forests with Long-Range Spatial Context for Organ Localization in CT Volumes. In: Proc. of MICCAI Workshop on Probabilistic Models for Medical Image Analysis, MICCAI-PMMIA (2009)
7. Doi, K.: Computer-aided diagnosis in medical imaging: Historical review, current status and future potential. Computerized Medical Imaging and Graphics 31, 198–211 (2007)
8. Donner, R., Birngruber, E., Steiner, H., Bischof, H., Langs, G.: Localization of 3D Anatomical Structures Using Random Forests and Discrete Optimization. In: Proc. MICCAI Workshop on Medical Computer Vision (2010)
9. Donner, R., Menze, B.H., Bischof, H., Langs, G.: Global Localization of 3D Anatomical Structures by Pre-filtered Hough Forests and Discrete Optimization. Medical Image Analysis (accepted, 2013)
10. Kelm, B.M., Zhou, S.K., Suehling, M., Zheng, Y., Wels, M., Comaniciu, D.: Detection of 3D Spinal Geometry Using Iterated Marginal Space Learning. In: Proc. MICCAI Workshop on Medical Computer Vision (2010)
11. Montillo, A., Shotton, J., Winn, J., Iglesias, J.E., Metaxas, D., Criminisi, A.: Entangled Decision Forests and Their Application for Semantic Segmentation of CT Images. In: Székely, G., Hahn, H.K. (eds.) IPMI 2011. LNCS, vol. 6801, pp. 184–196. Springer, Heidelberg (2011)
12. Pauly, O., Glocker, B., Criminisi, A., Mateus, D., Möller, A.M., Nekolla, S., Navab, N.: Fast Multiple Organ Detection and Localization in Whole-Body MR Dixon Sequences. In: Fichtinger, G., Martel, A., Peters, T. (eds.) MICCAI 2011, Part III. LNCS, vol. 6893, pp. 239–247. Springer, Heidelberg (2011)
13. Seifert, S., Barbu, A., Zhou, S., Liu, D., Feulner, J., Huber, M., Suehling, M., Cavallaro, A., Comaniciu, D.: Hierarchical Parsing and Semantic Navigation of Full Body CT Data. In: SPIE Medical Imaging (2009)
14. Shotton, J., Fitzgibbon, A., Cook, M., Sharp, T., Finocchio, M., Moorea, R., Kipman, A., Blake, A.: Real-Time Human Pose Recognition in Parts from a Single Depth Image. In: Proc. CVPR (2011)
15. Zheng, Y., Georgescu, B., Comaniciu, D.: Marginal Space Learning for Efficient Detection of 2D/3D Anatomical Structures in Medical Images. In: Prince, J.L., Pham, D.L., Myers, K.J. (eds.) IPMI 2009. LNCS, vol. 5636, pp. 411–422. Springer, Heidelberg (2009)

Oblique Random Forests for 3-D Vessel Detection Using Steerable Filters and Orthogonal Subspace Filtering[*]

Matthias Schneider[1], Sven Hirsch[1], Gábor Székely[1], Bruno Weber[2],
and Bjoern H. Menze[1]

[1] Computer Vision Laboratory, ETH Zurich, Switzerland
[2] Institute of Pharmacology and Toxicology, University of Zurich, Zurich, Switzerland

Abstract. We propose a machine learning-based framework using oblique random forests for 3-D vessel segmentation. Two different kinds of features are compared. One is based on orthogonal subspace filtering where we learn 3-D eigenspace filters from local image patches that return task optimal feature responses. The other uses a specific set of steerable filters that show, qualitatively, similarities to the learned eigenspace filters, but also allow for explicit parametrization of scale and orientation that we formally generalize to the 3-D spatial context. In this way, steerable filters allow to efficiently compute oriented features along arbitrary directions in 3-D. The segmentation performance is evaluated on four 3-D imaging datasets of the murine visual cortex at a spatial resolution of $0.7\,\mu\text{m}$. Our experiments show that the learning-based approach is able to significantly improve the segmentation compared to conventional Hessian-based methods. Features computed based on steerable filters prove to be superior to eigenfilter-based features for the considered datasets. We further demonstrate that random forests using oblique split directions outperform decision tree ensembles with univariate orthogonal splits.

Keywords: vessel segmentation, orthogonal subspace filtering, steerable filters, oblique random forest.

1 Introduction

Blood vessel enhancement and segmentation play a crucial role for numerous medically oriented applications and has attracted a lot of attention in the field of medical image processing. The multiscale nature of vessels, image noise and contrast inhomogeneities make it a challenging task. In this context, a large variety of methods have been developed exploiting photometric and structural properties of tubular structures. Extensive reviews on various state-of-the-art vessel segmentation techniques can be found in the literature [14,15]. Rather simple methods, e.g., absolute or locally adaptive thresholding, are in fact regularly used in practice due to their conceptual simplicity and computational efficiency but they are a serious source of error and require careful parameter selection [20,22]. More sophisticated segmentation techniques such as optimal filtering and Hessian-based approaches commonly rely on idealized appearance

---

[*] Supplementary material for this article is available at
http://www.vision.ee.ethz.ch/ReCoVa

B.H. Menze et al. (Eds.): MCV 2012, LNCS 7766, pp. 142–154, 2013.

and noise models. The former includes optimal edge detection [2], and steerable filters providing an elegant theory for computationally efficient ridge detection at arbitrary orientations [12,9]. The latter is based on the eigenanalysis of the Hessian capturing the second order structure of local intensity variations [4,24]. The Hessian is commonly computed by convolving the image patch with the partial second order derivatives of a Gaussian kernel as the method of choice for noise reduction and to tune the filter response to a specific vessel scale. This basic principle has already been used by Canny for edge and line detection [2]. The differential operators involved in the computation of the Hessian are well-posed concepts of linear scale-space theory [16]. Modeling vessels as elongated elliptical structures, the eigendecomposition of the Hessian has a geometric interpretation, which can be used to define a "vesselness" measure as a function of the eigenvalues [4,24]. Due to the multi-scale nature of vascular structures, Hessian-based filters are commonly applied at different scales. Besides, the eigenvector corresponding to the largest eigenvalue of the Hessian computed at the most discriminative scale is a good estimate for the local vessel direction. In practice, vesselness filters tend to be prone to noise and have difficulty in detecting vessel parts such as bifurcations not complying with the intrinsic idealized appearance model. Vesselness filters have also been successfully applied for global vessel segmentation in X-ray angiography using ridge tracking [26] and graph cut theory [10].

In this paper, we devise a machine learning approach for vessel segmentation based on the 2-D filament detection framework proposed by Gonzalez et al. [9] using steerable filters [5,12]. In our application, we aim at efficient classification of 3-D high-resolution imaging datasets ($> 10^{10}$ voxels) of the murine visual cortex (see Figure 1), which is of great interest for the analysis of the cerebrovascular system [22,11]. Due to the considerable computational challenge that comes with our application, we focus on a fast classification approach using local linear filters rather than complex non-local spatial models incorporating prior knowledge and regularization [26,10]. We compare different features computed from, respectively, orthogonal subspace filtering [17,23] and steerable filters using Gaussian derivatives [5,8]. In contrast to the framework proposed by Gonzalez et al. [9,8], we use oblique random forests (RF) for efficient classification We test "elastic net" node models that combine ℓ_1 and ℓ_2 regularization leading to sparser node models than the ℓ_2 regularized oblique splits proposed in [18].

2 Methods

In this section, we first introduce two different sets of features based on (1) orthogonal subspace filtering and (2) steerable filters computed at different scales and orientations in order to achieve rotational invariance. These features are then used to train an oblique random forest (RF) classifier that is well adapted to correlated feature responses from local image filters [18]. Different from standard discriminative learning algorithms such as support vector machines, RF classifiers return continuous probabilities when predicting vessel locations, which allows to choose an operating point by adapting the decision threshold. Moreover, RF is capable of coping with high dimensional feature vectors and tolerate false training labels. It is fast to train with only very few parameters to be optimized and even faster to apply. Efficient prediction becomes particularly important in view of our specific application using high-resolution image data at μm resolution.

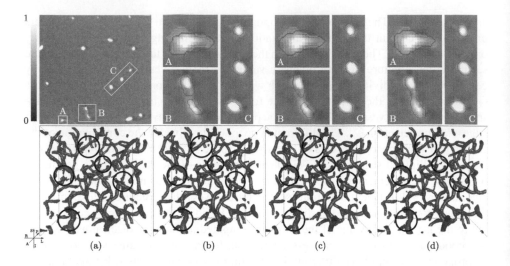

Fig. 1. Visualization of segmented cerebrovascular network for single axial slice (top) and whole 3-D test ROI (bottom) using different segmentation techniques. (a) Ground truth. (b) Frangi [4]. (c) RF-OSF ($d = 102$). (d) RF-SFT ($M = 4$). The binary segmentation maps are computed at the corresponding F_1-optimal operating points marked in Figure 4(b). The results are rendered in 3-D (bottom) and outlined in red (top) along with the ground-truth contours in blue for three subregions within the axial slice (A-C). Red contours in (a) mark the Otsu labels [20] used for RF training. Black circles in the 3-D plots highlight prominent differences in the segmentation. More results for the other datasets are provided in the supplementary material.

2.1 Orthogonal Subspace Filters (OSF)

Matched filters (MF) have widely been used in signal processing. They allow to detect a signal of known shape (template) by cross-correlation and perform provably optimal under additive Gaussian white noise conditions [19]. In terms of image processing, this corresponds to the convolution of the image with the MF. From a learning and classification perspective, matched filtering (signal detection) is closely related to linear regression for binary classification between background and pattern (vessel) [17]. Considering the image as a composition of local image patches with each pixel in the patch representing a feature, MF defines a 1-D linear subspace (regression coefficients) of this feature space which allows for separation of the pattern from background. Instead of an optimal 1-D subspace assuming linear separability in the feature space as implied by using a single matched filter, we use a less restrictive dimensionality reduction similar to [17], namely (linear) principal component analysis (PCA), in order to define a subspace of higher dimensionality. More formally, let $p_i \in \mathbb{R}^{P^3}$ denote a (cubic) image patch of size $P \times P \times P$. A d-dimensional subspace ($d \leq P^3$) capturing the most important modes of variation in the image patches can then be defined using PCA [13]:

$$\forall 1 \leq k \leq d \leq P^3 : \quad \boldsymbol{\alpha_k} \quad = \quad \underset{\substack{\boldsymbol{\alpha} \in \mathbb{R}^{P^3}, \ \|\boldsymbol{\alpha}\|=1, \\ \forall 1 \leq i < k: \ \text{cov}(\boldsymbol{\alpha_i}, \boldsymbol{\alpha})=0}}{\arg\max} \quad \text{var}(\boldsymbol{\alpha}^{\mathrm{T}} P_{\text{OSF}}) \quad , \tag{1}$$

where $P_{\text{OSF}} = [\boldsymbol{p_i}]_{1 \leq i \leq N_{\text{P}}} \in \mathbb{R}^{P^3 \times N_{\text{P}}}$ is the data matrix assembling N_{P} patches labeled as vessel. The principal axes $\boldsymbol{\alpha_k}$ form an orthonormal basis of the d-dimensional subspace and are ordered according to their preserved variance. They can be computed efficiently as the d eigenvectors corresponding to the largest eigenvalues of the covariance matrix of P_{OSF} after mean centering using singular value decomposition. Projecting an arbitrary image patch $\boldsymbol{p} \in \mathbb{R}^{P^3}$ onto the PCA subspace yields its d principal components (PC). The PCs of the image patches centered at pixels $\boldsymbol{x}$ in image I can thus be computed by d independent convolution operations of the image with each (properly reshaped) principal axis $\tilde{\boldsymbol{\alpha}}_k \in \mathbb{R}^{P \times P \times P}$:

$$\boldsymbol{f}_{\text{OSF}}(I, \boldsymbol{x}) = \left[(\tilde{\boldsymbol{\alpha}}_k * I)(\boldsymbol{x}) - \boldsymbol{\alpha}_k^{\mathrm{T}} \frac{1}{N_{\text{P}}} \sum_{i=1}^{N_{\text{P}}} \boldsymbol{p_i} \right]_{1 \leq k \leq d} \in \mathbb{R}^d \quad . \tag{2}$$

The (reshaped) principal axes will also be referred to as orthogonal subspace filters (OSF). The PCs, i.e., the OSF response of an image patch, are used as features along with a non-linear decision rule for vessel segmentation as described in Section 2.3.

2.2 Steerable Filter Templates (SFT)

The OSF eigenfilters learned from image patches as described in the previous section turn out to be highly structured (see Figure 2(a)). Instead of learning the structured filter kernels, we hence attempt to explicitly parametrize them. For this, we choose a steerable filter model based on Gaussian derivatives, which allows for efficient directional filtering at different scales and, most importantly, implicates rotational invariance [12]. Similar to [8], we define the filter templates as normalized derivatives of Gaussians up to order M [16]:

$$\forall \, m \geq 1 \, \wedge \, 0 \leq b \leq a \leq m \leq M : \ G^{\sigma}_{m,a,b}(\boldsymbol{x}) = \sigma^m \frac{\partial^{m-a} \partial^{a-b} \partial^b}{\partial_x^{m-a} \partial_y^{a-b} \partial_z^b} G^{\sigma}(\boldsymbol{x}) \quad , \tag{3}$$

where $G^{\sigma}(\boldsymbol{x}) = \frac{1}{(\sqrt{2\pi}\sigma)^3} \exp(-\frac{\|\boldsymbol{x}\|}{2\sigma^2})$ denotes the 3-D symmetric Gaussian kernel with variance σ and zero mean. As in Equation (2), each template induces a single feature by convolution with image I. They can be assembled to a feature vector of dimension $d_{\text{M}} = 1/6(M^3 + 6M^2 + 11M)$ at a fixed scale σ:

$$\boldsymbol{f}^{\sigma}(I, \boldsymbol{x}) = \left((G^{\sigma}_{1,0,0}, G^{\sigma}_{1,1,0}, G^{\sigma}_{1,1,1}, \dots, G^{\sigma}_{M,M,M})^{\mathrm{T}} * I \right)(\boldsymbol{x}) \in \mathbb{R}^{d_{\text{M}}} \quad . \tag{4}$$

We enhance the features by concatenating feature vectors at different scales $\sigma_1, \dots, \sigma_{\text{S}}$:

$$\boldsymbol{f}_{\text{SFT}}(I, \boldsymbol{x}) = \left(\boldsymbol{f}^{\sigma_1}(I, \boldsymbol{x}), \dots, \boldsymbol{f}^{\sigma_{\text{S}}}(I, \boldsymbol{x}) \right)^{\mathrm{T}} \in \mathbb{R}^{d_{\text{M}} S} \quad . \tag{5}$$

The steerability of Gaussian derivatives has been derived for the 2-D case in [12] and can readily be extended to 3-D [5,8]. Steerability refers to the property that the convolution of an image with a rotated version of the steerable filter template (SFT) can be expressed by a linear combination of the filter response of the image with the SFT without rotation:

$$I * G^{\sigma}_{m,a,b}(R\boldsymbol{x}) = \sum_{i=0}^{m} \sum_{j=0}^{i} \omega^{i,j}_{m,a,b} \underbrace{\left(I * G^{\sigma}_{m,i,j}\right)(\boldsymbol{x})}_{\boldsymbol{f}^{\sigma}_{m,i,j}(I,\boldsymbol{x})} \quad , \tag{6}$$

where $R \in SO(3)$ denotes a 3-D rotation matrix and $\omega^{i,j}_{m,a,b}$ the uniquely defined co-efficients that can be computed in closed form [12].[1] This formalism allows to efficiently evaluate the feature vector $\boldsymbol{f_{SFT}}$ for an arbitrary rotation without any additional costly convolution. We use a restricted set of rotations in our application considering the tubular structure of vessels. The local vessel direction $\boldsymbol{d} = (d_x, d_y, d_z)^T \in \mathbb{R}^3$, $\|\boldsymbol{d}\| = 1$ can be parametrized using spherical coordinates (θ, ϕ) with unit radius, elevation $\theta = \arctan\left(d_z / \sqrt{d_x^2 + d_y^2}\right)$, and azimuth $\phi = \arctan(d_y / d_x)$ relative to the x-y plane ($z = 0$). It is sufficient to restrict the parametrization to the positive hemisphere ($z > 0$), i.e., $0 \le \theta \le \pi/2$ and $-\pi < \phi \le \pi$. The vessel can then be transformed to the normalized pose $\boldsymbol{d_0} = (1, 0, 0)^T$ by applying the rotation matrix

$$R_{\theta,\phi} = \begin{pmatrix} \cos\theta\cos\phi & \cos\theta\sin\phi & \sin\theta \\ -\sin\phi & \cos\phi & 0 \\ -\sin\theta\cos\phi & -\sin\theta\sin\phi & \cos\theta \end{pmatrix} \quad . \tag{7}$$

The SFT features evaluated for this rotation according to Equation (6) hence describe the intensity variation characteristics of different order along the vascular structure as well as in the orthogonal plane. Assuming a symmetric vessel (intensity) profile perpendicular to the local vessel direction $\boldsymbol{d}$, restricting the set of rotations is reasonable as the vessel appearance is (locally) invariant under rotation about $\boldsymbol{d}$.

2.3   Vessel Classification - Shape Learning and Prediction

The OSF and SFT features as defined in Equations (2) and (5), respectively, are each used along with a non-linear decision rule for vessel segmentation. We train separate classifiers for the different feature types as follows: A representative set S of $2N_S$ tuples (image I_k, location $\boldsymbol{x_k}$, vessel orientation $\boldsymbol{d_k}$, class label y_k) is randomly sampled from a labeled set of images corresponding to N_S foreground ($y_k = 1$) and background ($y_k = -1$) samples, respectively: $S = \{(I_k, \boldsymbol{x_k}, \boldsymbol{d_k}, y_k) \mid 1 \le k \le 2N_S\}$. For these samples, the features $\boldsymbol{f}(I, \boldsymbol{x})$ can be extracted as defined in Equations (2) and (5). The SFT features are additionally rotated to the normalized orientation according to Equations (6) and (7) w.r.t. the local vessel direction $\boldsymbol{d}$. This defines the training set $\mathcal{T} = \{(\boldsymbol{f_k} = \boldsymbol{f}(I_k, \boldsymbol{x_k}), y_k) \mid 1 \le k \le 2N_S\}$ that is ultimately used to train a random forest (RF) classifier [1]. RF consists of an ensemble of decision trees used to model the posterior probability of each class (vessel/background). During training, each tree is fully grown from bootstrapped datasets using stochastic discrimination. For this, the data is split at each tree node by a hyperplane in the feature (sub-)space. In contrast to traditional bagging, the split is based on a small number of randomly selected

---

[1] Further details are provided in the supplementary material.

features only. We investigated both "orthogonal" and "oblique" trees. As proposed in Breiman's original paper [1], the former is based on optimal thresholds for randomly selected single features in every split, i.e., mutually orthogonal 1-D hyperplanes. The latter uses multidimensional hyperplanes to separate the feature space, e.g., by choosing randomly oriented hyperplanes [1] or applying linear discriminative models [18]. For the oblique RFs in this work, we employ a linear regression with an elastic net penalty [6] in order to learn multivariate (optimal) split directions w at each node:

$$\hat{w} = \underset{w \in \mathbb{R}^{N_F}}{\arg\min} \frac{1}{2|\mathcal{T}|} \sum_{k=1}^{|\mathcal{T}|} \left(y_k - w^T \tilde{f}_k\right)^2 + \lambda P_\alpha(w) \quad , \tag{8}$$

where $\tilde{f}_k \in \mathbb{R}^{N_F}$ are randomly selected (but fixed) features and $\lambda > 0$ is the regularization parameter for the elastic net penalty $P_\alpha(w) = (1 - \alpha)\frac{1}{2}\|w\|_{\ell_2}^2 + \alpha\|w\|_{\ell_1}$ as a compromise between the ridge regression ($\alpha = 0$) and the lasso penalty ($\alpha = 1$), where $\|\cdot\|_{\ell_1}$ and $\|\cdot\|_{\ell_2}$ denote the ℓ_1 and ℓ_2-norm, respectively. The advantage is joint regularization of the coefficients and sparsity — coefficients are both encouraged to be small, and to be zero if they are very small. The latter lasso property reduces the dimensionality of the split space, which is desirable for memory and robustness purposes. With $\alpha = 1$ (and $\lambda \gg 0$) we will get a single non-zero coefficient, i.e., RF with univariate splits, whereas choosing $\alpha = 0$ we have ridge regression as in [18].

The decision trees are grown separately as follows:

1. For each tree, a new set of samples is randomly drawn from the training data $\mathcal{T}$ with replacement, i.e., $\frac{2}{3}|\mathcal{T}|$ bootstrapped samples.
2. For every node, N_F features are randomly sampled without replacement from the feature pool of size $N_F^0 = d$ for OSF features and $N_F^0 = d_M S$ for SFT features, respectively (see Equations (2) and (4)).
3. The selected features of the bootstrapped samples are normalized to zero mean and unit variance at every split in order to enhance the stability of the linear model.
4. Finding optimal split
   a) Orthogonal split ($N_F = 1$): The feature values of all samples are tested as threshold to split the data w.r.t. the selected feature.
   b) Oblique split ($N_F = \lceil\sqrt{N_F^0}\rceil$): The optimal split direction is computed according to Equation (8) for $\alpha = 0.5$ using covariance updates [6].
5. Steps $2-4$ are repeated $\lceil\sqrt{N_F^0}\rceil$ times. The optimal split and threshold are ultimately selected w.r.t. the information gain as a result of the split. The samples are split accordingly and passed on to the child nodes.
6. For each of the N_T trees, steps $2-5$ are repeated until (1) all samples in a (leaf) node belong to the same class, (2) the maximum tree depth has been reached, or (3) there are too few samples to further split the data (avoid excessive overfitting).
7. Each leaf node is assigned a class label according to the majority vote of the training samples ending up in the considered leaf.

Previously unseen samples (images) can be classified by pushing the extracted features down all N_T decision trees of the ensemble. Thus, each tree assigns a class label

$\hat{y}_i \in \{0, 1\}$ associated with the leaf node in which the tested sample ends up. The ensemble confidence can then be defined as $\frac{1}{N_\mathrm{T}} \sum_{i=1}^{N_\mathrm{T}} \hat{y}_i$ as an estimate of the posterior. The binary class label $\hat{y}$ can finally be assigned using a majority vote or any other decision threshold.

In the case of OSF features, a single RF is trained for all vessel orientations. Therefore, the intrinsic orientation-induced structure in the OSF feature space has to be captured in the training set both for RF training and learning the OSF eigenfilters. In contrast, SFT features allow for explicit parametrization of the orientation. The expected filter response for an arbitrary orientation can efficiently be computed from the set of stationary base features f_SFT as defined in Equations (5) and (6). As the corresponding RF classifiers are trained on SFT features extracted from vessels with normalized orientation only, we sample the space of possible vessel orientations (half sphere) and compute the corresponding (rotated) SFT features in order to build an orientation independent predictor. The classification result with the maximum confidence is ultimately assigned as proposed in [9]. In contrast to OSF features, this allows to not only estimate the class posteriors but also a probability distribution on the vessel orientation.

3   Experiments

We have evaluated the performance of our method on four 3-D datasets $\mathcal{D}_{1-4}$ obtained from synchrotron radiation X-ray tomographic microscopy (srXTM) of cylindrical samples of the murine somatosensory cortex (volume size $2048\,\mathrm{px} \times 2048\,\mathrm{px} \times 4000\,\mathrm{px}$, isotropic voxel spacing $0.7\,\mathrm{\mu m}$, grayscale 16 bit) [22]. In a preprocessing step we applied anisotropic diffusion filtering in order to reduce image noise while preserving edge contrast [21]. From each (preprocessed) dataset we extracted two disjoint regions of interest (ROI) of size $(256\,\mathrm{px})^3$ for training and testing, respectively. In the following, we will refer to these non-overlapping ROIs as test and train data/ROI, respectively (see Figure 1(a)). For each test ROI, ground truth labels were manually generated by an expert assisted by a semi-automatic segmentation tool [27] on 15 evenly distributed slices along each reference direction (axial, coronal, sagittal). Thus, 125 slices have been labeled containing 7.3×10^4 foreground and 2.7×10^6 background labels in average ($\pm 3.9 \times 10^4$) corresponding to a vascular volume fraction of $2.6 \pm 1.4\,\%$.

In a first baseline experiment, all ROIs were segmented using both Otsu's method [20] and multiscale vessel enhancement filtering [4,24]. For the latter, we have performed an exhaustive grid search to optimize the vesselness scale on the test ROIs w.r.t. maximum area under the ROC curve using the ground-truth labels of the test ROIs. In the majority of the cases five logarithmically spaced scales performed best for both Frangi's and Sato's vesselness: $\sigma \in \{2.00, 3.09, 4.76, 7.35, 11.33\}\,[\mathrm{px}]$.

In a next step, we computed the OSF eigenfilters introduced in Section 2.1 from 3000 randomly sampled patches centered at voxels labeled as vessel in the Otsu label map. In particular, background patches were not considered during OSF learning. Besides the original vessel patches, five randomly rotated versions of each patch have been added to the set of patches P_OSF used in Equation (1) in order to account for rotational symmetry of vessel structures while keeping the total number of patches at a moderate level ($N_\mathrm{P} = 1.8 \times 10^4$). As in [17], the OSF patch size P was assessed from the random forest feature importance and set to $P = 19$.

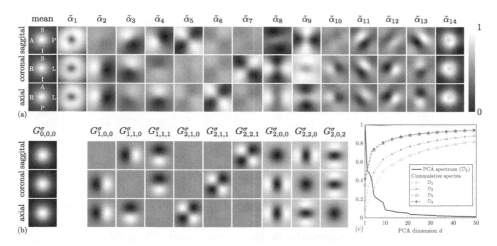

Fig. 2. (a) Visualization of the mean pattern and the most significant (reshaped) eigenfilters $\tilde{\alpha}_k$ along centered sagittal, coronal, and axial slices as learned from dataset $\mathcal{D}_2$ ($P = 19$). (b) Normalized Gaussian derivatives $G^{\sigma}_{m,a,b}$ at a fixed scale σ up to order $M = 2$ as defined in Equation (3). (c) Normalized PCA spectrum λ_k / λ_1 and variance preservation as measured by the cumulative spectrum $\sum_{k=1}^{d} \lambda_k / \sum_{k=1}^{P^3} \lambda_k$ for different datasets, where λ_k denotes the k-th eigenvalue of the data covariance matrix.

As for the SFT model, we performed a small parameter study to optimize the SFT scales similar to the multiscale vesselness parameters. In order to avoid overfitting, however, we used the train ROIs for the parameter optimization along with the Otsu labels considered as ground truth in this case. We ultimately select $S = 3$ logarithmically spaced scales $\sigma \in \{2.00, 3.65, 6.67\}$. The SFT model hence defines $d_{\mathrm{M}} S = 9$ (27, 57, 102) features for maximum Gaussian derivative order $M = 1$ (2, 3, 4), respectively (see Equations (4) and (5)). For a fair comparison of the SFT and OSF feature models, the PCA subspace dimension d of the OSF models, i.e., the number of OSF features, was chosen accordingly.

Different RF classifiers consisting of $N_{\mathrm{T}} = 256$ decision trees have been trained separately on the train ROI of a single dataset using OSF and SFT features along with orthogonal and oblique splits, respectively, as explained in Section 2.3. The training was repeated for each dataset using $N_{\mathrm{S}} = 4000$ foreground (vessel) and background samples, respectively, randomly drawn from the Otsu label map. The local vessel direction was estimated from the eigenanalysis of the Hessian computed at the most discriminative scale as defined by Frangi's multiscale vesselness [4]. Note that the training labels were computed fully automatically without any user interaction. The manually annotated ground-truth labels have been used for RF validation only.

Finally, the different RF models were applied to the test ROIs of each dataset. The classification performance was evaluated on the uniformly aligned slices with ground-truth labels available (see above). In this way, the generalization of the individual

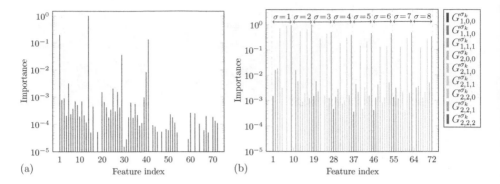

Fig. 3. Variable importance [1] of the (a) RF-OSF model ($P = 19$, $d = 57$) and (b) RF-SFT model ($M = 2$, $d_M = 9$, $S = 8$ scales $\sigma \in \{1, \ldots, 8\}$) on a logarithmic scale (oblique splits). The prominent peaks in (b) correspond to the Gaussian derivatives $G^\sigma_{2,0,0}$, $G^\sigma_{2,2,0}$, and $G^\sigma_{2,2,2}$.

classifiers is investigated (test ROIs of datasets not used for training) as well as the prediction quality for unseen samples from the dataset used for training (train ROI) but from a different subvolume (test ROI).

4 Results and Discussion

The learned OSF filter templates are highly structured (see Figure 2(a)). The ball-shaped mean shows a Gaussian-like pattern. The most significant principal axis captures the average image intensity in the vicinity of the sample. Patches $\alpha_2, \ldots, \alpha_4$ capture first order derivatives along the right-left (R-L), superior-inferior (S-I), and anterior-posterior (A-P) direction, respectively. Similar first-order patterns at a smaller scale appear in $\alpha_{10}, \ldots, \alpha_{13}$. Differently oriented second order derivatives are described by $\alpha_5, \ldots, \alpha_9$. The corresponding PCA spectra show a sharp profile as indicated in Figure 2(c). These observations can be made for all OSF models regardless of the considered patch size. For comparison of the structural similarities, the parameterized Gaussian derivatives up to order $M = 2$ as used for the SFT feature extraction are shown in Figure 2(b).

The normalized RF feature relevance score, i.e., the permutation importance from [1], for the RF-OSF and RF-SFT model using oblique splits are shown in Figure 3. The OSF patches describing the average image intensity in the local neighborhood (α_1, α_{14}) show high variable importance as compared to the patches capturing higher order derivatives $\alpha_2, \ldots, \alpha_{13}$. It also becomes clear that the OSF feature importance (discrimination capability) is not correlated to the PCA spectrum (variance preservation). This makes it difficult to choose a proper cutoff for the PCA subspace dimension. The variable importance of the SFT features indicates that the second order derivatives parallel and orthogonal to the vessel direction ($G^\sigma_{2,0,0}$, $G^\sigma_{2,2,0}$, $G^\sigma_{2,2,2}$) are most significant for the classification. Note that the Hessian-based segmentation approaches also rely on these features [4,24]. For larger scales σ, the importance values tend to decline.

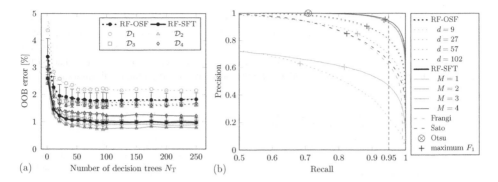

Fig. 4. Comparison of the classification performance. (a) Out of bag (OOB) error of the RF-OSF ($d = 102$) and RF-SFT ($M = 4$, $d_M = 34$) classifiers trained on dataset $\mathcal{D}_k$ for varying number of trees N_T (oblique splits). The average error is plotted in black with error bars indicating the standard deviation. (b) Precision-recall curves (PRC) and optimal operating points w.r.t. F_1 measure for RF-OSF and RF-SFT models ($N_T = 256$, oblique splits, trained on $\mathcal{D}_2$) with varying parameters d and M, respectively, in comparison to (optimized) Frangi's/Sato's vesselness, and Otsu thresholding [20] evaluated on test ROI of $\mathcal{D}_2$.

Figure 4(a) visualizes the out of bag (OOB) error of the RF-OSF and RF-SFT classifiers for different number of decision trees N_T. In both cases the OOB error declines rapidly for increasing N_T. The SFT model consistently shows smaller error rates compared to the OSF features. Moreover, the RF-SFT classifier is more robust across different datasets as indicated by the smaller standard deviation. Also note that the absolute values of the OOB error estimates may be somewhat overoptimistic due to the spatial correlation between the training samples.

Comparing the overall classification performance of the proposed learning-based approaches with different model parameters to standard segmentation approaches reveals the superior performance of the SFT features as indicated by the precision-recall curves (PRC) in Figure 4(b). The RF-based segmentation outperforms Frangi's/Sato's vesselness filters even for a small number of features ($d = 27$, $M = 2$). Note that the reported results for the vesselness-based segmentation have to be considered as upper bound as the scale parameters have been optimized on the test data (overfitting). The analysis also shows that for $M > 1$ the performance of the RF-SFT model hardly changes anymore, which is consistent with the observation of the second order derivatives being the most discriminative features (see Figure 3(d)).

A more detailed numerical analysis of the classification performance of the different approaches is summarized in Table 1 and confirms the superior performance of the RF-SFT model over the OSF features and the multiscale vesselness filters. Otsu's method [20] tends to underestimate the global threshold and hence results in an inaccurate segmentation of the vessel boundaries as indicated by the increased balanced error rate [3]. In order to assess the robustness of the learning-based segmentation approaches, we apply "intra-dataset" and "inter-dataset" cross-validation, i.e., choosing the (non-overlapping) train and test ROIs from the same (intra) or different (inter) datasets, respectively. The average segmentation performance for "totally" unseen data

Table 1. Detailed evaluation of classification performance of different RF-OSF ($d = 102$) and RF-SFT ($M = 4$, $d_M = 34$) classifiers ($N_T = 256$) using orthogonal and oblique splits, respectively. The performance is evaluated using "intra-dataset" and "inter-dataset" cross-validation (see text). The operating point was selected at the 95 % recall level (see Figure 4(b)). The partial area under the precision-recall curve (AUC-PR) has been computed on the recall interval $[0.5, 1]$.

	Method	Validation	Precision [%]	Specificity [%]	Error Rate [%]	AUC-PR [×10⁻²]	OOB Error [%]	Tree Depth
orthogonal	RF-OSF	intra-data	74.32 ± 7.26	99.20 ± 0.13	2.92 ± 0.06	45.29 ± 1.74	2.02 ± 0.44	9.02 ± 0.45
		inter-data	70.99 ± 7.55	98.97 ± 0.62	3.06 ± 0.33	44.35 ± 2.09		
	RF-SFT	intra-data	89.43 ± 1.19	99.70 ± 0.14	2.70 ± 0.09	48.35 ± 0.20	1.35 ± 0.22	7.42 ± 0.38
		inter-data	88.25 ± 2.05	99.67 ± 0.14	2.70 ± 0.07	48.13 ± 0.41		
oblique	RF-OSF	intra-data	78.96 ± 5.81	99.37 ± 0.16	2.84 ± 0.07	46.38 ± 1.19	1.82 ± 0.25	6.26 ± 0.21
		inter-data	78.35 ± 4.39	99.33 ± 0.26	2.87 ± 0.15	45.95 ± 1.15		
	RF-SFT	intra-data	93.53 ± 1.47	99.83 ± 0.07	2.62 ± 0.05	48.96 ± 0.22	0.96 ± 0.19	5.85 ± 0.24
		inter-data	92.80 ± 1.94	99.82 ± 0.06	2.62 ± 0.03	48.84 ± 0.31		
	Sato	average	62.15 ± 2.71	98.46 ± 0.75	3.27 ± 0.37	42.34 ± 0.64	n/a	n/a
	Frangi	average	59.61 ± 2.09	98.26 ± 0.90	3.37 ± 0.45	41.66 ± 0.53	n/a	n/a
	Otsu	average	99.96 ± 0.03	100.00 ± 0.00	14.59 ± 1.38	n/a	n/a	n/a

(inter-dataset) slightly decreases compared to the (still unseen) test data in the case of intra-dataset validation. The figures also reveal that oblique splits, as compared to orthogonal splits, yield both better classification performance and smaller (average) tree depth. The advantage of oblique over orthogonal splits may result from the highly correlated features [18]. Further experiments would be required to investigate the influence of the elastic net penalty of Equation (8) in more detail.

Figure 1 compares the binary segmentation of the cerebrovascular networks for the different approaches applied to the test data $\mathcal{D}_2$ using the F_1-optimal operating points marked in Figure 4(b). Visually, the Frangi filter and partly also the RF-OSF model generate very smooth networks missing some of the details on the vessel surface. The ideal elliptical appearance model underlying the Hessian-based vesselness filters produces many false negatives at bifurcations, in particular, where the model assumptions do not hold. Here the classification approach is able to consider more complex geometries, that are in accordance with higher order filter responses in the training data. As already indicated by the precision-recall analysis, the axial views reveal that the Frangi segmentation varies significantly from the ground-truth labels in many cases, whereas the RF-OSF and especially the RF-SFT results are in much better agreement to the reference segmentation.

5   Conclusions and Future Work

We have compared two kinds of features for 3-D vessel segmentation using a machine learning approach. Starting from orthogonal subspace filtering, we learn an orthogonal basis from vessel patches to describe the local vessel appearance in a low-dimensional feature space. In a second step, we parametrize and approximate the highly structured base filters by Gaussian derivatives, which allows to efficiently decompose the image into a multiscale rotational basis using steerable filter theory [12,8]. Both kinds of features are used to train random forest classifiers for vessel segmentation. The steerable filters in fact allow to train a single classifier on normalized (canonically oriented) vessel samples as proposed in [9] for 2-D filament detection. Our experiments on 3-D high-resolution srXTM imaging data of the murine visual cortex demonstrate that the steerable filter features outperform the orthogonal subspace features. Moreover, the machine learning approach proves to be superior to Hessian-based segmentation approaches, especially for vessel structures, such as bifurcations, that cannot easily be modeled explicitly and violate the common cylindrical appearance assumption. The RF classifiers show excellent classification performance on the 3-D datasets even for imperfect and incomplete training data as obtained by Otsu's method in our experiments. The proposed segmentation framework hence allows to fully automatically learn RF models for 3-D vessel segmentation on new datasets.

The choice of the type of splits to be used in the decision tree ensembles of the RF classifier turned out to have a major impact on the classification performance. For our task, oblique splits using linear regression are clearly favorable over univariate orthogonal splits. Besides a more comprehensive study on the choice of the elastic net penalty, it would be interesting to investigate if more complex information such as vessel caliber or centerline can be learned and predicted in a general and computationally cheap fashion on different types of 3-D angiographic datasets by extending the framework using Hough forests [7]. These additional data on the vessel morphology and topology may allow to ultimately reconstruct physiologically consistent full-fledged cerebrovascular networks possibly in combination with proper methods to replace or extend missing or faulty regions by synthetic vasculatures [25] in order to overcome shortcomings of the reconstruction technique or limitations of the imaging modality.

Acknowledgements. This work has been funded by the Swiss National Center of Competence in Research on Computer Aided and Image Guided Medical Interventions (NCCR Co-Me) supported by the Swiss National Science Foundation.

References

1. Breiman, L.: Random forests. Mach. Learn. 45, 5–32 (2001)
2. Canny, J.: Finding edges and lines in images. Tech. rep., Massachusetts Institute of Technology, Cambridge, MA, USA (1983)
3. Chen, Y.W., Lin, C.J.: Combining SVMs with various feature selection strategies. In: Guyon, I., Nikravesh, M., Gunn, S., Zadeh, L. (eds.) Feature Extraction. STUDFUZZ, vol. 207, pp. 315–324. Springer, Heidelberg (2006)
4. Frangi, A.F., Niessen, W.J., Vincken, K.L., Viergever, M.A.: Multiscale Vessel Enhancement Filtering. In: Wells, W.M., Colchester, A.C.F., Delp, S.L. (eds.) MICCAI 1998. LNCS, vol. 1496, pp. 130–137. Springer, Heidelberg (1998)
5. Freeman, W.T., Adelson, E.H.: The design and use of steerable filters. IEEE Trans. Pattern Anal. Mach. Intell. 13(9), 891–906 (1991)
6. Friedman, J.H., Hastie, T., Tibshirani, R.: Regularization paths for generalized linear models via coordinate descent. J. Stat. Softw. 33(1), 1–22 (2010)
7. Gall, J., Yao, A., Razavi, N., Van Gool, L., Lempitsky, V.: Hough forests for object detection, tracking, and action recognition. IEEE Trans. Pattern Anal. Mach. Intell. 33(11), 2188–2202 (2011)
8. González, G., Aguet, F., Fleuret, F., Unser, M., Fua, P.: Steerable Features for Statistical 3D Dendrite Detection. In: Yang, G.-Z., Hawkes, D., Rueckert, D., Noble, A., Taylor, C. (eds.) MICCAI 2009, Part II. LNCS, vol. 5762, pp. 625–632. Springer, Heidelberg (2009)

9. González, G., Fleurety, F., Fua, P.: Learning rotational features for filament detection. In: CVPR 2009, pp. 1582–1589 (June 2009)
10. Hernández-Vela, A., Gatta, C., Escalera, S., Igual, L., Martin-Yuste, V., Radeva, P.: Accurate and Robust Fully-Automatic QCA: Method and Numerical Validation. In: Fichtinger, G., Martel, A., Peters, T. (eds.) MICCAI 2011, Part III. LNCS, vol. 6893, pp. 496–503. Springer, Heidelberg (2011)
11. Hirsch, S., Reichold, J., Schneider, M., Székely, G., Weber, B.: Topology and hemodynamics of the cortical cerebrovascular system. J. Cereb. Blood Flow Metab (April 2012)
12. Jacob, M., Unser, M.: Design of steerable filters for feature detection using canny-like criteria. IEEE Trans. Pattern Anal. Mach. Intell. 26(8), 1007–1019 (2004)
13. Jolliffe, I.T.: Principal Component Analysis, 2nd edn. Springer (2002)
14. Kirbas, C., Quek, F.: A review of vessel extraction techniques and algorithms. ACM Comput. Surv. 36, 81–121 (2004)
15. Lesage, D., Angelini, E.D., Bloch, I., Funka-Lea, G.: A review of 3D vessel lumen segmentation techniques: models, features and extraction schemes. Med. Image Anal. 13(6), 819–845 (2009)
16. Lindeberg, T.: Edge detection and ridge detection with automatic scale selection. Int.J. Comput. Vis. 30, 465–470 (1996)
17. Menze, B.H., Kelm, B.M., Hamprecht, F.A.: From eigenspots to fisherspots - latent spaces in the nonlinear detection of spot patterns in a highly varying background. In: Decker, R., Lenz, H.J. (eds.) Advances in Data Analysis. Studies in Classification, Data Analysis, and Knowledge Organization., vol. 33, pp. 255–262. Springer (2006)
18. Menze, B.H., Kelm, B.M., Splitthoff, D.N., Koethe, U., Hamprecht, F.A.: On Oblique Random Forests. In: Gunopulos, D., Hofmann, T., Malerba, D., Vazirgiannis, M. (eds.) ECML PKDD 2011, Part II. LNCS, vol. 6912, pp. 453–469. Springer, Heidelberg (2011)
19. Moon, T., Stirling, W.: Mathematical methods and algorithms for signal processing. Prentice Hall (2000)
20. Otsu, N.: A threshold selection method from gray-level histograms. IEEE T. Syst. Man Cyb. 9(1), 62–66 (1979)
21. Perona, P., Malik, J.: Scale-space and edge detection using anisotropic diffusion. IEEE Trans. Pattern Anal. Mach. Intell. 12, 629–639 (1990)
22. Reichold, J., Stampanoni, M., Keller, A.L., Buck, A., Jenny, P., Weber, B.: Vascular graph model to simulate the cerebral blood flow in realistic vascular networks. J. Cereb. Blood Flow Metab. 29(8), 1429–1443 (2009)
23. Rigamonti, R., Türetken, E., González Serrano, G., Fua, P., Lepetit, V.: Filter learning for linear structure segmentation. Tech. rep., Swiss Federal Institute of Technology, Lausanne (EPFL) (2011)
24. Sato, Y., Nakajima, S., Atsumi, H., Koller, T., Gerig, G., Yoshida, S., Kikinis, R.: 3D Multi-Scale Line Filter for Segmentation and Visualization of Curvilinear Structures in Medical Images. In: Troccaz, J., Mösges, R., Grimson, W.E.L. (eds.) CVRMed-MRCAS 1997. LNCS, vol. 1205, pp. 213–222. Springer, Heidelberg (1997)
25. Schneider, M., Hirsch, S., Weber, B., Székely, G.: Physiologically Based Construction of Optimized 3-D Arterial Tree Models. In: Fichtinger, G., Martel, A., Peters, T. (eds.) MICCAI 2011, Part I. LNCS, vol. 6891, pp. 404–411. Springer, Heidelberg (2011)
26. Schneider, M., Sundar, H.: Automatic global vessel segmentation and catheter removal using local geometry information and vector field integration. In: ISBI 2010, pp. 45–48 (April 2010)
27. Yushkevich, P.A., Piven, J., Hazlett, H.C., Smith, R.G., Ho, S., Gee, J.C., Gerig, G.: User-guided 3D active contour segmentation of anatomical structures: Significantly improved efficiency and reliability. NeuroImage 31(3), 1116–1128 (2006),
http://www.itksnap.org

Pipeline for Tracking Neural Progenitor Cells

Jacob S. Vestergaard[1], Anders L. Dahl[1], Peter Holm[2], and Rasmus Larsen[1]

[1] Department of Informatics and Mathematical Modelling,
Technical University of Denmark
[2] Department of Basic Animal and Veterinary Sciences, Faculty of Life Sciences,
Copenhagen University

Abstract. Automated methods for neural stem cell lineage construction become increasingly important due to the large amount of data produced from time lapse imagery of *in vitro* cell growth experiments. Segmentation algorithms with the ability to adapt to the problem at hand and robust tracking methods play a key role in constructing these lineages. We present here a tracking pipeline based on learning a dictionary of discriminative image patches for segmentation and a graph formulation of the cell matching problem incorporating topology changes and acknowledging the fact that segmentation errors do occur. A matched filter for detection of mitotic candidates is constructed to ensure that cell division is only allowed in the model when relevant. Potentially the combination of these robust methods can simplify the initiation of cell lineage construction and extraction of statistics.

1 Introduction

Tracking of neural stem cells (NSCs) is fundamental in understanding the causes for cell fate outcomes in *in vitro* cell growth experiments. Previous studies of stem cells have used manually constructed cell lineages of a limited population to analyze, e.g., the developmental potential [7] or the morphological properties during cell division [5] and clearly show the benefit and importance of cell lineage construction. The development of automated methods for cell lineage construction is a key ingredient in processing large amounts of time lapse imagery and extracting meaningful statistics, previously not possible due to the need for extensive manual interaction.

We present a data driven pipeline for tracking pig neural progenitor cells in phase microscopy time lapse imagery using a supervised segmentation method, accommodating for small imprecisions in the manual annotation, and a completely data driven approach to tracking cells between time points. This pipeline enables for segmentation and tracking thousands of cells from a manual annotation of only 288 cells. The contribution includes novel approaches to mitosis detection, automatic correction of segmentation errors and data driven parameter estimation for the cell matching cost function.

The proposed mitosis detector is based on the observation that a NSC about to undergo mitosis becomes circular and moves out of focus of the imaging device,

B.H. Menze et al. (Eds.): MCV 2012, LNCS 7766, pp. 155–164, 2013.

making it easily detectable. A similar behavior is observed by [5] for human neural progenitor cells.

Previously, systems aiming to accomplish the same have been proposed, including LEVER [8] incorporating published methods for segmentation and lineaging [1,2]. A limitation by this and other systems is the sensitivity to image data with a slightly different appearance. We explore the possibilities of overcoming this limitation by driving the analysis by simple manual annotation of the image data. This allows the segmentation algorithm to adapt to the problem at hand.

Manual annotation of neural progenitor cells are tedious and difficult even for an expert. A single image cannot be annotated without preceding and following images from the time series. The inherent inaccuracy in these annotations are accommodated for by the choice of segmentation algorithm, namely dictionary learning from image patches. This method exploits the property that the textural appearance of neural progenitor cells can be condensed to a number of typical image patches.

Tracking of the cells during the time lapse image sequence is reduced to match the cells between two time frames. This is accomplished by a modification of the bipartite graph formulation of the matching problem proposed by [6]. The modifications introduced are 1) restricting topology changes to ensure cell division occur during cell mitosis and 2) acknowledging that segmentation errors *are* present and minimizing their disruptions to the cell lineage construction.

The methods applied have been chosen based on the problems arising from analysis of an approximately 83 hours time lapse image sequence with 5 minutes between acquisitions. This sequence consists of 1000 phase contrast microscopy images of neural progenitor cells with very irregular shapes and movement patterns. An example of such an image can be seen in Figure 1a. In the following sections the methodology embedded in the proposed pipeline is outlined and results are reported.

2   Dictionary Learning for Robust Segmentation

The cell segmentation is based on a trained dictionary of image and label patches [3]. Each intensity patch in the dictionary has a corresponding label patch. The dictionary is build from manually annotated image exemplars by randomly sampling a set of intensity patches with corresponding label patches. In the training phase the aim is to find a dictionary that well represents the image texture and simultaneously have unique label patches. The label patches have the same spatial resolution as the intensity patches and in each pixel they store the probability of the labels in the training set. A label patch that has high probability for one class and low for other classes in each pixel is considered unique. To optimize the dictionary a weighted k-means procedure is employed where weights are updated in each step based on the uniqueness criterion.

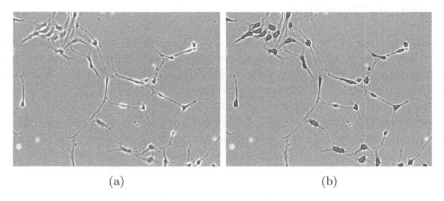

(a)   (b)

Fig. 1. a) Phase contrast microscopy image approximately 17 hours into the timeseries. b) Manual annotation (red) together with learned dictionary segmentation (blue) overlaid image.

Segmentation of an unknown image is computed using the trained dictionary. For each pixel an image patch is extracted and the label patch corresponding to the closest match in the intensity dictionary is assigned. The patches are overlapping, so the obtained probabilities are averaged.

In this experiment we chose the parameters for the segmentation based on a training and a test set. We had 15 manually annotated image where 8 were used for training and 7 were used for test. Our initial experiments suggested that we needed relatively large image patches, so we chose to downscale the images to half the size giving a spatial resolution of 300×400. The results of our experiments are shown in Table 1. Dice's coefficient denotes how well the segmentation captures the area and the ratio reported is the number of cells detected versus the number manually annotated. Thus a value above one is over segmentation and below one is under segmentation. The performance improves slightly going from a patch size of 7 to 9 but only little improvement is obtained by going from 9 to 11. We chose 9 as a good tradeoff between segmentation performance and computation time. It should be noted that it is a difficult task to manually annotate these images, so the results should be seen together with visual inspection of the segmentations as shown in Figure 1.

Table 1. Segmentation results obtained by varying patch sizes

	Training			Test		
Patch size	7	9	11	7	9	11
Dice's coefficient	0.80	0.81	0.81	0.78	0.79	0.80
$N_{\text{detected}}/N_{\text{true}}$	1.13	1.05	0.96	1.25	1.12	1.02

3   Mitosis Detection

Visual inspection of the time lapse imagery revealed that when a neural progenitor cell is about to undergo mitosis, it separates itself from the gel in the petri dish, floating up a bit and out of focus. When a cell is out of focus it has a very distinct pattern due to the imaging process.

This pattern can be derived analytically [10], but requires knowledge of the internal microscope parameters, which have not been available in this case. Therefore a model has been constructed from an image containing the pattern of interest. The image and extracted sample is shown in Figures 2a–b.

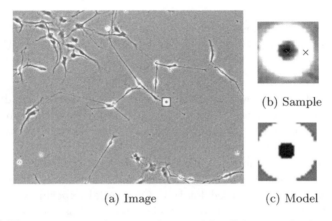

(a) Image   (c) Model

(b) Sample

Fig. 2. a) Phase contrast microscopy image with cell in pre-mitotic stage. b) Sample of out-of-focus cell extracted from phase contrast image. Intensity values are extracted from the marked points to transfer the contrast between the halo, center and background to the model. c) Constructed model.

The model is constructed by initializing an image of size 27×27, which is approximately the same size as the sample. The donut-like center of the sample is modeled by a 27×27 disk filter, where the hole in the donut is a 7×7 disk. The intensity values in these three regions are extracted from the sample as marked in Figure 2b. The resulting filter h, shown in Figure 2c is normalized by the maximum response from a convolution of the constructed model $\hat{h}$ with the sample S , such that $h_i = \frac{\hat{h}_i}{\max\{\hat{h}*S\}}$, $i \in \{1, \ldots, 27^2\}$ whereby subsequent filtering can be interpreted as "percentage of perfect response".

The constructed model is used for matched filtering of every phase contrast image. Connected components with a response above 0.9 and an eccentricity below 0.6 is marked as a mitotic candidate. The eccentricity is here the ratio of the distance between the foci of the ellipse and its major axis length. Examples of these detections can be seen in Figure 3.

This detector enables the tracking pipeline to detect and handle cell mitosis, which will be described in Section 4.

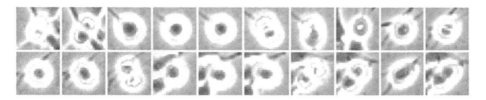

Fig. 3. 20 examples of detected mitotic candidates using the constructed model

4   Tracking

Finding the best match for each cell between two time points is needed to construct cell lineages. Here we employ a tracking method based on initially segmenting the cells, as described above, and subsequently matching the cells between two frames. This is opposed to integrating segmentation and tracking in a single scheme, such as the model evolution approach [4,9,11] where level sets are leveraged as a framework.

The goal is to match N cells $\{\mathcal{C}_i^{t-1}\}_{i=1}^N$ detected at the $t-1$'th time point to the M cells $\{\mathcal{C}_j^t\}_{j=1}^M$ at the t'th time point. Each of these cells are described with a feature vector $\mathbf{f}$ of length K, such that the feature vector for the j'th cell at time t will be denoted $\mathbf{f}_j^t$. Specifically we choose to describe each cell with its x- and y-coordinates and area, whereby $K = 3$.

To match the cells in a way that accounts for all cell features, the matching of cells between two time points can be formulated as a minimum cost problem. We adopt the formulation of the matching problem suggested by [6] where a bipartite graph with coupled edges is set up to accommodate for topology changes.

Tracking by acknowledging segmentation errors. Given the difficulty of the segmentation problem the tracking algorithm needs to accommodate for segmentation errors. The possible four types of segmentation errors are:

1. Undetected cell (false negative).
2. Two cells are mistakenly segmented as a single cell.
3. One cell is mistakenly segmented as two cells.
4. Cell detected where none is present (false positive).

It is assumed that any of these segmentation errors are only temporary, i.e., a cell is only undetected or mistakenly segmented for one or a few consecutive time points.

The model by [6] is modified to honor only the biologically possible topology changes, namely that a cell can only split into two if it is undergoing mitosis. A cell is marked as a mitotic candidate if it in the near-past (15 time points = 75 minutes) has been detected as in the pre-mitotic stage using the detector described in Section 3. The graph illustrating the possible topology changes between two time points is shown in Figure 4.

160   J.S. Vestergaard et al.

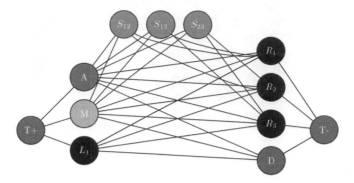

Fig. 4. Graph formulation of the matching problem. In this example there is one cell M detected as undergoing mitosis, wherefore allowed to split. The other cell L_1 can only move to cells R_1, R_2, R_3 or disappear.

Cell merging has not been included in the model as it is not possible for neural progenitor cells to merge with each other. Thereby the possibilities remaining for a cell – not marked as a mitotic candidate – are to move, appear or disappear between frames. The "appear" and "disappear" events include the cases where a cell enters or leaves the image frame, as suggested originally, but also covers the option for a cell to disappear or appear anywhere in the image. This is necessary to accommodate for the segmentation errors listed above.

In the case where a cell from time point $t - 1$ is found to disappear, without being near the image border, a phantom (a copy) of the cell is included in the set of cells at time point t and these are coupled as an ordinary "move" event. If no match is found for the phantom for a few time steps (here we choose 2 as the limit), the cell is finally marked as disappeared. For the first two cases listed above, the effect is obviously that the gap between detections is filled with the phantom. For the third and fourth cases, the spurious detection of a new cell in a few images will result in a very short cell track which can easily be detected during post-processing of the lineages. This approach effectively accommodates for the segmentation errors and allows for a robust tracking.

Edge costs. Calculation of the edge costs in the graph problem is inspired by [1]. The assigned cost $a(\mathcal{C}_i^{t-1}, \mathcal{C}_j^t)$ for matching the i'th cell at time point $t - 1$ to the j'th cell at time point t is the Mahalanobis distance

$$a(\mathcal{C}_i^{t-1}, \mathcal{C}_j^t) = \sqrt{(\mathbf{d}_{ij} - \boldsymbol{\mu})^T \boldsymbol{\Sigma}(\mathbf{d}_{ij} - \boldsymbol{\mu})} \quad \text{where} \quad \mathbf{d}_{ij} = \mathbf{f}_j^t - \mathbf{f}_i^{t-1} \qquad (1)$$

from the proposed change feature difference vector $\mathbf{d}_{ij}$ to a reference distribution described by the mean $\boldsymbol{\mu}$ and covariance matrix $\boldsymbol{\Sigma}$.

In [1] this reference distribution is estimated by manually supervising and correcting the tracks from a number of time points. Here we employ a purely data driven approach for estimating this distribution. Specifically, cells are matched over a period of 100 time points with a matching criterion specified as the nearest

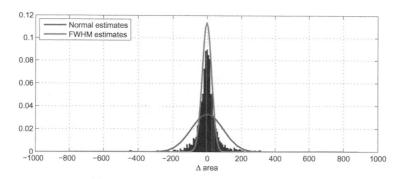

Fig. 5. Illustration of the FWHM principle when estimating parameters for the distribution describing change in area from a one-to-one nearest neighbor tracking

neighbor, with the constraint that only one-to-one correspondences are accepted, i.e., the nearest neighbor for cell i at time point $t - 1$ must also have this cell as its own nearest neighbor. Thereby only the very most obvious matches are included. The feature differences for these P matches are extracted and collected in the $P \times K$ matrix from which the mean μ and covariance Σ of the reference distribution are estimated.

However, with this approach a few erroneous matches are inevitably still included, whereby the parameter estimates are corrupted. To ensure that this does not happen, the principle of full-width-at-half-maximum (FWHM) is used to extract the dominant distribution for each feature difference. Figure 5 illustrates the difference in parameter estimates for the reference Gaussian distribution. It is clear that this is approach is necessary in order to extract viable parameters in a data driven context.

The cost for a cell to appear or disappear is set as the cost of moving from or to a cell with 1) a position of 10 standard deviations of the change in coordinates away and 2) its area set to the mode of the manually annotated cells' area. This forces the model to only let a cell appear or disappear if no suitable match is found in its proximity.

Splitting a cell into two has the cost of moving the cell to the convex hull of the resulting two cells. While there exist $\binom{M}{2}$ pairs of potential split candidates, this number can be heavily reduced by selecting only the top β percent pairs sorted according to mutual distance as proposed by [6].

5   Results

The methodology outlined above is applied to the entire time lapse image sequence of 1000 phase contrast microscopy images with 5 minutes between acquisitions. The images were captured using a Nikon BioStation IMQ with a magnification level of 10, an exposure time of 1/125s and a resolution of 600×800 pixels. The microscope acquires images in a 4×4 grid, but the images analyzed here are only from a single data point and therefore only 1/16 of the available scene. Thus this analysis should be seen as a proof-of-concept rather than a full analysis.

The mitosis detector described in Section 3 only allows cell division when cells undergo mitosis. Examples of the automatically detected mitotic cells can be seen in Figure 6. From these sequences it is seen that the detector successfully detects the out-of-focus shape characterizing the mitotic candidates, allowing the cell to divide within the near-future (chosen as 15 time points). The examples illustrate how the mitoses can be detected even in highly confluent areas. A total of 29 mitoses were detected during the entire time lapse sequence using this method. For completeness it should be mentioned that only 62% were true positive detections.

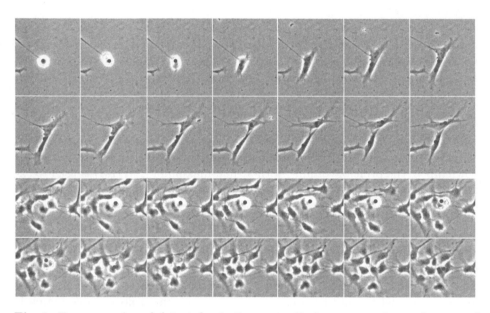

Fig. 6. Two examples of detected mitotic events. Each sequence shows the area of interest from −10 to +3 time points around the detected cell division. The dots indicate the centroids of the detected cells.

While the pipeline enables us to follow cells over time, direct interpretation of the cell trajectories is of limited value compared to statistics derived from these. In Figure 7 cell count and step lengths are documented as a function of time. The time series has been divided into ten equally sized periods, wherefore each statistic can be visualized as ten boxes. It is seen that the number of cells increase slightly in the beginning of the period followed by a decrease. Over the entire time period a definite increase in cell count is seen, which is expected given that mitosis occur.

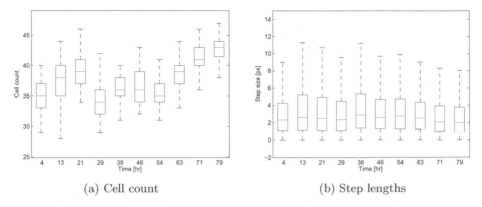

(a) Cell count   (b) Step lengths

Fig. 7. Simple statistics for the segmented and tracked time series. Each box represents 1/10 of the 83 hour period. The red line indicates the median, the edges of the box the 25th and 75th percentiles and the whiskers extend to the most extreme data points not considered outliers. Outliers are omitted. a) Cell count as a function of time. b) Cell step length between frames as a function of time.

The step length is reasonably constant over the period, except for a reduction in the last 16 hours. Visual inspection of the time lapse imagery confirms that the cells are less mobile towards the end of the time series.

Statistics concerning individual cells' tendency to undergo mitosis, i.e., whether it is the daughters of the same cell that continuously divides, are interesting, but the number of of mitotic events are too few to state anything with regards to this. To answer this question and similar, a large scale study using the proposed pipeline will be carried out in the near future.

6   Conclusions

A tracking pipeline based on a few manual annotations has been proposed. The pipeline accommodates for imprecisions in the manual annotation, by choice of segmentation method, and segmentation errors in the tracking model. Parameters for the tracking model were chosen using the principle of full-width-at-half-maximum to ensure meaningful extraction of parameters in a data driven context. A detector for mitotic candidate cells enables the model to restrict topology changes to those valid for a neural progenitor cell.

Validation of the segmentation algorithm was performed using a division into training and test set of 8 and 7 fully annotated images respectively. It was shown that a Dice's coefficient of 0.79 could be achieved while preserving a slight over-segmentation using a dictionary atom size of 9×9 in an image down sampled to 50% of the original size.

The pipeline was applied to a sequence of 1000 phase contrast microscopy images of moving and proliferating neural progenitor cells of very irregular shapes and movement patterns and varying confluence. A total of 30 mitotic events were detected and simple statistics were extracted from the cell lineages. While leaving room for improvements, this work shows that dictionary learning of discriminative image patches combined with a topology change enabling graph formulation is a flexible pipeline that can be applied even to very difficult tracking problems.

Acknowledgments. The authors would like to thank laboratory technician Jytte Nielsen from Department of Basic Animal and Veterinary Sciences, Faculty of Life Sciences, Copenhagen University, for manual annotation of cells and pleasant collaboration.

References

1. Al-Kofahi, O., Radke, R., Goderie, S., Shen, Q.: Automated Cell Lineage Construction. Cell Cycle 5(3), 327–335 (2006)
2. Cohen, A.R., Gomes, F.L.F., Roysam, B., Cayouette, M.: Computational prediction of neural progenitor cell fates. Nature Methods 7(3), 213–218 (2010)
3. Dahl, A., Larsen, R.: Learning dictionaries of discriminative image patches. In: Proceedings of the British Machine Vision Conference, BMVA (2011)
4. Dzyubachyk, O., van Cappellen, W.A., Essers, J., Niessen, W.J., Meijering, E.: Advanced level-set-based cell tracking in time-lapse fluorescence microscopy. IEEE Transactions on Medical Imaging 29(3), 852–867 (2010)
5. Keenan, T.M., Nelson, A.D., Grinager, J.R., Thelen, J.C., Svendsen, C.N.: Real time imaging of human progenitor neurogenesis. PloS One 5(10), e13187 (2010)
6. Padfield, D., Rittscher, J., Roysam, B.: Coupled minimum-cost flow cell tracking for high-throughput quantitative analysis. Medical Image Analysis 15(4), 650–668 (2011)
7. Ravin, R., Hoeppner, D., Munno, D., Carmel, L.: Potency and fate specification in CNS stem cell populations in vitro. Cell Stem Cell 3(6), 670–680 (2008)
8. Winter, M., Wait, E., Roysam, B., Goderie, S.K., Ali, R.A.N., Kokovay, E., Temple, S., Cohen, A.R.: Vertebrate neural stem cell segmentation, tracking and lineaging with validation and editing. Nature Protocols 6(12), 1942–1952 (2011)
9. Yang, F., Mackey, M.A., Ianzini, F., Gallardo, G., Sonka, M.: Cell Segmentation, Tracking, and Mitosis Detection Using Temporal Context. In: Duncan, J.S., Gerig, G. (eds.) MICCAI 2005. LNCS, vol. 3749, pp. 302–309. Springer, Heidelberg (2005)
10. Yin, Z., Li, K., Kanade, T., Chen, M.: Understanding the Optics to Aid Microscopy Image Segmentation. In: Jiang, T., Navab, N., Pluim, J.P.W., Viergever, M.A. (eds.) MICCAI 2010, Part I. LNCS, vol. 6361, pp. 209–217. Springer, Heidelberg (2010)
11. Zimmer, C., Labruyère, E., Meas-Yedid, V., Guillén, N., Olivo-Marin, J.-C.: Segmentation and tracking of migrating cells in videomicroscopy with parametric active contours: a tool for cell-based drug testing. IEEE Transactions on Medical Imaging 21(10), 1212–1221 (2002)

Automatic Heart Isolation in 3D CT Images

Hua Zhong[1], Yefeng Zheng[1], Gareth Funka-Lea[1], and Fernando Vega-Higuera[2]

[1] Imaging and Computer Vision, Siemens Corporate Technology, Princeton, NJ, USA
[2] Healthcare Sector, Siemens AG, Forchheim, Germany
hua.zhong@gmail.com, yefeng.zheng@siemens.com

Abstract. In this chapter, we present an automatic heart segmentation algorithm for the diagnosis of coronary artery diseases (CAD). The goal is to visualize the heart from a cardiac CT image with irrelevant tissues such as the lungs, rib cage, pulmonary veins, pulmonary arteries and left atrial appendage hidden so that doctors can clearly see the major coronary artery trees, aorta and bypass arteries if they exist. The algorithm combines a model-based detection framework with data-driven post-refinements to create a mask for a given cardiac CT image that contains only the relevant part of the heart. The marginal space learning [1] technique is used to localize mesh model or landmark points of different cardiovascular structures in the CT volume. Guided by such detected models, local data-driven voxel-based refinements are employed to produce precise boundaries of the heart mask. The algorithm is fully automatic and can process a 3D cardiac CT volume within a few seconds.

1 Introduction

Coronary Artery Disease (CAD) or Coronary Heart Disease (CHD) is the leading cause of death in the world [2]. Computed tomography (CT) is often used for diagnosis and treatment planing of CAD/CHD. Usually, 2D images from the stack of acquired axial images are used for diagnosis. However, only a small portion of a coronary artery is visible in a single 2D axial image. A 3D visualization provides a global and intuitive view for physicians to identify suspicious coronary segments (which are then verified on 2D slices). However, in cardiac CT images, the whole chest is imaged: both the heart and surrounding anatomical structures, which usually block the direct view of the heart in a 3D visualization. Figure 1 (a) shows an image from a CT scan. Ribs, sternum, and other structures block any direct view of the heart. Manual segmentation of the heart is tedious and error-prone. Here, we introduce a fully automatic system based on machine learning algorithms to reliably isolate the heart from 3D CT images. Figure 1 (b) presents a 3D visualization of the heart after segmenting it from the surrounding non-cardiac tissues. With this result, physicians can easily see detailed heart structures. However, the left atrial appendage (LAA), the pulmonary arteries (PA) and pulmonary veins (PV) still block the left coronary artery (LCA) tree. Figure 1 (c) is the improved result with the LAA, PA and PV being removed. Now, the left coronary artery tree can be clearly seen without any occlusion. Such a 3D view can greatly help physicians to perform CAD/CHD diagnosis.

B.H. Menze et al. (Eds.): MCV 2012, LNCS 7766, pp. 165–180, 2013.

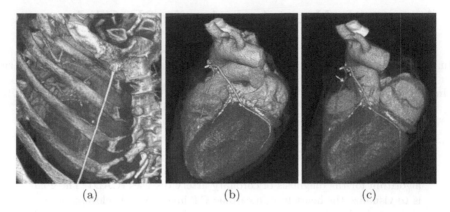

(a)   (b)   (c)

Fig. 1. Heart isolation visualization. (a) The original CT scan. Note that bones blocked any direct view of the heart. (b) The result of the pericardial isolation which only isolates the whole heart. Still, the pulmonary artery (PA), the pulmonary veins (PV) and the left atrial appendage (LAA) occlude the left coronary artery (LCA). (c) The result of final heart isolation. The PA, PV and LAA are removed automatically and the LCA (green arrow) is easily seen. After heart isolation, the plaques that block the left coronary artery tree can be easily identified. Note that in this case, there are two bypass arteries (white and blue arrows). The algorithm reliably keeps them intact.

There are a couple of other applications of heart isolation, e.g., radiotherapy planning and calcium scoring. In radiotherapy planning for the treatment of lung or liver tumors, the heart needs to be identified as part of the effort to reduce the radiation to it. Normally, a non-contrasted volume, as shown in the bottom row of Figure 2, is used for radiotherapy planning. A non-contrasted scan is used for calcium scoring as well. A calcium score is a well-established biomarker to predict future cardiac events [3]. To calculate a calcium score, the calcified coronary artery plaques (appearing as bright voxels in CT) need to be segmented. However, other bright tissues (e.g., the rib cage and sternum) need to be excluded. Heart isolation can provide a region of interest for detecting coronary calcifications.

Heart isolation is a hard problem due to the following challenges.

1. The boundary between the heart and some of the neighboring tissues (*e.g.*, liver and diaphragm) is quite weak in a CT volume.
2. The heart is connected to other organs by several major vessel trunks (*e.g.* aorta, vena cava, pulmonary veins, and pulmonary arteries). We must cut those trunks somewhere (normally at the position where the vessels connect to the heart), though there is no visible boundary.
3. The deformation of the whole heart in a cardiac cycle is more complicated than each individual chamber. This brings a large variation in the heart shape. Furthermore, there are quite a few scans with a part of the heart missing in the captured volume, especially at the top or bottom of the heart, which introduces extra shape variation.

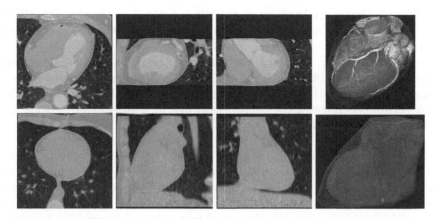

Fig. 2. Cardiac pericardium segmentation for a contrasted scan (top row) and a non-contrasted scan (bottom row). The first three columns show orthogonal cuts of the volume with green contours showing the automatically segmented heart surface mesh. The last column is 3D visualization of the segmented heart.

4. We are targeting both contrasted and non-contrasted data (as shown in Figure 2), instead of just one homogeneous set (*e.g.*, [4] for contrasted data and [5] for non-contrasted data). This presents an additional challenge.

While most previous work on heart segmentation focuses on segmenting heart chambers [1], there are only a limited number of papers on heart isolation. Atlas based methods are often used to segment the heart. For example, Rikxoort *et al.* [6] presented an adaptive, local multi-atlas based approach. It took about 30 minutes to segment a scan. Lelieveldt *et al.* [7] proposed another atlas based approach, segmenting several organs (*e.g.*, lung, heart, and liver) in a thoracic scan using a hierarchical organ model. Their approach only provided a rough segmentation and an error as large as 10 mm was regarded as a correct segmentation. It took 5 to 20 minutes to process one volume. Gregson *et al.* [8] proposed to segment the lungs first and the heart was approximated as a sphere between the left and right lungs. Moreno *et al.* [5] presented a more thorough model for the geometric relationship between lungs and the heart. Funka-Lea *et al.* [4] proposed an automatic approach based on a graph cut segmentation. They used the volumetric barycenter weighted by intensity as an initial estimate of the heart center. A small ellipsoid was put at the estimated heart center and progressively grown until it touched the transition between heart and lung (which was easy to detect in a CT volume). Graph cut was then applied to achieve the final detailed boundary delineation. It took about 20 seconds to process one volume, which was still slow for a clinical application.

In this chapter, we present an efficient and fully automatic approach for heart isolation. It contains two steps:

1. Pericardial Isolation. In this step, the whole heart (including the PA, PV and LAA) is isolated from surrounding structures. Most of the right coronary artery (RCA) tree can be seen after this step.
2. Removal of the PA, PV and LAA. Based on the pericardial isolation result, the PA, PV and LAA are automatically segmented and removed from the image. After that, the left coronary artery (LCA) tree is clearly visible. This step is not necessary for the radiotherapy planning and calcium scoring using non-contrasted scans.

We describe the two steps in details in the following sections. However, it is worth noting that all the algorithms used in both steps heavily rely on machine learning algorithms to reliably estimate the heart or the heart components' location, orientation and size. Because of this, the machine learning based component segmentation algorithm is briefly described first, followed by detailed description of the two steps of the heart isolation algorithm.

2 Marginal Space Learning Based Object Segmentation

Marginal space learning (MSL) [1] has been proposed as an efficient and robust method for 3D anatomical structure detection/segmentation in medical images. In MSL, object detection or localization is formulated as a binary classification problem: whether an image block contains the target object or not. For detection, an object can be found by testing exhaustively all possible combinations of locations, orientations, and scales using a trained classifier. However, exhaustive searching is very time consuming. The idea of MSL is not to learn a monolithic classifier, but split the estimation into three steps: position estimation, position-orientation estimation, and position-orientation-scale estimation. Each step can significantly prune the search space, therefore resulting in an efficient object detection algorithm. Please refer to [1] for more details of MSL.

After MSL based object pose estimation, a mean shape (which is trained on a set of example shapes of the object to be segmented) is aligned with the estimated translation, rotation, and scale as an initial shape. The mean shape is generally calculated as the average of the normalized shapes in an object-centered coordinate system. Therefore, the mean shape depends on the definition of the object-centered coordinate system, which is often set heuristically [1]. After initialization, we deform the shape for more accurate boundary delineation under the guidance of shape prior and a learning based boundary detector.

The MSL based object segmentation algorithm is extensively used by the heart isolation algorithm to segment the pericardial surface, the left atrium, the pulmonary artery trunk, the aortic root, and many landmark points as described in the following sections. Each object has its own trained pose detector, mean shape and boundary detector. With a reasonable amount of training data, these objects can be reliably segmented within a fraction of a second. In the following sections we will describe the two-step heart isolation algorithm in details.

3   Cardiac Pericardium Segmentation

The segmentation of the pericardial surface is based on the MSL algorithm. However, the mean shape generation process is modified to better fit the requirement
for an accurate initialization for hearts. The MSL segmentation result is a smooth
3D mesh. However, such smooth meshes cannot capture the details of the heart
surface around the rib cage or sternum. We introduce a post-processing step to
fix this.

3.1   Optimal Mean Shape for Accurate Shape Initialization

In MSL segmentation, after the initial pose of the object is estimated, a mean
shape based on training data is fit to the image as an initial shape for later
boundary delineation. In [1], the orientation of a heart chamber is defined by
its long axis; the position and scale are determined by the bounding box of the
chamber surface mesh. Although working well in applications with relatively
small shape variations, the mean shape derived using the previous methods is
not optimal for this application.

Here, we present an approach to searching for an optimal mean shape $\bar{m}$ that
represent the whole population well. A group of shapes, $M_1, M_2, \ldots, M_N$ are
supposed to be given and each shape is represented by J points $M_i^j, j = 1, \ldots, J$.
The optimal mean shape $\bar{m}$ should minimizes the residual errors after alignment,

$$\bar{m} = arg \min_m \sum_{i=1}^{N} \|\mathcal{T}_i(m) - M_i\|^2 . \tag{1}$$

Here, $\mathcal{T}_i$ is the corresponding transformation from the mean shape $\bar{m}$ to each
individual shape M_i. This procedure is called generalized Procrustes analysis [9]
in the literature. An iterative approach can be used to search for the optimal
solution. We first randomly pick an example shape as a mean shape. We then
align each shape to the current mean shape. The average of the aligned shapes
(the simple average of the corresponding points) is calculated as a new mean
shape. The iterative procedure converges to an optimal solution after a few
iterations.

Previously, the similarity transformation (with isotropic scaling) has often
used as the transformation $\mathcal{T}$. MSL can estimate the anisotropic scales of an
object efficiently. By removing more deformations, the shape space after alignment is more compact and the mean shape can represent the whole population
more accurately. Therefore, we use an anisotropic similarity transformation to
represent the transformation between two shapes,

$$\hat{T}, \hat{R}, \hat{S} = arg \min_{T,R,S} \sum_{j=1}^{J} \left\| \left(R \begin{bmatrix} S_x & 0 & 0 \\ 0 & S_y & 0 \\ 0 & 0 & S_z \end{bmatrix} M_1^j + T \right) - M_2^j \right\|^2 . \tag{2}$$

To the best of our knowledge, there are no closed-form solutions for estimating
the anisotropic similarity transformation. In this work, we propose a two-step
iterative approach to searching for the optimal transformation. Suppose there is

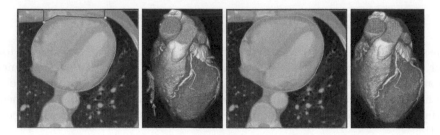

Fig. 3. Post-processing to exclude the rib cage from the heart mask. **Left**: Cross-section and 3D visualization of the result before post-processing. **Right**: After post-processing.

a common scale $s = (S_x + S_y + S_z)/3$, let $S'_x = S_x/s$, $S'_y = S_y/s$, and $S'_z = S_z/s$. Equation (2) can be re-written as

$$\hat{T}, \hat{R}, \hat{S} = arg \min_{T, R, S} \sum_{j=1}^{J} \left\| \left(Rs \begin{bmatrix} S'_x & 0 & 0 \\ 0 & S'_y & 0 \\ 0 & 0 & S'_z \end{bmatrix} M_1^j + T \right) - M_2^j \right\|^2 . \tag{3}$$

In the first step, suppose the anisotropic scales S'_x, S'_y, and S'_z are known. (At the beginning, we can assume the scaling is isotropic, $S'_x = 1$, $S'_y = 1$, and $S'_z = 1$.) We can calculate the isotropic similarity transformation using a closed-form solution [9]. In the second step, assuming that the isotropic similarity transformation (T, R, s) is given, we estimate the optimal anisotropic scales S'_x, S'_y, and S'_z. Simple mathematic derivation gives us the following closed-form solution,

$$\hat{S}'_x = \frac{\sum_{j=1}^{J} M_1^j(x) P_2^j(x)}{\sum_{j=1}^{J} M_1^j(x)^2} \quad \hat{S}'_y = \frac{\sum_{j=1}^{J} M_1^j(y) P_2^j(y)}{\sum_{j=1}^{J} M_1^j(y)^2} \quad \hat{S}'_z = \frac{\sum_{j=1}^{J} M_1^j(z) P_2^j(z)}{\sum_{j=1}^{J} M_1^j(z)^2}, \tag{4}$$

where

$$P_2^j = \frac{1}{s} R^{-1}(M_2^j - T). \tag{5}$$

The above two steps iterate a few times until they converge.

With a module solving the anisotropic similarity transformation between two shapes, we can plug it into the generalized Procrustes analysis method to search for the optimal mean shape $\bar{m}$. Besides the optimal mean shape, the optimal alignment $\mathcal{T}_i$ from the mean shape to each example shape is also obtained as a by-product. The transformation parameters of the optimal alignment provide the pose ground truth that MSL can learn to estimate.

3.2 Excluding Rib Cage from Heart Mask

For most cases, good segmentation results can be achieved after 3D heart pose detection and boundary delineation. However, for a few cases, a part of the rib cage (sternum and ribs) may be included in the heart mask (left columns of Figure 3) since the heart boundary is quite weak around that region. A post-processing step is further applied to explicitly segment the sternum and ribs based on adaptive thresholding and connected component analysis. We first detect three landmarks, namely the sternum (red dot), the left (yellow dot) and right (cyan dot) lung tips on each slice, as shown in the left columns of Figure 3. These landmarks determine a region of interest (ROI) (indicated by a blue polygon in Figure 3). A machine learning based technique is used to detect the landmarks on each slice. To be specific, 2D Haar wavelet features and the probabilistic boosting tree (PBT) [10] are used to train a detector for each landmark.

After landmark detection, we extract the ROI on each slice. Stacking the ROIs on all slices, we get a volume of interest (VOI). Normally, bones are brighter than the soft tissues in a CT volume, therefore, we can use intensity thresholding to extract the rib cage. However, due to the variations in the scanners, patients, and scanning protocols, a predefined threshold does not work for all cases. An adaptive optimal threshold [11] is automatically determined by analyzing the intensity histogram of the VOI. For some cases, a part of a chamber may be included in the VOI, however this is rare. Three dimensional connected component analysis of the bright voxels is performed and only the large components are preserved as the rib cage. We then adjust the heart mesh to make sure the rib cage is completely excluded from the mask (see the right columns of Figure 3).

3.3   Pericardium Segmentation Results

The method has been tested on 589 volumes (including both contrasted and non-contrasted scans) from 288 patients. The scanning protocols are heterogeneous with different capture ranges and resolutions. Each volume contains 80 to 350 slices and the slice size is 512×512 pixels. The resolution inside a slice is isotropic and varied from 0.28 mm to 0.74 mm, while slice thickness is generally larger than the in-slice resolution and varied from 0.4 mm to 2.0 mm.

For training and evaluation purposes, the pericardium surface of the heart was annotated, using a semi-automatic tool, with a triangulated mesh of 514 points and 1024 triangles. The cross-volume point correspondence was established using the rotation-axis based resampling method [1]. The point-to-mesh error, E_{p2m}, was used to evaluate the segmentation accuracy. For each point in a mesh, we search for the closest point in the other mesh to calculate the minimum distance. We calculate the point-to-mesh distance from the detected mesh to the ground-truth mesh and vice versa to make the measurement symmetric. A four-fold cross-validation was used to evaluate the performance of the algorithm.

First, we evaluate the shape initialization error of the optimal mean shape and the heuristic bounding-box based mean shape [1]. After MSL based heart pose estimation, we align the mean shape with the estimated position, orientation, and anisotropic scales. We then calculate the error E_{p2m} of the aliged mean shape w.r.t. the ground truth mesh. As shown in Table 1, the optimal mean shape is more accurate than the heuristic bounding-box based mean shape. It reduces the mean initialization error from 4.35 mm to 3.60 mm (a 17% reduction). After shape initialization, we deform the mesh under the guidance of a learning based boundary detector, which further improves the boundary delineation accuracy. As shown in Table 1, the mean error is 2.12 mm if we start from the bounding-box based mean shape. Using the proposed optimal shape initialization, we can reduce the final mean error

172   H. Zhong et al.

Table 1. Comparison of the proposed optimal mean shape and the heuristic bounding-box based mean shape [1] on shape initialization and final heart isolation errors. The point-to-mesh error (in millimeters) is used to measure the accuracy in the boundary delineation.

	Shape Initialization		Final Segmentation	
	Bounding-Box Mean Shape	Optimal Mean Shape	Bounding-Box Mean Shape	Optimal Mean Shape
Mean Error	4.35	**3.60**	2.12	**1.91**
Std Deviation	1.43	1.05	0.89	0.71
Median Error	4.11	**3.52**	1.89	**1.77**

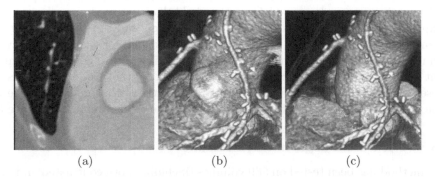

(a)   (b)   (c)

Fig. 4. Directly applying the model-based machine-learning algorithm from [1] on the PA root usually result in a thin layer of the PA (green arrow) remaining in the image (b), even though the mesh looks accurate in (a). That's because the mesh model's resolution cannot capture the voxel-level details of the shape. For comparison, our algorithm can create a clean mask with the PA removed (c).

further to 1.91 mm (a 10% reduction). Our method works well on both contrasted and non-contrasted scans. The mean and median errors on the contrasted data are 1.85 mm and 1.71 mm, respectively. The corresponding errors increase moderately on the non-contrasted data to 2.22 mm and 2.11 mm, respectively.

We also compared our approach with the graph cut based approach proposed by Funka-Lea *et el.* [4], which was used for 3D visualization of the heart. Tissues darker than the myocardium (e.g., lung) included in the heart mask does not effect the visualization since the intensity window can be tuned to hide these extra tissues. Consequently the outputs of the two methods are not likely to be identical and whe should expect more accuracy in our proposed method. Keeping this in mind, the mean and median errors achieved by the graph-cut based method are 4.60 mm and 4.00 mm, respectively (our method is 1.85 mm and 1.71 mm). Furthermore, our method is about 10-20 times faster than the graph-cut based method.

4 Removal of the PA, PV and LAA

The pericardial isolation can separate the heart from surrounding non-cardiac structures such as the lungs and ribs. However, it is not sufficient for the 3D visualization of coronary arteries since some heart structures such as the PA, PV and LAA still remain and cover the proximal left coronary artery (LCA) tree in many cases. In this step, we segment and remove these heart structures to reveal the LCA.

Since the PA, PV and LAA are very close to the coronary artery tree and they are all connected to heart chambers we want to keep, pure data-driven algorithms such as region growing cannot segment them cleanly without leaking into nearby chambers or the aorta. Though the model-based segmentation algorithm[1] can reliably detect the anatomies based on mesh models, it has some limitations. First, it works well for anatomies with relatively smaller variations, like the four chambers, but not highly variable structures like the LAA and PV, which can hardly be represented by a single-part mesh model. Second, note that standard local refinements based on a statistical shape model [12] and mesh smoothing algorithms [13] are used by the algorithm to generate a smoothed mesh. However, such a smoothed mesh, when converted to a voxel mask, may not cover all the voxels of the detected anatomy and consequently will generate visible artifacts (Figure 4).

To overcome these problems, we combine a local region growing algorithm with the global shape model to solve the PA, PV and LAA segmentation problems. We use slightly different segmentation algorithms for each of the PA, PV and LAA. However, the frameworks of all these algorithms are similar: a global shape-model detected by the MSL [1] and local refinement based on the statistics of voxel intensities. After global shape model (either mesh based or fiducial control point based) based detection/segmentation, we use constrained local intensity based region growing algorithms to refine the shapes and generate a detailed voxel mask of the objects. In order to avoid any removal of the aorta and LA which we want to keep for context, we also use a model-based algorithm to explicitly segment them and the segmented mask is used as a "protection" zone where no removal is allowed. Using the proposed method, we can achieve a fully-automatic, efficient and clean removal of the PA, PV, and LAA for 3D visualization of the LCA.

4.1   Globe Shape Segmentation

Pulmonary Artery Model: The PA trunk root, the portion of the PA from the pulmonary valve to the bifurcation, is modeled as a tubular mesh. From the bifurcation, it is difficult to approximate the shape with a tube. In this case, we use five fiducial control points: one at the bifurcation, two at the left PA branch and two at the right PA branch as shown in Figure 5 (a). We first describe how the PA trunk mesh is detected.

For the PA trunk mesh, we use the MSL algorithm [1]. The shape model, the bounding box detector and the boundary detector were trained with 320 manually annotated volume data. After the the PA trunk is detected, the detection of the five fiducial points from the PA bifurcation is a mixture of a statistical shape model and individual fiducial point detectors using the MSL algorithm [1] trained on 120 manually labeled volumes. The reason for this mixture is that in

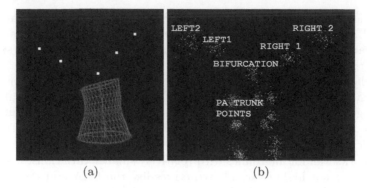

(a)   (b)

Fig. 5. PA model: (a) the mesh and five fiducial point model. (b) the statistical shape model for detecting the fiducial points (bifurcation, left 1 and 2, right 1 and 2). Based on 120 manually labeled data, we select nine points from the PA trunk mesh and combine them together with the five PA fiducial points to create a statistical shape model.

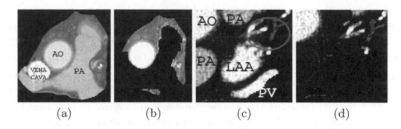

(a)   (b)   (c)   (d)

Fig. 6. Voxel-based refinement for the PA, PV, and LAA. (a) Before removal, the bypass arteries are highlighted by the red circle. (b) the PA and the vena cava are removed by region growing while bypass right adjacent to PA is kept intact. (c) before removal, we can see the small isolated chambers of the LAA very close to the coronary arteries highlighted by the red circle. (d) the LAA, PA and PV are removed cleanly while the coronary arteries are intact.

many cases, the PA fiducial points are not inside the image, or are very close to the image borders. Thus, the MSL-based bounding box detector may fail since it relies on image features which are not available outside an image. However, the statistical shape model method can handle this out-of-boundary situations well. In our method, we build a statistical shape model [12] containing nine PA trunk points selected from the PA trunk mesh and the five PA fiducial points: bifurcation, left 1 and 2, right 1 and 2 as shown in Figure 5 (b). When the PA trunk is detected, we extract the nine PA trunk points from the detected mesh. We then use the statistical shape model to estimate the optimal location of the five PA fiducial points given the nine PA trunk points' locations. The statistical shape model can estimate the location of a fiducial point even if it is outside the volume. We select only nine PA trunk points instead of all the mesh points because we want the statistical shape model to capture variations for both the PA trunk and the left/right PA branches in a balanced way. If all the PA trunk

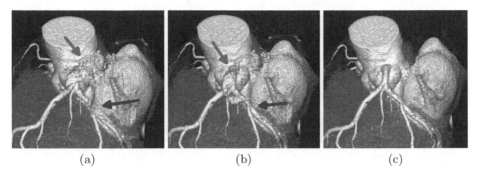

Fig. 7. LAA removal: (a) With LAA mesh model only: some LCA is cut (blue arrow) while some LAA is not removed (red arrow). (b) First pass of connected component analysis: only the largest connected region in the bounding box of LAA mesh is removed. LCA is intact (blue arrow) however still some small isolated regions of LAA remain (red arrow). (c) Second pass of connected component analysis: run in the whole image and any isolated pieces that are entirely within the LAA bounding box are removed. The result is a clean removal of all LAA voxels.

mesh points are included, the statistical shape model will be dominated by the shape variations of the PA trunk, and makes the estimation of the left and right PA less accurate. We found that with nine PA trunk mesh points the algorithm works very well for our purpose. Next, we use the learned MSL detectors to refine each of the five estimated PA fiducial points. The MSL detectors will only search a small neighborhood around the current estimated locations thus it is reliable and fast. If MSL detectors failed because a fiducial point is close to or out of the image border, the statistical shape model result will be used as the final detection result. Otherwise the MSL detector's result will be used.

Pulmonary Vein Model: The PV's shape varies too much to be represented by a single mesh model. Instead, we use two fiducial points defined on the detected left atrium (LA) mesh model to locate the root of the left and the right pulmonary veins. In practice, they are defined as two specified vertices on the LA mesh. The detailed mask for the PV is handled by a region growing method described in the next section.

Left Atrial Appendage Model: We model the LAA using the same mesh model as a heart chamber. The mesh is designed to capture the outer boundary of LAA. However, the LAA's shape varies much more than any heart chambers both for its topology and size. This mesh model usually cannot capture the exact boundary of the LAA. Instead, we only use this model to locate the LAA's bounding box so that the exact boundary can be segmented using the intensity based refinement described in the next section.

4.2 Local Voxel-Based Refinement

As we have stated before, the global shape model usually cannot generate the exact voxel mask for the PA, PV and LAA. A local refinement is necessary

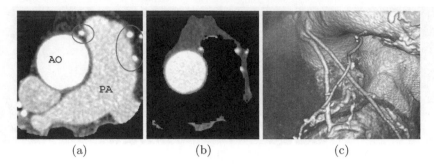

(a)   (b)   (c)

Fig. 8. Protection of vessels while removing the PA. (a) One case where bypass is deeply embedded in the PA as shown with the red circles. (b) Region growing constrained by vesselness classification can reliably remove any voxels belong to the PA while keep the bypass arteries untouched. Also the aorta is protected by segmentation. (c) 3D visualization of the case, the bypass arteries are intact and clearly visible.

for our heart isolation application. For the PA, PV and LAA, we use different refinement strategies. However, the goals are the same: to find clear boundaries without cutting into any of the CA or bypass.

Pulmonary Artery: For the PA, the global shape model contains two parts: the PA trunk mesh and the five fiducial points. For the mesh, we first close its openings and then mask out any voxels inside the mesh. As shown in Figure 4, usually a thin layer of the PA trunk still remains due to the mesh smoothing. We then use the region growing algorithm to dilate the mask out-ward for 2-3 millimeters. The region growing algorithm's threshold is determined by the mean and standard deviation of the voxels which are already in the mask. With an adaptive threshold, region growing can work for images with or without contrast agent in the PA to successfully remove the thin layer left by the PA trunk mesh. For the left PA, right PA and the PA bifurcation regions, we start region growing from each of the five fiducial points. In this step, the range for region growing is limited to 15 mm since the PA fiducial points are defined as less than 15 mm apart from each other. The region growing from the fiducial points thus can cover all the voxels of the PA bifurcation and the two branches. However, it tends to leak into surrounding objects, especially to nearby bypass arteries or the LCA as it only relies on local information. To prevent such "leaks" and protect the coronary arteries, we use a learning-based vesselness measurement to create a forbidden zone, which will be described later.

Pulmonary Vein: For the PV, we apply the same region growing algorithm from the two root fiducial points of left and right PV as for the PA fiducial points. The intensity threshold is based on the statistics of voxel intensities within the detected LA mesh model. To prevent leakage into nearby structures, we limit the growing range to 25 mm.

Left Atrial Appendage: The LAA is more complex. First, the LAA mesh model only gives an approximate boundary: it may not cover the whole LAA and it may include some LCA segment or other structures. This is due to the high variation of the LAA's shape. Second, there usually are many small chambers in the LAA which make the LAA not look like a single connected region in the image. To deal with these challenges, we design an algorithm composed with model-based mesh detection and connected component analysis (CCA). The algorithm consists of three steps (as illustrated in Figure 7):

1. The LAA mesh is detected. It gives us an initial estimation of the LAA's location and shape. We then create a bounding box slightly larger than the mesh to make sure we cover the whole LAA regions as the LAA mesh may be smaller than the exact LAA region.
2. The first CCA pass is run *within the bounding box* and the largest connected region is removed. We assume it is the largest chamber of the LAA. However, smaller isolated chambers still remain and they are difficult to be separated from LCA pieces within the bounding box.
3. The second CCA pass is run on the *whole image*. The LCA pieces in the LAA bounding box in this pass should be connected to the whole LCA tree and eventually to the aorta and LV. Thus, they should form a large connected region spanning across the LAA bounding box. The remaining LAA pieces form smaller isolated regions that are *entirely within* the bounding box. We remove all such small regions.

4.3   Chamber and Vessel Protection

Sometimes pieces of the important structures such as the aorta, LA or CA are removed by the leakage of the region growing process because of similar voxel intensities of them to the PA, PV or LAA. To prevent this, we introduce several measures to protect these structures. First, we use the segmentation results of the aorta and the LA to mask them as "not possible to grow." The region growing algorithms for the PV and PA and the connected component analysis for the LAA then will ignore any such regions.

It is more difficult to protect the CA and the bypass arteries since they are small and usually very close to the PA, PV and LAA. Furthermore, we do not have a clean mask of the CA tree as we have for the aorta and the LA. Here, we use a machine-learning based vesselness protection algorithm. As described in [14], the idea is to train a voxel classifier based on image context to tell the probability of the voxel being in a vessel. This algorithm is capable of quickly classifying a voxel to be vessel or not by applying a threshold to the returned vesselness probability. We found that a threshold equal to 75% works well for our purpose. However, there would be a waste of computation power if we classify all voxels in an image. Instead, we confine the classification to only those voxels around the PA trunk, LAA and PV where cutting of the CA or bypass arteries by the region-growing or CCA algorithms could happen.

For arteries around the PA trunk, any voxels within 3 mm to the PA trunk mesh will be classified for vesselness. For regions around the LAA and PV, usually only the LCA may be cut. In order to efficiently identify the LCA region

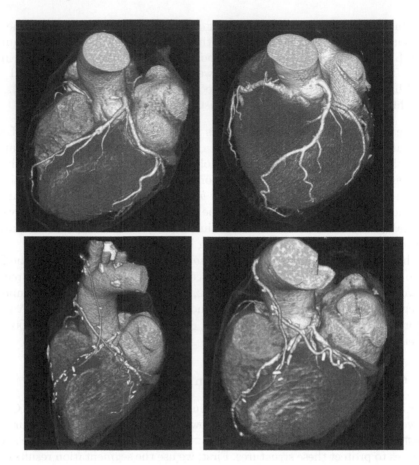

Fig. 9. Heart isolation results on normal (top row) and bypass (bottom row) cases. It shows that our algorithm can reliably remove the PA, PV and LAA while keeping coronary arteries and bypass intact. Such 3D visualization provides a global and intuitive view for physicians to identify suspicious coronary segments.

around LAA and PV, we build a similar fiducial point model as the PA trunk: it contains the left coronary ostium point, the point where left main (LM) coronary artery bifurcated into the left anterior descending artery (LAD) and left circumflex artery (LCX), 20 control points along LCX and 20 selected points from the LA mesh. We then train a statistical shape model for these 42 points based on a manually labeled training database. During the detection, the 20 LA points from the detected LA mesh, the detected left coronary ostium and the bifurcation point (using [15]) are used to estimate the positions of the 20 LCX points based on the learned statistical model. We then run vesselness classification around the region of this estimated LCA control points.

In our test, the vesselness classification in the regions described above takes only 0.02 seconds on a 4-core Xeon 2.53 GHz CPU. After the vesselness classification, we can create a vessel protection mask. This vesselness protection method

Table 2. Subjective score of the heart isolation quality on the test dataset. Score 1 is failed, 2 is acceptable, 3 is good, 4 is very good and 5 is perfect. Our algorithm achieves an average score of 3.73.

Score	1	2	3	4	5
Percentage	0.00%	13.33%	13.33%	60.00%	13.33%

can preserve LCA, RCA and bypass very well in our application, as shown in Figure 8.

5 Evaluation

The goal of the algorithm is to remove most of the LAA, PA and PV so that the coronary arteries and bypass can be clearly seen in 3D visualization. The removal should not touch any coronary arteries or bypass arteries. The algorithm is tested on a database containing 120 cardiac CT images and most of them are bypass cases. The result is then visually examined by experienced testers and a score of 1-5 is given for each case:

1. **Fail:** Major CA cut or bypass cut, important structures removed.
2. **Acceptable:** Large pieces of un-wanted structures are not removed, some minor shave or cut on the CA or the bypass arteries.
3. **Good:** Un-wanted structures are largely removed, no cut on CA or bypass.
4. **Very good:** Only very little of un-wanted structures remained, no cut on CA or bypass.
5. **Perfect:** Clean mask of the heart, no CA or bypass cut.

A score of 3 is thought to be useful, a score of 4 is very good and 5 is perfect. Score 1 is not useful and regarded as failed. Our algorithm's average score is 3.73 and there are no failed cases. The distribution of scores is shown in Table 2. Some examples of our result images are shown in Figure 9. We tested the speed on 80 cardiac CT scans. The size of the scans varies from $512 \times 512 \times 419$ to $512 \times 512 \times 667$ voxels. Resolution of the scans is around $0.4mm \times 0.4mm \times 0.4mm$. The longest processing time is less than 5 seconds on a 2.53 GHz Xeon E5630 CPU.

6 Conclustion

In this chapter, we presented an algorithm that can reliably remove both non-cardiac structures and pulmonary artery, the pulmonary veins and the left atrial appendage for 3D visualization of the coronary arteries from CT. The approach combines global shape models recovered through machine learning techniques with local intensity-based region growing to segment the important anatomical structures. The approach also provides important structural preservation mechanisms to ensure that native or bypass coronary arteries are not cut. The test results demonstrate that this approach can achieve the goal well and this is useful for an efficient CAD/CHD daignosis and treatment planning.

References

1. Zheng, Y., Barbu, A., Georgescu, B., Scheuering, M., Comaniciu, D.: Four-chamber heart modeling and automatic segmentation for 3D cardiac CT volumes using marginal space learning and steerable features. IEEE Trans. Medical Imaging 27(11), 1668–1681 (2008)
2. Lloyd-Jones, D., Adams, R., Carnethon, M., et al.: Heart disease and stroke statistics. Circulation 119(3), 21–181 (2009)
3. Blaha, M., Budoff, M., DeFilippis, A., Blankstein, R., Rivera, J., Agatston, A., O'Leary, D., Lima, J., Blumenthal, R., Nasir, K.: Associations between C-reactive protein, coronary artery calcium, and cardiovascular events: implications for the JUPITER population from MESA, a population-based cohort study. The Lancet 378(9792), 684–692 (2011)
4. Funka-Lea, G., Boykov, Y., Florin, C., Jolly, M.P., Moreau-Gobard, R., Ramaraj, R., Rinck, D.: Automatic heart isolation for CT coronary visualization using graph-cuts. In: Proc. IEEE Int'l Sym. Biomedical Imaging, pp. 614–617 (2006)
5. Moreno, A., Takemura, C.M., Colliot, O., Camara, O., Bloch, I.: Using anatomical knowledge expressed as fuzzy constraints to segment the heart in CT images. Pattern Recognition 41(8), 2525–2540 (2008)
6. van Rikxoort, E.M., Isgum, I., Staring, M., Klein, S., van Ginneken, B.: Adaptive local multi-atlas segmentation: Application to heart segmentation in chest CT scans. In: Proc. of SPIE Medical Imaging (2008)
7. Lelieveldt, B.P.F., van der Geest, R.J., Rezaee, M.R., Bosch, J.G., Reiber, J.H.C.: Anatomical model matching with fuzzy implicit surfaces for segmentation of thoracic volume scans. IEEE Trans. Medical Imaging 18(3), 218–230 (1999)
8. Gregson, P.H.: Automatic segmentation of the heart in 3D MR images. In: Canadian Conf. Electrical and Computer Engineering, pp. 584–587 (1994)
9. Dryden, I.L., Mardia, K.V.: Statistical Shape Analysis. John Wiley, Chichester (1998)
10. Tu, Z.: Probabilistic boosting-tree: Learning discriminative methods for classification, recognition, and clustering. In: Proc. Int'l Conf. Computer Vision, pp. 1589–1596 (2005)
11. Otsu, N.: A threshold selection method from gray-level histograms. IEEE Trans. Sys., Man., Cyber. 9(1), 62–66 (1979)
12. Cootes, T.F., Taylor, C.J., Cooper, D.H., Graham, J.: Active shape models—their training and application. Computer Vision and Image Understanding 61(1), 38–59 (1995)
13. Taubin, G.: Curve and surface smoothing without shrinkage. In: Proc. Int'l Conf. Computer Vision, pp. 852–857 (1995)
14. Zheng, Y., Loziczonek, M., Georgescu, B., Zhou, S.K., Vega-Higuera, F., Comaniciu., D.: Machine learning based vesselness measurement for coronary artery segmentation in cardiac CT volumes. In: Proc. of SPIE Medical Imaging, pp. 1–12 (2011)
15. Zheng, Y., John, M., Liao, R., Boese, J., Kirschstein, U., Georgescu, B., Zhou, S.K., Kempfert, J., Walther, T., Brockmann, G., Comaniciu, D.: Automatic aorta segmentation and valve landmark detection in C-arm CT: Application to aortic valve implantation. In: Proc. Int'l Conf. Medical Image Computing and Computer Assisted Intervention, pp. 1–8 (2010)

Randomness and Sparsity Induced Codebook Learning with Application to Cancer Image Classification

Quannan Li[1,2], Cong Yao[2,3], Liwei Wang[2,4], and Zhuowen Tu[1,2]

[1] Lab of Neuro Imaging, University of California, Los Angeles
[2] Microsoft Research Asia
[3] Huazhong University of Science and Technology
[4] The Chinese University of Hong Kong
{quannan.li,yaocong2010,wlwsjtu1989,zhuowen.tu}@gmail.com

Abstract. Codebook learning is one of the central research topics in computer vision and machine learning. In this paper, we propose a new codebook learning algorithm, Randomized Forest Sparse Coding (RFSC), by harvesting the following three concepts: (1) ensemble learning, (2) divide-and-conquer, and (3) sparse coding. Given a set of training data, a randomized tree can be used to perform data partition (divide-and-conquer); after a tree is built, a number of bases are learned from the data within each leaf node for a sparse representation (subspace learning via sparse coding); multiple trees with diversities are trained (ensemble), and the collection of bases of these trees constitute the codebook. These three concepts in our codebook learning algorithm have the same target but with different emphasis: subspace learning via sparse coding makes a compact representation, and reduces the information loss; the divide-and-conquer process efficiently obtains the local data clusters; an ensemble of diverse trees provides additional robustness. We have conducted classification experiments on cancer images as well as a variety of natural image datasets and the experiment results demonstrate the efficiency and effectiveness of the proposed method.

Keywords: Sparsity, Randomness, Codebook Learning, Cancer Image Classification.

1 Introduction

A large number of applications in machine learning, medical image classification, and computer vision deals with the fundamental representation problem where the data are high-dimensional and live in complex manifolds. With their intrinsic and mathematical properties gradually unfolded, research in three general directions has led to significant progress on classification, recognition, and compression: (1) ensemble learning, (2) divide-and-conquer, and (3) sparse coding. More specifically, four concepts have emerged as being essential to the three directions: (1) voting, (2) randomizing, (3) partitioning, and (4) sparsity.

B.H. Menze et al. (Eds.): MCV 2012, LNCS 7766, pp. 181–193, 2013.

Ensemble learning approaches such as bagging [2], boosting [11], and random forests [3] have shown to be among the best choices for classifiers [6,5]. The randomness in the data and feature selection stage leads to robustness in classification, as shown in the random forests [3] where trees are learned from randomly drawn subsets with the splitting criterion being locally optimal on some features randomly chosen. In Extremely Randomized Trees [14] and Random Projection Trees [7], the full data sets are used as the randomization in both feature/basis and threshold selection can provide sufficient diversities.

As real data are of high dimension and they typically do not live in a well-regularized space, the Gaussian type distribution leads to limited representational power [26] and a divide-and-conquer strategy is more appropriate. In machine learning, decision tree [23] is a standard approach where training data are recursively partitioned into subsets. The random projection tree [7] also has recursive data partition based on randomly generated bases.

More recently, sparse representations such as compressed sensing [4] and LASSO [25] have gained a great deal of popularity. One message emerging from sparse representation is that high-dimensional data within intrinsic lower dimension can be well represented by sparse samples of high dimension. The robustness of the sparse representation often assumes a subspace of certain regularity, e.g. well-aligned data [29].

In this paper, we tackle the problem of codebook learning for high dimensional visual data. Inspired by the above observations, we propose a randomized forest sparse coding (RFSC) method. Given a large set of visual data, we train an ensemble of random splitting/projection trees (when we are not sure about the form of the whole data population, it is desirable to perform random partition with certain local optimality); for each leaf node in the tree, we learn a set of bases to best represent the data with sparse coefficients. The overall codebook is a collection of all the bases from all the tree leaves. RFSC carries the ideas of voting, randomizing, partitioning, and sparse coding in a natural way. Its applicable to applications such as Modern cancer diagnosis, which largely benefits from high resolution histopathology images providing distinctive and reliable cues for discriminating abnormal tissues from normal ones.

2   Related Works

As we have discussed, our approach is inspired by the literature in ensemble learning [2,11,3], divide-and conquer approaches [23,14,7], and sparse representation [4,25,29,19]. Two types of work are particularly related to our approach: tree based splitting/projection methods, e.g., Extremely Randomized Trees [14] and Random Projection Trees [7], and sparse coding based codebook learning techniques [30,15,13].

Extremely Randomized Tree (ERT) [14] is a variant of random forest. ERTs randomize both the feature selection and the quantization threshold searching process, making the trees less correlated. When used for visual codebook learning (ERC-Forest) in [20], the generated trees are not treated as an ensemble of decision trees, instead, they are referred to as an ensemble of hierarchical spatial partitioners. The samples (image patches) in each leaf node are assumed to form a small cluster in the feature space. The leaves in the forest are uniquely indexed and serve as the codes for the codebook. When a query sample reaches a leaf node, the index of that leaf is assigned to the query sample. A histogram is formed by accumulating the indices of the leaf nodes, which serves as a Bag of Words (BOA) representation. Similar to ERC-Forest, [24] introduces a semantic texton forest using ERT to perform image classification and segmentation.

Random Projection Tree [7] is a variant of k-d tree. The k-d tree splits the data set along one coordinate at the median and recursively builds the tree. Though widely used for spatial partitioning, it suffers from the curse of dimensionality problem. Based on the realization that, high dimensional data often lies on low-dimensional manifold, RPT splits the samples into two roughly balanced sets according to a randomly generated direction. This randomly generated direction approximates the principal component direction, and can adapt to the low dimensional manifold. The RPT naturally leads to tree-based vector quantization and an ensemble of RPTrees can be used as a codebook.

We use Extremely Randomized Trees/Random Projection Trees to partition the samples. But instead of splitting the samples till we cannot split any more, we stop early according to certain criterion and find some bases that can best reconstruct all the samples in that node. These bases serve as codes of the codebook.

There are already some methods using sparse coding for codebook learning. In [30], the authors generalize vector quantization to sparse coding, and construct the histogram using multi-scale spatial max pooling. Each patch can be assigned to several (sparse) codes, and thus the reconstruction error can be reduced. Also, this method extends the Spatial Pyramid Matching method [15] to a linear SPM kernel. In [13], Laplace sparse coding preserves the consistency in the sparse representation and alleviates the problem in [30] that similar patches may be assigned to different codes. In [28], a locality-constrained linear coding scheme is proposed that utilizes the locality constraints to project descriptors to their local-coordinate system. This scheme can preserve the property of local smooth sparsity. Compared with these methods, the advantages of RFSC is obvious. One advantage is the efficiency. Utilizing techniques such as ERT and RPT, the sparse coding is performed only in subspaces and the computational burden is greatly reduced. The second advantage is the potential promotion of the discriminative ability. The label information can easily be used into the tree splitting process (ERT) and the codebook created could have more discriminative power.

3   Randomized Forest Sparse Coding

3.1   Problem Formulation

Suppose we are given a set of training data $S = \{\mathbf{x}_i\}_{i=1}^{n}$ and $\mathbf{x}_i \in \mathbb{R}^D$ (in a supervised setting, each $\mathbf{x}_i$ is also associate with a label $y_i \in \mathcal{Y} = \{0, ..., K\}$ and thus $S = \{(\mathbf{x}_i, y_i)\}_{i=1}^{n}$), our goal is to learn a codebook (a set of bases) $\mathbf{B} = \{\mathbf{b}_i\}_{i=1}^{m}$ and $\mathbf{b}_i \in \mathbb{R}^D$ such that

$$\min_{\mathbf{B},\mathbf{w}} \sum_{i=1}^{n} \left\| \mathbf{x}_i - \sum_{j=1}^{m} w_{ij} \mathbf{b}_j \right\|_2^2$$
$$s.t. \ \forall i, \sum_j |w_{ij}| \leq \tau \tag{1}$$

The first term in Eqn. (1) minimizes the reconstruction error and the second term gives the sparsity constraints on the reconstruction coefficients. Eqn. (1) actually includes two coupled optimization problems: (1) given $\mathbf{w}$, find the optimal codebook $\mathbf{B}$; (2) given a codebook $\mathbf{B}$, find the best reconstruction coefficients $\mathbf{w}$. A similar formulation appears in [30]. After an optimal basis set $\mathbf{B}^*$ is found, for a new sample $\mathbf{x}$, we can compute its reconstruction coefficients $\mathbf{w}$ via:

$$\min_{\mathbf{w}} \left\| \mathbf{x} - \sum_{j=1}^{m} w_j \mathbf{b}_j \right\|_2^2$$
$$s.t. \ \sum_j |w_j| \leq \tau \tag{2}$$

The vector $\mathbf{w}$ can be used to characterize the sample $\mathbf{x}$. In codebook learning, each $\mathbf{b}_j$ serves as a code, and the reconstruction coefficients with respect to the codes are pooled to form a histogram.

In Eqn. (1), the norm of $\mathbf{b}_j$ can be arbitrarily large, making w_{ij} arbitrarily small. Further constraints should be made on $\mathbf{b}_j$. In our paper, we make a reasonable constraint that all the bases in the codebook should be from the training set S, i.e., $\mathbf{B} \subset S$. With this constraint, Eqn. (1) can be transformed into

$$\min_{\mathbf{v},\mathbf{w}} \sum_{i=1}^{n} \left\| \mathbf{x}_i - \sum_{j=1}^{n} w_{ij} v_j \mathbf{x}_j \right\|_2^2 \tag{3}$$
$$s.t. \ \sum_j v_j \leq m, v_j \in \{0,1\}$$
$$\forall i, \ \sum_j |w_{ij}| \leq \tau \tag{4}$$

Here, v_j serves as an indicator value $\in \{0,1\}$ and $\mathbf{B} = \{\mathbf{x}_j : \mathbf{x}_j \in S, \ v_j = 1\}$. Eqn. (3) is seemingly more complex than Eqn. (1) with the introduction of $\mathbf{v}$. However, it can be solved more efficiently since the search space for the bases is greatly reduced.

Learning a codebook of size greater than e.g. $5,000$ from tens of thousands of samples is computationally demanding. As motivated before, we could perform a divide-and-conquer strategy to partition the data space with complex manifolds into local subspaces. Within a subspace, it is then much more efficient to learn bases for a sparse representation.

3.2   Randomized Forest Data Partition

In this section, we take the Extremely Randomized Tree (ERT) [14] and Random Projection Trees (RPT) as examples to illustrate the data projection process. Both ERT and RPT partition the samples recursively in a top-down manner. ERT adopts the label information and uses normalized Shannon entropy as the criterion to select features. RPT is unsupervised and it does not need any label information; it splits the data via hyper-planes normal to the randomly generated projection bases.

Discriminative Partition via Extremely Randomized Tree. Given a labeled sample set $S = \{(\mathbf{x}_i, y_i)\}_{i=1}^n$, ERT proceeds by randomly selecting a subset of features from the feature pool $\{f_i, 1 \leq i \leq D\}$. For each selected feature f_i, a threshold θ_i is sampled according to a uniform distribution. Based on the features selected and thresholds sampled, boolean tests $\{T_i : \mathbf{x}(i) < \theta_i\}$ can be used to split the set S. If T_i = true, $\mathbf{x}$ goes to the left branch S_1; otherwise, $\mathbf{x}$ goes to the right branch S_2.

To select the best boolean test for splitting, the normalized Shannon entropy was used:

$$Score(S, T_i) = \frac{2 \cdot I_{\mathcal{Y}, T_i}(S)}{H_{\mathcal{Y}}(S) + H_{T_i}(S)} \tag{5}$$

where, $I_{\mathcal{Y}, T_i}(S) = H_{\mathcal{Y}}(S) - \sum_{p=1}^{2} \frac{n_p}{n} H_{\mathcal{Y}}(S_p)$. $I_{\mathcal{Y}, T_i}(S)$ is the information gain; $H_{\mathcal{Y}}(S) = -\sum_{y \in \mathcal{Y}} \frac{n_y}{n} \log_2(\frac{n_y}{n})$ denoting the entropy of class distribution of the original set S. $H_{T_i}(S) = -\sum_{p=1}^{2} \frac{n_p}{n} \log_2(\frac{n_p}{n})$ denotes the entropy for the test T_i that splits the data into two branches. The T_i with the largest $Score(S, T_i)$ is selected.

The use of $H_{T_i}(S)$ as a normalization term in Eqn. (5) will favor uneven splitting, making the forest more unbalanced. In our randomized forest sparse coding scheme (RFSC), it is desirable to have balanced trees, so we use a slightly modified form of Eqn. (5):

$$Score(S, T_i) = \frac{2 \cdot I_{\mathcal{Y}, T_i}(S)}{H_{\mathcal{Y}}(S) + 1 - H_{T_i}(S)} \tag{6}$$

Since $H_{T_i}(S)$ is a concave function and it achieves the maximum value 1 when the numbers of samples in S_1 and S_2 are the same, this criterion can make the trees more balanced.

Unsupervised Splitting via Random Projection Tree (RPT). At each node, RPT chooses a random unit projection direction $\mathbf{b} \in \mathbb{R}^D$, and splits the samples into two roughly equal-sized sets. The random projection and thresholding also serve as a type of boolean test. We use the splitting criterion as

$$T := \mathbf{x}^T \mathbf{b} \leq \left(median(\mathbf{z}^T \mathbf{b} : \mathbf{z} \in S) + \delta \right).$$

Here δ is a random perturbation that adapts to the structure of S. Splitting around the median value makes the splitting balanced while the perturbation δ introduces certain randomness [7].

Since RPTs can automatically adapt to the low dimensional manifold of the dataset S, the samples in the leaf nodes observe local subspaces. The local structures of all the leaf nodes thus collectively comprise the global structure of the data set S (Fig. 1 (b)).

Basis Pursuit at the Leaf Nodes. Both ERT and RPT build the trees to the fine scale and use the leaf nodes as the codes. Instead of building the trees of very deep level, RFSC stops at some relatively higher level (e.g., when the number of samples is less than M). At such nodes, the local manifold structure is assumed

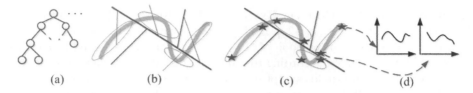

Fig. 1. Illustration of the idea of RFSC using Random Projection Tree (best viewed in color). (a) The forest consists of ensemble of random projection trees; (b) The spatial partition of the dataset by one tree (A copy from [10]). A cell stands for a leaf node. The width of the separation line indicates the level of the tree. (c) For RFSC, it does not build the tree to fine level. At certain level when local manifold structures are found, bases (indicated by the red stars) are learned for the local structure in each cell. (d) For the samples in each cell, their reconstruction coefficients with respect to the bases are different.

to be relatively simple and regularized. RFSC seeks a set of bases to sparsely represent the subspaces at those nodes. This process can be illustrated using Random Projection Tree in Fig. 1 in which a visualization is displayed and RPT tends to split the data along the principal component direction (Fig. 1 (b)). For RFSC, when the local structure is relatively regularized, it seeks some bases (the red stars) to sparsely represent the local subspace. Different from RPT or ERT that use the mean of the local subspace or a single index to represent the cell, the information conveyed via the reconstruction coefficients with respect to each basis (Fig. 1 (d)) is richer and more informative. Note that the bases in different clusters could be spatially close to each other. As an illustration, see the two bases on the bottom right in Fig. 1(c). From this point of view, the number of bases and the redundancy would increase. However, according to Theorem 1 in the justification part, the total number of bases in all the leaf nodes is bounded. Since at each node when the splitting process stops, there are generally $80 \sim 200$ samples (depending on the codebook size) and $3 \sim 10$ bases, the computational overhead of subspace learning is not significant compared with directly pursuing bases from the entire sample set.

3.3   Optimization Scheme

The constraint that $v_j \in \{0, 1\}$ makes Eqn. (3) a hard problem. In this subsection, we present two schemes to solve this optimization problem. The first one is to relax v_j to a real value and use coordinate descent algorithm to optimize on **w** and **v** iteratively. The second one is a greedy pursuit approach that selects the bases one by one.

Convex Relaxation. The first optimization scheme is to relax the values of v_j to real numbers and use ℓ^1 constraint $\sum_j |v_j| \leq m$ instead of ℓ^0 like constraint in Eqn. (3). Putting this constraint as a regularization term, we can transform this problem into an equivalent form:

$$\frac{1}{2}\sum_{i=1}^{n}\left\|\mathbf{x}_i - \sum_{j=1}^{n}w_{ij}v_j\mathbf{x}_j\right\|_2^2 + \lambda_1\sum_{i,j}|w_{ij}| + \lambda_2\sum_{j}|v_j| \tag{7}$$

Here, $v_j \in \mathbb{R}$. λ_1 and λ_2 are regularization parameters that make the trade-offs between the residue and the norms of the weight vectors.

There are two sets of variables $\mathbf{w}$ and $\mathbf{v}$ in Eqn. (7). To optimize Eqn. (7), we adopt an EM-like algorithm that iterates by fixing one set of variables and optimize on the other set using coordinate descent algorithm [12].

Greedy Pursuit Approach. Starting from an empty basis collection, the greedy pursuit approach selects the bases one by one. Suppose some l samples $\mathbf{B}_l = \{\mathbf{x}_{s_i}, 0 \le i \le l, 1 \le s_i \le n\}$ have been selected from the n samples, i.e., $v_{s_i} = 1$. To select the $(l+1)$th basis, we optimize the following function:

$$s_{l+1} = \min_{k \notin \{s_i\}} \frac{1}{2}\sum_{i=1}^{n}\left\|\mathbf{x}_i - \sum_{j\in\{s_i\}}w_{ij}\mathbf{x}_j - w_{ik}\mathbf{x}_k\right\|_2^2$$

$$+ \lambda_1\sum_{i=1}^{n}\sum_{j\in\{s_i\}}|w_{ij}| + \lambda_1\sum_{i=1}^{n}|w_{ik}| \tag{8}$$

According to Eqn. (8), the sample that reconstructs all the n patches together with the first l selected bases is selected as the $(l+1)$th basis.

The greedy approach finds suboptimal solution to Eqn. (3). But it's more efficient than the convex relaxation approach, and in practice, we find that its performance is comparable with the convex relaxed solution. Thus in some of our experiments, we only use this greedy approach.

3.4 Theoretical Justification

In this section, we give some theoretical justification to our approach. Our intuition is to show that the three steps in randomized forest sparse coding: (1) ensemble of trees, (2) randomized projection tree, and (3) sparse coding leads to the same complexity level in the number of bases as to the original data.

Given $S = \{\mathbf{x}_i, i = 1..n\}$ with $\mathbf{x}_i \in \mathbb{R}^D$, assume that $\mathbf{x}_i$ lives in the intrinsic lower dimension $d \ll D$. It can be seen that the number of bases needed to reconstruct S is bounded. Following the definition of Assouad dimension [1] [7]:

Definition: For any point $\mathbf{x} \in \mathbb{R}^D$ and $r > 0$, let $B(\mathbf{x}, r) = \{\|\mathbf{x} - \mathbf{z}\| \le r\}$ denote the closed ball of radius r centered at $\mathbf{x}$. The Assouad dimension of $S \in \mathbb{R}^D$ is the smallest integer d such that for any ball $B(\mathbf{x}, r) \in \mathbb{R}^D$, the set $B(\mathbf{x}, r) \cap S$ can be covered by 2^d balls of radius $r/2$.

Theorem 1. *The number of bases needed to reconstruct S by Randomized Forest Sparse Coding (RFSC) is $O(2^{d\log d})$.*
Proof:
    Fixing radius r, suppose we want to create a codebook such that each basis function covers $r/2$, a size of $O(2^d)$ codebook is required to cover the entire dataset S, according to the definition of Assouad dimension.

The main result in [7] shows that $O(d \log d)$ levels of a random projection/partition tree would reach cells with radius $r/2$. Therefore, the number of cells is $O(2^{d \log d})$. Suppose there are k trees in the forest, and in each leaf node, l bases are found, then the number of the bases becomes $O(kl2^{d \log d})$. As k and l are generally small and can be kept constant, the bound still reduces to:

$$O(2^{d \log d}).$$

Although RFSC slightly increases the size of the codebook compared to $O(2^d)$, since d is generally small $(d \ll D)$, this is reasonably bounded.

4   Experiments

To evaluate the effectiveness of the proposed codebook learning algorithm, we conducted extensive classification experiments on a collection of cancer images and a variety of natural image datasets: Graz-02 image set, and the PASCAL 2005 image set.

As the baselines, we obtained the source code for ERC-Forest from the authors of [20] and implemented the RPTs according to [7]. In our experiments, the feature vectors are used without any normalization, which is sometimes done in subspace learning and sparse coding (we found that performing normalization does not affect the overall performance in the experiments reported here). For each leaf node, 5 bases are learned. For the Graz-02 image set, $\lambda_1 = 2$ and $\lambda_2 = 6$, while for the PASCAL 2005 image set, $\lambda_1 = 15$ and $\lambda_2 = 6$. To solve the subspace learning problem via sparse coding defined in Eqn. (3), 10 iterations between $\mathbf{w}$ and $\mathbf{v}$ are enough to find a good sparse solution.

In the following, we use RFSC to denote subspace learning via sparse coding under Extremely Randomized Trees; RPT-SC denotes subspace learning on Random Projection Trees. For RFSC and RPT-SC, the postfix "-Cvx" refers to using the convex relaxation version and "-Gdy" regards to using the greedy basis pursuit version. For the classification task of Cancer Images, the performance is measured using the Area under the curve of the ROC curve, while for natural image classification, the performance is measured using the classification accuracy at the equal error rate and the reported accuracies are the averages of 10 rounds of execution.

4.1   Experiments on Cancer Images

Dataset: We used a histopathology image data set with 60 colon images (30 cancer images and 30 non-cancer images). Sample images are shown in Fig. 2. The images are labeled as cancer or non-cancer by two pathologists independently. If disagreement happens for a certain image, these two pathologists together with a third senior pathologist will carefully examine and discuss until final agreement.

Experimental Setup: Before feature extraction, the original images are downsampled with a factor of 2. As no obvious spatial regularities are observed from the images (Fig. 2), instead of using the Bag-of-Features (BOF) vectors, we

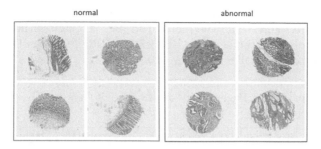

Fig. 2. Cancer image examples. The images in the green box are normal samples. i.e. there are no cancerous cells. The images in the red box are abnormal samples, i.e. there are cancerous cells.

randomly sample $N = 200$ local patches (32×32) for each image. Each patch is represented by Lab color histogram, Local Binary Pattern [21], and SIFT [18]. For the proposed method, each patch is encoded by the proposed coding schemes RFSC or RPT-SC; for the baseline, we use the raw feature. Random Forests [3] is adopted as the strong classifier for its simplicity and high performance. The overall classification score of an image is the mean of the scores of all the patches. Half of the images in the dataset are chosen randomly for training and the rest for testing. We run the experiments 5 times for each method and report the averaged performance. For RFSC and RPT-SC, the convex relaxation versions are used. The Area Under Curve (AUC) for the methods are RPT-SC 0.98, RFSC 0.987, RPT 0.927, ERC-Forest 0.95, and raw feature 0.967 respectively; our method performs better than the alternatives.

4.2 Experiments on Natural Images

The reconstruction coefficients are pooled in the natural image classification task. To pool the reconstruction coefficients, unless otherwise stated, max-pooling is used as in [30]. The reconstruction coefficients of the trees are pooled and concatenated to form a histogram leaving the voting process till the classification step; Linear SVM is used in the image classification stage. In all the following image classification experiments, we do not include the adaptive saliency map process. This makes the image classification performance of ERC-Forest slightly worse than that reported in [20]. However, this performance degeneration is reasonable and in accordance with the case illustration in [20].

GRAZ-02 Dataset [22]. GRAZ-02 image set consists of three object categories and one counter-category. For each category, the categorization task is to distinguish the object category from the counter-category, None. Similar to [20], we also pick the two hardest cases: Cars vs. None and Bikes vs. None.

To make a direct comparison with [20] and [22], we conduct the experiment according to the setting in [20] using the first 300 images of each category for training. We use the greedy version of RFSC and vary the codebook size from

5000 to 9000. From Table 1 and Table 2, we observe that, RFSC-Gdy performs better than ERC-Forest and the method in [22]. Though without the adaptive saliency map process, the accuracy (83.9%) of RFSC-Gdy on the case of Bikes vs. None approaches that reported in [20] (84.4%).

Table 1. Comparison of the accuracy on the case of Cars vs. None in the GRAZ-02 images [22]

size of codebook	5000	6000	7000	8000	9000
[22]	70.5%				
ERC-Forest	71.3%	73.5%	74.5%	74.7%	74.8%
RPT	66.5%	66.6%	65.3%	67.7%	66.9%
RFSC-Gdy	73.4%	74.3%	**75.7%**	74.9%	74.3%
RPT-SC-Gdy	68%	69.8%	69%	69.5%	68.2%

Table 2. Comparison of the accuracy for Bikes vs. None in the GRAZ-02 images [22]

size of codebook	5000	6000	7000	8000	9000
[22]	77.8%				
ERC-Forest	78.8%	78%	78.5%	78.5%	78.5%
RPT	73.3%	74.3%	74.1%	75.1%	74.4%
RFSC-Gdy	80.7%	**83.9%**	80.8%	81.3%	80%
RPT-SC-Gdy	76.5%	76.8%	76.1%	76.7%	76%

We also conduct the experiments using all the images instead of the first 300 images. Average-pooling is adopted here and the results are reported in Table 3 and Table 4. The performance of the two optimization schemes is similar. RFSC-Cvx-1tree refers to using one randomized tree instead of the forest, an ensemble of trees. It performs worse than RFSC. This justifies the benefit of using ensembles.

Table 3. Comparison of the accuracy using all the images for Cars vs. None in the GRAZ-02 images [22]

size of codebook	5000	6000	7000	8000	9000
ERC-Forest	67.2%	67%	68.6%	68.8%	71.3%
Leaf-Kmeans	68.2%	70.9%	73%	72.6%	73.2%
RFSC-Cvx-1tree	72.6%	72.2%	71.4%	75%	75%
RFSC-Cvx	75%	75%	73.7%	73.1%	75.2%
RFSC-Gdy	74.3%	75.5%	74.5%	74.8%	**75.5%**

We do not compare RFSC and RPT-SC with directly performing dictionary learning on the image classification task since solving Eqn. (1) directly when $m = 5,000$ or $9,000$ is time consuming. However, benefiting from the divide-and-conquer process, it takes less than 1 hour for RFSC and RPT-SC to build a

Table 4. Comparison of the accuracy using all the images for Bikes vs. None in the GRAZ-02 images [22]

size of codebook	5000	6000	7000	8000	9000
ERC-Forest	77.8%	78.3%	78.3%	79.1%	78.8%
Leaf-Kmeans	75.1%	74.4%	79.7%	78.7%	79.5%
RFSC-Cvx-1tree	77.8%	78.2%	78.6%	79.5%	79.5%
RFSC-Cvx	80%	82.2%	**82.6%**	81.4%	81.8%
RFSC-Gdy	81.5%	80.3%	81.5%	80.8%	80.9%

forest with 5 trees and 9,000 codes. This improvement in efficiency stems from seeking a small amount of bases from hundreds of patches instead of seeking thousands of bases from tens of thousands of training patches. Other efficient algorithms such as [16] can be used to solve Eqn. (1), but the conclusion of the improvement in efficiency induced by the divide-and-conquer process still holds. RFSC and RPT-SC are also very efficient at the testing stage. It takes about 0.5 second to process an image and pooling the reconstruction coefficients. As a comparison, it would take around 30 seconds for K-Means to assign patches to the codes for an image when the feature vector is of dimension 768 and the codebook size K is 5,000.

PASCAL 2005 Image Set [8]. We also compare our method with ERC-Forest on PASCAL 2005 image set. The results are shown in Table 5. RFSC-Gdy achieves better results on all of the 4 categories than ERC-Forest.

Table 5. Comparison of the accuracy on PASCAL 2005 image set [8]

method	motobikes	cars	bikes	person
ERC-Forest	96%	95%	89%	90.9%
RFSC-Gdy	**96.4%**	**95.3%**	**90.6%**	**91.4%**

5   Conclusion

In this paper, we have introduced a codebook learning method called randomized forest sparse coding that integrates three concepts: ensemble, divide-and-conquer and sparse coding. Justifications for the effectiveness and efficiency of our method are also provided. The proposed scheme is applied to both the Cancer Image Classification and natural image classification and observes significant improvement in performance.

Acknowledgment. This work is supported by Office of Naval Research Award N000140910099 and NSF CAREER award IIS-0844566.

References

1. Assouad, P.: Plongements lipschitziens dans rn. Bull. Soc. Math. France (4), 429–448 (1983)
2. Breiman, L.: Bagging predictors. Machine Learning 24(2), 123–140 (1996)
3. Breiman, L.: Random forests. Machine Learning 45(1), 5–32 (2001)
4. Candes, E., Tao, T.: Near-optimal signal recovery from random projections: universal encoding strategies. IEEE Trans. Inform. Theory 52(2), 5406–5425 (2005)
5. Caruana, R., Karampatziakis, N., Yessenalina, A.: An empirical evaluation of supervised learning in high dimensions. In: ICML, pp. 96–103 (2008)
6. Caruana, R., Niculescu-Mizil, A.: An empirical comparison of supervised learning algorithms. In: ICML, pp. 161–168 (2006)
7. Dasgupta, S., Freund, Y.: Random projection trees and low dimensional manifolds. In: STOC, pp. 537–546 (2008)
8. Everingham, M., Zisserman, A., Williams, C.K.I., Van Gool, L., Allan, M., Bishop, C.M., Chapelle, O., Dalal, N., Deselaers, T., Dorkó, G., Duffner, S., Eichhorn, J., Farquhar, J.D.R., Fritz, M., Garcia, C., Griffiths, T., Jurie, F., Keysers, D., Koskela, M., Laaksonen, J., Larlus, D., Leibe, B., Meng, H., Ney, H., Schiele, B., Schmid, C., Seemann, E., Shawe-Taylor, J., Storkey, A.J., Szedmak, S., Triggs, B., Ulusoy, I., Viitaniemi, V., Zhang, J.: The 2005 PASCAL Visual Object Classes Challenge. In: Quiñonero-Candela, J., Dagan, I., Magnini, B., d'Alché-Buc, F. (eds.) MLCW 2005. LNCS (LNAI), vol. 3944, pp. 117–176. Springer, Heidelberg (2006)
9. Ferrari, V., Jurie, F., Schmid, C.: Accurate Object Detection with Deformable Shape Models Learnt from Images. In: CVPR (2007)
10. Freund, Y., Dasgupta, S., Kabra, M., Verma, N.: Learning the structure of manifolds using random projections. In: NIPS, vol. 20 (2007)
11. Freund, Y., Schapire, R.E.: A decision-theoretic generalization of on-line learning and an application to boosting. J. of Comp. and Sys. Sci. 55(1) (1997)
12. Friedma, J., Hastie, T., Hofling, H., Tibshirani, R.: Pathwise Coordinate Optimization. The Annals of Applied Stat. (2007)
13. Gao, S., Tsang, I.W.H., Chia, L.T., Zhao, P.: Local features are not lonely - laplacian sparse coding for image classification. In: CVPR (2010)
14. June, P.G., Ernst, D., Wehenkel, L.: Extremely Randomized Trees. In: Machine Learning, vol. 36 (2003)
15. Lazebnik, S., Schmid, C., Ponce, J.: Beyond bags of features: Spatial pyramid matching for recognizing natural scene categories. In: CVPR (2006)
16. Lee, H., Battle, A., Raina, R., Ng, A.Y.: Efficient sparse coding algorithms. In: NIPS (2007)
17. Li, Y., Osher, S.: Coordinate descent optimization for ℓ^1 minimization with application to compressed sensing; a greedy algorithm. CAM Report (2009)
18. Lowe, D.G.: Distinctive image features from scale-invariant keypoints. International Journal of Computer Vision 60(2), 91–110 (2004)
19. Mairal, J., Bach, F., Ponce, J.: Task-driven dictionary learning. IEEE Trans. on PAMI (to appear)
20. Moosmann, F., Nowak, E., Jurie, F.: Randomized clustering forests for image classification. IEEE Trans. on PAMI 30(9), 1632–1646 (2008)
21. Ojala, T., Pietikäinen, M., Mäenpää, T.: Multiresolution gray-scale and rotation invariant texture classification with local binary patterns. IEEE Trans. Pattern Anal. Mach. Intell. 24(7), 971–987 (2002)

22. Opelt, A., Pinz, A., Fussenegger, M., Auer, P.: Generic Object Recognition with Boosting. IEEE Trans. on PAMI 28(3), 416–431 (2006)
23. Quinlan, J.R.: Induction of decision trees. Machine Learning 1 (1986)
24. Shotton, J., Johnson, M., Cipolla, R.: Semantic texton forests for image categorization and segmentation. In: CVPR (2008)
25. Tibshirani, R.: Regression shrinkage and selection via the lasso. J. Royal. Statist. Soc B. 56(1), 267–288 (1996)
26. Turk, M.: Eigenface for recognition. Journal of Cognitive Neuroscience (1991)
27. Vedaldi, A., Fulkerson, B.: Vlfeat: an open and portable library of computer vision algorithms. In: ACM Multimedia, pp. 1469–1472 (2010)
28. Wang, J., Yang, J., Yu, K., Lv, F., Huang, T., Gong, Y.: Locality-constrained linear coding for image classification. In: CVPR (2010)
29. Wright, J., Yang, A., Ganesh, A., Sastry, S., Ma, Y.: Robust face recognition via sparse representation. IEEE Trans. on PAMI 31(2) (2009)
30. Yang, J., Yu, K., Gong, Y., Huang, T.: Linear spatial pyramid matching using sparse coding for image classification. In: CVPR (2009)

Context Enhanced Graphical Model for Object Localization in Medical Images

Yang Song[1], Weidong Cai[1], Heng Huang[2], Yue Wang[3],
and David Dagan Feng[1]

[1] BMIT Research Group, School of IT, University of Sydney, Australia
[2] Computer Science and Engineering, University of Texas at Arlington
[3] Bradley Department of Electrical and Computer Engineering,
Virginia Polytechnic Institute and State University

Abstract. Object localization is an important step common to many different medical applications. In this Chapter, we will review the challenges and recent approaches tackling this problem, and focus on the work by Song et.al. [20]. In [20], a new graphical model with additional contrast and interest-region potentials is designed, encoding the higher-order contextual information between regions, on the global and structural levels. A discriminative sparse-coding based interest-region detector is also integrated as one of the context prior in the graphical model. This object localization method is generally applicable to different medical imaging applications, in which the objects can be distinguished from the background mainly based on feature differences. Successful applications on two different medical imaging applications – lesion dissimilarity on thoracic PET-CT images and cell segmentation on microscopic images – are demonstrated in the experimental results.

1 Introduction

A wide variety of medical applications comprise object localization as an important step for discovering the anatomical or pathological information from images. For example, region-of-interest (ROI) detection is helpful for early screening of diseases; and lesion segmentation is useful for treatment planning. We consider object localization as a generalization of both detection and segmentation, with both automatic identification of ROI, and a good delineation of its boundary.

We focus on medical imaging problems in which objects can be localized based on local-level features and feature differences between the objects and background. For example, in positron emission tomography – computed tomography (PET-CT) images, abnormalities typically show higher uptakes than normal tissues. In fluorescence microscopic images, the cell nuclei normally depict darker colors then the other cell structures and the background. In brain magnetic resonance imaging (MRI), the white and gray matter display quite different intensities and spatial patterns.

Local features are usually not sufficient for a good localization, because of large inter-subject variations causing same anatomical structures appearing quite

B.H. Menze et al. (Eds.): MCV 2012, LNCS 7766, pp. 194–205, 2013.
© Springer-Verlag Berlin Heidelberg 2013

differently across images. The problem is further complicated due to low feature differences between different tissue types and especially for the boundary areas between the objects and background. In addition, pathologies often lead to larger imaging variations, and an accurate object localization is thus more challenging.

For such imaging problems, while lots of work have been reported [25,16,19,5,18,4,21,15], they are mostly designed to be domain specific; and often rely on sophisticated feature sets, which can be computational-intensive and difficult to adapt to other imaging problems. Furthermore, because such features are usually designed based on domain knowledge and empirical studies, their effectiveness may be restricted to the limited scenarios available in the datasets.

Therefore, in [20], we proposed an object localization method that can be generally applicable, requires simpler feature sets, and addresses low feature differences and large inter-subject variations. With region-based labeling, each image region is classified as the object or background to produce the localization output. In summary, our main contributions are the following: (i) the discriminative capability of the basic conditional random field (CRF) is enhanced with two contextual priors, namely the contrast and interest-region potentials, to encode the global contrast information and region-based feature similarities, for improving the boundary delineations; (ii) a sparse-coding classification method is proposed for interest-region detection, with improved discriminative power of the learned dictionaries; and (iii) the design is kept general with simple feature sets configurable for the specific application, and has been successfully applied to both lesion dissimilarity on thoracic PET-CT images and cell segmentation on microscopic images.

Related Work. We focus our review on CRF-based localization methods in both medical and general imaging domains. As an undirected graphical model, CRF is now one of the most successful trends in object class image segmentation [6]. The basic and most commonly used formulation is to have local features represented as graph nodes and consistency constraints between neighboring regions as edge connections [17]. However, comparing to the non-graphical discriminative approach, generally such models add advantages little more than spatial smoothing of labelings [25].

Higher-level features, i.e. contexts in images, are often acknowledged as important discriminative factors [6,4]. In particular, relationship information on a larger scale, such as those across image slices [8], relating to reference objects [2], or between distant image regions [7], can be modeled as pairwise connections to encourage labeling consistency or enhance the discriminative power of local features. Such ideas of connecting beyond immediate neighbors are inspiring; however, choosing the related pairs and describing their interactions are rather application specific. To explore multi-scale region interactions, hierarchical models have been proposed [11,3]; however, they are normally created based on region clustering, without considering the actual object structures. At a more structural level, object detectors with bounding box outputs have been incorporated into CRFs as consistency constraints [12,6]. Although the idea is sound, such methods are normally built based on well-established object detectors and thus require only simple interaction modeling; but both assumptions are not suitable for our problem domain.

2   Object Localization

Given an image I, we first oversegment it into a set of regions $\{r_p\}$, using quick-shift clustering [24], to incorporate superpixel-level information around the pixels. The objective of object localization is then to derive a binary mask $L = \{l_p\}$, with each $l_p \in \{0, 1\}$ indicating whether the region r_p belongs to the object.

2.1   The Proposed CRF Model

We formulate the object localization problem as a binary labeling task using a new CRF model, with the following energy function:

$$E(L|I) = \underbrace{\sum_p \phi_L(l_p)}_{\text{local}} + \underbrace{\sum_{(p,q)\in N_S} \psi_S(l_p, l_q)}_{\text{smooth}} + \underbrace{\sum_{(p,c)\in N_C} \psi_C(l_p, l_c)}_{\text{contrast}} + \underbrace{\sum_{(p,i)\in N_R} \psi_R(l_p, l_i)}_{\text{interest-region}} \tag{1}$$

where the set of random variables or nodes of the graph is denoted by $L = \{\{l_p\} \cup \{l_c\} \cup \{l_i\}\}$, including the new auxiliary nodes from the contrast (l_c) and interest-region (l_i) potentials. The probability of a certain configuration is a conditional distribution on the energy function $E(L|I)$, and the optimal labeling is derived by minimizing the total energy using the graph cut [10].

The local potential $\phi_L(l_p)$ describes the cost of r_p labeled as 0 or 1:

$$\phi_L(l_p) = 1 - P(r_p = l_p|f_p) \tag{2}$$

where f_p is the local feature vector of r_p, and $P(.)$ is the probability estimate of labeling obtained using a binary support vector machine (SVM).

The smooth potential $\psi_S(r_p, r_q)$ penalizes the differences in labeling of the neighboring regions r_p and r_q based on their feature distances with a Potts model:

$$\psi_S(l_p, l_q) = \exp(-\frac{\| f_p - f_q \|^2}{2\beta_S})\mathbf{1}(l_p \neq l_q) \tag{3}$$

where β_S is the normalization factor as the average of all L2 distances between neighboring feature vectors in I. The regions r_p and r_q are considered neighbors if they share some common border in I, and the set of all neighboring pairs is denoted by N_S.

While the first two potentials follow the standard CRF constructs (Figure 1a), we describe the contrast and interest-region potentials (ψ_C, ψ_R, N_C and N_R) in the following.

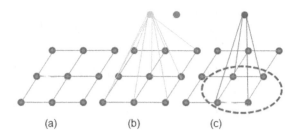

Fig. 1. The proposed CRF model. (a) The standard CRF construct, with nodes representing the image regions and edges linking the neighboring regions. (b) Introducing two auxiliary nodes (object and background) for the contrast potential, with edges linking the image regions and the auxiliary nodes (showing only one set of edges for easier viewing). (c) Based on the detected interest region (purple circle), an auxiliary node for the interest-region potential is added, with edges linking all image regions in the interest-region and the added node.

2.2   Contrast Potential

To improve the labeling accuracy, we want to explore the contrast information in the image I, with the following motivations. Across different images, there are often large inter-subject variations, causing overlaps between the feature ranges and hence misclassifications. Nevertheless, within one image, there is always a certain degree of contrast between the objects and background; and the contrast information helps to discriminate between the two types. To encode the contrast information, two additional nodes corresponding to the object and background, namely the contrast nodes l_c^o and l_c^b, are then added to the graph. A pairwise connection between the image region l_p and each of the two nodes is also established (Figure 1b), and N_C denotes the set of all such pairwise connections. With such a construct, we expect to encourage the same labelings between the image region and contrast nodes if they exhibit similar features, and also different labelings otherwise.

To do this, we first define the unary potentials of the two contrast nodes:

$$\phi_C(l_c^{o/b}) = \begin{cases} 0 & \text{if } l_c^{o/b} = 1/0 \\ C & \text{otherwise} \end{cases} \tag{4}$$

where C is a large constant, so that large costs are assigned to $l_c^o \neq 1$ and $l_c^b \neq 0$ and 0 costs otherwise, to effectively fix the labelings of the two nodes in the inference results.

We then define the pairwise potentials for the edges (l_p, l_c) with the following. First, based on the labeling outputs with local features only (Eq. (2)), we obtain the initial estimation of the objects and background areas, and two feature vectors f_c^o and f_c^b are then derived for the estimated objects and background (details of feature derivation in Sec 4). Next, we compute the contrast features between r_p and the objects and background as $g_p = \{f_p, f_p/f_c^o, f_p/f_c^b\}$, and classify the feature g_p to two classes – likely or unlikely to represent the object, denoted as $likely(1)$ and $unlikely(1)$ – using a binary SVM. Then, based on the probability estimates γ_p of class $likely(1)$, the pairwise costs are computed as:

$$\psi_C(l_p, l_c^o) = \begin{cases} 0 & \text{if } l_p = 1, \text{ and } likely(1) \\ 1 - \gamma_p & \text{if } l_p = 1, \text{ and } unlikely(1) \\ \gamma_p & \text{if } l_p = 0 \end{cases} \tag{5}$$

$$\psi_C(l_p, l_c^b) = \begin{cases} 0 & \text{if } l_p = 0, \text{ and } unlikely(1) \\ \gamma_p & \text{if } l_p = 0, \text{ and } likely(1) \\ 1 - \gamma_p & \text{if } l_p = 1 \end{cases} \tag{6}$$

Note that because of the *likely* and *unlikely* terms, the above pairwise potentials no longer follow the Potts model, and penalize labeling consistency if the features of the image regions and the contrast nodes are actually dissimilar. The total energy of the contrast potential can however, be rewritten in the following format, to keep it submodular (binary and with pairwise term encouraging consistency) for efficient graph-cut energy minimization:

$$\sum_{(p,c)\in N_C} \psi_C(l_p, l_c) = \sum_c \phi_C(l_c) + \\ \sum_p \alpha_p \mathbf{1}(unlikely(l_p)) + \sum_{(p,c)\in N_C} \alpha_p \mathbf{1}(l_p \neq l_c) \tag{7}$$

where $\alpha_p = \gamma_p$ if $l_p = 0$, and $\alpha_p = 1 - \gamma_p$ otherwise.

2.3   Interest Region Potential

Although the contrast nodes represent the object and background regions of an image I on a global scale, the structural information between image regions is not explored. An obviously important structural information is that, regions that are likely parts of the same anatomical or pathological structure should take the same labelings. In our formulation, the hypothesis is that, if we can detect a set of structures, i.e. interest regions R_i, the comprising regions $r_p \in R_i$ should preferably be assigned to the same category, but also depending on their individual suitability of such an labeling. The advantage of such an approach is that, we can employ a totally different method to detect the interest regions (e.g. non-CRF and different features), so the generated regions can serve as a second opinion to refine the object localization.

Assume a set of interest regions R_i are detected from an image I (details in Sec 3), and each interest region is characterized by its feature f_i, most probable label $l_i^* \in \{0, 1\}$ and a set of image regions r_p covered. Note that r_p might partially overlap with R_i especially around the boundary areas of R_i, and hence not all r_p covered by R_i should have the same label as l_i^*. To determine the the probability of $l_p = l_i^*$, we first compute the following feature vector:

$$v_p = \{\cap(r_p, R_i)/r_p, \| f_p - f_i \|, f_{i-p}/f_i\} \tag{8}$$

which represents the degrees of area overlap and feature homogeneity between r_p and R_i, with f_{i-p} denoting the feature of R_i excluding r_p. Then a binary SVM is trained to classify v_p into *same* or *diff* categories, indicating if $l_p = l_i^*$ or otherwise, and the probability estimate of $l_p = l_i^*$ is denoted by $\theta_{p,i}$.

Next, to integrate the interest-region detection hypothesis into the CRF formulation, for each R_i detected, a node l_i is added to the graph, with the unary potential $\phi_R(l_i)$ defined similarly to Eq. (4). An edge is then connected between each pair of (l_p, l_i) for all $r_p \in R_i$ (Figure 1c) with N_R denoting all such edges for image I, and we define the pairwise potential as:

$$\psi_R(l_p, l_i) = \theta_{p,i}\mathbf{1}(l_p \neq l_i) \tag{9}$$

Since $r_p \in R_i$ is quite likely to exhibit the same labeling as R_i, we choose to use the Potts model to encourage such consistency. The cost of different labelings is directly related to the probability of $l_p = l_i^*$, and hence we use $\theta_{p,i}$ as the pairwise cost. If r_p is less likely to be labeled as l_i^*, the use of $\theta_{p,i}$ is also able to lessen the consistency constraint.

With the above definitions, the total energy term of the interest-region potential is thus rewritten as the following:

$$\sum_{(p,i)\in N_R} \psi_R(l_p, l_i) = \sum_i \phi_R(l_i) + \sum_{(p,i)\in N_R} \theta_{p,i}\mathbf{1}(l_p \neq l_i) \tag{10}$$

2.4 Graph Inference

All energy terms are given equal weights (based on our empirical evaluation), and piecewise learnings of the probability estimates used in the local, contrast and interest-region potentials are conducted first. The binary inference problem $L^* = \text{argmin } E(L|I)$ is then solved efficiently using the graph cut.

3 Detection for Interest Region Potential

Due to our motivation of detecting the interest regions in a totally different way from the graph-based approach to support the interest-region potential (Sec 2.3), we choose to design a sparse-coding based classification method for interest-region detection. Besides its popularity and widely demonstrated effectiveness [14], we believe sparse coding can be particularly suitable for our problem because of the large variations in the dataset.

3.1 Sparse Coding for Classification

Let Y be a set of n-dimensional data samples $Y = \{y_j : j = 1, ..., J\}$ and $Y \in R^{n \times J}$. A representative dictionary for Y with K atoms is denoted as $D = \{d_k : k = 1, ..., K\} \in R^{n \times K}$. Each y_j can then be represented as a linear combination of a few (i.e. $\leq T$) atoms in D with minimum reconstruction error, and the corresponding coefficient vector x_j is the sparse code. Denoting the set of sparse codes of the data samples Y as $X = \{x_j : j = 1, ..., J\} \in R^{K \times J}$, both the dictionary D and sparse coding X can be learned with K-SVD [1] by solving the following problem:

$$\langle D, X \rangle = \underset{D,X}{\operatorname{argmin}} \ \|Y - DX\|_2^2 \quad s.t. \forall j, \|x_j\|_0 \leq T \qquad (11)$$

where $\|Y - DX\|_2^2$ represents the reconstruction error.

Once the dictionary D is learned, a given data sample y can then be represented as a sparse code x by solving the following using the OMP algorithm [23]:

$$x = \underset{x}{\operatorname{argmin}} \ \|y - Dx\|_2^2 \quad s.t. \ \|x\|_0 \leq T \qquad (12)$$

A classifier (e.g. SVM) can then be trained based on a set of such sparse codes, so that x and hence y can be classified.

In our context, an image I is divided into grid-based patches, and each image patch is represented by its feature descriptor y. The dictionary D is generated with a training set Y, and each image patch is then classified as interest region or otherwise ($h \in \{1, 0\}$) based on its sparse code x.

3.2 Discriminative Sparse Learning

A shortcoming with the above approach is the separation of the dictionary learning and classifier training, hence the learned dictionary might not produce discriminative sparse codes for the classification. Several approaches have thus been proposed to integrate the two steps of learning [9]. However, it is observed that such an integrated approach is still largely optimized for the reconstruction term, which may affect the discriminative power of W. Therefore, we suggest that the integrated learning for dictionary D should not totally replace the separate classifier training, and propose a different method as follows.

First, for the data samples $Y \in R^{n \times J}$, we create a corresponding labeling vector $H = \{h_j\} \in \{-1, 1\}^{1 \times J}$, with 1 for interest region. Based on linear-kernel SVM, the optimization objective of the weight vector $w \in R^{1 \times K}$ is:

$$\operatorname{argmin}_{w,\xi,b} \ \tfrac{1}{2}\|w\|^2 + C \sum_j \xi_j$$
$$s.t. \ \forall j, h_j(w * x_j + b) \geq 1 - \xi_j, \ \xi_j \geq 0 \qquad (13)$$

Combining Eq. (11) and (13), and by simplifying the complexities caused by the inequality constraints on ξ_j and the signed h_j, we relax the formulation based on least squares SVM (LS-SVM) [22] as:

$$\langle D, X, w \rangle = \operatorname{argmin}_{D,X,w} \ \|Y - DX\|_2^2 + \|w\|^2 + \sum_j \xi_j^2$$
$$s.t. \ \forall j, \|x_j\|_0 \leq T, \ h_j(w * x_j + b) = 1 - \xi_j \qquad (14)$$

By combining w and b, and substituting ξ_j, the problem is then equivalent to the following:

$$\langle D', X', w' \rangle = \operatorname{argmin}_{D', X', w'} \|Y - D'X'\|_2^2 + \|w'\|^2 +$$

$$\|H - w'X'\|_2^2 \qquad s.t. \ \forall j, \|x'_j\|_0 \leq T \tag{15}$$

where $w' = [w, b] \in R^{1 \times (K+1)}$ and $X' \in R^{(K+1) \times J}$ appended an addition dimension with constant value 1 to absorb b, and $D' \in R^{n \times (K+1)}$ with an additional atom to be dimensionally compatible with X'. To solve Eq. (15), an alternative approach is used, as detailed in [20].

4 Experimental Results

4.1 Results on Lesion Dissimilarity

Measuring lesion similarity is important in many medical applications, such as content-based image retrieval for diagnosis referencing. In our approach, first, lesions (i.e. lung tumors and abnormal lymph nodes) in thoracic PET-CT images are localized in each image slice with the proposed method. Second, their textural and spatial features are extracted in 3D. Lastly, a weighted histogram-intersection is used to compute the feature distance. The actual implementation details are referred to [20]. The datasets comprise of 40 thoracic PET-CT 3D image sets from non-small cell lung cancer studies. A total of 64 lesions including lung tumors and abnormal lymph nodes are annotated, and the similarity/dissimilarity relationships between each pair of 3D image sets are marked as the ground truth. Three image sets showing typical thoracic characteristics are selected for training, and testing is performed on all image sets.

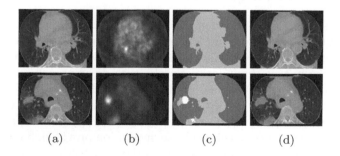

(a)   (b)   (c)   (d)

Fig. 2. Two example localization outputs. (a) Transaxial CT image slices (showing the thorax after preprocessing). (b) Co-registered PET image slices. (c) The labeling outputs using standard CRF, with dark gray for lung field, light gray for mediastinum and white for lesion. (d) Our localization outputs with the two additional potentials, with lesions highlighted in orange.

Figure 2 shows examples of the lesion localization. The first example illustrates the benefits of the contrast potential, in which the lesion is initially not detected with standard CRF, due to the relatively low PET intensities. The interest-region potential is particularly useful in refining the lesion boundaries, which tend to be underestimated with the standard CRF, as shown in the second example. It is observed that, the standard CRF tends to produce a large number of either totally undetected or underestimated lesions. Based on the measured 3D object-level localization results, we summarize the localization recall, precision and F-score in Table 1.

The localized lesions are then used to retrieval images with similar lesions. The retrieval tests are performed by using each 3D image set as a query image, and the remaining 39 images are ranked accordingly. We compare the retrieval performance with three other approaches: (i) state-of-the-art of thoracic PET-CT image retrieval [18]; (ii) spatial pyramid matching (SPM) with local intensity features extracted from grid-based image patches; and (iii) bag-of-words with SIFT descriptor. As shown in Figure 3, our proposed method exhibits the highest retrieval precisions for all recall levels.

Table 1. The localization performances comparing our proposed method with standard CRF

	Recall (%)	Precision (%)	F-score (%)
Ours	97.0	95.4	96.2
CRF	76.6	94.2	84.5

4.2 Results on Cell Segmentation

Cell nucleus segmentation is one of the most important tasks in analyzing and quantifying fluorescence microscopic images. In our approach, the cell nucleus is localized using the proposed method; and since the localization results also tend to delineate the nucleus boundaries closely, such an approach can be directly used for segmentation. The actual implementation details are referred to [20]. The serous database [13] is used to evaluate the cell segmentation. The database contains 10 microscopic images. A total of 254 cell nuclei are present in the images, with ground truth of cell nuclei segmentation provided. Same as [4], half of the images are used for training and the others for testing.

To evaluate the segmentation performance, we compute the PASCAL VOC criteria of pixel- and object-level accuracies, both as $TP/(TP+FN+FP)$. We also compare our results with three approaches: (i) L+S, the standard CRF with local and smooth potentials; (ii) L+S+C, with additional contrast potential; (iii) L+S+R, with additional interest-region potential; and (iv) the state-of-the-art discriminative labeling method [4] reported for the same database. As listed in Table 2, our method achieves the highest pixel- and object-level accuracies.

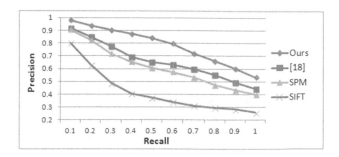

Fig. 3. The retrieval precision and recall

Table 2. The segmentation results comparing various methods

	Ours	L+S	L+S+C	L+S+R	[4]
Pixel Acc (%)	85.6	82.0	83.1	84.6	85.1
Obj Acc (%)	89.3	84.5	86.2	88.7	84.0

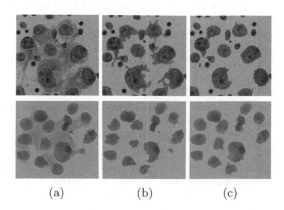

(a)   (b)   (c)

Fig. 4. Two example segmentation results. (a) Cropped microscopic images, with orange circles delineating the segmentation ground truth. (b) The segmentation results with L+S. (c) The segmentation results of our proposed method.

The improvements of having the contrast and potential terms are evident. The performance difference between L+S and [4] suggests that if we incorporate the feature set of [4], the segmentation accuracies would be further improved. By replacing the interest-region detection with standard sparse-coding classification, it is found that our proposed method exhibits on average 1.1% improvement for both pixel- and object-level measurements with the new approach.

The first example shown in Figure 4 indicates that our method is quite effective in removing the cytoplasm areas that connect the cell nuclei. As shown in the second example, lighter intensities of the cell nuclei cause many false negatives with the standard CRF approach; and our result shows more accurate delineations of the actual contours.

5   Summary

In this Chapter, we describe a new method for object localization in medical images [20]. A new CRF model with additional contrast and interest-region potentials is proposed for effective object localization, addressing large inter-subject variations and low feature differences between the objects and background. A new sparse-coding classification approach is also designed for the interest-region detection, with enhanced discriminative power of the learned dictionaries. The proposed method is applied to lesion dissimilarity on thoracic PET-CT images, and cell segmentation on microscopic images, and shows higher performance compared to the state-of-the-art techniques.

References

1. Aharon, M., Elad, M., Bruckstein, A.: K-SVD: an algorithm for designing over-complete dictionaries for sparse representation. IEEE Trans. Signal Process. 54(1), 4311–4322 (2006)
2. Ben Ayed, I., Punithakumar, K., Garvin, G., Romano, W., Li, S.: Graph Cuts with Invariant Object-Interaction Priors: Application to Intervertebral Disc Segmentation. In: Székely, G., Hahn, H.K. (eds.) IPMI 2011. LNCS, vol. 6801, pp. 221–232. Springer, Heidelberg (2011)
3. Bauer, S., Nolte, L.-P., Reyes, M.: Fully Automatic Segmentation of Brain Tumor Images Using Support Vector Machine Classification in Combination with Hierarchical Conditional Random Field Regularization. In: Fichtinger, G., Martel, A., Peters, T. (eds.) MICCAI 2011, Part III. LNCS, vol. 6893, pp. 354–361. Springer, Heidelberg (2011)
4. Cheng, L., Ye, N., Yu, W., Cheah, A.: Discriminative Segmentation of Microscopic Cellular Images. In: Fichtinger, G., Martel, A., Peters, T. (eds.) MICCAI 2011, Part I. LNCS, vol. 6891, pp. 637–644. Springer, Heidelberg (2011)
5. Feuerstein, M., Glocker, B., Kitasaka, T., Nakamura, Y., Iwano, S., Mori, K.: Mediastinal atlas creation from 3-d chest computed tomography images: application to automated detection and station mapping of lymph nodes. Med. Image Anal. 16(1), 63–74 (2011)
6. Gonfaus, J., Boix, X.: Harmony potentials for joint classification and segmentation. In: CVPR, pp. 3280–3287 (2010)
7. Guo, R., Dai, Q., Hoiem, D.: Single-image shadow detection and removal using paired regions. In: CVPR, pp. 2033–2040 (2011)
8. Jagadeesh, V., Vu, N., Manjunath, B.S.: Multiple Structure Tracing in 3D Electron Micrographs. In: Fichtinger, G., Martel, A., Peters, T. (eds.) MICCAI 2011, Part I. LNCS, vol. 6891, pp. 613–620. Springer, Heidelberg (2011)
9. Jiang, Z., Lin, Z., Davis, L.: Learning a discriminative dictionary for sparse coding via label consistent K-SVD. In: CVPR, pp. 1697–1704 (2011)
10. Kolmogorov, V., Zabih, R.: What energy functions can be minimized via graph cuts? IEEE Trans. Pattern Anal. Mach. Intell. 26(2), 147–159 (2004)

11. Ladicky, L., Russell, C., Kohli, P., Torr, P.H.S.: Associative hierarchical CRFs for object class image segmentation. In: ICCV, pp. 739–746 (2009)
12. Ladický, Ľ., Sturgess, P., Alahari, K., Russell, C., Torr, P.H.S.: What, Where and How Many? Combining Object Detectors and CRFs. In: Daniilidis, K., Maragos, P., Paragios, N. (eds.) ECCV 2010, Part IV. LNCS, vol. 6314, pp. 424–437. Springer, Heidelberg (2010)
13. Lezoray, O., Cardot, H.: Cooperation of color pixel classification schemes and color watershed: a study for microscopical images. IEEE Trans. Image Process. 11(7), 783–789 (2002)
14. Liu, M., Lu, L., Ye, X., Yu, S., Salganicoff, M.: Sparse Classification for Computer Aided Diagnosis Using Learned Dictionaries. In: Fichtinger, G., Martel, A., Peters, T. (eds.) MICCAI 2011, Part III. LNCS, vol. 6893, pp. 41–48. Springer, Heidelberg (2011)
15. Lu, C., Chelikani, S., Jaffray, D.A., Milosevic, M.F., Staib, L.H., Juncan, J.S.: Simultaneous nonrigid registration, segmentation, and tumor detection in MRI guided cervical cancer radiation therapy. IEEE Trans. Med. Imag. 31(6), 1213–1227 (2012)
16. van Ravesteijin, V.F., van Wijk, C., Vos, F.M., Truyen, R., Peters, J.F., Stoker, J., van Vliet, L.J.: Computer-aided detection of polyps in CT colonography using logistic regression. IEEE Trans. Med. Imag. 29(1), 120–131 (2010)
17. Shotton, J., Winn, J.M., Rother, C., Criminisi, A.: *TextonBoost*: Joint Appearance, Shape and Context Modeling for Multi-class Object Recognition and Segmentation. In: Leonardis, A., Bischof, H., Pinz, A. (eds.) ECCV 2006. LNCS, vol. 3951, pp. 1–15. Springer, Heidelberg (2006)
18. Song, Y., Cai, W., Eberl, S., Fulham, M.J., Feng, D.: Discriminative Pathological Context Detection in Thoracic Images Based on Multi-level Inference. In: Fichtinger, G., Martel, A., Peters, T. (eds.) MICCAI 2011, Part III. LNCS, vol. 6893, pp. 191–198. Springer, Heidelberg (2011)
19. Song, Y., Cai, W., Eberl, S., Fulham, M., Feng, D.: Thoracic image case retrieval with spatial and contextual information. In: ISBI, pp. 1885–1888 (2011)
20. Song, Y., Cai, W., Huang, H., Wang, Y., Feng, D.D.: Object localization in medical images based on graphical model with contrast and interest-region terms. In: CVPR Workshop, pp. 1–7 (2012)
21. Song, Y., Cai, W., Kim, J., Feng, D.D.: A multistage discriminative model for tumor and lymph node detection in thoracic images. IEEE Trans. Med. Imag. 31(5), 1061–1075 (2012)
22. Suykens, J., Vandewalle, J.: Least squares support vector machine classifiers. Neural Process. Letters 9(3), 293–300 (1999)
23. Tropp, J.: Greed is good: algorithmic results for sparse approximation. IEEE Trans. Inf. Theory 50(10), 2231–2242 (2004)
24. Vedaldi, A., Soatto, S.: Quick Shift and Kernel Methods for Mode Seeking. In: Forsyth, D., Torr, P., Zisserman, A. (eds.) ECCV 2008, Part IV. LNCS, vol. 5305, pp. 705–718. Springer, Heidelberg (2008)
25. Wu, D., Lu, L., Bi, J., Shinagawa, Y., Boyer, K., Krishnan, A., Salganicoff, M.: Stratified learning of local anatomical context for lung nodules in CT images. In: CVPR, pp. 2791–2798 (2010)

A Cascade Learning Method
for Liver Lesion Detection in CT Images

Dijia Wu[1], David Liu[1], Michael Suehling[1], Kevin S. Zhou[1],
and Christian Tietjen[2]

[1] Siemens Corporate Research, Princeton NJ 08544, USA
[2] Siemens Healthcare, Siemensstr. 1, Forchheim 91301, Germany

Abstract. The automatic detection and segmentation of liver lesion is useful in many clinical application, whereas it remains a challenging task due to the largely varied shape, size and texture of the diseased masses. In this paper, we present a cascade learning approach comprising multiple classifiers for the detection of two different types of solid liver lesions, hypodense and hyperdense lesions. In particular, we propose an efficient gradient based locally adaptive segmentation method for the solid lesions, where the segmentation results are used to extract shape features to boost up the detection performance. The proposed method is validated on a total of 660 volumes with 1,302 hypodense lesions, and 234 volumes with 328 hyperdense lesions. The experimental results show a resulting 90% detection rate at 1.01 false positives per volume for hypodense lesion and 1.58 false positives per volume for hyperdense lesion, respectively, using three fold cross validation.

1 Introduction

Detection and segmentation of abnormal hepatic masses is important to liver disease diagnosis, treatment planning and follow-up monitoring. As a significant part of clinical practice in radiology, liver tumors are usually examined and tracked every several weeks or months to assess the cancer staging and therapy response based on 3D Computed Tomography (CT) data. However, manually finding these lesions is tedious and time consuming, and highly dependent on the observer's experiences. Hence, a system of automatic lesion detection and measurement is desirable.

There is a limited amount of previous work directed to automatic liver lesion detection, compared with lesion segmentation. Ye et al. proposed the use of gray-level statistical features and temporal enhancement pattern of different contrast phases to classify the liver tissues with SVM, however, it required experienced radiologists to draw region of interest in advance and multi-phase enhanced CT images [1]. Moltz et al. presented a simple threshold filtering method followed by circular structure detection with Hugh transform to locate matching lesions in follow-up CT examinations [2]. It assumes that the lesion mask of the baseline scan is available, hence the tumor location is known coarsely and detection can be restricted to a local area in the follow up scans. A multi-level Otsu's method with

B.H. Menze et al. (Eds.): MCV 2012, LNCS 7766, pp. 206–214, 2013.
© Springer-Verlag Berlin Heidelberg 2013

level set algorithm was used in [3] to segment complicated liver lesion but the user has to first manually select several points covering the whole lesion inside the liver area. Other lesion segmentation methods dependent on user interactions include random walker [4], graph cut and watershed [5], and seeded region growing [6].

In this work, we present a fully automated method to detect two most common types of hepatic lesions, *hypodense* (darker) and *hyperdense* (brighter) lesions, from single 3D CT image of any contrast phase. It generates lesion candidates with a learning based approach as opposed to simplistic thresholding or painstaking local minimum point clustering [7,8]. Because lesion detection is usually a highly unbalanced classification problem where negative samples, i.e., healthy tissues or other structures such as vessels, are many more than positive samples, a cascade learning framework [9] is employed to speed up the detection and improve the classification result for unbalanced data problems [10]. This differentiates our method from other learning based liver lesion segmentation approaches such as ensemble segmentation using AdaBoost [11] or iterative Bayesian approach [12]. In addition, we propose a new gradient based locally adaptive lesion segmentation method. The aim of the segmentation is not to perfectly locate the lesion boundaries, but provide fast and reasonable segmentation results from which geometric and statistical features can be extracted to improve detections. The idea of coupling segmentation and detection was proposed in [13] and later applied in lymph node detection problem [14]. Our work uses a much simpler segmentation method than the Gaussian MRF and gradient descent in [14] and extracts different segmentation based features.

The rest of the paper is organized as follows. Section 2 describes this cascade learning system for liver lesion detection and outlines the gradient based locally adaptive segmentation method. It will be explained how the unsupervised constructed segmentation can be used to improve the supervised detection performance. In Section 3, experimental validation results on two particular types of liver lesions, hypodense and hyperdense lesions, are presented. We conclude with a review of our contribution and potential extensions in Section 4.

2   Liver Lesion Detection and Segmentation

2.1   Liver Segmentation and Liver Lesion Annotation

To constrain the search, the liver is first automatically segmented using a hierarchical learning based method described in [15]; the liver subvolume is then cropped and resampled to 1.5 mm isotropic resolution. Each liver lesion of size at least 10 mm in the dataset is annotated by placing a bounding box around it as shown in Fig.1. The voxels within a predefined distance from the bounding box centers are used as positive samples and voxels out of the boxes as negative samples in training. The lesions are labeled as hypodense (darker) or hyperdense (brighter) depending on the enhancement pattern difference between normal liver parenchyma and lesions.

2.2   Detection and Segmentation

Like many other Computer Aided Diagnosis (CAD) problems, lesion detection data sets are large and extremely unbalanced between positive and negative classes, given the fact that liver lesions are generally a few and small compared with the whole liver volume. Therefore, we use a cascade classification framework for lesion detection as shown in Fig.2. The coarse-to-fine cascade structure has been shown effective in speeding up the detection process by discarding many negative samples with fewer simple features before more complex classifiers are called upon to further reduce the false positives [9]. The cascade framework can also be used to simplify the difficult unbalanced classification problem into a sequence of linear programs, each of which separates only a subset of negative samples from the positives [10].

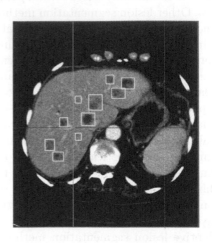

Fig. 1. The liver lesions are annotated with bounding boxes. The segmented liver is overlaid on the original volume in light red.

As shown in Fig.2, the proposed liver lesion detection system comprises four classifiers from simple to complex. First, we use a Haar based detector to generate lesion candidates followed by bootstrapping to prune these candidates also with Haar features. Then lesion segmentation is performed and the resulting segmentation is used to obtain geometric and statistical features to verify the candidates and reject the negative ones. Finally, a more informative set of steerable features [16] are extracted from the segmentation to further reduce false positives.

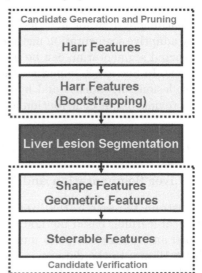

Fig. 2. Liver lesion detection system

Lesion   Candidate   Generation.
Liver lesion center candidates are detected from all voxels in the liver subvolume in two stages. The initial set of candidates are generated using a fast Haar-based detector. It is a cascade of two AdaBoost classifiers [17], the first classifier has 100 weak learners and the second has 200. They are trained using

138,464 3D Haar features [18] with all positive voxels and 1% negative voxels randomly sampled. This stage achieves 100% detection rate with an average false positive rate about 0.4% on training data.

A second Haar detector is trained for bootstrapping, using the same set of features and classifier configuration but with all positives and all negatives passing through the first stage. This stage achieves about 25% false positive rate on the average at 100% detection rate on training data. The significantly increased false positive rate suggests that Haar features are not enough to further reduce the false detections. More complicated features such as texture features or shape features are often used to distinguish various lesions, e.g., gray-level co-occurrence matrix [1], local binary pattern [19] or Hessian eigen-system based filters [20]. However, these features are computationally expensive. In this work, we employ geometric and statistical features which embed the shape and texture information and can be efficiently computed from the lesion segmentation. From the perspective of marginal space learning [16], segmentation provides extra information about object size and orientation that improves the detection performance.

Lesion Segmentation. Many liver lesion segmentation methods have been proposed as mentioned in Section 1. We choose adaptive thresholding because it is fully automatic, very simple and precise segmentation is not our target. However, all previous works use single threshold for filtering the lesions, which is selected with different methods such as histogram analysis [2,21], or cross-entropy minimization [22]. However, single threshold is subject to the constraint of inhomogeneous lesions in one liver. To solve this problem, we present a multi-thresholding method based on local surface gradients as given in Algorithm 1. This method presents a connected component tree structure which is similar to maximally stable extremal regions (MSER) [23] approach used in stereo matching and object recognition. But we select the optimal threshold based on maximum gradient response rather than area stability criterion in [23]. The example segmentation results of the proposed multi-threshold method are given and compared with single threshold [2] in Fig.3. It is clear that the proposed

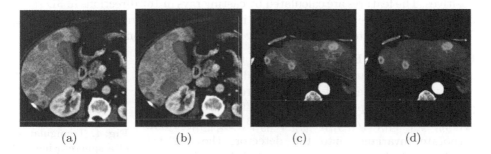

(a)   (b)   (c)   (d)

Fig. 3. (a) (c) single threshold segmentation; (b) (d) proposed multi-threshold segmentation. Note that for hyperdense lesion, the original volume should be inverted before applying algorithm 1.

Algorithm 1. Gradient based locally adaptive segmentation method

---

Input: Liver volume $I(x,y,z)$ and number of thresholds n.
Output: Threshold $\Omega(x,y,z)$, binary segmentation $S(x,y,z) = 1$ if $I(x,y,z) <$ $\Omega(x,y,z)$ and 0 otherwise.

---

1. Run liver intensity histogram analysis and obtain the peak value τ and standard deviation σ. Set $\tau_{min} = \tau - n\sigma, \tau_{max} = \tau$ and $\Delta\tau = \sigma$.
2. Start from single threshold $\omega = \tau_{max}$ and obtain initial binary segmentation S.
3. Run 3D connected component labeling on S. Each connected component is denoted as C_i and its surface as R_i.
4. Calculate the mean surface gradient norm of C_i: $G_i = \Sigma_{(x,y,z)\in R_i}|\nabla I(x,y,z)|/|R_i|$.
5. For C_i, use threshold $\omega' = \omega - \Delta\tau$ to obtain new segmentation and connected components C_i', R_i' and G_i'.
6. $\Omega(x,y,z) = \omega$ if $G_i \geq G_i'$ and ω' otherwise, $\forall(x,y,z) \in C_i$, then update S.
7. Set $\omega = \omega'$ and $\omega' = \omega' - \Delta\tau$ and repeat step 3 to 7 until $\omega = \tau_{min}$.

---

method achieves better segmentation results. Finally, watershed transform [24] is performed on the segmentation results to separate closely connected lesions.

Lesion Candidate Verification. The segmentation is used to derive more informative features for further evaluation of the liver lesion candidates. The candidate verification consists of two coarse-to-fine detectors as shown in Fig.2. The first detector calculates 28 geometric features and 6 statistical features of each connected component obtained in the segmentation. The geometric features include diameter, volume size, surface area, compactness, rectangularity, elongation, central moments and so on; the statistical features comprise min, max, mean, variance, skewness and kurtosis of intensities. Because some structures in the liver show similar intensities to the lesions, for instance, vessels and hyperdense lesions are both enhanced in the arterial phase, many segmented objects are not lesions. Therefore, we use these shape and statistical descriptors to identify and reject the obvious non-lesion segmentations.

The second candidate verification detector uses much more dense steerable features [14,16] computed from the segmentation to further remove difficult false positives. The features are calculated by casting rays in 162 directions in 3D space from each candidate location as shown in Fig.4. In each direction, the following features are calculated at the boundary of the segmentation:

Intensity Based Features: Assume the intensity and gradient at boundary (x,y,z) is I and $g = (g_x, g_y, g_z)$, respectively. For each of the 162 directions, we compute 24 feature types, including I, $\sqrt{(I)}$, I^2, I^3, $\log I$, g_x, g_y, g_z, $||g||$, $\sqrt{(||g||)}$, $||g||^2$, $||g||^3$, $\log ||g||$. To incorporate invariance into the detector, the 162 values for each feature type are sorted by value. This not only ensures rotational invariance, but invariance

Fig. 4. Triangulation of a sphere using 162 vertices and 320 triangles

to all permutations, including mirroring. Additionally, for each of the 24 feature types, the 81 sums of feature values at the pairs of opposite vertices are computed and sorted by value.

Geometry Features: The 81 diameters (distances between opposite vertices relative to the segmentation center) are sorted. For each diameter the following features are computed: (a) The value of each diameter. (b) Asymmetry of each diameter, i.e. the ratio of the larger radius over the smaller radius. (c) The ratio of the i-th sorted diameter and the j-th diameter for all $1 \leq i < j \leq 81$. (d) For each of the 24 feature types, the max or min of the feature values at the two diameter ends. (e) For each of the 24 feature types, the max or min of the feature values half way to the diameter ends.

In total there are about 17,000 features. Using these features, a cascade of two AdaBoost classifiers with 70 and 140 weak learners each is trained. Because multiple candidates can be detected in a single lesion, all the remaining candidates at the final stage are clustered using non-maximal suppression [14]. To accommodate to lesions of vastly different sizes, the above process is repeated with different resolutions in a pyramid manner.

3   Experimental Results and Discussion

Data Collection. In the experiment, we collected 661 liver CT subvolumes from 564 subjects with 1,302 hypodense lesions, and 234 volumes from 198 subjects with 328 hyperdense lesions. The annotations were obtained as described in Section 2.1 by two radiologists based on visual assessment and consensus review. In this work, we target tumors of moderate size with diameter between 10 mm to 100 mm, therefore all the annotated lesions are of size in this range. Data were collected from multiple hospitals.

Evaluation Methodology. A lesion is considered as detected if there exists a detection with its center inside this lesion bounding box, whereas a detection is considered as false positive if its center outside any annotated lesion bounding boxes.

Results. The liver subvolumes are split into training and testing data via three-fold cross validation which is repeated for 5 times and all results presented here are the averages over 5 runs. The volumes of the same patient are always put into the same folder. The resulting ROC curves are given in Fig.6. The proposed detection system reaches 1.01 false positives per volume and 1.58 false positives per volume at 90% sensitivity for hypodense and hyperdense lesion, respectively. The detection performance based on single threshold segmentation method [2] and without watershed transform is also compared in Fig.6.

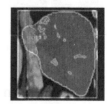

Fig. 5. False positive of hyperdense lesion detection

The hypodense lesion detection is better than hyperdense detection because we have less annotations of hyperdense lesions and more importantly, hyperdense lesions detection is more easily confused with other bright structures especially the vessels as shown in Fig.5. In this example, the aorta is falsely truncated and segmented as a part of liver, which is then misclassified as a hyperdense lesion.

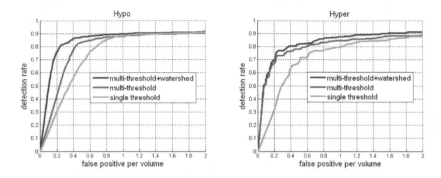

Fig. 6. Lesion detection ROC curves

Examples of detected true positives are shown in Fig.7. The bounding box of a detected lesion is obtained from the segmentation. Note that not all segmented objects are lesions. For hyperdense lesion, the liver segmentation is also given. As shown in Fig.7, the proposed system can detect lesions of highly different sizes, shapes, intensities and positions in the liver. The average running time is 20-30 seconds per volume.

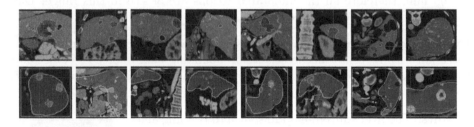

Fig. 7. Example detection and segmentation results. Top row: hypodense lesions. Bottom row: hyperdense lesion.

4   Conclusion

In this paper, we presented a cascade learning system for automated liver lesion detection based on a novel multi-threshold segmentation method. We discussed how the segmentation results can be used to extract shape and intensity features to improve the detection performance. Ongoing work will include improvement of hyperdense lesion detection, particularly separation from the vessels. As liver lesions exhibit various appearances in different contrast phases, the prior knowledge of the contrast phase can also potentially benefit the detection performance. Also, because both hyperdense and hypodense lesions possess similar shapes and structures, they might be used in training together to improve each other's detection with techniques such as transfer learning.

References

1. Ye, J., Sun, Y., Wang, S., Gu, L., Qian, L., Xu, J.: Multi-Phase CT Image Based Hepatic Lesion Diagnosis by SVM. In: Proc. iCBBE, vol. 1, pp. 1–5 (2009)
2. Moltz, J.H., Schwier, M., Peitgen, H.O.: A General Framework for Automatic Detection of Matching Lesions in Followup CT. In: Proc. ISBI, vol. 1, pp. 843–846 (2009)
3. Luo, Z., Wu, X., Cen, R., Ou, S.: Segmentation of Complicated Liver Lesion Based on Local Multiphase Level Set. In: Proc. iCBBE, vol. 1, pp. 1–4 (2009)
4. Grady, L., Jolly, M.P.: 3D General Lesion Segmentation in CT. In: Proc. ISBI (2008)
5. Stawiaski, J., Decencire, E., Bidault, F.: Interactive Liver Tumor Segmentation Using Graph-cuts and Watershed. In: Proc. MICCAI Workshop (2008)
6. Wong, D., Liu, J., Yin, F., Tian, Q., Xiong, W.: A Semi-Automated Method for Liver Tumor Segmentation Based on 2D Region Growing with Knowledge-Based Constraints. In: Proc. MICCAI Workshop (2008)
7. Hame, Y.: Liver Tumor Segmentation Using Implicit Surface Evolution. In: Proc. MICCAI Workshop (2008)
8. Kubota, T.: Efficient Automated Detection and Segmentation of Medium and Large Liver Tumors: CAD Approach. In: Proc. MICCAI Workshop (2008)
9. Viola, P., Jones, M.J.: Robust Real-Time Face Detection. Int J. Comput. Vision 57, 137–154 (2004)
10. Bi, J., Periaswamy, S., Okada, K., Kubota, T., Fung, G., Salganicoff, M., Rao, B.: Computer Aided Detection via Asymmetric Cascade of Sparse Hyperplane Classifiers. In: Proc. SIGKDD (2006)
11. Shimizu, A., Narihira, T., Furukawa, D., Kobatake, H., Nawano, S., Shinozaki, K.: Ensemble Segmentation Using AdaBoost with Application to Liver Lesion Extraction from a CT Volume. In: Proc. MICCAI Workshop (2008)
12. Taieb, Y., Eliassaf, O., Freiman, et al.: An Iterative Bayesian Approach for Liver Analysis: Tumors Validation Study. In: Proc. MICCAI Workshop (2008)
13. Leibe, B., Leonardis, A., Schiele, B.: Robust Object Detection with Interleaved Categorization and Segmentation. Int J. Comput. Vision 77, 259–289 (2008)
14. Barbu, A., Suehling, M., Xu, X., Liu, D., Zhou, S.K., Comaniciu, D.: Automatic Detection and Segmentation of Axillary Lymph Nodes. In: Jiang, T., Navab, N., Pluim, J.P.W., Viergever, M.A. (eds.) MICCAI 2010, Part I. LNCS, vol. 6361, pp. 28–36. Springer, Heidelberg (2010)
15. Ling, H., Zheng, Y., Georgescu, B., Zhou, S.K., Suehling, M.: Hierarchical Learning-Based Automatic Liver Segmentation. In: Proc. CVPR (2008)
16. Zheng, Y., Barbu, A., Georgescu, B., Scheuering, M., Comaniciu, D.: Four-Chamber Heart Modeling and Automatic Segmentation for 3-D Cardiac CT Volumes Using Marginal Space Learning and Steerable Features. IEEE Trans. Med. Imag. 27(11), 1668–1681 (2008)

17. Tu, Z.: Probabilistic Boosting-Tree: Learning Discriminative Models for Classification, Recognition, and Clustering. In: Proc. ICCV, vol. 2, pp. 1589–1596 (2005)
18. Tu, Z., Zhou, X.S., Barbu, A., Bogoni, L., Comaniciu, D.: Probabilistic 3D Polyp Detection in CT Images: The Role of Sample Alignment. In: Proc. CVPR (2006)
19. Zhou, J., Chang, S., Metaxas, D., Zhao, B., Schwartz, L.H., Ginsberg, M.S.: Automatic Detection and Segmentation of Ground Glass Opacity Nodules. In: Larsen, R., Nielsen, M., Sporring, J. (eds.) MICCAI 2006. LNCS, vol. 4190, pp. 784–791. Springer, Heidelberg (2006)
20. Wu, D., Lu, L., Bi, J., Shinagawa, Y., Boyer, K., et al.: Stratified Learning of Local Anatomical Context for Lung Nodules in CT Images. In: Proc. CVPR (2010)
21. Moltz, J.H., Bornemann, L., Dicken, V., Peitgen, H.O.: Segmentation of Liver Metastases in CT Scans by Adaptive Thresholding and Morphological Processing. In: Proc. MICCAI Workshop (2008)
22. Choudhary, A., Moretto, N., Ferrarese, F.P., Zamboni, G.A.: An Entropy Based Multi-Thresholding Method for Semi-Automatic Segmentation of Liver Tumors. In: Proc. MICCAI Workshop (2008)
23. Matas, J., Chum, O., Urba, M., Pajdla, T.: Robust Wide Baseline Stereo from Maximally Stable Extremal Regions. In: Proc. BMVC, pp. 384–396 (2002)
24. Vincent, L., Soille, P.: Watersheds in Digital Spaces: An Efficient Algorithm Based on Immersion Simulations. IEEE Trans. Pattern Anal. Mach. Intell. 13(6), 583–598 (1991)

Automatic Event Detection within Thrombus Formation Based on Integer Programming

Loic Peter[1], Olivier Pauly[1,2], Sjoert B.G. Jansen[3,4], Peter A. Smethurst[3,4],
Willem H. Ouwehand[3,4,5], Nassir Navab[1]

[1] Computer Aided Medical Procedures, Technische Universitaet Muenchen,
Munich, Germany
[2] Institute of Biomathematics and Biometry, Helmholtz Zentrum Muenchen,
Munich, Germany
[3] Department of Haematology, University of Cambridge, Cambridge,
United Kingdom
[4] National Health Service Blood and Transplant, Cambridge, United Kingdom
[5] The Wellcome Trust Sanger Institute, Hinxton, United Kingdom

Abstract. After a blood vessel injury, blood platelets progressively aggregate on the damaged site to stop the resulting blood loss. This natural mechanism called thrombosis can however be prone to malfunctions and lead to the complete obstruction of the blood vessel. Thrombosis disorders play a crucial role in coronary artery diseases and the identification of genetic risk predispositions would therefore considerably help their diagnosis and therapy. *In vitro* experiments are conducted in this purpose by perfusing blood from several donors over a surface of collagen fibres, which results in the progressive attachment of platelets. Based on the segmentation over time of these aggregates called thrombi, we propose in this paper an automatic method combining tracking and event detection which allows the extraction of characteristics of interest for each thrombus growth individually, in order to find a potential correlation between these growth features and blood donors genetic disorders. We demonstrate the benefits of our approach and the accuracy of its results through an experimental validation.

Keywords: Microscopy image analysis, thrombus segmentation, multi-target tracking, event detection.

1 Introduction

Thrombosis denotes the abnormal coagulation of platelets that may occur after a blood vessel injury and eventually leads to the complete obstruction of the blood circulation. In addition to the identification of environmental risk factors such as smoking, obesity, and physical inactivity, the study of possible genetic predispositions to thrombosis is becoming increasingly important to improve the diagnosis and the therapy of coronary artery diseases. Genome-wide association studies identified some potential novel genes as being correlated with thrombosis. Experimental analyses are conducted to confirm their involvement in thrombosis

B.H. Menze et al. (Eds.): MCV 2012, LNCS 7766, pp. 215–224, 2013.

malfunction, either *in vivo* on zebrafish larvae [1] or *in vitro* by perfusing freshly collected human blood through a chamber filled with collagen fibres. In the latter case, the progressive attachment of platelets leads to the formation of individual thrombi observed through a phase-contrast microscopic system. The growth rate of each individual thrombus over time is a measure of interest as well as the time to attachment of their first platelet. The high number of required experiments raises the need of a tool able to automatically segment and track the different thrombus areas over time to derive their individual growth characteristics.

The tracking of multiple objects within microscopic videos is a challenging problem for which many methods exist in the litterature. It often follows a first step where objects of interest are detected. Based on these detections, objects are matched from frame to frame using optimisation methods as for example the Hungarian algorithm for linear assignment [2] or the branch and bound algorithm for binary integer programming [3]. Other approaches are based on model evolution like particle filtering generalised for the tracking of several objects [4]. Most of the tracking methods follow one of these two kinds of approaches, or try to combine them [5]. A first attempt has been presented in [6] for the segmentation and tracking of thrombi in a similar experimental setup. Authors introduced three complementary gradient-based features that were learned on a video of reference. Then, by feeding these features into a decision tree, they could demonstrate promising segmentation results. Each thrombus was defined by the first platelet and tracked over the whole video to ultimately obtain the growth curve of each thrombus over time. However, the fact that thrombi grow at many different locations often results in merging events. The blood flow regularly causes the detachment of platelets, which can also result in splitting of thrombi. Several tracking methods able to follow objects along videos despite split and merge conditions emerged from the computer vision community [7,8,9]. They assume however that each object is well defined all along the scene. In our case, the integrity of each thrombus vanishes as soon as it exchanges platelets with other thrombi, e.g during merging or splitting. Moreover, such events disrupt the measured growth by inducing artificial changes of size without any biological meaning. Being able to identify such events is a major requirement since it permits to compute reliable growth rates to perform a meaningful comparison between blood donors. We introduce in this paper a new method which is able, from a segmented video, to match objects between two consecutive frames to identify appearance, disappearance, splitting and merging events. Thereby we can extract the relevant information to our application.

2   Methods

In this section, we first introduce our method for the thrombus segmentation (Section 2.1). We describe afterwards our automatic method to identify special events by assigning objects between two consecutive frames (Section 2.2).

2.1   Thrombus Segmentation

We propose to formulate the thrombus segmentation problem as a binary classification task in which each pixel of a given frame is assigned to one of these
two classes of objects: background (B) or thrombus (T). The segmentation is
performed independently within each frame. More formally, let us consider a
frame represented by the intensity function $\mathbf{I} : \Omega \to \mathbb{R}$, where $\Omega \subset \mathbb{N}^2$ represents the pixel lattice in the image domain. We denote by $\mathbf{x} = (x, y)$ a
pixel of coordinates $(x, y) \in \Omega$ in the frame $\mathbf{I}$. Our goal is to assign a la-
bel $\mathbf{c} \in \{\mathrm{background}(B), \mathrm{thrombus}(T)\}$ to each pixel $\mathbf{x}$ of the frame $\mathbf{I}$. In a
probabilistic fashion, this could be done by modeling the posterior distribution
$P(\mathbf{c}|\mathbf{x}, \mathbf{I})$ and using maximum a posteriori:

$$\hat{\mathbf{c}} = \operatorname*{argmax}_{\mathbf{c} \in \{B, T\}} P(\mathbf{c}|\mathbf{x}, \mathbf{I}) \tag{1}$$

The posterior $P(\mathbf{c}|\mathbf{x}, \mathbf{I})$ quantifies the probability of observing the class $\mathbf{c}$ at the
pixel $\mathbf{x}$ given the information available over the frame. To model this posterior,
we propose to use a classification forest as described in [10]. Therefore, we generate a training set from a set of pixels extracted at different frames. Each training
instance is a pair $(\mathbf{X}^{(n)}, \mathbf{c}^{(n)})$, where $n = \{1, \cdots, N_{\mathrm{train}}\}$, that represents a pixel
$\mathbf{x}^{(n)}$ from a given frame described by a feature vector $\mathbf{X}^{(n)}$ and its corresponding class label $\mathbf{c}^{(n)}$. To characterize the visual context of a pixel, we extract
at different scales a set of gradient-based features [6]. Following a "divide and
conquer" strategy, each tree of a forest $\{\mathbf{T}_i\}_{i=1}^{N_{\mathrm{trees}}}$ provides a piece-wise approxi-
mation $P_i(\mathbf{c}|\mathbf{x}, \mathbf{I})$ by: (1) creating a partition over the feature space using simple
decision functions and (2), estimating the posterior in each cell of this partition.
Tree posteriors can be aggregated over the whole forest using averaging:

$$P(\mathbf{c}|\mathbf{x}, \mathbf{I}) = \frac{1}{N_{\mathrm{trees}}} \sum_{i=1}^{N_{\mathrm{trees}}} P_i(\mathbf{c}|\mathbf{x}, \mathbf{I}) \tag{2}$$

The final segmentation is obtained by thresholding this posterior, with a threshold chosen to maximise the performance with respect to manually delineated
videos. Each connected component of the segmented image is called object. We
also apply some post-processing operations (morphological opening to discard
objects whose shape is too elongated and we remove the objects or holes smaller
than the size of a platelet).

2.2   Event Detections

Given the segmentation at frames t and $t + 1$, we want to identify the events
that occur between these two frames. The segmentation at frame t is a collection
of binary objects $(\mathcal{O}_{t,k})_{1 \le k \le N_t}$. Between t and $t + 1$, the possible events are the
following:

- **Appearance**: A new object (generally a single platelet) appears in the frame $t + 1$. Such appearances can occur anywhere within the field of view.
- **Disappearance**: An object of the frame t cannot be seen anymore in the frame $t + 1$. It often corresponds to isolated platelets that detach.
- **Merge**: Several objects of the frame t merge into an object of the frame $t + 1$.
- **Split**: An object of the frame t splits in several objects in the frame $t + 1$.
- **Normal growth**: A thrombus grows undisrupted between the two frames.

The identification of these events is seen as an **assignment problem**. Similarly as for a multi-target tracking problem, each object in a frame must be associated to one, several or no objects in the next (or previous) one. The possibility to assign an object to several objects (resp. none) allows us to identify splitting and merging (resp. appearance and disappearance). Assignments are found globally through the resolution of a binary integer programming problem minimising a cost function especially designed for this application. We start the description of our method by the definition of two types of distances we will use. We then identify candidate regions for splitting and merging events by clustering thrombi that are close to each other. Finally, we explain in details our formalism with the help of a concrete example and the associated optimisation problem.

Distances between Two Objects. Distances between objects are an essential quantity to estimate the cost of each association of objects. In the following, we define two types of distances : the **static** and **dynamic** distances between two objects.

Static distance: Within a same frame, we define the static distance between two objects $\mathcal{O}_{t,i}$ and $\mathcal{O}_{t,j}$ by

$$d_S(\mathcal{O}_{t,i}, \mathcal{O}_{t,j}) = \min_{(\mathbf{x}_i, \mathbf{x}_j) \in \mathcal{O}_{t,i} \times \mathcal{O}_{t,j}} d(\mathbf{x}_i, \mathbf{x}_j) \tag{3}$$

where d is the classical Euclidean distance between two points.

Dynamic distance: To define a distance between an object $\mathcal{O}_{t,i}$ at frame t and an object $\mathcal{O}_{t+1,j}$ at frame $t + 1$, we could use the distance we have just defined. However, we propose to introduce some additional knowledge. In our controlled experiment, we assume the blood flow to be laminar and constant through the chamber, i.e horizontally from left to right in our images. Therefore, objects can physically only move towards the right of the field of view with a significantly low vertical component. Anticipating the fact that the distance between objects $\mathcal{O}_{t,i}$ and $\mathcal{O}_{t+1,j}$ will be used as a cost to link $\mathcal{O}_{t,i}$ and $\mathcal{O}_{t+1,j}$, we propose to forbide physically impossible motions by assigning an infinite distance between the two objects if $\mathcal{O}_{t+1,j}$ is located "behind" $\mathcal{O}_{t,i}$. More precisely, the (asymmetric) dynamic distance is defined as

$$d_D(\mathcal{O}_{t,i}, \mathcal{O}_{t+1,j}) = \min_{(\mathbf{x}_i, \mathbf{x}_j) \in \mathcal{O}_{t,i} \times \mathcal{O}_{t+1,j}} d'_\theta(\mathbf{x}_i, \mathbf{x}_j) \tag{4}$$

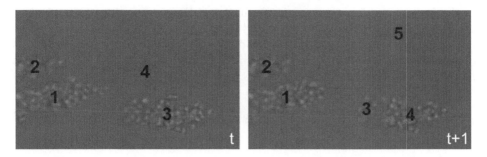

Fig. 1. Two consecutive frames from a video. The frames have been spatially cropped to reduce the number of objects and facilitate the visualisation. Please note that the labels of the objects are arbitrarily generated within each frame and do not symbolise any tracking.

where $d'_\theta(\mathbf{x}_i, \mathbf{x}_j)$ is the classical Euclidean distance between two points if $\mathbf{x}_j$ is located in the cone whose apex is $\mathbf{x}_i$, whose aperture is θ and horizontally oriented towards the right. If not, $d'_\theta(\mathbf{x}_i, \mathbf{x}_j)$ is set to infinity (a very high number in practice).

Potential Splitting and Merging Regions. Let us assume that N_t objects are segmented in the frame t, where N_t rarely goes above 30 in such experiments. We start our analysis by clustering objects that are close to each other in order to identify candidate regions where merging or splitting might occur. We define a maximum distance $d^{\mathrm{SM}}_{\max}$ stating the maximum possible static distance between two objects at frame t that are susceptible to merge. For each object $\mathcal{O}_{t,i}$, we define its candidate objects for splitting and merging as the objects $\mathcal{O}_{t,j}$ verifying $d_S(\mathcal{O}_{t,i}, \mathcal{O}_{t,j}) \le d^{\mathrm{SM}}_{\max}$. The identification of these candidate regions reduces thereby the number of events we consider in our assignment problem and makes it more tractable (the theoretical number of all possible combinations would be exponential with respect to N_t).

Assignment Using Binary Representation. Let us denote N_m and N_s respectively the number of possible merges and the number of possible splits computed as we just described. Our goal is to assign to each object the type of event it is involved in and to link it to the right object(s) in the other frame. We represent the assignment of all objects by a binary matrix X of size $K_t \times K_{t+1}$ with $K_t = N_t + N_m + 1$ and $K_{t+1} = N_{t+1} + N_s + 1$. The optimal assignment matrix X is found as the solution of a minimisation binary integer programming problem under equality constraint.

Before going in details into the construction of this minimisation problem, we illustrate on an example how a matrix X encodes the assignments. Let us consider the situation shown in Figure 1, taken from a real video but cropped to reduce the number of objects and increase the readability. 4 objects are seen in the frame t and 5 objects in the frame $t + 1$. By constructing the equivalent classes of thrombi in the frame t, we find the merge $M\{1, 2\}$ as the only possible one. Similarly, looking at the equivalence classes in the frame $t + 1$ informs us about the possible splits: only $S\{1, 2\}$ and $S\{3, 4\}$. The expected assignment matrix is the following:

	$\mathcal{O}_{t+1,1}$	$\mathcal{O}_{t+1,2}$	$\mathcal{O}_{t+1,3}$	$\mathcal{O}_{t+1,4}$	$\mathcal{O}_{t+1,5}$	$S\{1, 2\}$	$S\{3, 4\}$	Disappearance
$\mathcal{O}_{t,1}$	1	0	0	0	0	0	0	0
$\mathcal{O}_{t,2}$	0	1	0	0	0	0	0	0
$\mathcal{O}_{t,3}$	0	0	0	0	0	0	1	0
$\mathcal{O}_{t,4}$	0	0	0	0	0	0	0	1
$M\{1, 2\}$	0	0	0	0	0	0	0	0
Appearance	0	0	0	0	1	0	0	0

We can reformulate the information included in this matrix as follows. The objects 1 and 2 of the frame t are normally growing without being involved in any particular event. They are respectively linked to the objects 1 and 2 in the frame $t + 1$. Although the labelling number of these objects remains the same between the two frames in this case, please note that labels are independently assigned at each frame. The object 3 in the frame t splits into two objects labelled 3 and 4 in the frame $t + 1$. Finally, the object 4 of the frame t is disappearing, while an object labelled 5 appears in the frame $t + 1$. These two objects are not linked to each other since the trajectory which this link would form is unrealistic from a physical point of view (the vertical component is too high).

We can see with this example how X summarises in the general case all the assignments. The rows correspond to the frame t and the columns to the frame $t + 1$. More precisely, the N_t first rows correspond to the objects of the frame t, the N_m following rows correspond to the possible merge events and the last one corresponds to appearances. Similarly, the columns correspond to objects in the frame $t + 1$, splits and disapperances. We propose to estimate the assignment matrix X as the solution of this optimisation problem:

$$\min_{X \in \mathcal{M}_{K_t, K_{t+1}}(\{0,1\})} \|C.X\|_1 \tag{5}$$

where C is a cost matrix and . denotes the pointwise product. C summarizes the cost associated to each possible assignment and the way it is computed is described later in the paper. We add a linear equality constraint on X stating that there is one and only one positive assignment for every object. This can be formalised as

$$\forall k \in \{1, \ldots, N_t\} \sum_{i \in \phi(k)} \sum_{j=1}^{K_{t+1}} X(i, j) = 1 \tag{6}$$

and

$$\forall k \in \{1, \ldots, N_{t+1}\} \sum_{j \in \psi(k)} \sum_{i=1}^{K_t} X(i, j) = 1 \tag{7}$$

where $\phi(k)$ (resp. $\psi(k)$) denotes the set of the indices of the rows (resp. columns) where the object $\mathcal{O}_{t,k}$ (resp. $\mathcal{O}_{t+1,k}$) is involved. Our minimisation problem belongs to the class of binary integer programming problems. We classically propose to solve it with the branch and bound algorithm [11].

Cost Matrix. We define the cost of each assignment as follows:
- The cost of disappearance of an object $\mathcal{O}_{t,i}$ is set to γ size$(\mathcal{O}_{t,i})$
- The cost of appearance of an object $\mathcal{O}_{t+1,j}$ is set to γ size$(\mathcal{O}_{t+1,j})$
- The cost of linking an object $\mathcal{O}_{t,i}$ to an object $\mathcal{O}_{t+1,j}$ is set to $d_D(\mathcal{O}_{t,i}, \mathcal{O}_{t+1,j})$ $+ \alpha$ |size$(\mathcal{O}_{t,i})$ − size$(\mathcal{O}_{t+1,j})$|
- The cost of merging several objects $(\mathcal{O}_{t,i_k})_k$ into an object $\mathcal{O}_{t+1,j}$ is set to β max$_k$ $d_D(\mathcal{O}_{t,i_k}, \mathcal{O}_{t+1,j}) + \alpha$ |size$(\sum_k \mathcal{O}_{t,i_k})$ − size$(\mathcal{O}_{t+1,j})$|
- The cost of splitting an object $\mathcal{O}_{t,i}$ into several objects $(\mathcal{O}_{t+1,j_k})_k$ is set to β max$_k$ $d_D(\mathcal{O}_{t,i}, \mathcal{O}_{t+1,j_k}) + \alpha$ |size$(\sum_k \mathcal{O}_{t+1,j_k})$ − size$(\mathcal{O}_{t,i})$|

All the other costs of the matrix are set to infinity. Let us give some intuitions about these choices of costs. Appearance and disappearance events concern only small objects (mostly single platelets) since bigger objects are more robustly attached. We thus set the cost of appearance or disappearance as proportional to the size of the object. The cost of matching two objects, in the case of normal growth, is set as the dynamic distance between them (which takes into account the direction of the flow). Since the growth between two frames is always low, an additional cost comparing the sizes of the two objects is added to prevent unrealistic matchings. To compute the cost of several objects to merge into a single one, we compute for each of them the dynamic distance to this object and take the biggest of them as cost. If an object within a set of merging objects is unrelevant, the whole merging event is thus penalised and ultimately a merging set involving only relevant objects will be preferred. We also assume that there is not any motion of the objects involved in a merging event. The coefficient β is therefore taken high to penalise the distance term. Finally, the consistency in size is also checked. The cost for splitting events is similar than for merging. α, β and γ are coefficients balancing the relative weight of each term.

3   Experiments and Results

Random Forest Training. 7 videos were available to both learning and evaluating steps. One frame every 10 seconds, giving approximately 15 test frames for each video, was manually delineated to provide a reference for the learning and the evaluation. We trained the random forest using a "leave-one-video-out" approach: each video is segmented by learning the random forest on the 6 others. For each frame, we draw randomly points within background and thrombus. A subset of the points representing the background is purposely constrained to the neighbourhood of thrombi to perform a better robustness around thrombus edges. The number of trees in the forest is fixed at 50 and the optimal depth 20 has been tuned experimentally. The gradient-based features are computed at 13 different scales ($r \in \{8, \ldots, 20\}$).

Table 1. Evaluation of the segmentation performance

	Video 1	Video 2	Video 3	Video 4	Video 5	Video 6	Video 7
F-measure	0.89	0.90	0.89	0.895	0.89	0.86	0.85

Table 2. Evaluation of the performance of our event detection method

	Normal growth	Merging	Splitting	Disappearance	Appearance
TP	4159	164	138	188	253
FP	2	7	11	5	4
FN	12	0	0	3	9
Precision	0.9995	0.96	0.93	0.97	0.98
Recall	0.997	1.00	1.00	0.98	0.97
F-measure	0.998	0.98	0.96	0.98	0.975

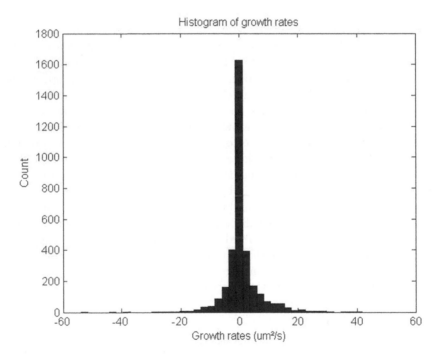

Fig. 2. The identification of normal growth events, i.e where no splitting and merging occurs, permits a reliable measurement of growth rates. We can then plot them as an histogram for each video. It is expected that the histograms are correlated with the genetic disorders of the blood donors.

Segmentation. We choose the F-measure to quantify the performance of the thrombus segmentation. The results for each video are briefly summarised in Table 1. These results show that our segmentation method is accurate enough to build our event analysis upon it.

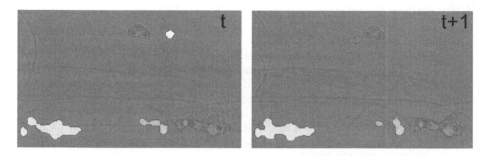

Fig. 3. Example of results of event detection between two consecutive frames. A code based on colour has been chosen for a better visualisation. A thrombus in yellow (resp. green) merges (resp. splits) between the two frames. A thrombus in white (resp. blue) disappears (resp. appears) between t and $t + 1$. Thrombi that do not have any colour are evolving between the two frames without any interaction with other thrombi.

Event Detection. The parameters in the cost function are experimentally set to $\alpha = 0.1$, $\beta = 3$ and $\gamma = 0.2$. We test our event detection method on 2 videos entirely labeled. Please note that although the number of videos on which we test is very low, this represents within each video at least 100 pairs of frames for which the assignments are independant. We count for each kind of event how many times this event has been correctly identified (TP), how many times it has been by mistake detected (FP) and how many times it has not been identified (FN). We also compute for each event the precision, recall and F-measure. The results are summarised in Table 2 and demonstrate the accuracy of our method. In particular, the precision is extremely high for the normal growth events. This allows us to reliably measure growth rates by excluding splitting and merging events. Resulting growth rates can be plotted as histograms (Figure 2) to visualise the thrombotic characteristics of a given blood donor.

4   Conclusion

In this paper, we tackled the problem of measuring growth rates and time to attachment of thrombi under splitting, merging, appearance and disappearance conditions. We proposed a matching method between each pair of consecutive frames which is able to recognise such undesired events in order to measure growth rates only in normal conditions of growth. We modeled this situation as a binary integer programming problem which is tractable and solvable with the branch and bound algorithm. We showed through a quantification of performance the efficiency of the approach. The extracted characteristics of growth could be compared between blood donors and potentially allow to identify possible genetic risk predispositions of thrombosis.

References

1. Brieu, N., Navab, N., Serbanovic-Canic, J., Ouwehand, W.H., Stemple, D.L., Cvejic, A., Groher, M.: Image-based characterization of thrombus formation in time-lapse dic microscopy. Medical Image Analysis 16(4), 915–931 (2012)
2. Jaqaman, K., Loerke, D., Mettlen, M., Kuwata, H., Grinstein, S., Schmid, S.L., Danuser, G.: Robust single-particle tracking in live-cell time-lapse sequences. Nature Methods 5(8), 695–702 (2008)
3. Li, F., Zhou, X., Ma, J., Wong, S.: Multiple nuclei tracking using integer programming for quantitative cancer cell cycle analysis. IEEE Transactions on Medical Imaging 29(1), 96–105 (2010)
4. Smal, I., Draegestein, K., Galjart, N., Niessen, W., Meijering, E.: Particle filtering for multiple object tracking in dynamic fluorescence microscopy images: Application to microtubule growth analysis. IEEE Transactions on Medical Imaging 27(6), 789–804 (2008)
5. Li, K., Miller, E.D., Chen, M., Kanade, T., Weiss, L.E., Campbell, P.G.: Cell population tracking and lineage construction with spatiotemporal context. Medical Image Analysis 12(5), 546–566 (2008); Special issue on the 10th international conference on medical imaging and computer assisted intervention - MICCAI 2007
6. Peter, L., Brieu, N., Jansen, S., Smethurst, P.A., Ouwehand, W.H., Navab, N.: Automatic segmentation and tracking of thrombus formation within in vitro microscopic video sequences. In: IEEE International Symposium on Biomedical Imaging: From Nano to Macro (2012)
7. Nillius, P., Sullivan, J., Carlsson, S.: Multi-target tracking - linking identities using bayesian network inference. In: IEEE Conference on Computer Vision and Pattern Recognition, vol. 2, pp. 2187–2194 (2006)
8. Bose, B., Wang, X., Grimson, E.: Multi-class object tracking algorithm that handles fragmentation and grouping. In: IEEE Conference on Computer Vision and Pattern Recognition, pp. 1–8 (June 2007)
9. Khan, Z., Balch, T., Dellaert, F.: Mcmc-based particle filtering for tracking a variable number of interacting targets. IEEE Transactions on Pattern Analysis and Machine Intelligence 27(11), 1805–1819 (2005)
10. Criminisi, A., Shotton, J., Konukoglu, E.: Decision Forests: A Unified Framework for Classification, Regression, Density Estimation, Manifold Learning and Semi-Supervised Learning. In: Foundations and Trends in Computer Graphics and Vision, vol. 7 (2012)
11. Wolsey, L.A.: Integer Programming. John Wiley and Sons, Inc. (1998)

Automatic Extraction of the Curved Midsagittal Brain Surface on MR Images

Hugo J. Kuijf, Max A. Viergever, and Koen L. Vincken

Image Sciences Institute, University Medical Center Utrecht, The Netherlands

Abstract. Many methods exist for the automatic extraction of the midsagittal plane from neuroimages, assuming bilateral symmetry. However, this assumption is incorrect owing to brain torque and the possible presence of pathology. In this paper, a method for extracting the curved midsagittal surface from brain images is presented.

First, the method localizes the interhemispheric fissure with an existing technique for midsagittal plane extraction. Next, the plane is modelled as a bicubic spline and the configuration of the control points is optimized to obtain the midsagittal surface.

The midsagittal surface results in a better segmentation of the cerebral hemispheres. Not only is the result visually more appealing, the absolute volume of misclassified tissue decreases significantly.

1 Introduction

Bilateral symmetry is an important concept in biology and many animal species, including humans. Our appearance exhibits bilateral symmetry and some organs in our body come in symmetrical pairs, for example our brain. The cerebrum is divided into two hemispheres, separated by the interhemispheric fissure (IF). Comparison of the two hemispheres and detection of differences has been a topic of discussion for many years. Besides the lateralization of brain function, anatomical differences can suggest the presence of pathology (like a brain mass or tumour), indicate schizophrenia [1], or various other diseases.

The midsagittal plane is a geometric plane that separates the two hemispheres and coincides with the IF. In the past years, multiple methods have been published to extract the midsagittal plane from neuroimages. Assuming bilateral symmetry, most of the methods work by optimizing a symmetry metric between the neuroimage and a reflected version of itself.

However, the human brain has no perfect bilateral symmetry. The left occipital and right frontal lobe are larger than their counterparts in the other hemisphere are, which is known as brain torque. Besides brain torque, the presence of brain masses could induce asymmetries in the cerebrum. Existing techniques to extract the midsagittal plane from neuroimages do not take these asymmetries into account and might therefore fail to correctly segment the two hemispheres.

The midsagittal surface is a curved surface following the IF. In the presence of asymmetries, either owing to natural variation or pathology, the midsagittal surface will correctly segment the two hemispheres, whereas a midsagittal plane

B.H. Menze et al. (Eds.): MCV 2012, LNCS 7766, pp. 225–232, 2013.
© Springer-Verlag Berlin Heidelberg 2013

would intersect or misclassify some brain tissue. It is therefore likely that the midsagittal surface will result in more accurate analysis of interhemispherical differences.

In the present study, a novel method for extracting the curved midsagittal surface will be presented, based on an existing method for extracting the midsagittal plane.

2   Methods and Materials

2.1   Participants and MRI

A total of 50 consecutive participants (mean age: 59 years, sd: 10 years) from the SMART study [2] have been included for evaluation of the method. The SMART study was approved by the Medical Ethics Committee and written informed consent was given by all participants.

MRI acquisition was performed on a 1.5T whole-body system (Gyroscan ACS-NT, Philips Medical Systems, Best, the Netherlands). The protocol included, among others, a transversal T1-weighted gradient-echo sequence (repetition time (TR)/echo time (TE): 235/2 ms); a transversal T2-weighted fluid-attenuated inversion recovery (FLAIR) (TR/TE/inversion time (TI): 6000/100/2000 ms), and a transversal inversion recovery (IR) (TR/TE/TI: 2900/22/410 ms), all with a reconstructed voxel size of $0.9 \times 0.9 \times 4.0$ mm.

For extraction of the midsagittal plane and surface, the T1-weighted sequence was used.

2.2   Midsagittal Plane

Many methods exist for the automatic extraction of the midsagittal plane, which can be roughly divided into two categories: symmetry-based methods (e.g. [3–10]) and fissure-based methods ([11–13]). Symmetry-based methods work with the implicit assumption that the brain possesses bilateral symmetry. These methods try to align the image with a reflected version of itself, while optimizing a symmetry-metric. However, due to the asymmetric nature of the brain, these techniques sometimes fail.

Fissure-based methods try to detect the IF, based on its distinctive characteristics visible in the image. With imaging modalities as CT and MRI, the cerebrospinal fluid (CSF) located in the IF gives a high visual contrast with the surrounding gray and white matter of both hemispheres. This contrast is clearly visible in Figures 1(a), (d), and (g), and can be used to extract the midsagittal plane and surface. A fissure-based method for extracting the midsagittal plane is described by Volkau *et al.* [12] and Nowinski *et al.* [13] and was used in the present study. The approach of this method, as will be explained below, allows for extension to extract the midsagittal surface and thus formed an ideal candidate for the present study.

First, two reference planes were taken 2 cm apart from the central sagittal slice of the image. As the method assumes that the brain is approximately located in the centre of the image, these reference planes consist mostly of gray and white matter. A single probability distribution of the gray values present in the two references slices was created.

Next, all slices in-between the two reference slices were inspected. For each slice, a probability distribution of the gray values was created. The Kullback-Leibler (KL) divergence was computed using the reference probability distribution and the probability distribution of the current slice. This resulted in a measure of the difference between the two probability distributions (the KL-value). As the reference slices contains mostly gray and white matter and the IF contains mostly CSF, the slice containing (a large part of) the IF would result in a relatively large KL-value.

The sagittal slice with the largest KL-value was taken as an initial guess for the MSP. As the brain can be rotated, the IF will not always perfectly align with a sagittal slice in the image. Therefore, three random corner points of the MSP were taken and shifted along the left/right axis of the scan. The location of these three corner points could be optimized in terms of the KL-value. For each new location, the KL-value was computed and the rotated slice with the largest difference to the reference distribution was taken as the final MSP. This process is summarized in Figure 1.

2.3   Midsagittal Surface

The midsagittal plane computed in the previous section was used to initialize the method for extracting the midsagittal surface. The surface was represented as a bicubic spline, as implemented in ALGLIB [14]. Control points for the spline were placed in a regular $m \times n$ grid on the computed MSP, having m be the number of control points in the anterior-posterior direction and n in the head-feet direction. The values of m and n were user-defined. An example is shown in Figure 2(a)

An optimization method was used to determine the optimal configuration of the control points. The control points could only be moved along the left/right axis of the scan during optimization. The Kullback-Leibler's divergence was used as a cost function that needed to be maximized. It used the previously computed reference probability distribution and generated a probability distribution of the bicubic spline during optimization.

A limited-memory Broyden-Fletcher-Goldfarb-Shanno quasi-newton method (L-BFGS), as implemented in the dlib C++ library [15], was used to determine the direction of the search. This method required gradient information of the cost function to be optimized, which was numerically approximated. The step size of each control point in each iteration was scaled with the gradient at each control point, allowing subvoxel accuracy in the configuration. The optimization method was terminated when the cost function converged: two consecutive optimization steps had a difference in KL-value of 1×10^{-5} or less. An example of this procedure can be seen in Figure 2.

228   H.J. Kuijf, M.A. Viergever, and K.L. Vincken

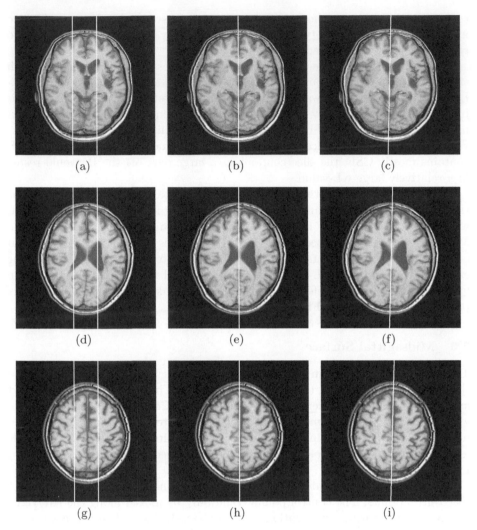

Fig. 1. Extraction of the midsagittal plane shown on three slices taken from one scan. Left: lines indicate the two initial reference planes. Middle: line indicates the sagittal slice with the largest KL-value. Right: line indicates the midsagittal plane.

2.4 Experiments and Validation

The quality of the midsagittal plane and surface extraction was evaluated visually and quantitatively in the cerebrum, ignoring the cerebellum. The cerebellum was ignored, since a left/right segmentation is ambiguous and ill-defined. This is commonly done in segmentation algorithms. [16] For the quantitative validation, the brain tissue volume in the cerebrum that was classified as either left or right was assessed automatically and compared to a ground truth. First, reasonable settings for m and n were determined heuristically on a smaller subset of

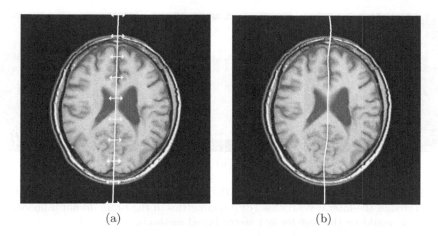

(a)   (b)

Fig. 2. Left: Figure 1(f) is shown with the control points for the optimization. The arrows indicate the direction in which the control points could move. Right: Optimal configuration according to the KL-divergence is shown. The error that the midsagittal plane made at the left occipital lobe was corrected by the computed surface.

participants. The influence of these parameters was assessed visually and fixed for the quantitative analysis.

Second, a gray and white matter segmentation was obtained with a probabilistic k-Nearest Neighbour classification segmentation method. This method used the T1-weighted, IR, and FLAIR sequences, as described by Anbeek *et al.* [17]

Using the MNI152 template [18, 19], a ground truth left/right segmentation was created. For this template, a true left/right atlas of the cerebrum is available. By computing a deformable registration of the MNI152 template to the T1-weighted scan, the left/right atlas could be propagated to the gray and white matter segmentation. Registrations were computed with elastix [20], with registration parameters taken from Van der Lijn *et al.* [21] The quality of the registration was assessed visually by an experienced observer and all registrations were considered accurate.

3 Results

Values for m and n were set at 10 and 5. Lower values were unable to capture the curvature of the IF and higher values resulted in overfitting of the spline.

The results of the extraction of the midsagittal plane were visually inspected for correctness. In all cases, the midsagittal plane was found correctly and aligned with the IF, as was also previously reported by Volkau and Nowinski. [12, 13] However, small errors were made by the method, mostly at the left occipital lobe (as visible in Figure 1) and the right frontal lobe. This was to be expected, owing to the possible presence of brain torque.

The midsagittal surface showed a visually more appealing result than the midsagittal plane. The surface followed the interhemispheric fissure at locations

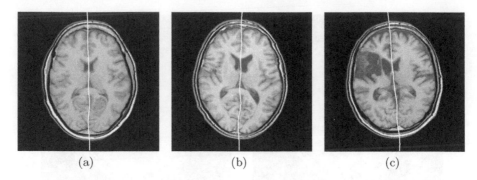

(a)   (b)   (c)

Fig. 3. Example results of the method. (b) The midsagittal surface was sometimes fitted through the lateral ventricles. (c) Asymmetries in the brain do not influence the results, as would be the case for symmetry-based methods.

where the midsagittal plane would cut through tissue. An example of this was shown in Figure 2(b) and more results are shown in Figure 3.

For the quantitative validation, the absolute volume of tissue in the cerebrum that was misclassified (i.e. classified as left where it should be right, or vice versa) was assessed automatically. In the ideal case, this error would be zero. The average error (mean $\pm$ sd) of the midsagittal plane was 1.06 ± 0.89 ml and the average error of the midsagittal surface was 0.59 ± 0.63 ml. The difference between the midsagittal plane and the midsagittal surface was statistically significant, using a one-sided, paired, Student's t-test, with a p-value of 1.0×10^{-6}.

Computation time of the midsagittal plane was approximately 2 seconds. Depending on the number of iterations required, the computation of the midsagittal surface was 2 to 10 seconds.

4 Discussion

The implementation of the midsagittal surface shows a clear improvement over the midsagittal plane. Not only does the midsagittal surface show a visually more correct and appealing result, the improvement in the absolute volume of misclassified tissue is statistically significant. Besides the statistical significance, the absolute reduction in the error with 0.5 ml on average is relevant in many applications. Although a volume 0.5 ml is relatively small compared to the whole brain volume, it is a considerable amount of tissue in the vicinity of the IF. Next to the average reduction in error, the standard deviation of the error also decreases. This indicates that the midsagittal surface gives a more robust estimate of the left-right segmentation than the midsagittal plane does.

An error sometimes made by the midsagittal surface is found at the location of the lateral ventricles. During optimization, the cost function will try to avoid the septum pellucidum, the membrane separating the lateral ventricles, and fit the spline through the CSF-filled ventricles. This will give a more optimal solution in terms of KL-value, although it is not the most logical separation at that location.

However, it has no influence on the left/right segmentation of the tissue in the cerebrum. An example was shown in Figure 3(b).

The quantitative validation of the method required an atlas-registration of the MNI152 template to each individual image. By doing this, the quality of the ground truth depends on the quality of the registration. Thorough inspection of the registration results by an experienced observer did not reveal any errors in the left-right segmentation of the cerebrum generated by the registration.

Of course, one could argue that having a left-right segmentation available by means of registration with the MNI152 template already solves the problem of extracting the midsagittal surface. However, the registration of the MNI152 template to the scans required 7 minutes per scan. The computation of the midsagittal surface required, at most, 12 seconds, making an expensive atlas registration superfluous.

The method works without adaptation on other image contrasts, such as FLAIR and IR, and higher field strengths, such as 3.0T or 7.0T. The only prerequisite for the method is a visible contrast between the interhemispheric fissure and surrounding tissue. The method can be applied to other imaging modalities, such as CT, as well. [22]

Besides segmentation of the cerebrum into the left and right hemispheres, there is a possibility to use this method for the detection of midline shift. Techniques for this application have been published before [23], using the midsagittal plane and a Bézier curve. The midsagittal surface could be used instead, without the limited degrees of freedom of a Bézier curve.

References

1. Crow, T.: Schizophrenia as an anomaly of cerebral asymmetriy. In: Imaging of the Brain in Psychiatry and Related Fields, pp. 1–17 (1993)
2. Simons, P., Algra, A., van de Laak, M., Grobbee, D., van der Graaf, Y.: Second manifestations of arterial disease (smart) study: Rationale and design. European Journal of Epidemiology 15, 773–781 (1999)
3. Junck, L., Moen, J.G., Hutchins, G.D., Brown, M.B., Kuhl, D.E.: Correlation methods for the centering, rotation, and alignment of functional brain images. Journal of Nuclear Medicine 31(7), 1220–1226 (1990)
4. Minoshima, S., Berger, K.L., Lee, K.S., Mintun, M.A.: An automated method for rotational correction and centering of three-dimensional functional brain images. Journal of Nuclear Medicine 33(8), 1579–1585 (1992)
5. Ardekani, B.A., Kershaw, J., Braun, M., Kanno, I.: Automatic detection of the midsagittal plane in 3-d brain images. IEEE Transactions on Medical Imaging 16(6), 947–952 (1997)
6. Smith, S., Jenkinson, M.: Accurate Robust Symmetry Estimation. In: Taylor, C., Colchester, A. (eds.) MICCAI 1999. LNCS, vol. 1679, pp. 308–317. Springer, Heidelberg (1999)
7. Liu, Y., Collins, R., Rothfus, W.E.: Robust midsagittal plane extraction from normal and pathological 3d neuroradiology images. IEEE Transactions on Medical Imaging 20(1), 175–192 (2001)
8. Prima, S., Ourselin, S., Ayache, N.: Computation of the mid-sagittal plane in 3-d brain images. IEEE Transactions on Medical Imaging 21(2), 122–138 (2002)

9. Hu, Q., Nowinski, W.L.: A rapid algorithm for robust and automatic extraction of the midsagittal plane of the human cerebrum from neuroimages based on local symmetry and outlier removal. NeuroImage 20(4), 2153–2165 (2003)
10. Tuzikov, A.V., Colliot, O., Bloch, I.: Evaluation of the symmetry plane in 3d mr brain images. Pattern Recognition Letters 24(14), 2219–2233 (2003)
11. Brummer, M.E.: Hough transform detection of the longitudinal fissure in tomographic head images. IEEE Transactions on Medical Imaging 10(1), 74–81 (1991)
12. Volkau, I., Prakash, K.B., Ananthasubramaniam, A., Aziz, A., Nowinski, W.L.: Extraction of the midsagittal plane from morphological neuroimages using the kullback-leibler's measure. Medical Image Analysis 10(6), 863–874 (2006)
13. Nowinski, W.L., Prakash, B., Volkau, I., Ananthasubramaniam, A., Beauchamp Jr, N.J.: Rapid and automatic calculation of the midsagittal plane in magnetic resonance diffusion and perfusion images. Academic Radiology 13(5), 652–663 (2006)
14. Bochkanov, S., Bystritsky, V.: Alglib, www.alglib.net
15. King, D.E.: Dlib c++ library, www.dlib.net
16. Liang, L., Rehm, K., Woods, R.P., Rottenberg, D.A.: Automatic segmentation of left and right cerebral hemispheres from mri brain volumes using the graph cuts algorithm. NeuroImage 34(3), 1160–1170 (2007)
17. Anbeek, P., Vincken, K.L., van Bochove, G.S., van Osch, M.J., van der Grond, J.: Probabilistic segmentation of brain tissue in mr imaging. NeuroImage 27(4), 795–804 (2005)
18. Fonov, V., Evans, A., McKinstry, R., Almli, C., Collins, D.: Unbiased nonlinear average age-appropriate brain templates from birth to adulthood. NeuroImage 47(suppl.1) (2009); S102 Organization for Human Brain Mapping 2009 Annual Meeting.
19. Fonov, V., Evans, A.C., Botteron, K., Almli, C.R., McKinstry, R.C., Collins, D.L.: Unbiased average age-appropriate atlases for pediatric studies. NeuroImage 54(1), 313–327 (2011)
20. Klein, S., Staring, M., Murphy, K., Viergever, M., Pluim, J.: elastix: A toolbox for intensity-based medical image registration. IEEE Transactions on Medical Imaging 29(1), 196–205 (2010)
21. van der Lijn, F., de Bruijne, M., Hoogendam, Y., Klein, S., Hameeteman, R., Breteler, M., Niessen, W.: Cerebellum segmentation in mri using atlas registration and local multi-scale image descriptors. In: IEEE International Symposium on Biomedical Imaging: From Nano to Macro, ISBI 2009, pp. 221–224 (2009)
22. Puspitasari, F., Volkau, I., Ambrosius, W., Nowinski, W.: Robust calculation of the midsagittal plane in ct scans using the kullbackleibler measure. International Journal of Computer Assisted Radiology and Surgery 4, 535–547 (2009)
23. Liao, C.C., Xiao, F., Wong, J.M., Chiang, I.J.: Automatic recognition of midline shift on brain ct images. Computers in Biology and Medicine 40(3), 331–339 (2010)

Identification of Malignant Breast Tumors Based on Acoustic Attenuation Mapping of Conventional Ultrasound Images

Sivan Harary and Eugene Walach

IBM Research - Haifa, Israel

Abstract. Although breast cancer imaging techniques continue to improve rapidly, about 75% of all breast biopsies turn out to be benign. These unnecessary biopsies are expensive and very stressful for the patients. In this paper we propose a new method for reducing the number of unnecessary biopsies. Our approach consists of transforming conventional ultrasonic images into corresponding attenuation maps. These maps are then analyzed, yielding automatic classification of malignant tumors. We provide a proof of concept for this approach by testing it on a benchmark of clinical images from three different image acquisition systems. Our tests show excellent sensitivity and specificity, indicating that up to four-fold reduction in the number of unnecessary biopsies may be possible. Moreover, we demonstrate the system robustness by working on all the images without any system-specific tuning.

Keywords: Acoustic Attenuation, Breast Cancer, Computer-Aided Diagnosis, Ultrasound Imaging.

1 Introduction

Worldwide, breast cancer comprises just under 30% of all diagnosed cancers in women. Mammography is currently the most common modality for screening and detecting breast cancer. However, a large portion of the breast lesions found in mammograms are benign. In order to improve the specificity, doctors often examine the suspicious lesions using ultrasound (US) imaging. Nevertheless, even when using both mammography and US, about 80% of the biopsies turn out to be benign. Clearly, the unnecessary biopsies cause both physical pain and emotional stress. They also result in a significant waste of health-care resources.

Accordingly, a great deal of effort has been devoted to improving breast cancer diagnostic tools. A technological review of commonly used methods and new experimental techniques was conducted in [1]. Many of the newly developed techniques are based on US due to its non-ionizing nature, low cost, and mobility. US is often used for guidance during the biopsy itself, so it is only natural to use it as a final diagnostic tool before inserting the needle. A review of US techniques was compiled in [2].

The improvements to diagnostic tools can be divided into two categories: enhancements to the imaging equipment and the introduction of computerized

B.H. Menze et al. (Eds.): MCV 2012, LNCS 7766, pp. 233–243, 2013.
© Springer-Verlag Berlin Heidelberg 2013

image analytics. The first category includes solutions such as Elastography [3], which produces images of the breast stiffness or strain by applying compression or vibration using US waves. Another approach is to introduce tomographic 3D US images, which provide a more comprehensive view of the tumor in question [4]. In the second category, there are several computer-aided diagnosis (CAD) systems. A survey of CAD systems for breast US was conducted in [5]. These systems typically compute a variety of breast image features and use a variety of classification techniques to distinguish between malignant and benign tumors. These features include the shape of the tumor, its texture, and sometimes acoustic properties. Unfortunately, in many cases, the efficacy of US CAD systems tends to be limited due to high dependency on the specific image acquisition system.

Our work focuses on a specific acoustic feature, namely the acoustic tissue attenuation. Studies, such as [6,7], show that acoustic attenuation measurements can distinguish between malignant and benign tissues, and can therefore be used as an effective basis for a CAD system. Tissue attenuation can be calculated using transmission US in a tomographic manner [4]. However, clinical US systems produce B-scans, which are based on backscattering rather than transmission. Consequently, the authors of [8] developed a system for attenuation estimation that uses B-scans but with an additional metal plate. Other methods that use only B-scans with no alteration of the hardware setting are available [7,9,10]. These techniques produce one global attenuation measure either for the entire breast or for a pre-specified region of interest (ROI).

In this paper we propose a new technique for the estimation of local acoustic attenuation. This method uses conventional B-scan images so there is no need to modify the image acquisition process or hardware. Moreover, we have no dependency on a specific US system. Rather than computing the average attenuation for the entire ROI, as described in [7,9], we calculate the local attenuation of each pixel in the region and create an attenuation map. This map is more informative than a global measurement and is therefore more effective for differentiating between malignant and benign lesions. The attenuation map can be presented as is to the doctor, similar to what is usually done with Elastography images. However, to reduce the burden on the examining doctor, we also introduce an automatic analysis of the attenuation map to classify the breast tumors. This analysis can be used either as a stand-alone CAD system or in combination with other CAD systems.

Testing the algorithm on a benchmark of clinical images showed excellent sensitivity and specificity. Moreover, it demonstrated the system robustness by working on images from three deferent image acquisition systems without any system-specific tuning. Although promising, these are only preliminary results on a moderate benchmark that provide only a proof of concept for our approach. Our future work will focus on more extensive testing and clinical trials of this method.

Our method for attenuation estimation draws on earlier techniques for attenuation mapping of the liver [11]. However, we introduce significant changes to the method in order to enable reliable estimation of attenuation in breast tissue, which is highly inhomogeneous. In Section 2, we present both the attenuation estimation algorithm and the subsequent module for tumor classification. Section 3 presents the results of our tests on clinical data. Finally, Section 4 concludes this work.

2   The Method

In this section we describe our proposed system for classifying breast tumors based on local acoustic attenuation estimation. We apply our processing on the same B-scan images that are displayed on the physician's screen. This renders our technique transparent to the image acquisition hardware, making it very convenient for the users. Unfortunately, this also means that we work with inherently distorted images. One of the major sources of such distortions is the Time Gain Compensation (TGC). All state-of-the-art US systems use TGC to compensate for the loss of echo amplitude with depth [12]. Images produced using TGC are more uniform and have an effective attenuation of zero. Although these images are easier for doctors to interpret, the TGC distorts our attenuation maps and prevents reliable quantitative analysis. Nevertheless, the attenuation maps are still useful as they show the relative attenuation difference between healthy and malignant tissue areas.

Since the proposed method is aimed at assisting doctors in the evaluation of suspicious lesions, the segmentation of the lesion is preformed manually by the doctor. This approach is very common in US CAD systems; see for instance [13].

Accordingly, we propose the following process:

1. The doctor marks the suspicious area (ROI) on the image.
2. The attenuation map is estimated inside and around the ROI.
3. The attenuation map is analyzed by the CAD algorithm to determine whether the marked tissue is benign or malignant.
4. The results are superimposed on the original US image.

To accommodate the above process, our system consists of two main complementary modules, which are described in the following sections. The first module computes the attenuation map and the second one provides classification of the attenuation results.

2.1   Acoustic Attenuation Map Estimation

Our proposed algorithm for attenuation mapping is a modification of the algorithm proposed in [11] for attenuation mapping of the liver. In [11], the attenuation is estimated for each pixel by looking at a small surrounding block. The attenuation in this block is assumed to be uniform, except for outliers (i.e., pixels that significantly differ from the central one), which are removed. Accordingly, the block average attenuation is computed using the least squares method. This approach works quite well for relatively uniform tissues such as liver. For highly heterogeneous tissues, such as breast, the uniformity assumption no longer holds.

Therefore, our modified algorithm identifies for each block a uniform subregion (mask) with properties similar to that of the central pixel. The modified algorithm is presented in Table 1. Below is an elaboration of its steps.

Table 1. Creating the attenuation map

For each pixel in and around the ROI:
1. Define a block of size $L \times P$ around the pixel.
2. Define a mask (a subregion) of the block.
3. Estimate the attenuation in the block using only the pixels in the mask.
4. Assign the block's attenuation value to the central pixel.

Following [12], we express the intensity of the pixel in the nth column and mth row of the US image as follows:

$$E_{m,n} = E_0 \sigma_{m,n} \exp\left(- 2\Delta \sum_{k=1}^{m-1} \alpha_{k,n} \right), \tag{1}$$

where E_0 is the initial amplitude, Δ is the size of the pixels, and $\sigma_{m,n}, \alpha_{k,n}$ are the backscattering and attenuation coefficients, respectively. Without loss of generality we assume that $\Delta = 1$. This is equivalent to simply changing the unit of measure of the attenuation.

We are interested in estimating $\alpha_{k,n}$ for each pixel in and around the ROI. To that end we assume that in a small vicinity of each pixel the attenuation and backscatter coefficients are constant. In order to define this vicinity, first we define a small block of constant size $L \times P$ around each pixel. For example, we use 65×17 pixels. If the attenuation was uniform in this block, then (1) would reduce to:

$$E_{j,i} = E_i \exp\left(- 2 \sum_{k=1}^{j-1} \alpha \right) = E_i e^{-2(j-1)\alpha}, \tag{2}$$

where $E_{j,i}$ is the intensity in the j, i pixel in the block, and α is the block's constant attenuation, which we are looking for. However, since the breast tissue is not homogeneous enough, the block's attenuation is not necessarily uniform. Therefore, instead of using all of its pixels, in the second step of the algorithm we identify a subregion (mask) of the block where the constant attenuation assumption is reasonable. Then, equation (2) is applied only to pixels on this mask.

We identify this mask in two stages. First, we find the mask for all in-range pixels, i.e., pixels in the block with intensity within 3dB proximity to the central pixel. Then, we remove peripheral blobs (connected nonzero pixels) from the mask. That is, any blob whose distance from the main blob exceeds 4 is removed. Note that we refer to 2D blobs in contrast to [11], where each column is processed separately. In case the remaining mask contains too few pixels, we can not rely on it for the estimation. Thus, we assign an attenuation value of zero, and move on to the next pixel. Fig. 1 presents an example for a block and its mask. As can be seen the mask indicates all pixels of the same tissue type as the central pixel.

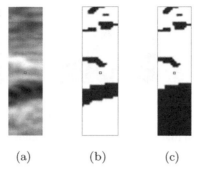

(a)   (b)   (c)

Fig. 1. Block masking. (a) is the block defined for the central pixel (marked in red). (b) is the initial in-range mask. (c) is the final mask, after removing peripheral blobs.

Since the mask indicates a subregion with homogeneous attenuation, the model in (2) holds for all pixels indicated by the mask. Therefore, we define our cost function to be the sum over all those pixels of the squared differences between the actual and the theoretical intensities. That is:

$$C(E_i, \alpha) = \sum_{i=1}^{P} \sum_{j \in \Omega_i} \left(E_{j,i} - E_i e^{-2(j-1)\alpha} \right)^2, \tag{3}$$

where Ω_i is the ith column of the mask. The goal is to find E_i and α that minimize this cost function. Algorithms for solving similar least-squares problems exist in the literature, for example [14,15]. However, since this is a nonlinear problem, those algorithms tend to be iterative. To avoid the computational complexity involved, instead of using those methods we limit the solution to its first order approximation. This way the problem becomes linear and its solution can be expressed in a closed form. This limitation is appropriate under the assumption that $\alpha << 1$ such that the exponential in (3) is small. Since the attenuation value of most biological tissues is rarely above 0.01 nepers/pixel, in our case this assumption is quite valid. The first order approximation of (3) is:

$$C(E_i, \alpha) = \sum_{i=1}^{P} \sum_{j \in \Omega_i} \left(E_{j,i} - E_i(1 - 2(j-1)\alpha) \right)^2. \tag{4}$$

Let k_i denote the number of nonzero pixels on the ith column of the mask, and define:

$$a_i = \frac{2}{k_i} \sum_{j \in \Omega_i} (j-1) \quad , \quad b_i = \frac{1}{k_i} \sum_{j \in \Omega_i} E_{j,i} \quad , \quad c_i = \frac{1}{k_i} \sum_{j \in \Omega_i} (j-1) E_{j,i} - a_i b_i$$

Using this notation it is easy to see that setting to zero the derivative of $C(E_i, \alpha)$ according to E_i, and using fist order approximation yields:

$$\hat{E}_i - b_i - 2c_i \alpha. \tag{5}$$

238   S. Harary and E. Walach

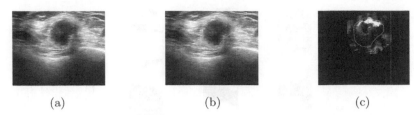

(a)   (b)   (c)

Fig. 2. Mapping example. (a) is the original US image. (b) presents the doctor's annotation of the ROI, as a green line. (c) is the attenuation map of the ROI and its vicinity.

Substituting (5) into (4) and keeping only first order of α yields a simple square function of α, whose single global minimum is in:

$$\hat{\alpha} = \frac{\sum_{i=1}^{P} D_i^T B_i}{\sum_{i=1}^{P} B_i^T B_i},$$ (6)

where $\Omega_{j,i}$ is the j,i pixel in the mask and

$$D_i = (b_i - E_{1,i}, \ldots, b_i - E_{L,i})^T \quad , \quad B_i = 2(\Omega_{1,i}c_i, \ldots, \Omega_{L,i}(c_i - (L-1)b_i)\ldots)^T$$

The estimated attenuation value $\hat{\alpha}$ is assigned only to the central pixel and not to the entire block. Performing this calculation for each pixel in and around the ROI yields the attenuation map. Fig. 2 presents an example of an US image and its associated attenuation map, estimated by the proposed method.

2.2   Attenuation Analysis

As discussed above, due to the TGC, attenuation maps are relative rather than absolute. In general, we expect zero attenuation for healthy tissue and higher attenuation values for malignant tumors. Fig. 3 presents some examples of attenuation maps of benign and malignant tumors. As can be observed in Fig. 3, malignant tumors have relatively large patches of high attenuation, while the overall structure is inhomogeneous. This fact fits well with our expectations based on the known morphology of cancerous tumors. Based on this insight we developed several features for classification between malignant and benign tumors, which are described in Table 2.

In order to quantify features number 1 and 2 in Table 2 we first smooth the attenuation map using the H-maxima transform, which suppresses mild maxima. For feature number 1, the regions of relatively high attenuation are identified by applying a fixed threshold (say of 10^{-3} nepers/pixel) on the smoothed map, while dismissing blobs with too small area. For feature number 2 we look for two regions with uniform attention in the smoothed map. The first region consists of all the pixels whose value equals the median value of the smoothed attenuation map. The second region is defined similarly as all the pixels whose value equals the median of the pixels that are not in the first region. Figure 4 presents an example for such uniform attenuation regions.

Table 2. Features of the attenuation map

	The Feature	Description
1	The portion of the tumor that is covered by regions of relatively high attenuation.	A small portion may indicate a benign tumor.
2	The portion of the tumor that is covered by uniform attenuation regions.	A large portion may indicate a benign tumor, since malignant tumors usually have inhomogeneous structure.
3	The maximal attenuation in the tumor.	Malignant tumors tend to have higher attenuation.
4	The portion of the tumor with attenuation close to the maximum from feature 3.	A small portion may indicate a benign tumor.
5	The portion of the tumor with negative attenuation.	A large portion may indicate a benign tumor.

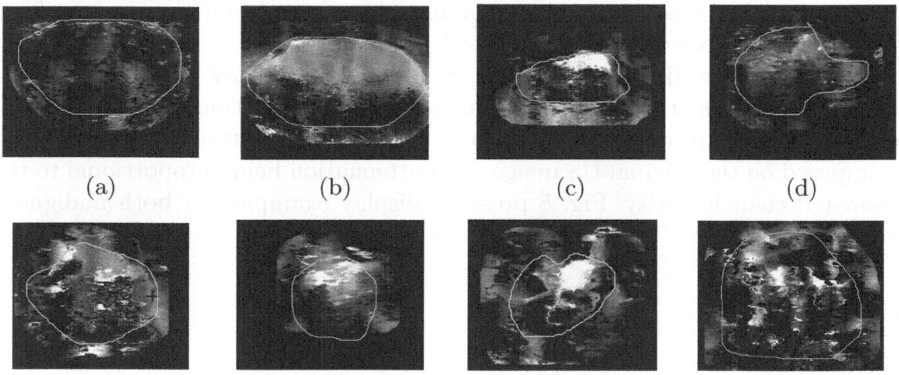

Fig. 3. Examples of attenuation maps. (a)-(d) are maps of benign tumors, (e)-(g) are maps of malignant ones. The gray-levels in the images correspond to the attenuation values. ROI marked in cyan.

In some benign cases the maximal attenuation value (feature number 3) is high due to artifacts. However, in those cases, this maximum value occurs only for small number of isolated pixels. Accordingly, we have introduced feature number 4 which examines the area where the attenuation is close to the maximum.

Another important feature is the size of the tumor, which can influence the assessment of the remaining features. For instance, our tests showed that the minimal acceptable intensity for feature number 3 and the parameter of the H-maxima transform should be smaller when dealing with smaller tumors. This is due the fact that for small tumors the attenuation estimation accuracy is lower.

Since the purpose of this work is to provide a proof of concept, in order to use these features for classification we had manually set thresholds and relation between them. Our future work will focus on using these features in a more sophisticated machine learning method, such as support vector machine classifier, on a much larger benchmark.

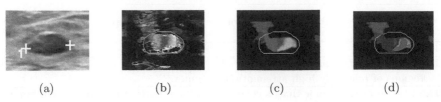

(a)	(b)	(c)	(d)

Fig. 4. Example for uniform attenuation regions. (a) is an US image of a benign tumor. (b) is the attenuation map. The green line marks the tumor's boundaries. (c) and (d) are the smoothed attenuation map, where the colored regions on (d) mark two uniform attenuation regions.

Special care should be taken of dark regions in the US image. Some doctors set the dynamic range such that those dark regions are saturated (i.e. the intensity level equals zero). Clearly, such regions yield false zero attenuation estimate. In order to mitigate this artifact we estimate the tumor attenuation and preform the classification based on non-saturated pixels only.

To facilitate the diagnostic process, we adopted a display combining the attenuation map and the original US image. If the given tumor is classified as benign, its attenuation map is discarded. Otherwise, the attenuation map is superimposed on the original US image with attenuation being proportional to the yellow-red color intensity. Fig. 5 presents display examples for both malignant and benign cases.

3   Results

To evaluate the efficacy of the above approach, we applied it to a diverse clinical benchmark including a total of 233 images of 80 different lesions. In all cases, the examining physician performed standard diagnostic procedure and decided to send the patient for a biopsy. We used the results of the biopsy as a gold standard to classify the benchmark into 46 benign and 34 malignant tumors. Most of the malignant tumors in our benchmark are IDC, while few are DCIS and ILC. Most of the benign lesions are fibroadnoma or fibrotic tissue, while the rest are: fat necrosis, PSH, cyst, tubular adenoma, hematoma, and abscess. The size of the tumors in the benchmark ranges from 3 to 40mm.

In should be noted that our database does not include mucinous (colloid) carcinoma which is a rare type of tumor that is, by nature, softer and has lower attenuation. Therefore, mucinous tumors are not likely to be detected by the proposed method. In order to detect such tumors our method should be applied together with a CAD system that processes the original US image, as apposed to the attenuation map.

We tested the robustness of our approach by acquiring the images using three different US systems, with no system-dependent tuning. All the images were processed using the aforementioned technique. Clearly, attenuation mapping provided additional information that, presently, is invisible to the examining physician. However, for the sake of objective quantitative testing, we limited our

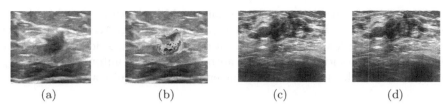

(a)   (b)   (c)   (d)

Fig. 5. Display examples. (a) is an US image of a malignant tumor. (b) is the output image. The green line marks the ROI. The color indicates attenuation intensity ranging from yellow (mild) to dark red (high). (c) is an US image of a benign tumor. (d) is the output image; no attenuation map is visible, only the ROI is marked.

evaluation to the correctness of our malignant/benign classification. We performed our analysis on a per-case basis, which is crucial from the clinical point of view. In other words, the tumor was deemed to be benign only if the algorithm classified all its images as benign.

The summary of the results is presented in Table 3. As indicated by the results in the table, our algorithm identified all the malignant tumors - without exception. This corresponds to 100% sensitivity. Moreover, only 12 benign tumors were misdiagnosed yielding specificity of 74%. Thus, our results indicate that it may be possible to drastically cut down the number of unnecessary biopsies by a factor of 4 without any significant deterioration in the system sensitivity.

Table 3. Performance evaluation

	Images	Tumors	Marked as Malignant	Marked as Benign
Malignant	113	34	34	0
Benign	120	46	12	34

4   Discussion and Conclusions

We presented an algorithm for transforming conventional B-scan images into their corresponding attenuation maps. The algorithm is valid for inhomogeneous tissue such as breast and does not require any modifications in the US image acquisition hardware or software. The attenuation map can help physicians distinguish between benign and malignant tumors and thus reduce the number of redundant biopsies currently being carried out. The proposed scheme also includes an automatic classification algorithm, whose preliminary results indicate that the number of unnecessary biopsies may be rapidly reduced.

As future work, it is important to substantiate the results by significantly increasing the tested benchmark. A larger benchmark will allow us to replace the current CAD algorithm with a machine learning algorithm (for instance support vector machines), that will automatically find the best classification using our features. Moreover, we believe that our results can be further enhanced by additional CAD features. One such example could be features aimed at detecting fibrotic cases, which are benign but highly attenuating. Accordingly, fibrotic cases cause quite a few false detections in our benchmark. Additional improvement would be the introduction of an automatic or semi-automatic tumor segmentation. This addition would make attenuation CAD fully automatic.

5 Patent Disclosure

The method described in this paper is the subject of two pending patent applications: 13/151303 and 13/558372.

Acknowledgments. The images used for this work were produced by Dr. Scott Fields from Hadassah Medical Organization in Jerusalem, and Dr. Ora Moskovitz from Or Breast Center in Haifa.

References

1. Nover, A.B., Jagtap, S., Anjum, W., Yegingil, H., Shih, W., Shih, W., Brooks, A.D.: Modern Breast Cancer Detection: A Technological Review. International Journal of Biomedical Imaging (2009)
2. Sehgal, C.M., Weinstein, S.P., Arger, P.H., Conant, E.F.: A Review of Breast Ultrasound. Journal of Mammary Gland Biology and Neoplasia 11(2) (2006)
3. Hall, T.: AAPM/RSNA Physics Tutorial for Residents: Topics in US: Beyond The Basics: Elasticity Imaging With US. Radiographics, 1657–1671 (2003)
4. Li, C., Duric, N., Huang, L.: Breast Imaging Using Transmission Ultrasound: Reconstructing Tissue Parameters of Sound Speed and Attenuation. In: BMEI (2008)
5. Chenga, H.D., Shana, J., Jua, W., Guo, Y., Zhang, L.: Automated Breast Cancer Detection and Classification Using Ultrasound Images: A Survey. Pattern Recognition 43(1), 299–317 (2010)
6. Goss, S.A., Johnston, R.L., Dunn, F.: Compilation of empirical ultrasonic properties of mammalian tissues II. Journal of The Acoustical Society of America 68(1), 93–108 (1980)
7. Chang, C.H., Huang, S.W., Li, P.C.: Attenuation Measurements for Ultrasonic Breast Imaging: Comparisons of Three Approaches. In: IEEE Ultrasonics Symposium, pp. 1306–1309 (2008)
8. Chang, C.H., Huang, S.W., Yang, H.C., Chou, Y.H., Li, P.C.: Reconstruction of Ultrasonic Sound Velocity and Attenuation Coefficient Using Linear Arrays: Clinical Assessment. Elsevier Ultrasound. Med. BioL. 33(11), 1681–1687 (2007)
9. Berger, G., Laugier, P., Thalabard, J.C., Perrin, J.: Global Breast Attenuation: Control Group and Benign Breast Diseases. Ultrasonic Imaging 12(1), 47–57 (1990)
10. Zheng, Y., Greenleaf, J.F., Gisvold, J.J.: Reduction of Breast Biopsies With a Modified Self Organizing Map. IEEE TNN 8(6), 46–56 (1997)
11. Walach, E., Shmulewitz, A., Itzchak, Y., Heyman, Z.: Local Tissue Attenuation Images Based on Pulsed-Echo Ultrasound Scans. IEEE Trans. Biomed. Eng. 36(2), 211–221 (1989)

12. Hughes, D.I., Duck, F.A.: Automatic Attenuation Compensation for Ultrasonic Imaging. Ultrasound in Medicine and Biology 23(5), 651–664 (1997)
13. Chen, D., Hsiao, Y.: Computer-aided Diagnosis in Breast Ultrasound. Elsevier Journal of Medical Ultrasound 16(1), 46–56 (2008)
14. McDonough, R., Huggins, W.: Best Least-Squares Representation of Signals by Exponentials. IEEE Trans. Autom. Control 13(4), 408–412 (1968)
15. Xie, W., Cai, C., Wang, Y.: Best Least Squares Solution for Prony Model. In: ISPACS, pp. 292–295 (2007)

What Genes Tell about Iris Appearance

Stine Harder[1], Susanne R. Christoffersen[1], Peter Johansen[2], Claus Børsting[2],
Niels Morling[2], Jeppe D. Andersen[2], Anders L. Dahl[1], and Rasmus R. Paulsen[1]

[1] Technical University of Denmark
DTU Informatics - Informatics and Mathematical Modelling
2800 Lyngby, Denmark
[2] University of Copenhagen
Section of Forensic Genetics - Department of Forensic Medicine
Faculty of Health and Medical Sciences
2100 Copenhagen O, Denmark

Abstract. Predicting phenotypes based on genotypes is generally hard,
but has shown good results for prediction of iris color. We propose to
correlate the appearance of iris with DNA. Six single-nucleotide polymor-
phisms (SNPs) have previously been shown to correlate with human iris
color, and we demonstrate that especially one of the six SNPs are correlated with iris appearance. To perform this analysis we need a method to
model the iris appearance, and we suggest an iris characterization based
on a bag of visual words, which gives us a similarity measure between
images of eyes. We have a dataset of 215 eye images with corresponding
SNP types, where the image of the iris has been segmented. We perform
two experiments based on the iris characterization. An agglomerative
clustering is performed and the result is that one SNP – rs12913832
(HERC2) is highly correlated with the image clustering. Furthermore
subspace projections are performed supporting that this SNP is very
important for eye color expression. With the suggested image characterizations we are able to investigate the correlation between the phenotypic
iris appearance and specific SNPs. This has potential for further investigation of the relation between DNA and iris appearance, especially with
focus on iris texture.

Keywords: Iris color, Iris texture, Image analysis, Image clustering,
Canonical discriminant analysis, DNA.

1 Introduction

Predicting complex human phenotypes from genotypes has great potentials in
application areas like personalized medicine [2, 6] or forensic genetics [7]. Personalized medicine does already exist for monogenetic disorders such as Huntington
disease [6], but finding the etiology of more complex diseases is not an easy task.
Liu et al. [11] did however demonstrate that genetic prediction of complex phenotypes is possible. Liu et al. [11] investigated 37 SNPs, representing all currently
known genetic variants with statistically significant eye color association, and

B.H. Menze et al. (Eds.): MCV 2012, LNCS 7766, pp. 244–253, 2013.
© Springer-Verlag Berlin Heidelberg 2013

found that six SNPs were the major predictors. The six SNPs are rs12913832 (HERC2), rs1800407 (OCA2), rs12896399 (SLC24A4), rs16891982 (SLC45A2), rs1393350 (TYR), and rs12203592 (IRF4). Prediction of human phenotypes from genotypes is of large interest in forensic genetics, where externally visible characteristics (EVCs) could be used as a "biological witness" in forensic cases. The cases of interest are e.g. when a DNA profile from a crime scene does not match either the possible suspects or DNA profiles in the criminal database. Then it would be a great advantage to be able to predict the appearance of the suspect.

The six SNPs found by Liu et al. [11] have also been used by Walsh et al. [15] to build a tool, called IrisPlex, for iris color prediction. Their investigations also revealed that rs12913832 is the main determinant for blue or brown colored eyes. This SNP is however not a vey precise predictor for the human iris color, because it varies continuously from the darkest brown to the lightest blue and is not clearly separable into the discrete expressions of the investigated SNPs. Our work is a step towards a more precise prediction of the human eye appearance based on DNA by investigating the correlation between our proposed image characterisations and the six SNPs found by Liu et al. [11]. This approach avoids subjective evaluation of iris color, partitioning of iris color into classes and it enables us to investigate overall iris appearance including iris structures.

2   Data

The study was approved by the Danish Ethical Committee of the Capital Region (H-4-2009-125) for samples conducted at Section of Forensic Genetics, Department of Forensic Medicine, Faculty of Health and Medical Sciences, University of Copenhagen, or as part of the Danish Blood Donor Study for samples conducted at the Blood Bank, Glostrup Hospital. The data consist of 215 high resolution eye images and corresponding DNA types. The images were subsampled to a spatial resolution of 639×426 pixels in RGB color.

The camera was equipped with a Twin flash, which ensured precise and repeatable acquisition and uniform illumination. The Twin flash gave two overexposed square regions in the iris and pupil area, which were removed in our segmentation procedure. Image examples are shown in Fig. 1.

From the DNA sample the SNPs [11]: rs12913832, rs1800407, rs12896399, rs16891982, rs1393350 and 12203592 were typed. The SNPs have three expressions or layers, i.e. there are three types of each SNP, however not all combinations were identified.

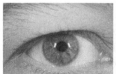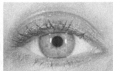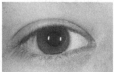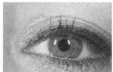

Fig. 1. Eye image examples

3   Iris Characterization

To construct an image characterization based on the iris we first need to segment
the image. After the segmentation we preform a radial image transformation
giving us the iris as a square image. We represent this image both by its color
as a histogram of RGB values and as a combined histogram of color and image
descriptors – a bag of visual words (BOW), which also contains information
about the iris texture.

Iris segmentation. The iris segmentation is performed by fitting a circle to the
inner and outer boundaries of the iris and fitting a spline to the upper and lower
eyelid boundaries, similar to the method proposed by Daugman [4].

    The eye images have a large gradient from the pupil to the iris and also
from the iris to the sclera. Utilizing this we propose an optimization scheme
where we look for a circle with maximum radial gradient. For a circle with
center at $\mathbf{x} = [x, y]^T$ and radius r, the image intensity of a point is given by
$f_\theta(\mathbf{x}, r) = I([x + r\cos(\theta), y + r\sin(\theta)]^T)$, where I is the image intensity and θ is
an angle. We estimate the radial gradient $\frac{df_\theta}{dr}$ using finite differences. We wish
to find the parameters of the circle that maximizes the gradient along the circle

$$
\underset{\mathbf{x},r}{\arg\max} \int_0^{2\pi} \left| \frac{df_\theta}{dr} \right| d\theta \approx \underset{\mathbf{x},r}{\arg\max} \sum_{i=0}^{n-1} \left| \frac{df_{i\Delta\theta}}{dr} \right|,
\tag{1}
$$

where $\Delta\theta = \frac{2\pi}{n}$. The solution to Eq. 1 is found using a coarse to fine sampling
strategy. The search for the center coordinate is performed by sampling in a
regular grid and choosing a finer sample grid around the position with the highest
gradient sum. This is repeated until single pixel accuracy is obtained. The radial
search is performed by calculating the gradient sum for a number of equally
spaced radii and then limiting the search area to a region around the radius
with the highest gradient sum. The search for radius and center coordinate is
performed simultaneously and the process is continued until single pixel accuracy
is obtained. To avoid detection of fine structures such as eyelashes we initially
smooth the image using a Gaussian kernel with a standard deviation of $\sigma = 3$
and we use $n = 36$ sample points.

    While the optimization works well for the pupil, it has problems with the iris
since the eyelids often covers part of the iris. To avoid this we choose only to
sum the gradient in the intervals $\theta \in [-\pi/4, \pi/4] \cup [3\pi/4, 5\pi/4]$, which is similar
to the approach in [3]. Therefore $n = 20$ for the iris. The small square spots from
the flash are removed using a simple threshold.

Eyelid Boundaries. The eyelid boundaries are located using a Markov Random
Field (MRF) based segmentation [10]. The segmentation is performed on the
second HSV component of the eye images, since this color component shows the

largest difference in pixel value between skin and inner eye regions. The chosen labels are sclera, eyelashes, skin and iris, and the iris label is divided into blue and brown. The statistics used in the MRF segmentation is calculated from manually annotated exemplars.

Let g be a label configuration and I the image. We estimate the posterior energy, $E(g|I)$, as

$$E(g|I) = \sum_i \left(\sum_{j \in \mathcal{N}_i} \delta(g_i, g_j) + \frac{1}{2} \log(\sigma_l^2) + \frac{(I_i - \mu_l)^2}{2\sigma_l^2} \right) (-log(Q(g_i))), \qquad (2)$$

where i is a site (pixel position) in the image. The neighborhood $\mathcal{N}_i$ is the four nearest sites. We assume the pixel intensities of the different labels to be normally distributed with $N(\mu_l, \sigma_l)$. Q is a probability matrix modeling the prior knowledge of position of the different classes based on 50 manually annotated images. The prior, $\delta(g_i, g_j)$, is modeled by

$$\delta(g_i, g_j) = \begin{cases} \beta, & \text{if } g_i \neq g_j \\ 0, & \text{if } g_i = g_j \end{cases}. \qquad (3)$$

The segmentation problem using MRF is solved using Graph Cut with α-expansion [8]. The three parameters in Eq. 2 are chosen experimentally. The final eyelid boundaries are found by fitting splines to the segmentation of the upper and lower eyelid boundaries.

The final iris image (the iris map) is obtained by radially sampling the segmented iris along lines going through the center of the pupil. The samples are chosen equidistantly along these lines from the circle fitted to the inner boundary of the iris to the circle on the outer boundary. The lines are sampled tangentially at equal angle steps. The number of angular steps is 720 and the number of radial steps is 120. The resulting image is therefore 120×720. We employ a mask to avoid the eyelid and highlight regions in our analysis. A result of the entire iris extraction procedure can be seen in Fig. 2. A few eye images was not precisely segmented, so for these samples we adjusted the segmentation manually.

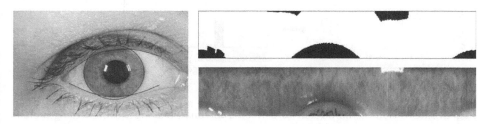

Fig. 2. Left: Final result for the detection of the eyelid boundaries, Right top: mask for iris map, Right bottom: iris map

Color characterization. The first image characterization is purely based on color. From a representative set of training images containing both blue and brown irises, we partition the three dimensional RGB color space into 852 color bins. This is done using a hierarchical binary separation of color channels based on the same principle as building a balanced kd-tree [1]. Hereby we ensure that each color bin contains approximately the same number of samples. The 852 color bins are used for constructing iris histograms, which are normalized using the L_1 norm.

BOW iris characterization. The second iris characterization is based on a bag of visual words (BOW) [13] in addition to color. We chose to use DAISY features [14] to represent the texture appearance because these features are computed in all pixels very efficiently and have shown similar performance as SIFT [12]. The resulting DAISY feature is a 100 dimensional vector $\mathbf{d}_d = [d_1, ..., d_{100}]^T$ and we represent the RGB value as the vector $\mathbf{d}_c = [R, G, B]^T$. These two vectors are L_2 normalized and concatenated to obtain a 103 dimensional descriptor vector $\overline{\mathbf{d}} = \sqrt{\frac{1}{2}}[\overline{\mathbf{d}}_d, \overline{\mathbf{d}}_c]^T$. We obtain a dictionary of visual words using k-means clustering into 400 clusters with cluster centers as visual words from 40000 randomly chosen training samples. Each image feature is labeled by assigning it to the nearest visual word using the L_2 norm. An overview of the process can be seen in Fig. 3. To include spatial information in the image characterization we perform a spatial weighting of the visual words using Gaussians distributed at 12 positions as illustrated in Fig. 4. Based on this representation we can estimate the similarity of iris maps as histogram differences.

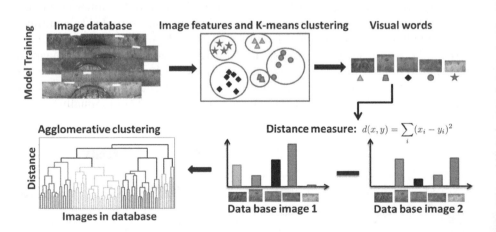

Fig. 3. Illustration of the bag of words model for images along with the images clustering procedure

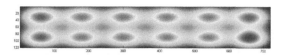

Fig. 4. Spatial Gaussian weighting used for building the explanatory histograms

4 Analysis and Results

Based on the color and combined color and texture characterization our aim is to compare the genotypes with the visual appearance. We perform two explorative experiments – the first based on hierarchical agglomerative clustering [9] of the image characterizations and compare this to the genetic expression, and the second is subspace projection based on canonical discriminant analysis [5].

Agglomerative Clustering. The image characterizations based on respectively color and combined color and texture are used to generate an agglomerative clustering. The agglomerative clustering is based on the L_2 distance between the histograms, and similar histograms are clustered together. The result is a dendrogram for respectively color and combined color and texture, as seen in Fig. 5. The lower part of the figures show the six SNPs defined in Sec. 2. Each bin in a dendrogram, corresponding to an eye image, has the six SNPs represented with color below. The different layers of the SNPs are colored with respectively red, green or blue. It is clear that the image clustering results for both color and a combination of color and texture corresponds very well with the genotypes of rs12913832.

Subspace projections. We have performed a subspace projection of the iris descriptor histograms shown in Fig. 6 using principal component analysis (PCA) and canonical discriminant analysis (CDA). The first principal or canonical direction is horizontal and the second is vertical. We treat the three genetic expressions of rs12913832 as classes. To account for the rank deficiency of the estimated covariance matrices we initially perform a data projection using PCA where we keep the first 100 principal components. This corresponds to 98.8% of the variance of the color descriptor and 86.2% of the variance of the combined color and texture descriptor.

The iris maps are overlapping and in the overlapping regions their color is averaged. This gives a blurring effect where the iris maps are overlapping. Using PCA the iris maps are mainly sorted according to color, whereas the CDA clearly separates the iris maps into the three distinct groups according to the three expressions of the rs12913832 SNP.

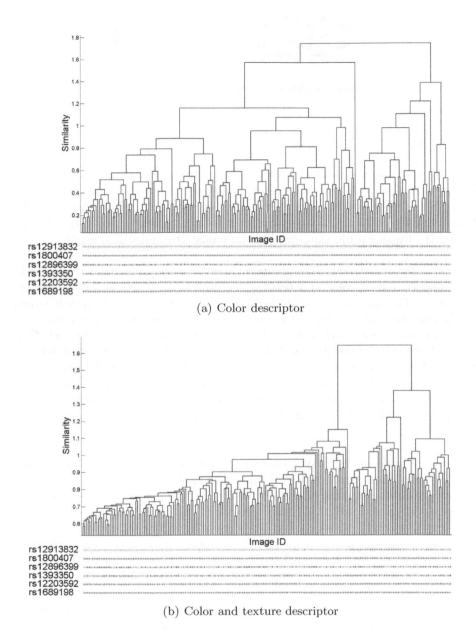

(a) Color descriptor

(b) Color and texture descriptor

Fig. 5. Top part shows a dendrogram obtained using agglomerative clustering based on (a) the color descriptor and (b) the combined color and texture descriptor histograms. The dendrograms are based on the L_2 distance between the histograms explained in Sec. 3. Below each bin in a dendrogram the expressions of the six SNPs are represented by a color.

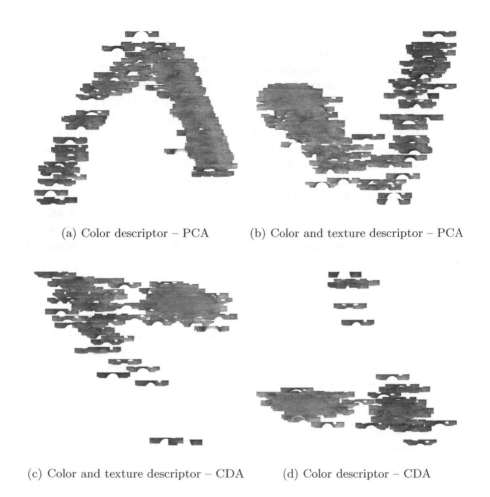

(a) Color descriptor – PCA   (b) Color and texture descriptor – PCA

(c) Color and texture descriptor – CDA   (d) Color descriptor – CDA

Fig. 6. Iris maps projected to the first two (a,b) principal components and (c,d) the first two canonical dimensions based on (a,c) the color descriptor histograms and (b,d) the combined color and texture descriptor histograms. Classes in the canonical discriminant analysis are based on the genetic expression of rs12913832.

5   Discussion

The agglomerative clustering based on the image characterization for respectively color and a combination of color and texture showes a large correlation with rs12913832. rs12913832 seems to be the major explanation for iris appearance and the contribution from the remaining five SNPs seem to be minor. The dendrograms obtained for color and combined color and texture reveal very similar results. This indicates that iris color is the main contributor to the image characterization and that the texture is not expressed in the analysed SNPs.

We only present the subspace projection analysis based on rs12913832 as class labels. The other SNPs also separate nicely using CDA, but with PCA only rs12913832 was sorted according to its expression. This further underlines the observation from the clustering experiment, that rs12913832 is very important for the iris color, but there is only little influence on the iris texture. Our investigations so far do not support that any of the included SNPs influence iris texture, but the texture is an important element in the iris appearance. However with the suggested image descriptors we are able to analyze this further.

The radial transformation performed after the iris extraction consist of a radial sampling, where the inner part of the iris is sampled more densely than the outer part. The sampling procedure entail that the features close to the pupil will have a greater impact than features located in the periphery of the iris. This property is similar for all eye images and the distance measure is therefore not affected. A great advantage with the sampling method is that the new coordinate system becomes invariant to the size of the iris and to pupil dilation as explained by Daugman [4].

6   Conclusion

We have analyzed the genetic expression of six SNPs in relation to iris appearance. To perform this investigation, we have suggested a representation of the iris appearance based on color and texture from a radial warped eye image. The image representation is a histogram of image features. We perform an explorative analysis in the form of an image based clustering and a subspace projection. Our investigations show that especially rs12913832 is closely correlated with the iris color, whereas the other SNPs show a less clear pattern. We do not see a relation between iris texture and the investigated SNPs, but our descriptors clearly show that texture is an important part of the iris appearance. The proposed methodology enables us to investigate this further.

Acknowledgments. We thank Section of Forensic Genetics, Department of Forensic Medicine, Faculty of Health and Medical Sciences, University of Copenhagen and the Blood Bank, Glostrup Hospital for collecting data.

References

[1] Bentley, J.L.: Multidimensional binary search trees used for associative searching. Communications of the ACM 18(9), 509–517 (1975)
[2] Brand, A., Brand, H., et al.: The impact of genetics and genomics on public health. European Journal of Human Genetics 16(1), 5–13 (2007)
[3] Daugman, J.G.: High confidence visual recognition of persons by a test of statistical independence. IEEE Transactions on Pattern Analysis and Machine Intelligence 15(11), 1148–1161 (1993)
[4] Daugman, J.G.: How iris recognition works. IEEE Transactions on Circuits and Systems for Video Technology 14(1), 21–30 (2004)

[5] Fisher, R.A.: The use of multiple measurements in taxonomic problems. Annals of Human Genetics 7(2), 179–188 (1936)

[6] Janssens, A.C.J.W., Van Duijn, C.M.: Genome-based prediction of common diseases: advances and prospects. Human molecular genetics 17(R2), R166–R173 (2008)

[7] Kayser, M., Schneider, P.M.: Dna-based prediction of human externally visible characteristics in forensics: motivations, scientific challenges, and ethical considerations. Forensic Science International: Genetics 3(3), 154–161 (2009)

[8] Kolmogorov, V., Zabin, R.: What energy functions can be minimized via graph cuts? IEEE Transactions on Pattern Analysis and Machine Intelligence 26(2), 147–159 (2004)

[9] Krishnamachari, S., Abdel-Mottaleb, M.: Image browsing using hierarchical clustering. In: Proceedings of IEEE International Symposium on Computers and Communications, pp. 301–307. IEEE (1999)

[10] Li, S.Z.: Markov random field modeling in image analysis. Springer-Verlag New York Inc. (2009)

[11] Liu, F., van Duijn, K., Vingerling, J.R., Hofman, A., Uitterlinden, A.G., Janssens, A., Kayser, M.: Eye color and the prediction of complex phenotypes from genotypes. Current Biology 19(5), R192–R193 (2009)

[12] Lowe, D.G.: Distinctive image features from scale-invariant keypoints. International Journal of Computer Vision 60(2), 91–110 (2004)

[13] Sivic, J., Zisserman, A.: Video google: A text retrieval approach to object matching in videos. In: Proceedings of the Ninth IEEE International Conference on Computer Vision, pp. 1470–1477. IEEE (2003)

[14] Tola, E., Lepetit, V., Fua, P.: Daisy: An efficient dense descriptor applied to wide-baseline stereo. IEEE Transactions on Pattern Analysis and Machine Intelligence 32(5), 815–830 (2010)

[15] Walsh, S., Lindenbergh, A., Zuniga, S.B., Sijen, T., de Knijff, P., Kayser, M., Ballantyne, K.N.: Developmental validation of the irisplex system: determination of blue and brown iris colour for forensic intelligence. Forensic Science International: Genetics 5(5), 464–471 (2011)

Robust Dense Endoscopic Stereo Reconstruction for Minimally Invasive Surgery

Sylvain Bernhardt[1], Julien Abi-Nahed[2], and Rafeef Abugharbieh[1]

[1] Biomedical Signal and Image Computing Lab, University of British Columbia,
Vancouver, Canada
[2] Qatar Robotic Surgery Centre, Qatar Science and Technology Park, Qatar
sylvainb@ece.ubc.ca

Abstract. Robotic assistance in minimally invasive surgical interventions has gained substantial popularity over the past decade. Surgeons perform such operations by remotely manipulating laparoscopic tools whose motion is executed by the surgical robot. One of the main tools deployed is an endoscopic binocular camera that provides stereoscopic vision of the operated scene. Such surgeries have notably garnered wide interest in renal surgeries such as partial nephrectomy, which is the focus of our work. This operation consists of the localization and removal of tumorous tissue in the kidney. During this procedure, the surgeon would greatly benefit from an augmented reality view that would display additional information from the different imaging modalities available, such as pre-operational CT and intra-operational ultrasound. In order to fuse and visualize these complementary data inputs in a pertinent way, they need to be accurately registered to a 3D reconstruction of the imaged surgical scene topology captured by the binocular camera. In this paper we propose a simple yet powerful approach for dense matching between the two stereoscopic camera views and for reconstruction of the 3D scene. Our method adaptively and accurately finds the optimal correspondence between each pair of images according to three strict confidence criteria that efficiently discard the majority of outliers. Using experiments on clinical in-vivo stereo data, including comparisons to two state-of-the-art 3D reconstruction techniques in minimally invasive surgery, our results illustrate superior robustness and better suitability of our approach to realistic surgical applications.

Keywords: stereovision, rectification, dense matching, 3D reconstruction, stereo camera, stereo vision, partial nephrectomy, augmented reality, robotic assisted surgery.

1 Introduction

The past decade witnessed an ever-increasing number of reports on robot-assisted surgical interventions where the surgeon remotely controls a robot that reproduces the motion of his/her hands on laparoscopic tools. Medical robots, such as the *da Vinci Surgical System* (Intuitive Surgical, Inc., Sunnyvale, CA, USA),

B.H. Menze et al. (Eds.): MCV 2012, LNCS 7766, pp. 254–262, 2013.

have for example been widely used in renal surgery due to similar or even better clinical outcomes than those of standard procedures [1].

The fact that the surgeon's view of the operated scene is digitized via a stereo camera has made augmented reality (AR) in minimally invasive surgery (MIS) an very active research area since the early 2000s [2][3]. The aim is to grant the surgeon the ability to see "beyond" the visible surface by overlaying visual information from other available intra-operative and pre-operative data onto the endoscopic camera feed. However, registration of such data with the 3D scene remains a difficult problem since, particularly in abdominal MIS, the environment is mostly composed of soft tissue and organs that significantly deform due to the surgeon's actions as well as patient breathing and cardiovascular activity. One approach to solving this problem is to use the stereo stream from the camera to perform dense matching and provide a 3D model of the surgical scene that can then serve as a registration base for the other imaging data, e.g. as in [4]. Many methods for dense stereo matching have been proposed over the last decades [8][9], however, there are two main distinctions between the kind of data typical in MIS and the traditional reference datasets for dense stereo matching, such as the Middlebury images [10]. The first is that our binocular camera provides a video output, i.e. sequences of images with very little differences between two successive frames. Therefore, temporal smoothness gains more importance and can be enforced. Furthermore, since the MIS scenes are generally not static when captured, a significant amount of motion blur is typically introduced, which makes the stereo matching problem more difficult.

The second main difference is related to the content of the images. Datasets traditionally used in computer vision studies represent static scenes with a variety of rather simply shaped objects laid out at different depths. Moreover, the surfaces are most of time matte and the lighting is uniform, which does not induce complex lighting artifacts. On the other hand, intra-abdominal tissue is soft and presents complex reflections, due to the non-Lambertian nature of the surfaces, as well as irregular shapes, highly variable textures and various distortion . Additionally, there is a constant presence of surgical tools that severely occludes the scene with textureless plastic or highly reflective metallic parts (see figure 1). Overall, image sequences in MIS are very challenging to reconstruct and defy the robustness of current stereo matching techniques.

Few methods at dense reconstruction of stereo endoscopic images have been proposed. In [2], a method was presented for detecting and virtually removing the tools from the reconstructed scene. Later [12], Vagvolgyi et al proposed a method to overlay a kidney model onto the stereo display by registering the model to the kidney surface reconstructed from stereo data. More recently [5], Stoyanov et al presented a method to perform near real-time stereo reconstruction in MIS based on belief propagation. A similar work has been recently proposed in [6] where hybrid recursive matching was used.

All these previous methods are based on existing stereo matching algorithms that have not been designed for MIS data. For example, they all try to enforce spatial smoothness constraints, which is supposed to ensure homogeneous

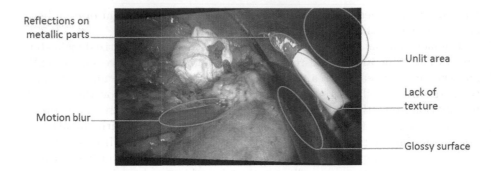

Fig. 1. Example image depicting a scene captured during a partial nephrectomy procedure. Commonly encountered artifacts are highlighted in orange.

disparities in regular areas. However, practical MIS images are more challenging, therefore mismatches are more prone to happen. If spatial smoothness is enforced, this will tend to spread errors into little clusters of homogeneous outliers, which are harder to discard than isolated ones. Also, the risk of getting rid of actual inliers is greater if they are in a group since a single pixel standing out from the rest of the depth map does not represent a realistic scene in world space. The work presented in this paper aims to address such issue by providing a 3D model of the surgical scene with emphasis on accuracy and robustness. The primary goal is to discard outliers and yet provide enough information across all frames of the video stream such that registration is still possible. To achieve this, we first detect only the most reliable matches by enforcing a series of strict criteria reflecting certainty of matching. We then enforce limited spatial smoothness to handle the few isolated outliers that still survive.

2   Methodology

2.1   Pre-processing

The output from our surgical binocular camera is an interlaced high definition video (1080i). To alleviate the problem of jagged edges in the de-interlaced images, each extracted frame is downsampled by a factor 2 down to 960×540 pixels. For each pair of frames, we then perform a sparse matching using the SIFT descriptor [13]. Occasional mismatches are discarded during the robust calculation of the fundamental matrix F using RANSAC as in [7]. The epipoles are calculated from F and used to rectify the images. This process aligns the two images into the same plane in the world space (see figure 2a-b). Then, according to the laws of epipolar geometry, every feature or pixel in one frame has its correspondence on the same row in the other frame, which greatly facilitates the matching (see figure 2b). We use polar rectification, as it is simple and guarantees minimal distortion of the images [14]. The matching of a feature yields the disparity d which is inversely proportional to the feature depth Z in

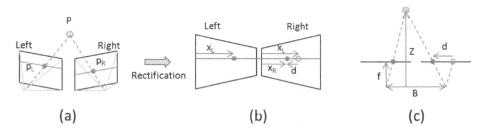

Fig. 2. Rectification and relation between depth and disparity. (a) shows the projection of a point P in world space onto the two image planes in p_L and p_R. In (b), the vertical alignment of this point in the rectified images gives the disparity d between its left and right locations, respectively x_L and x_R. The disparity d is also inversely proportional to the depth, as shown in (c) the top view of (b).

the world space (see figure 2c and equation 1, where f is the focal length and B the baseline between the two optical centers).

$$Z = -\frac{Bf}{d} \qquad (1)$$

Finally, the images are converted to grayscale by averaging the three color channels with different weights as recommended in [15] where it was shown that the use of color in dense stereo matching is not beneficial.

2.2   Robust Matching via Confidence Criteria

Our dense matching is based on calculating similarity between patches from the left and right images using normalized-cross correlation (NCC) as a metric, which is efficient even in the presence of brightness change. For a given point and window in the left image, the similarity profile is calculated across the same row in the right image, bounded by a range centered at the same position. The local maxima represent the location of candidates for matching with the best candidate chosen as the one with the highest similarity value. As robustness is paramount in our application, we ensure that each point pair matching satisfies strict confidence criteria that reflect three metrics of uncertainty in the matching in our approach:

First, blurry, unlit and textureless parts of the image present very little structural information, which makes the matching difficult if not impossible. To mitigate this problem, a simple and effective gradient dispersion metric γ is considered, in order to estimate the spatial structure. Let γ_L be its value for the considered patch I_p and γ_R the one for the best candidate patch I_c. Our **first criterion** is that both of these values have to be greater than a certain threshold γ_{min} (see equation 2). If this condition is not met, the matching is declared too risky.

$$\gamma_L = stdev(\nabla^2 I_p) > \gamma_{min} \quad \text{and} \quad \gamma_R = stdev(\nabla^2 I_c) > \gamma_{min} \qquad (2)$$

Second, the quality of a matching also appears in the difference of similarity score in the NCC profile between the two highest peaks, as illustrated by figure 3. The blue curve represents the matching from the left to right images, and the green one from right to left. The graph (a) of the figure reflects a patch of size of 7x7 pixels. As can be easily seen, the profile presents many peaks of approximatively the same score, which means the content of the patch is not discriminative enough and hence the window may be too small. On the graph (b) of the figure, the window size is 13x13 pixels, which allows the patch to contain more complex patterns. As a result, the correct solution stands out in the profile since the gap between the best and other peaks is significant. Our **second criterion** is thus that this difference δ has to be beyond a threshold δ_{min}. If this condition is not satisfied, the matching is declared not discriminative enough.

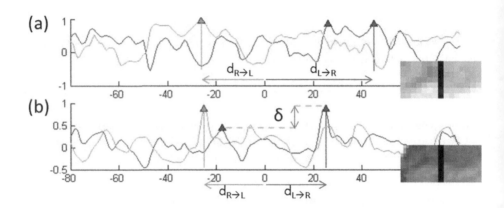

Fig. 3. Two example NCC profiles for the same point but with two different window sizes. The blue curve represents the matching from the left to right images, and the green one from right to left. On the y-axis is the similarity score and on the x-axis the disparity. The best peak is designated by a vertical line and its score difference with the second best peak is δ. The disparities of the best candidates from left to right and right to left are also displayed as $d_{L \to R}$ and $d_{R \to L}$, respectively. (b) here shows better discrimination.

Third, let us consider $d_{L \to R}$ and $d_{R \to L}$. If this correspondence is correct, then the inverse matching (from right to left) should yield the dual result: $d_{R \to L} = -d_{L \to R}$. Therefore, if both previous criteria are satisfied, then inverse matching is performed starting from the best candidate in the right image. Our **third criterion** is thus that $d_{R \to L}$ and $d_{L \to R}$ should cancel out within a threshold ϵ (see equation 3). If this is not true, the matching is then considered incorrect.

$$|d_{L \to R} + d_{R \to L}| < \epsilon \tag{3}$$

In case of failure in satisfying the above third criterion, the window is increased by a step dw in hope of providing a more discriminative matching. If the window

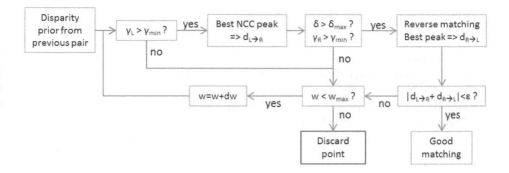

Fig. 4. Block diagram of our proposed dense matching method

size reaches a threshold w_{max} and still none of the criteria are satisfied, then this particular point in the image is discarded (see figure 4). This matching method is iterated through the image until completion.

2.3   Post-processing and Temporal Smoothness

Even though the previous criteria are very restrictive, it is still possible to have outliers slipping through. Fortunately, since spatial smoothness has not been enforced, the few surviving outliers are most of the time isolated and easy to identify. Therefore, our post-processing step consists of finding isolated pixels that are significantly different from their neighborhood. More specifically, in a window of size Δw around each point that has been matched, we consider the number N of disparities whose difference with the actual point disparity is less than a threshold Δd. If the ratio $N/\Delta w^2$ is smaller than a threshold μ, then the matching for this point is discarded. Once outliers are weeded out, one or two-pixel wide holes are filled with the median of their surrounding values. It is important to note that no other attempt at filling larger empty areas is needed, as subsequent frames will fill larger gaps (i.e. uncertain matching areas) locally across time. For computational considerations and due to the highly reliable matches, the disparities found for one image pair are used as priors for the next pair of frames by reducing the search range of a point matching around its previous disparity value, thus enforcing the temporal smoothness of the depth evaluations.

3   Results and Discussion

All experiments were carried on frames extracted from in-vivo videos recorded by our own high definition endoscopic stereo camera during four different partial nephrectomies assisted by a *da Vinci* robot. The sequences have a resolution of 1920×1080 pixels at a frame rate of 25 fps and the images color space is YCbCR.

Our experiments have shown that $\gamma_{min} = 0.5$, $\delta_{min} = 0.1$, $\epsilon = 5$, $\Delta d = 4$, $\Delta w = 5$, $\mu = 0.4$, a square window of initial width $w_{min} = 7$, maximum width $w_{max} = 30$ and step $dw = 4$, for frames of size 960×540, yield good results for a wide range of MIS scenes.

We compared our algorithm to the two latest methods in dense reconstruction from stereo in MIS – [5] and [6] – over various pair of frames from our data. Although their techniques often yielded accurate results, they would still present significant outliers in difficult areas as in figure 1. In contrast, our method has successfully discarded the vast majority of difficult areas (see figure 5), while still matching the easier parts of the image.

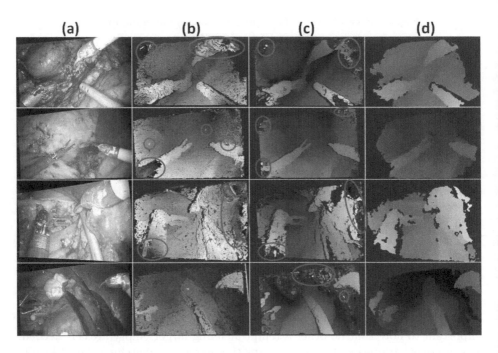

(a)   **(b)**   **(c)**   **(d)**

Fig. 5. Comparison with other methods. (a) Original image; (b) Depth map from [5]; (c) Depth map from [6] and (d) our method. Our method successfully dismisses error-prone areas while the two other methods present outliers (highlighted in red). In the depth maps, whiter is shallower.

Given that certain difficult areas may be discarded in our robust matching process which may result in occasional localized loss of reconstruction information, the temporal nature of our matching ensures that successful reconstruction is attained within a few frames. For example, in the central parts of the frame, most pixel reconstructions are updated within 10 frames which represent less than 0.5 seconds, as illustrated in figure 6. Therefore, the region of interest can always be successfully reconstructed locally in time.

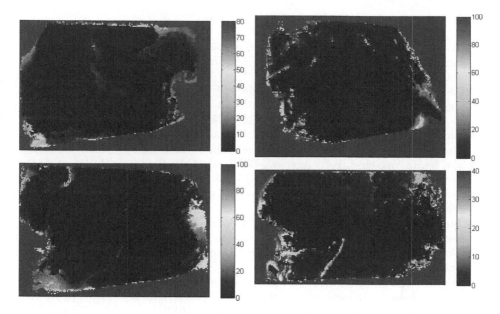

Fig. 6. Depth update with respect to image region. This figure presents four different sequences. For each graph, the pixel value represents the largest number of successive frames for the corresponding pixel reconstruction to be updated again in the sequence. The colormap scales from 0 to the total number of frames. Pixels with the maximum value (red) are those which have never been matched, either for being out of the rectified image or because of difficult regions. However, in all four example sequences shown, the central parts of the image is always blue i.e. these pixels are matched very regularly.

4   Conclusions

The purpose of this work was to provide an accurate and robust stereo dense matching method that is suited to surgical scene reconstruction. By enforcing strict matching confidence criteria and relaxing spatial smoothness, we have shown that our method is capable of discarding most outliers in frame pairs from real in-vivo clinical data where current state-of-the-art techniques fail.

Since all matchings are independent of each other, our method is highly parallelizable and will reach its full potential once implemented on GPU, which is our plan for the near future.

Acknowledgements. The author would like to thank Dr. Danail Stoyanov for providing the code of his method, Sebastian Roehl for submitting results from his program on our images, the Hamad Medical Corporation hospital for providing the surgical stereo sequences and Mitchell Vu for his help on compiling results.

References

1. Babbar, P., Hemal, A.K.: Robot-assisted partial nephrectomy: current status, techniques, and future directions. International Urology and Nephrology 44(1), 99–109 (2012)
2. Mourgues, F., Devernay, F., Coste-Maniere, E.: 3D Reconstruction of the Operating Field for Image Overlay in 3D-Endoscopic Surgery. In: International Symposium on Augmented Reality, pp. 191–192 (2001)
3. Sielhorst, T., Feuerstein, M., Navab, N.: Advanced Medical Displays: A Literature Review of Augmented Reality. Journal of Display Technology 4(4), 451–467 (2008)
4. Su, L.-M., Vagvolgyi, B.P., Agarwal, R., Reiley, C.E., Taylor, R.H., Hager, G.D.: Augmented reality during robot-assisted laparoscopic partial nephrectomy: toward real-time 3D-CT to stereoscopic video registration. Journal of Urology 73(4), 896–900 (2009)
5. Stoyanov, D., Visentini-Scarzanella, M., Pratt, P., Yang, G.-Z.: Real-time stereo reconstruction in robotically assisted minimally invasive surgery. In: International Conference on Medical Image Computing and Computer-Assisted Intervention, vol. 13(pt 1), pp. 275–282 (2010)
6. Roehl, S., et al.: Dense GPU-enhanced surface reconstruction from stereo endoscopic images for intraoperative registration. The International Journal of Medical Physics Research and Practice 39(3), 1632–1645 (2012)
7. Hartley, R.I., Zisserman, A.: Multiple View Geometry in Computer Vision, 2nd edn. Cambridge University Press (2004) ISBN: 0521540518
8. Scharstein, D., Szeliski, R., Zabih, R.: A taxonomy and evaluation of dense two-frame stereo correspondence algorithms. In: IEEE Workshop on Stereo and Multi-Baseline Vision, vol. (1), pp. 131–140 (2002)
9. Brown, M.Z., Burschka, D., Hager, G.D.: Advances in computational stereo. EEE Transactions on Pattern Analysis and Machine Intelligence 25(8), 993–1008 (2003)
10. http://vision.middlebury.edu/stereo/data/
11. Stoyanov, D., Elhelw, M., Lo, B.P., Chung, A., Bello, F., Yang, G.-Z.: Current Issues of Photorealistic Rendering for Virtual and Augmented Reality in Minimally Invasive Surgery. In: International Conference on Information Visualization, pp. 350–358 (2003)
12. Vagvolgyi, B.P., Su, L.-M., Taylor, R.H., Hager, G.D.: Video to CT Registration for Image Overlay on Solid Organs. In: Augmented Reality in Medical Imaging and Augmented Reality in Computer-Aided Surgery (AMIARCS), pp. 78–86 (2008)
13. Lowe, D.G.: Object recognition from local scale-invariant features. In: International Conference on Computer Vision, pp. 1150–1157 (1999)
14. Pollefeys, M., Koch, R., Van Gool, L.: A simple and efficient rectification method for general motion. In: International Conference on Computer Vision, pp. 496–501 (1999)
15. Bleyer, M., Chambon, S.: Does Color Really Help in Dense Stereo Matching? In: International Symposium on 3D Data Processing, pp. 1–8 (2010)

Model-Based Human Teeth Shape Recovery
from a Single Optical Image with Unknown Illumination

Aly Farag[1], Shireen Elhabian[1], Aly Abdelrehim[1],
Wael Aboelmaaty[2], Allan Farman[2], and David Tasman[2]

[1] Computer Vision and Image Processing Laboratory,
University of Louisville, Louisville, KY 40292
[2] School of Dentistry, University of Louisville, Louisville, KY, 40202, USA

Abstract. Several existing 3D systems for dental applications rely on obtaining an intermediate solid model of the jaw (cast or teeth imprints) from which the 3D information can be captured. In this paper, we propose a model-based shape-from-shading (SFS) approach which allows for the construction of plausible human jaw models *in vivo*, without ionizing radiation, using fewer sample points in order to reduce the cost and intrusiveness of acquiring models of patients teeth/jaws over time. The inherent relation between the photometric information and the underlying 3D shape is formulated as a statistical model where the effect of illumination is modeled using Spherical Harmonics (SH) and the partial least square (PLS) approach is deployed to carry out the estimation of dense 3D shapes. Moreover, shape and texture alignment is accomplished using a proposed definition of anatomical jaw landmarks which can be automatically detected. Vis-à-vis dental applications, the results demonstrate a significant increase in accuracy in favor of the proposed approach. In particular, our approach is able to recover geometrical details of tooth occlusal surface as well as mouth floor and ceiling as compared to SFS-based approaches.

1 Introduction

Object modeling from a single image, augmented with prior information, facilitates various studies and applications in art, design, reverse engineering, rapid prototyping and basic analysis of deformations and uncertainties. Without the use of ionizing radiation (e.g. X-ray and Computer Tomography - CT), object modeling involves constructing a 3D representation for the information conveyed in the given 2D images. This problem has been studied in the past four decades resulting in many solutions bundled under the name *shape-from-X*. In particular, techniques, such as shape-from-shading provide promise of image-based 3D reconstruction when the imaging environment is somewhat precise.

To motivate the contribution of this work, we consider a dental application; 3D reconstruction of the visible part of the human jaw. Dentistry usually require accurate 3D representation of the teeth and jaw for diagnostic and treatment purposes. For instance, orthodontic treatment involves the application, over time, of force systems to teeth for malocclusion correction. Several existing 3D systems for dental applications found in literature rely on obtaining an intermediate solid model of the jaw (cast or teeth imprints) and then capturing the 3D information from that model, e.g. [1]. There may

B.H. Menze et al. (Eds.): MCV 2012, LNCS 7766, pp. 263–272, 2013.
© Springer-Verlag Berlin Heidelberg 2013

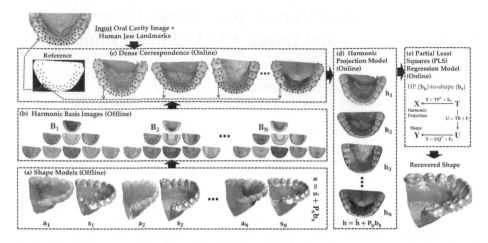

Fig. 1. Block diagram of the proposed model-based human jaw shape recovery: (a) An aligned ensemble of the shapes and textures (oral cavity images) of human jaws is used to build the 3D shape model. (b) Given the texture and surface normals (defining the shape) of a certain jaw in the ensemble, harmonic basis images are constructed. Given an input oral cavity image under general unknown illumination and a set of human jaw anatomical landmark points: (c) Dense correspondence is established between the input image and each jaw sample in the ensemble, where each pixel position within the convex hull of a reference jaw shape corresponds to a certain point on a sample jaw (shape and texture) and in the same time to a certain point on the input image. (d) The input image, in the reference frame, is projected onto the subspace spanned by the harmonic basis of each sample in the ensemble which are scaled (using the projection coefficients) and summed-up to construct the harmonic projection (HP) images which encodes the illumination conditions of the input image. Such images are then used to construct an HP model of the input image. (e) The inherit relation between the HP images and the corresponding shape is cast as a regression framework where partial least squares is used to solve for shape coefficients to recover the shape of the input image.

therefore be a demand for intraoral measurement that could be fulfilled by photogrammetry, which has been applied to the measurement of many small objects, even the measurement of dental replicas. Thus photogrammetry seems to offer a reduced cost technique while avoiding the need for castings.

Our argument of image-based approach for 3D reconstruction as an alternative to CT-scanning is based on the following. During the exposure to diagnostic imaging using x-ray (ionizing/ electromagnetic radiation), the patient body is penetrated by millions of x-ray photons whose ionization can damage the body's molecules especially DNA in chromosomes. Most DNA damage is repaired immediately, but rarely a portion of a chromosome may be permanently altered (a mutation) leading ultimately to the formation of a tumor [2]. While doses and risks for dental radiology are small, a number of epidemiological studies have provided evidence of an increased risk of brain [3], salivary gland [4] and thyroid tumors [5] for dental radiography. Also, pregnant mothers undergoing diagnostic or therapeutic procedures involving ionizing radiation, or who may be exposed to environmental radiation, there is a great potential for damage to the early embryo [6]. These effects are believed to have no threshold radiation dose below which they will not occur [7]. On the other hand, CT-scanning is considered expensive and not paid by insurance companies unless disease oriented. Meanwhile, dental offices in rural areas do not have such a luxury. Thus our intent is to develop a purely image-based reconstruction mechanism as a cost-effective information tool for the dentist.

In this paper we aim at making it easy and feasible for doctors, dentists, and researchers to obtain models of a person's jaw *in vivo*, without ionizing radiation, using fewer sample points in order to reduce the cost and intrusiveness of acquiring models of patients teeth/jaws over time. This is a challenging problem due to the "unfriendly" environment of taking measurements inside a person's mouth [8]. Further assumptions of the presence of distinct features or texture regions on the object in stereo images and the photo consistency in space carving are rarely valid in practice.

Due to the lack of surface texture, shape-from-shading (SFS) algorithms have been used to reconstruct the 3D shape of human teeth/jaw due to the significant shading cue presented in an intra-oral image, e.g. [9]. Nonetheless, in principle, SFS is an ill-posed problem, Prados and Faugeras [10] showed that constraining the SFS problem to a specific class of objects can improve the accuracy of the recovered shape. Thus the main objective of the presented work is to develop and validate a holistic approach for image-based 3D reconstruction of the human jaw based on statistical shape-from-shading (SSFS), covering regions which the classical SFS approach does not handle, using scanned molds and images of the oral cavity to estimate the shape of a human jaw in order to create a more accurate jaw 3D model. In specific, the structure of human jaw reveals what can be acquired in terms of prior information to enhance the SFS process where the upper and lower jaws are symmetric and lined up according to specific anatomical features and landmarks. We believe that this approach has the potential to greatly improve plausibility of the resulting shape from shading models.

2 Related Work

There has been a substantial amount of work regarding statistical shape recovery for human face modeling and biomedical structures with distinct shapes - e.g., modeling the corpus callosum, the kidney and spinal cord; it is an active research area under shape and appearance modeling (e.g., [11, 12]). Atick et al. [13] proposed the first statistical SFS method where principal component analysis (PCA) was used to parameterize the set of all possible facial surfaces. Scene parameters such as pose and illumination were estimated in the process of a morphable model fitting using a stochastic gradient descent-based optimization. By considering the statistical constraint of [13] and the geometric constraint of symmetry in [14], Dovgard and Basri [15] introduced a statistical symmetric SFS method. Smith and Hancock [11] modeled surface normals within the framework of statistical SFS. Based on active appearance models (AAM) concept of Cootes et al. [16], Castelan et al. [17] developed a coupled statistical model to recover the 3D shape from intensity images with frontal light source, where the 2D shape model in [16] is replaced with a 3D shape model composed of height maps. The main advantage of the Castelan approach over the 3D morphable model framework [18] is the straightforward recovery of the 3D face shape, without undergoing a costly optimization process.

One of the main challenges that confront SFS algorithms is dealing with arbitrary illumination. Basri and Jacobs [19] proved that images of convex Lambertian object taken under arbitrary distant illumination conditions can be approximated accurately using low-dimensional linear subspace based on spherical harmonics. This has also been validated for near illumination conditions [20]. Since then, SH was incorporated in SFS framework to tackle the problem of illumination [21–23, 12].

3   Contributions

In this paper, we propose to investigate the SSFS approach on the human jaw where face and jaw modeling carry similarities and differences. Facial images can be easily obtained and databases of various imaging conditions are already in place, along with a significant body of algorithmic development. Human faces are easy to annotate and automate the process of face cropping and feature extraction. On the other hand, the human jaw is not a friendly environment to image, as indicated before, while no databases exist to carry out a SSFS methodology.

Fig. 1 illustrates the SSFS problem for reconstruction of the human jaw using a series of textures and shapes (obtained from CT scans of molds) for a group of subjects. The process starts with annotating the jaw at the known anatomical landmarks, in order to co-register the shapes and textures needed to construct the corresponding models. We use spherical harmonics to provide the optimal basis for illumination representation, and the partial least square (PLS) approach to carry out the estimation of dense 3D shapes. Key requirements for successful SSFS are the availability of a comprehensive database that describe the teeth/jaw variability per age, gender and ethnic factors. Our work aims to undertake such a task and make the databases available for researchers worldwide.

Vis-à-vis dental applications, the results demonstrate a significant increase in accuracy in favor of the proposed approach. In particular, our approach is able to recover geometrical details of tooth occlusal surface as well as mouth floor and ceiling as compared to shape-from-shading based approaches.

4   Proposed Definition of Anatomical Jaw Landmarks

4.1   Landmarks Definition

In this work, we mainly focus on the reconstruction of the *clinical crowns* which are defined to be the portion of the teeth that is visible in the mouth. As such, we limit the jaw's anatomical landmarks to such a space as follows according to their location, i.e. on the tooth surface or on the interface between the tooth and the gum. Typically a landmark represents a distinguishable point which is present in most of the images under consideration, for example, the location of central grooves of each tooth. Fig. 2 illustrates the location of 72 landmark points for a fourteen-teeth jaw.

In case of posterior teeth (i.e. cuspids, premolars and molars) which are responsible for chewing food, we are interested in the coalescence of the crown lobes. In particular, a *central pit or groove* can be considered as a landmark which is the deepest portion of a tooth fossa. While anterior teeth (i.e. incisors) whose job is to rip food apart is identifiable by a convex elevation of the crown surface which forms the biting edge. Hence we consider the midpoint of the *incisal edge or ridge* as a landmark for an anterior tooth.

The fibrous tissue covering the alveolar bone and surrounds the necks of the teeth, i.e. the gum, forms what is denoted as *gingival line*. This line marks the level of termination of the non-attached soft tissue surrounding the tooth. It separates the clinical crown and the root. We define the *gingival line midpoint* to be the minimum or maximum point on the gingival line formed by a single tooth. On the other hand, *gingival embrasure* is the respective point in the open space between the proximal surfaces of two adjacent teeth in the same dental arch.

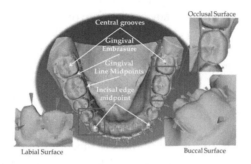

Fig. 2. Illustration of the proposed human jaw anatomical landmarks

4.2   Landmark Localization in Optical Images

In the online stage of our approach, a single image of the visible crowns is given from which the defined landmarks should be identified. This guides the alignment of the input image to the prior model, e.g. [24]. Hence, it is essential to automate the detection of such landmarks. In the training set, we manually annotate an ensemble of human jaws surfaces (based on CT-scanning of molds) in order to construct a sparse version of the jaw shape. These landmarks serve as a correspondence operator between individual training samples where we use the generalized Procrustes analysis [25] to filter out translation, scale and rotation. We deployed the Active Shape Model (ASM) by Cootes [26] to search for the landmarks in the given image. The ASM repeats the following two steps until convergence: (i) suggest a tentative shape by adjusting the locations of shape points by template matching of the image texture around each point (ii) conform the tentative shape to a global shape model. The individual template matches are unreliable and the shape model pools the results of the weak template matchers to form a stronger overall classifier. The entire search is repeated at each level in an image pyramid, from coarse to fine resolution. The initialization of the mean shape onto the given image is accomplished by segmenting the teeth region based on fitting a Gaussian mixture to the image intensity with two dominant classes; jaw and background.

5   Illumination-Invariant Statistical Shape from Shading

When the light source and the viewer are far from the object, the image intensity I at a pixel $\mathbf{x}$ can be obtained from the image irradiance of the corresponding surface point, which is defined as the surface radiance being modulated by the surface texture $a(\mathbf{x})$, i.e. $I(\mathbf{x}) = a(\mathbf{x})\mathcal{R}(n(\mathbf{x}))$. The classical brightness constraint in SFS measures the total brightness of the reconstructed image compared to the input image, it can be defined as;

$$\epsilon = \int \int \left(I(\mathbf{x}) - a(\mathbf{x})\mathcal{R}(n(\mathbf{x})) \right)^2 d\mathbf{x} \tag{1}$$

where $a(.)$ is the surface texture at point $\mathbf{x}$ while $\mathcal{R}(.)$ is the radiance of the surface patch with unit normal $n(\mathbf{x})$, also known as surface reflectance function.

The brightness constraint in (1) can be rewritten in the discrete domain as a linear combination of harmonic basis images resulted from the 2nd order SH approximation to the reflectance function [19]. Thus the image intensity I can be expressed as; $I(\mathbf{x}) = \sum_{i=0}^{n-1} \alpha_i b_i(\mathbf{x})$ where $b_i(\mathbf{x}) = f_i(a(\mathbf{x}), \mathbf{n}(\mathbf{x}))$ are the harmonic basis images which are functions of surface texture $a(\mathbf{x})$ and surface normals $\mathbf{n}(\mathbf{x})$ at pixel $\mathbf{x}$ (refer to [19] for their definition). The coefficient α_i denotes the ith coefficient in the illumination spectrum being modulated by the Lambertian kernel spectrum.

In matrix notation, let $I \in \mathbb{R}^{d \times 1}$ be an image vector with d pixels, $\mathbf{B} = [b_0(\mathbf{x}), ..., b_{n-1}(\mathbf{x})] \in \mathbb{R}^{d \times n}$ be the matrix of harmonic basis images as its columns, where n is the number of basis images, typically $n = 9$, and $\alpha \in \mathbb{R}^{n \times 1}$ vector of SH coefficients[1]. Hence the discrete version of the brightness constraint becomes,

$$\epsilon = \sum_{\mathbf{x}} \left(I(\mathbf{x}) - \mathbf{B}(\mathbf{x})\alpha \right)^2 = \| I - \mathbf{B}\alpha \| \tag{2}$$

Representing the surface reflectance function in terms of SH allow us to infer the illumination of a given image; given an input image I, the harmonic basis images $\mathbf{B}$ of a 3D object (a human jaw in particular), defined by its shape $\mathbf{s} = [\mathbf{n}(\mathbf{x}_0), ..., \mathbf{n}(\mathbf{x}_{d-1})]^T$ and texture $\mathbf{a} = [a(\mathbf{x}_0), ..., a(\mathbf{x}_{d-1})]^T)$, are obtained to deduce the coefficients $\widehat{\alpha}$ that best matches the input image. This results in an over-determined linear system of equations $I = \mathbf{B}\alpha$ which can be solved for $\widehat{\alpha}$ using singular value decomposition (SVD).

If the input image and the basis images used to compute the coefficients $\widehat{\alpha}$ belong to the same object, we can reconstruct the input image from these coefficients, i.e. $h = \mathbf{B}\widehat{\ell} = I$, where h denotes what we call *harmonics projection* (HP) image. However in the general case, the basis images $\mathbf{B}$ would belong to an object which is different from the one in the input image I, nonetheless they belong to the same object class e.g. different realizations of a human jaw. Thus the reconstructed image h provide a mean of encoding the illumination of the input image while maintaining the identity of the object whose basis images are used in the reconstruction process.

While (1) can be solved in an iterative manner to infer the underlying shape as in [22], the inherit relation between the HP images h and the corresponding shape s can be cast

---

[1] Since the information of this harmonic expansion mainly lies in the analytic form of the SH basis, we denote its coefficients as SH coefficients.

into a regression framework resulting into the HP-to-shape model. In this case, the shape is solved for using a series of matrix operations guaranteeing faster shape recovery when compared to its iterative counterpart. This was proven to yield comparable results in terms of reconstruction accuracy [12].

Dimensionality reduction is performed using PCA to construct 3D shape model (offline step) and HP model (online step) where the coefficients are used to build the regression model rather than the original shape and HP instances. In particular, the 3D shape model can be constructed by performing PCA on a set of aligned samples of 3D shapes, the resulting shape model is $s = \bar{s} + \mathbf{P_s b_s}$ where $\bar{s}$ is the mean shape, $\mathbf{P_s}$ are the shape eigenvectors and $\mathbf{b_s}$ is the set of shape coefficients. On the other hand, the HP model is trained online which incorporate the illumination conditions of the input image; given an image I and the basis images $\mathbf{B}_k$ of object instance k, the HP image h_k is obtained, where $h_k = \mathbf{B}_k \widehat{\alpha}_k$ with $\widehat{\alpha}_k$ obtained by solving the linear system of equations $I = \mathbf{B}_k \alpha_k$. After reconstructing the projection images of all the instances in the jaw database, we can model the HP images using PCA as $h = \bar{h} + \mathbf{P_h b_h}$ where $\bar{h}$ is the mean HP image, $\mathbf{P_h}$ are the HP images eigenvectors and $\mathbf{b_h}$ is the set of HP coefficients. Thus, instead of using the high dimensional vectors s_k and h_k into the regression, they are replaced by their respective coefficients $\mathbf{b}_{sk}$ and $\mathbf{b}_{hk}$, where the HP coefficients are considered the independent variable while the shape coefficients are the dependent variables. We use partial least squares regression (PLS) instead of the classical least squares to avoid random noise which might exist in the dependent and independent variables. Fig. 1 shows a block diagram of the offline/online processes for the proposed shape recovery approach.

6 Experimental Results

In this section, we show experiments to evaluate the performance of the proposed framework in recovery 3D models for human jaws. Upper and lower jaw models are constructed from eight young-aged subjects using their oral cavity images and the CT-scan of their respective molds. There are two samples per subject, one pre-repair jaw and another post-repair jaw. The original 3D scans are converted into a Monge patch format which represents the surface as $(x, y, f(x, y))$. We use a landmark-based approach to establish the dense correspondence between database samples, where a set of sparse anatomical landmark points are manually annotated (refer to Fig. 1 for their illustration). Generalized Procrustes Analysis (GPA) is first performed to align the set of shapes to a common reference frame. The average of the aligned shapes define the reference shape which is crucial in establishing dense correspondence between the jaw samples, see Fig. 1. Each pixel within the convex hull of the reference shape corresponds to a certain point on each jaw sample scan through a physically motivated thin-plate splines warping function.

To evaluate the proposed approach, out-of-training jaw samples are reconstructed and compared against the ground truth CT-scan. Four types of samples are considered: (a) pre-repair and (b) post-repair lower jaw, (c) pre-repair and (d) post-repair upper jaw.

Fig. 3(c) shows a sample reconstruction of a human jaw based on the proposed approach. Notice that it is close to its ground truth shape, as illustrated in Fig. 3(b).

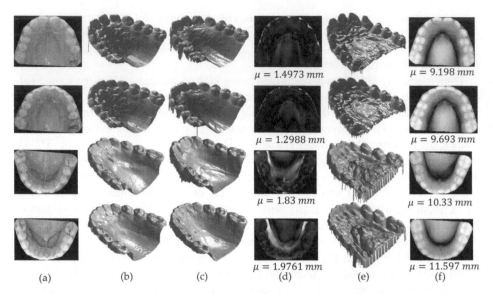

$\mu = 1.4973\ mm$ $\mu = 9.198\ mm$

$\mu = 1.2988\ mm$ $\mu = 9.693\ mm$

$\mu = 1.83\ mm$ $\mu = 10.33\ mm$

$\mu = 1.9761\ mm$ $\mu = 11.597\ mm$

(a)   (b)   (c)   (d)   (e)   (f)

Fig. 3. Sample reconstruction result of a single subject: (first row) upper, pre-repair jaw, (second row) upper, post-repair jaw, (third row) lower, pre-repair jaw, and (fourth row) lower, post-repair jaw. (a) Input image being masked using the convex hull of the jaw landmarks. (b) Ground truth shape from the CT-scanner. (c) Reconstructed shape based on our approach. (d) root-mean-squared error map with average error shown in mm. (e) Reconstructed shape based on SFS of [9]. (f) root-mean-squared error map of (e) with average error shown in mm.

While Fig. 3(e) shows inaccurate reconstructions based on SFS of [9] which was recently proposed for jaw shape recovery. This emphasizes the role of incorporating prior-information for shape recovery as well as illumination modeling.

Table 1 reports the root-mean-square error in mm between the 3D points from the CT scan and the corresponding reconstructed surface points. Notice that the error values are minimal when compared to SFS-based reconstruction. Post-repair error values are also smaller than pre-repair values in most of the samples, indicating that it is more difficult to reconstruct human jaws with irregular tooth shapes and locations. One can observe higher errors in case of SFS for the lower jaw when compared to the upper one where there is no occlusion due to the tongue.

A natural question to be asked is how to make use of SFS results and SSFS? Of course, SFS is based on the visible surface of the jaw; at best the crown would be

Table 1. Average surface reconstruction accuracy (RMS) in mm

Jaw type	SSFS	SFS
Upper, pre-repair	2.08999	8.80572
Upper, post-repair	2.02334	8.96832
Lower, pre-repair	3.11911	10.02804
Lower, post-repair	2.57112	11.42853

possibly constructed, while SSFS constructs the entire jaw. On the other hand, SFS provides the object-specific constructions. A logical thing would be to enhance the SSFS with SFS, by morphing the upper part of the model with the crown portion generated from SFS. With a good database of objects, credible SSFS models would be possible, which when morphed to the crown reconstructions would produce a more realistic jaw.

7 Conclusion and Future Work

In this paper, we presented an affordable, flexible, automatic dental tool for the reconstruction of the clinically visible part of the human jaw. It was based on a single captured optical image and a statistical shape recovery approach which makes use of a small number of measured points to construct a plausible 3D model through a learned correspondence based on a measured human jaw dataset. We expressed the surface reflectance function in terms of spherical harmonics to provide the optimal basis for illumination representation. The brightness constraint was then cast as a Partial Least Squares (PLS) regression problem, which allows for the rapid computation of the solution. The PLS algorithm is composed of a sequence of matrix operations; the approach in this work can recover 3D shapes much faster than its iterative counterpart, without compromising the integrity of the results. The results demonstrated the effect of adding statistical prior as well as illumination modeling on the accuracy of the recovered shape. The next step is to investigate the fusion of SFS and SSFS where SFS provides the object-specific constructions while SSFS is perform shape recovery based on partial information. This will lend benefits to tasks such as teeth restoration in dental applications.

References

1. Goshtasby, A.A., Nambala, S., de Rijk, W.G., Campbell, S.D.: A system for digital reconstruction of gypsum dental casts. IEEE Transactions on Medical Imaging 16, 664–674 (1997)
2. European Commission, European guidelines on radiation protection in dental radiology. Radiation Protection Issue number 136 (2004)
3. Maillie, H.D., Gilda, J.E.: Radiation-induced cancer risk in radiographic cephalometry. Oral Surg. Oral Med. Oral Pathol. 75, 631–637 (1993)
4. Horn-Ross, P.L., Ljung, B.M., Morrow, M.: Environmental factors and the risk of salivary gland cancer. Epidemiology 8, 414–419 (1997)
5. Hallquis, A., Hardell, L., Degerman, A., Wingren, G., Boquist, L.: Medical diagnostic and therapeutic ionizing radiation and the risk for thyroid cancer: a case-control study. Eur. J. Cancer Prevention 3, 259–267 (1994)
6. Wilson, K., Sun, N., Huang, M., Zhang, W., Lee, A., Li, A., Wang, S., Wu, J.: Effects of ionizing radiation on self renewal and pluripotency of human embryonic stem cells. Cancer Res. 70(13), 5539–5548 (2010)
7. European Commission, Low dose ionizing radiation and cancer risk. Radiation Protection Issue number 125 (2001)
8. Yamany, S.M., Farag, A.A., Tasman, D., Farman, A.G.: A 3-d reconstruction system for the human jaw using a sequence of optical images. IEEE Transactions on Medical Imaging 19, 538–547 (2000)

9. Abdelrahim, A.S., Abdelrahman, M.A., Abdelmunim, H., Farag, A., Miller, M.: Novel image-based 3d reconstruction of the human jaw using shape from shading and feature descriptors. In: Proceedings of the British Machine Vision Conference, pp. 41.1–41.11. BMVA Press (2011)

10. Prados, E., Faugeras, O., Camilli, F.: Shape from shading: a well-posed problem? RR 5297, INRIA Research (August 2004)

11. Smith, W.A.P., Hancock, E.R.: Recovering facial shape using a statistical model of surface normal direction. IEEE Trans. on Pattern Analysis and Machine Intelligence 28

12. Rara, H., Elhabian, S., Starr, T., Farag, A.: 3d face recovery from intensities of general and unknown lighting using partial least squares. In: 17th IEEE International Conference on Image Processing (ICIP 2010) (September 2010)

13. Atick, J.J., Griffin, P.A., Norman Redlich, A.: Statistical approach to shape from shading: Reconstruction of three-dimensional face surfaces from single two-dimensional images. Neural Comput. 8(6), 1321–1340 (1996)

14. Zhao, W.Y., Chellappa, R.: Symmetric shape-from-shading using self-ratio image. Int. J. Comput. Vision 45(1), 55–75 (2001)

15. Dovgard, R., Basri, R.: Statistical Symmetric Shape from Shading for 3D Structure Recovery of Faces. In: Pajdla, T., Matas, J(G.) (eds.) ECCV 2004. LNCS, vol. 3022, pp. 99–113. Springer, Heidelberg (2004)

16. Cootes, T.F., Edwards, G.J., Taylor, C.J.: Active appearance models. IEEE Transactions on Pattern Analysis and Machine Intelligence 23, 681–685 (2001)

17. Castelan, M., Smith, W., Hancock, E.: A coupled statistical model for face shape recovery from brightness images. IEEE Transaction on Image Processing 16, 1139–1151 (2007)

18. Blanz, V., Vetter, T.: Face recognition based on fitting a 3d morphable model. IEEE Trans. Pattern Anal. Mach. Intell. 25(9), 1063–1074 (2003)

19. Basri, R., Jacobs, D.W.: Lambertian reflectance and linear subspaces. IEEE Transactions on Pattern Analysis and Machine Intelligence 25(2), 218–233 (2003)

20. Frolova, D., Simakov, D., Basri, R.: Accuracy of Spherical Harmonic Approximations for Images of Lambertian Objects under Far and Near Lighting. In: Pajdla, T., Matas, J(G.) (eds.) ECCV 2004. LNCS, vol. 3021, pp. 574–587. Springer, Heidelberg (2004)

21. Ahmed, A., Farag, A.A.: A New Statistical Model Combining Shape and Spherical Harmonics Illumination for Face Reconstruction. In: Bebis, G., Boyle, R., Parvin, B., Koracin, D., Paragios, N., Tanveer, S.-M., Ju, T., Liu, Z., Coquillart, S., Cruz-Neira, C., Müller, T., Malzbender, T. (eds.) ISVC 2007, Part I. LNCS, vol. 4841, pp. 531–541. Springer, Heidelberg (2007)

22. Rara, H., Elhabian, S., Starr, T., Farag, A.: Model-based shape recovery from single images of general and unknown lighting. In: 16th IEEE International Conference on Image Processing (ICIP 2009), November 7-10, pp. 517–520 (2009)

23. Castelan, M., Van Horebeek, J.: Relating intensities with three-dimensional facial shape using partial least squares. Computer Vision, IET 3, 60–73 (2009)

24. Blanz, V., Mehl, A., Vetter, T., Seidel, H.P.: A statistical method for robust 3d surface reconstruction from sparse data. In: Int. Symp. on 3D Data Processing, Visualization and Transmission, pp. 293–300 (2004)

25. Gower, J.C.: Generalized procrustes analysis. Psychometrika 40(1), 33–51 (1975)

26. Taylor, C.J., Cootes, T.F.: Technical report: Statistical models of appearance for computer vision, The University of Manchester School of Medicine (2004), www.isbe.man.ac.uk/bim/refs.html

Brain Tumor Cell Density Estimation from Multi-modal MR Images Based on a Synthetic Tumor Growth Model

Ezequiel Geremia[1], Bjoern H. Menze[1,2,3], Marcel Prastawa[4], M.-A. Weber[5], Antonio Criminisi[6], and Nicholas Ayache[1]

[1] Asclepios Research Project, INRIA Sophia-Antipolis, France
[2] Computer Science and Artificial Intelligence Laboratory, MIT, USA
[3] Computer Vision Laboratory, ETH Zurich, Switzerland
[4] Scientific Computing and Imaging Institute, University of Utah, USA
[5] Diagnostic and Interventional Radiology, Heidelberg University Hospital, Germany
[6] Machine Learning and Perception Group, Microsoft Research Cambridge, UK

Abstract. This paper proposes to employ a detailed tumor growth model to synthesize labelled images which can then be used to train an efficient data-driven machine learning tumor predictor. Our MR image synthesis step generates images with both healthy tissues as well as various tumoral tissue types. Subsequently, a discriminative algorithm based on random regression forests is trained on the simulated ground truth to predict the continuous latent tumor cell density, and the discrete tissue class associated with each voxel. The presented method makes use of a large synthetic dataset of 740 simulated cases for training and evaluation. A quantitative evaluation on 14 real clinical cases diagnosed with low-grade gliomas demonstrates tissue class accuracy comparable with state of the art, with added benefit in terms of computational efficiency and the ability to estimate tumor cell density as a latent variable underlying the multimodal image observations. The idea of synthesizing training data to train data-driven learning algorithms can be extended to other applications where expert annotation is lacking or expensive.

1 Introduction

Brain tumors are complex patho-physiological processes representing a series of pathological changes to brain tissue [1]. Increasing effort is invested in modelling the underlying biological processes involved in brain tumor growth [2, 3]. As brain tumors show a large variety of different appearances in multi-modal clinical images, the accurate diagnosis and analysis of these images remains a significant challenge. We show in the example of gliomas, the most frequent brain tumor [4], how a *generative* patho-physiological model of tumor growth can be used in conjunction with a *discriminative* tumor recognition algorithm, based on random regression forests. Applied to real data the random forest is capable of predicting the precise location of the tumor and its substructures.

B.H. Menze et al. (Eds.): MCV 2012, LNCS 7766, pp. 273–282, 2013.

In addition, our model can also infer the spatial distribution of (unobservable) latent physiological features such as tumor cell densities, thus avoiding the need for expensive patho-physiological model inversion [5].

Generative probabilistic segmentation models of spatial tissue distribution and appearance proved to generalize well to previously unseen images [6–9]. In [6], tumors are modeled as outliers relative to the expected appearance of healthy tissue following a related approach for MS lesion detection [10]. Other methods [7, 8] provide explicit models for the tumor class. For instance, [8] builds a tumor appearance model for channel specific segmentation of the tumor, combining a tissue appearance model with a latent tumor class prior from [9]. Tumor growth models (*e.g.* reaction-diffusion models) have been used repeatedly to improve image registration [11] and, hence, atlas-based tissue segmentation [12]. Similarly, [13] relies on a bio-mechanical tumor growth model to estimate brain tissue loss and displacement. Generative approaches require a detailed formal description of the image generation process and may need considerable modifications when applied to slightly different tasks. These approaches also tend to be computationally inefficient.

In contrast, discriminative techniques focus on modeling the difference between *e.g.* a lesion and healthy tissues, directly [14–16]. A number of recent techniques based on decision tree ensembles have shown strong generalization capabilities and computational efficiency, even when applied to large data sets [17–19]. In [20], for example, a *classification* forest is used for segmenting multiple sclerosis lesions using long-range spatial features. In [15], the authors derived a constrained minimization problem suitable for min-cut optimization that incorporates an observation model provided by a discriminative Probabilistic Boosting Trees classifier into the process of segmentation. For multi-modal brain lesion segmentation, [16] propose a hierarchical segmentation framework by weighted aggregation with generic local image features. Unfortunately, fully supervised discriminative approaches may require large expert-annotated training sets. Obtaining such data is often prohibitive in many clinical applications.

This paper proposes a new way of combining the best of the generative and discriminative world. We use a generative model of glioma [21] to synthesize a large set of heterogeneous MR images complete with their ground truth annotations. Such images are then used to train a multi-variate *regression* forest tumor predictor [20, 22]. Thus given a previously unseen image the forest can perform an efficient, per-voxel estimation of both tumor infiltration density *and* tissue type. The general idea of training a discriminative predictor (a classifier or a regressor) on a large collection of synthetic training data is inspired by the recent success of the Microsoft Kinect for XBox 360 system [23]. This approach has great potential in different domains and especially for medical applications where obtaining extensive expert-labelled is nearly impossible.

2   Learning to Estimate Tissue Cell Density from Synthetic Training Data

This section describes the two basic steps of our algorithm: i) synthesizing heterogeneous MR images showing tumors, and ii) training a tumor detector which works on *real* patient images.

2.1   Generative Tumor Simulation Model

The automatic generation of our synthetic training dataset relies on the publicly available brain tumor simulator presented in [21]. It builds on an anisotropic glioma growth model [24] with extensions to model the induced mass-effect and the accumulation of the contrast agents in both blood vessels and active tumor regions. Then, multi-sequence MR images are synthesized using characteristic image textures for healthy and pathological tissue classes.

We generate synthetic pathological cases with varying tumor location, tumor count, levels of tumor expansion and extent of edema. The resulting synthetic cases successfully reproduce mass-effect, contrast enhancement and infiltration patterns similar to what observed in the real cases. The synthetic dataset contains 740 synthetic cases. It includes a large variability of brain tumors ranging from very diffusive tumors, showing a large edema-infiltration pattern without necrotic core, to bulky tumors with a large necrotic core surrounded by an enhanced vascularization pattern. For each case, the simulation provides four MR sequences (cf. Fig. 1) which offer different views of the same underlying tumor density distribution.

This synthetic ground truth provides a diverse view of the pathological process including mass-effect and infiltration, but also very detailed annotations for the healthy structures of the brain. The ground truth consists of voxel-wise annotations on the data that are: white matter (WM), gray matter (GM), cerebrospinal fluid (CSF), edema, necrotic tumor core, active tumor rim and blood vessels. Unlike binary annotations which provide a mask for each tissue class, the ground truth consists of a continuous scalar map for each tissue class. Each scalar map provides, for every voxel in the volume, the density of every tissue class.

2.2   Regression Forests for Estimating Tissue Cell Density

Problem setting. We adapt a regression forests similar to the one of [17] to train an estimator of tissue cell densities from visual cues in the multi-channel MR images. For each voxel $\mathbf{v}$, the ground truth provides the density $R_c(\mathbf{v}) \in [0,1]$ of each tissue class $c \in \mathcal{C}$. The density distribution R is normalized so that it satisfies $\sum_{c \in \mathcal{C}} R_c(\mathbf{v}) = 1$ in every voxel $\mathbf{v}$.

T1   T1+Gad   T2   FLAIR

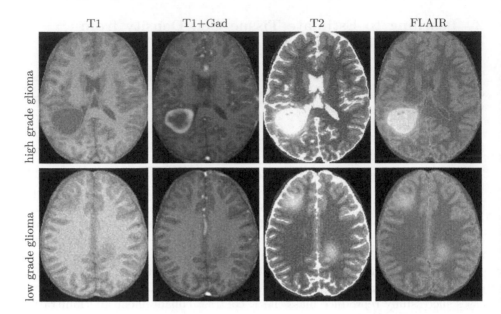

Fig. 1. Synthetic MR images. From left to right: T1, T1+Gad, T2, and FLAIR MR images. Top row: bulky tumor characterized by a large necrotic and a surrounding vascularization pattern. Bottom row: very infiltrating tumor characterized by the extended of the edema.

Feature representation. To calculate the local image features – both during training and for predictions – we sub-sample or interpolate all images to $1 \times 1 \times 2$ mm^3 resolution. We perform a skull-stripping and an intensity normalization [25] so that real MR images match the intensity distribution of synthetic MR sequences. Then image features are calculated for each voxel $\mathbf{v}$. Features include local multi-channel intensity (T1, T1+Gad, T2, Flair) as well as long-range displaced box features such as in [20]. In addition we also incorporate symmetry features, calculated after estimating the mid-sagittal plane [26]. In total, every voxel is associated with a $213-$long vector of feature responses.

Regression forest training. The forest consists of T trees indexed by t. During training observations of all voxels $\mathbf{v}$ are pushed through each of the trees. Each internal node p applies a binary test $t_p = \tau_{low} \le \theta(\mathbf{v}) < \tau_{up}$ implementing a double thresholding (τ_{low}, τ_{up}) of the visual feature $\theta(\mathbf{v})$ evaluated at voxel $\mathbf{v}$. The voxel $\mathbf{v}$ is then sent to one of the two child nodes based on the outcome of this test. As a result, each node p receives a partition of the input training data $\mathcal{T}_p = \{\mathbf{v}, R(\mathbf{v})\}_p$, composed of a voxel $\mathbf{v}$ and a vector $R(\mathbf{v}) \in [0,1]^{|C|}$ storing the cell density value for each tissue class. We model the resulting distribution via a multi-variate Gaussian $\mathcal{N}_p(\mu_p, \Gamma_p)$ where μ_p and Γ_p are the mean and covariance matrix of all $R(\mathbf{v}) \in \mathcal{T}_p$, respectively. During training, the parameters (τ_{low}, τ_{up}) of the node test function and the employed visual feature θ are optimized to maximize the information gain. We define the information gain $IG(t_p)$ to measure the quality of the test function t_p which splits $\mathcal{T}_p$ into $\mathcal{T}_p^{left}$ and $\mathcal{T}_p^{right}$. The information gain is defined as $IG(t_p) = -\sum_{k \in \{left, right\}} \omega_k log \rho_k$ with $\omega = |\mathcal{T}_p^k|/|\mathcal{T}_p|$ and $\rho_k = max|eig(\Gamma_k)|$ where eig denotes all matrix eigenvalues. In contrast to the more conventional information gain used in [17], our formulation gives a robust estimate of the dispersion. Indeed, the information gain presented in [17] models the dispersions as $|\Gamma_k|$ which evaluates to 0 in the case a tissue class is missing from the input partition $\mathcal{T}_p$. Our definition of the information gain focuses on the direction showing maximum dispersion, i.e. ρ_k, and ignores the missing information on tissue classes.

At each node p, the optimal test $t_p^* = \arg\max_\Lambda IG(t_p)$ is found by exhaustive search over a random subset of the feature space $\Lambda = \{\tau_{low}, \tau_{up}, \theta\}$. Maximizing the information gain encourages minimizing ρ_p, thus decreasing the prediction error when approximating $\mathcal{T}_p$ with $\mathcal{N}_p$. The trees are grown to a maximum depth D, as long as $|\mathcal{T}_p| > 100$.

After training, the random forest embeds a hierarchical piece-wise Gaussian model which captures the multi-modality of the training data. In fact, each leaf node l_t of every tree t stores the Gaussian distribution $\mathcal{N}_{l_t}$ associated with the partition of the training data arrived at that leaf $\mathcal{T}_{l_t}$.

The employed random regression forest approximates the multi-variate distribution R by a piece-wise Gaussian distribution $\hat{R}$.

Regression forest prediction. When applied to a previously unseen test volume $\mathcal{T}_{test} = \{\mathbf{v}\}$, each voxel $\mathbf{v}$ is propagated through all the trained trees by successive application of the relevant binary tests. When reaching the leaf node l_t in all trees $t \in [1..T]$, estimated cell densities $r_t(\mathbf{v}) = \mu_{l_t}$ are averaged together to compute the forest tissue cell density estimation $r(\mathbf{v}) = (\sum_{t \in [1..T]} r_t(\mathbf{v}))/T$. Note that in each leaf l_t we maintain an estimate of the confidence Γ_{l_t} associated to the cell density estimation μ_{l_t}.

3   Experiments

We conducted two main experiments. First, as a proof of concept, we tested how well the learned forest reproduces the tissue cell densities in the synthetic model. In a second experiment we applied our method to real, previously unseen, clinical images and measured accuracy by comparing the detected and ground truth tumor outlines.

We evaluate the predictions for every test case using two complementary metrics: a segmentation metric and a robust regression metric. The segmentation metric compares binary versions of the physiological maps, independently normalized for each tissue class. The binary masks are obtained by thresholding the prediction and the ground truth at the same value. Then, we evaluate the true postive rate $TPR = TP/(TP + FN)$, the false positive rate $FPR = TP/(TP + FP)$ and the positive predictive value $PPV = TP/(TP + FP)$, where

TP, FP, and FN are the number of true positives, false positives, and false negatives, respectively. Finally, we compute the area under the ROC and the one precision-recall curves to measure how well the prediction fits the ground truth.

The robust regression metric evaluates the estimation error between the predicted continuous map and the ground truth. For every tissue class c, we compute the mean over the voxels v of the estimation error, defined as $E_c(v) = |R_c(v) - r_c(v)|$. In order to avoid artificial decrease of the mean error, we make this metric robust by only considering regions of the physiological map showing at least 10% signal in either the prediction or the ground truth.

In both experiments, we used the same forest containing $T = 160$ trees of depth $D = 20$ trained on 500 synthetic cases. The values of these meta-parameters were tuned by training and testing on a different synthetic set.

3.1   Experiment 1: Estimating Cell Density in Synthetic Cases

We tested the random forest on a previously unseen synthetic dataset with 240 cases. Results (Fig. 2) show a good qualitative match between predicted and ground truth physiological maps. As a segmentation metric we calculate the true and false positive rates as well as the positive predictive value for each possible

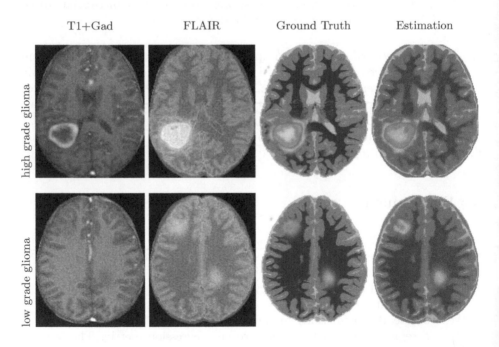

Fig. 2. Estimation of tissue cell densities. From left to right: T1+Gadolinium, FLAIR image, the ground truth provided by the simulator, the estimation of our random regression forest. Each voxel of the ground truth maps displays the mixed density between predefined tissue classes: WM (dark blue), GM (light blue), CSF (cyan), edema (green), blood vessels (orange), and necrotic core (yellow).

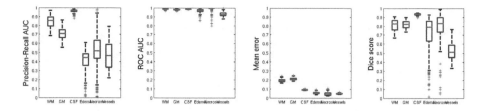

Fig. 3. Evaluation of the predictions on the synthetic dataset for each cell density map. Each label in the x-axis represents a tissue class: WM, GM, CSF, edema, necrotic core, blood vessels, respectively. We show from left to right: the area under the precision-recall curve, the area under the ROC curve, the estimation of the mean prediction error, and the dice score Each point of the ROC and precision-recall curves is built by thresholding the prediction and the ground truth at the same value. The ground truth and the prediction density maps were thresholded at the same value, i.e. 0.3.

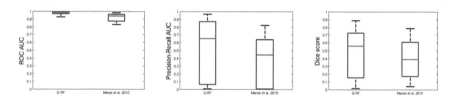

Fig. 4. Evaluation of the predictions on the clinical dataset. Box plots of the area under the ROC curve (left), under the precision-recall curve (right), and the dice score. Comparison of the proposed method (G-RF) with the method presented in [8].

threshold jointly on r and R and summarize it through ROC and precision-recall curves. For every tissue class c, we also compute the mean approximation error, defined as $E_c(v) = |R_c(v) - r_c(v)|$ (integrating over voxels with $> .001$ tumor cell density for tumor classes). Results in Fig. 3 show excellent results for WM, GM, CSF. The predicted tumor cell density is in good agreement with ground truth. A systematic bias leads to a slightly larger variance in the error metric due to the small size of the tumor classes compared to the healthy tissue classes.

3.2 Experiment 2: Segmenting Tumors in Clinical Images

We tested the same random forest on 14 clinical cases showing low and high grade glioma (Fig. 5) with T1, T1+Gad, T2 and FLAIR images. None of the clinical cases was used during training. Training was done exclusively on synthetic images. The manually-obtained ground truth consists of a binary tumor mask delineating the tumor+edema region. We calculated the same tumor outline from the predicted continuous physiological masks as done for the synthetic model [21]. Segmentation results (Fig. 4) are in excellent agreement with a

280   E. Geremia et al.

FLAIR   Expert Segmentation   Tumor cell density   Predicted Segmentation

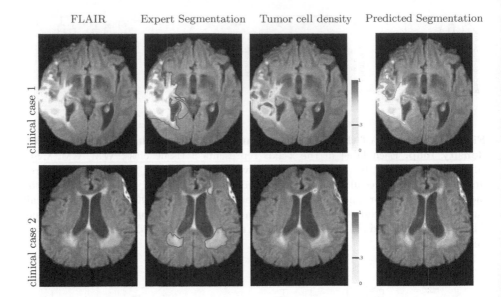

Fig. 5. Segmentation and tumor cell distribution. From left to right: preprocessed Flair MR image, FLAIR MR image overlayed with the segmentation of an
expert, the normalized tumor cell density, and the predicted tumor segmentation
(threshold at 0.3).

state-of-the-art unsupervised multimodal brain tumor segmentation method that
also outperformed standard EM segmentation in an earlier study [8]. Note that
the method presented in [8] significantly outperformed [6]. Interestingly, in a
qualitative evaluation (cf. Fig. 5), the tumor cell density map shows smooth
transition between the active rim of the tumor (red) and the edema (green).

4   Conclusions

This paper presented a new generative-discriminative algorithm for the automatic detection of glioma tumors in multi-modal MR brain images. A regression
forest model was trained on multiple synthetically-generated labelled images.
Then the system demonstrated to work accurately on previously unseen synthetic cases. It showed promising results on real patient images which led to
state of the art tumor segmentation results. Our algorithm can estimate continuous tissue cell densities both for healthy tissues (WM, GM, CSF) as well as
tumoral ones.

Acknowledgments. This work was partially funded by the ERC MedYMA
grant. We would like to thank Marc-André Weber from the Diagnostic and Interventional Radiology Group in Heidelberg University Hospital, Germany for
providing us with the clinical data.

References

1. Angelini, E.D., Delon, J., Bah, A.B., Capelle, L., Mandonnet, E.: Differential MRI analysis for quantification of low grade glioma growth. Medical Image Analysis 16, 114–126 (2012)
2. Cristini, V., Lowengrub, J.: Multiscale Modeling of Cancer: An Integrated Experimental and Mathematical Modeling Approach, pp. 185–205. Cambridge University Press (2010)
3. Deisboeck, T.S., Stamatakos, G.S.: Multiscale Cancer Modeling, pp. 359–406. CRC Press (2010)
4. Angelini, E.D., Clatz, O., Mandonnet, E., Konukoglu, E., Capelle, L., Duffau, H.: Glioma dynamics and computational models: A review of segmentation, registration, and in silico growth algorithms and their clinical applications. Cur. Med. Imag. Rev. 3, 262–276 (2007)
5. Menze, B.H., Van Leemput, K., Honkela, A., Konukoglu, E., Weber, M.-A., Ayache, N., Golland, P.: A Generative Approach for Image-Based Modeling of Tumor Growth. In: Székely, G., Hahn, H.K. (eds.) IPMI 2011. LNCS, vol. 6801, pp. 735–747. Springer, Heidelberg (2011)
6. Prastawa, M., Bullitt, E., Ho, S., Gerig, G.: A brain tumor segmentation framework based on outlier detection. Medical Image Analysis 8, 275–283 (2004)
7. Zou, K.H., Wells III, W.M., Kaus, M.R., Kikinis, R., Jolesz, F.A., Warfield, S.K.: Statistical Validation of Automated Probabilistic Segmentation against Composite Latent Expert Ground Truth in MR Imaging of Brain Tumors. In: Dohi, T., Kikinis, R. (eds.) MICCAI 2002, Part I. LNCS, vol. 2488, pp. 315–322. Springer, Heidelberg (2002)
8. Menze, B.H., van Leemput, K., Lashkari, D., Weber, M.-A., Ayache, N., Golland, P.: A Generative Model for Brain Tumor Segmentation in Multi-Modal Images. In: Jiang, T., Navab, N., Pluim, J.P.W., Viergever, M.A. (eds.) MICCAI 2010, Part II. LNCS, vol. 6362, pp. 151–159. Springer, Heidelberg (2010)
9. Riklin-Raviv, T., Leemput, K.V., Menze, B.H., Wells, W.M., Golland, P.: Segmentation of image ensembles via latent atlases. Medical Image Analysis 14, 654–665 (2010)
10. Leemput, K.V., Maes, F., Vandermeulen, D., Colchester, A.C.F., Suetens, P.: Automated segmentation of multiple sclerosis lesions by model outlier detection. IEEE Trans. Med. Imaging 20(8), 677–688 (2001)
11. Cabezas, M., Oliver, A., Lladó, X., Freixenet, J., Cuadra, M.B.: A review of atlas-based segmentation for magnetic resonance brain images. Comp. Meth. Prog. Biomed. 104, 158–164 (2011)
12. Gooya, A., Pohl, K.M., Bilello, M., Biros, G., Davatzikos, C.: Joint Segmentation and Deformable Registration of Brain Scans Guided by a Tumor Growth Model. In: Fichtinger, G., Martel, A., Peters, T. (eds.) MICCAI 2011, Part II. LNCS, vol. 6892, pp. 532–540. Springer, Heidelberg (2011)
13. Zacharaki, E.I., Hogea, C.S., Shen, D., Biros, G., Davatzikos, C.: Non-diffeomorphic registration of brain tumor images by simulating tissue loss and tumor growth. NeuroImage 46, 762–774 (2009)
14. Lee, C.-H., Wang, S., Murtha, A., Brown, M.R.G., Greiner, R.: Segmenting Brain Tumors Using Pseudo–Conditional Random Fields. In: Metaxas, D., Axel, L., Fichtinger, G., Székely, G. (eds.) MICCAI 2008, Part I. LNCS, vol. 5241, pp. 359–366. Springer, Heidelberg (2008)

15. Wels, M., Carneiro, G., Aplas, A., Huber, M., Hornegger, J., Comaniciu, D.: A Discriminative Model-Constrained Graph Cuts Approach to Fully Automated Pediatric Brain Tumor Segmentation in 3-D MRI. In: Metaxas, D., Axel, L., Fichtinger, G., Székely, G. (eds.) MICCAI 2008, Part I. LNCS, vol. 5241, pp. 67–75. Springer, Heidelberg (2008)

16. Corso, J.J., Sharon, E., Dube, S., El-Saden, S., Sinha, U., Yuille, A.L.: Efficient multilevel brain tumor segmentation with integrated bayesian model classification. IEEE Transactions on Medical Imaging 27, 629–640 (2008)

17. Criminisi, A., Shotton, J., Robertson, D., Konukoglu, E.: Regression Forests for Efficient Anatomy Detection and Localization in CT Studies. In: Menze, B., Langs, G., Tu, Z., Criminisi, A. (eds.) MICCAI 2010. LNCS, vol. 6533, pp. 106–117. Springer, Heidelberg (2011)

18. Montillo, A., Shotton, J., Winn, J., Iglesias, J.E., Metaxas, D., Criminisi, A.: Entangled Decision Forests and Their Application for Semantic Segmentation of CT Images. In: Székely, G., Hahn, H.K. (eds.) IPMI 2011. LNCS, vol. 6801, pp. 184–196. Springer, Heidelberg (2011)

19. Gray, K.R., Aljabar, P., Heckemann, R.A., Hammers, A., Rueckert, D.: Random Forest-Based Manifold Learning for Classification of Imaging Data in Dementia. In: Suzuki, K., Wang, F., Shen, D., Yan, P. (eds.) MLMI 2011. LNCS, vol. 7009, pp. 159–166. Springer, Heidelberg (2011)

20. Geremia, E., Clatz, O., Menze, B.H., Konukoglu, E., Criminisi, A., Ayache, N.: Spatial decision forests for ms lesion segmentation in multi-channel magnetic resonance images. NeuroImage 57, 378–390 (2011)

21. Prastawa, M., Bullitt, E., Gerig, G.: Simulation of brain tumors in MR images for evaluation of segmentation efficacy. Medical Image Analysis 13, 297–311 (2009)

22. Criminisi, A., Shotton, J., Konukoglu, E.: Decision forests for classification, regression, density estimation, manifold learning and semi-supervised learning. Technical report, Microsoft (2011)

23. Shotton, J., Fitzgibbon, A., Cook, M., Sharp, T., Finocchio, M., Moore, R., Kipman, A., Blake, A.: Real-time human pose recognition in parts from single depth images. In: Proc CVPR, pp. 1297–1304 (2011)

24. Clatz, O., Sermesant, M., Bondiau, P.Y., Delingette, H., Warfield, S.K., Malandain, G., Ayache, N.: Realistic simulation of the 3d growth of brain tumors in mr images coupling diffusion with mass effect. IEEE Transactions on Medical Imaging 24, 1334–1346 (2005)

25. Coltuc, D., Bolon, P., Chassery, J.M.: Exact histogram specification. IEEE TIP 15, 1143–1152 (2006)

26. Prima, S., Ourselin, S., Ayache, N.: Computation of the mid-sagittal plane in 3d brain images. IEEE Transactions on Medical Imaging 21, 122–138 (2002)

Current-Based 4D Shape Analysis
for the Mechanical Personalization of Heart Models

Loïc Le Folgoc[1], Hervé Delingette[1], Antonio Criminisi[2], and Nicholas Ayache[1]

[1] Asclepios Research Project, INRIA Sophia Antipolis, France
[2] Machine Learning and Perception Group, Microsoft Research Cambridge, UK

Abstract. Patient-specific models of the heart may lead to better understanding of cardiovascular diseases and better planning of therapy. A machine-learning approach to the personalization of an electro-mechanical model of the heart, from the kinematics of the endo- and epicardium, is presented in this paper. We use 4D mathematical currents to encapsulate information about the shape and deformation of the heart. The method is largely insensitive to initialization and does not require on-line simulation of the cardiac function. In this work, we demonstrate the performance of our approach for the joint estimation of three parameters on one heart geometry. We manage to retrieve parameters such that the model matches the 4D observations with an accuracy below the voxel size, in less than three minutes of computation.

Keywords: patient-specific heart model, mechanical personalization, currents, machine-learning.

1 Introduction

Patient-specific models may help better understand the role of biomechanical and electrophysiological factors in cardiovascular pathologies. They may also prove to be useful in predicting the outcome of potential therapeutic interventions for individual patients. In this paper we focus on the mechanical personalization of the Bestel-Clement-Sorine (BCS) model, as described in [2][4].

Model personalization aims at optimizing model parameters so that the behaviour of the personalized model matches the acquired patient-specific data (e.g. cine-MR images). Several approaches to the problem of cardiac model personalization have been suggested in the recent years, often formulating the inverse problem via the framework of variational data assimilation[6] or that of optimal filtering theory[14][13][3]. The output of these methods is dependent on the set of parameters used to initialize the algorithm; for this reason calibration procedures are introduced as a preprocessing stage, such as the one developed in [16]. Furthermore these approaches rely on on-line simulations, as an accurate estimation of the effect of parameter changes along several directions in the parameter space is required to drive the parameter estimation. Due to the complexity of the direct simulation these approaches are costly in time and computations.

In this paper, we explore a novel machine-learning approach, in which the need for initialization and on-line simulation is removed, by moving the analysis of the parameter effects on the kinematics of the model (and thus the bulk of the computations) to an

B.H. Menze et al. (Eds.): MCV 2012, LNCS 7766, pp. 283–292, 2013.

off-line learning phase. In this work we assume the tracking of the heart motion from images to be given (e.g. via [15]) and focus on the mechanical personalization of the cardiac function from meshes. Our work makes use of currents, a mathematical tool which was originally introduced to the medical imaging community in the context of shape registration[18][8] and offers a unified, correspondence-free statistical representation of geometrical objects. Our main contributions include the construction of 4D currents to represent, and perform statistics on $3D + t$ beating hearts and the proposal of a machine-learning framework to personalize electromechanical cardiac models.

The remaining of this article is organized as follows. In the first part we introduce the background on currents necessary to present the rest of our work. We develop our method in the following section, then present and discuss experimental results in the final sections.

2   Currents for Shape Representation

2.1   A Statistical Shape Representation Framework

Currents provide a unified representation of geometrical objects of any dimension, embedded in the Euclidean space $\mathbb{R}^n$, that is fit for statistical analysis. The framework of currents makes use of geometrically rich and well-behaved data spaces allowing for the proper definition of classical statistical concepts. Typically the existence of an inner product structure provides a straightforward way to define the mean and principal modes of a data set for instance, as in the Principal Component Analysis (PCA). These comments motivate an approach of currents from the perspective of kernel theory in this section, although currents are formally introduced in a more general way *via* the field of differential topology. The connection to differential topology is particularly relevant to outline the desirable properties of currents when dealing with discrete approximations of continuous shapes, in terms of convergence and consistence of the representation [7].

A well-known theorem due to Moore and Aronszajn[1] states that for any symmetric, positive definite (p.d.) kernel on a set $\mathcal{X}$, there exists a unique Hilbert space $\mathcal{H}_K \subset \mathbb{R}^{\mathcal{X}}$ for which K is a reproducing kernel. This result suggests a straightforward way of doing statistics on $\mathcal{X}$ as long as a p.d. kernel K can be engineered on this set, by mapping any point $x \in \mathcal{X}$ to a function $K(x, \cdot) \in \mathcal{H}_K$ and exploiting the Hilbert space structure in $\mathcal{H}_K$. Furthermore, practical computations can be efficiently tracted thanks to the *reproducing kernel* property - namely, for any $x, y \in \mathcal{X}$, we have

$$(K(x, \cdot) \mid K(y, \cdot))_{\mathcal{H}_K} = K(x, y) , \tag{1}$$

and more generally yet, for any $f \in \mathcal{H}_K$, $(K(x, \cdot) | f)_{\mathcal{H}_K} = f(x)$. Expanding on this, one can compute statistics on pairs of points and m-vectors $(x, \eta) \in \mathbb{R}^n \times \Lambda_m \mathbb{R}^n$ by mapping them to functions $K(x, \cdot)\eta$ and making use of the reproducing property

$$(K(x, \cdot)\eta | K(y, \cdot)\nu) = \eta^\top \nu K(x, y) . \tag{2}$$

Eq. 2 simply extends Eq. 1 to vector-valued functions, making use of the fact that the tensor product of two kernels is again a kernel over the product space. Expanding the framework even further, we can regard a discrete shape as a finite set $\{(x_i, \eta_i)\}_{1 \leq i \leq p}$, where η_i describes the tangent space at x_i, and associate to it a signature function $\sum_{1 \leq i \leq p} K(x_i, \cdot) \eta_i$. The correlation between two discrete shapes $\{(x_i, \eta_i)\}_{1 \leq i \leq p}$ and $\{(y_j, \nu_j)\}_{1 \leq j \leq q}$ can then be measured by the inner product

$$(\sum_i K(x_i, \cdot) \eta_i \mid \sum_j K(y_j, \cdot) \nu_j) = \sum_{i,j} \eta_i^\top \nu_j K(x_i, y_j) . \tag{3}$$

This construction may in fact be acknowledged as a special case of the convolution kernel on discrete structures described in [11] and [10]. The above defines a correspondence-free way to measure proximity between shapes, trading hard correspondences for an aggregation of the measures of proximity between each simplex of one shape with every simplex of the other shape in the sense of a kernel $K(\cdot, \cdot)$. We have yet to specify a choice of kernel K. In the following, we will consider the multivariate Gaussian kernel with variance Σ:

$$K_\Sigma(x, y) = \frac{1}{\{(2\pi)^n |\Sigma|\}^{1/2}} \exp -\frac{1}{2}(x - y)^\top \Sigma^{-1}(x - y) .$$

The choice of kernel width Σ can be interpreted as a choice of scale at which the shape of interest is observed: shape variations occurring at a lower scale are likely to be smoothed by the convolution and go unnoticed. This mechanism naturally introduces some level of noise insensitivity in the analysis. This parameter should thus be decided with regard to the mesh resolution and the level of noise in the data.

Finally, the linear pointwise-evaluation functional $\delta_x^\eta : \omega \mapsto \omega(x)(\eta)$ is continuous and dual to $K(x, \cdot) \eta$ by the reproducing kernel property. In the following we will refer to δ_x^η as a *delta-current* or a *moment*. To summarize, the discretized m-manifold $\{(x_i, \eta_i)\}_{1 \leq i \leq p}$ admits equivalent representations as the current $\sum_i \delta_{x_i}^{\eta_i}$, its dual differential m-form $\sum_{1 \leq i \leq p} K(x_i, \cdot) \eta_i^\top$ or its dual vector field $\sum_{1 \leq i \leq p} K(x_i, \cdot) \eta_i$.

2.2 Computational Efficiency and Compact Approximate Representations

This framework lends itself to an efficient implementation. Firstly, the inner product between two discrete shapes can be computed in linear time with respect to the number of momenta through the use of a translation invariant kernel. Indeed $\gamma(\cdot) = \sum_i K(x_i, \cdot) \eta_i$ may then be precomputed at any desired accuracy on a discrete grid by convolution, and rewriting $\sum_{i,j} \eta_i^\top \nu_j K(x_i, y_j)$ as $\sum_j \gamma(y_j)^\top \nu_j$ demonstrates the claim.

Secondly, if the mesh diameter is small with respect to the scale Σ, the initial delta-current representation will be highly redundant. Durrleman et al.[9] introduced an iterative method to obtain compact approximations of currents at a chosen scale and with any desired accuracy. We rely on this procedure at training time to fasten computations and reduce the memory load. This algorithm is inspired from the Matching Pursuit method[5]. A compact current is built from the current S to approximate (of dual field γ) by iteratively adding a single delta current $\delta_{x_n}^{\eta_n}$ to the previous approximation S_{n-1}, in such a way that the difference $\|S - S_n\|_{\mathcal{H}'_S}$ steadily decreases. This is achieved by greedily placing the moment at the maximum (in $\|\cdot\|_2$ norm) x_n of the residual field $\gamma(\cdot) - \gamma_{n-1}(\cdot)$, then choosing the optimal η, i.e. the one that minimizes

$\|\gamma - \{\gamma_{n-1} + K(\mathbf{x}_n, \cdot)\eta\}\|_{\mathcal{H}_\Sigma}^2$. It is shown in [9] that this algorithm is greedy in $\|\cdot\|_{\mathcal{H}_\Sigma}$ norm, and converges both in $\|\cdot\|_{\mathcal{H}_\Sigma}$ norm and $\|\cdot\|_\infty$ norm. The stopping criterion is on the residual norm $\|\gamma(\cdot) - \gamma_n(\cdot)\|_{\mathcal{H}_\Sigma}^2$. Our implementation uses a discrete kernel approximation of the Gaussian kernel, rather than an FFT based scheme, for fast local updates of the residual field.

3   Method

The workflow for the proposed machine-learning based parameter estimation method couples three successive processing steps: the first one aims at generating a current from an input sequence of meshes, so as to obtain a statistically relevant representation; the second one consists in a dimensionality reduction step, so as to derive a reduced shape representation in $\mathbb{R}^k$, which leads to computationally efficient statistical learning; the third step tackles the matter of finding a relationship between the reduced shape space and the (biophysical) model parameters. The three modules are mostly independent and can easily be adjusted in their own respect. As a machine learning based method, our work involves an off-line learning stage and an on-line testing stage: all three modules of the pipeline are involved during each stage. Fig. 1 gives a visual overview of our approach. The rest of this section describes the three afore-mentioned processing steps and their use during learning and testing stages.

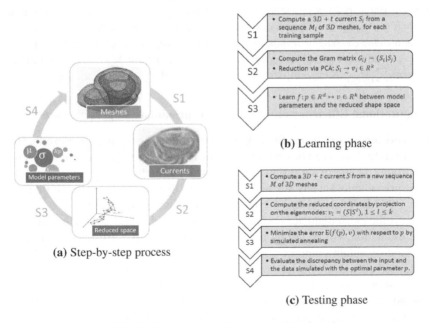

Fig. 1. Overview of the learning and testing phases

3.1 Current Generation from Mesh Sequences

Let us briefly describe the way we build a current from a time sequence of 3D meshes. We first extract surface meshes from the volumetric meshes. This choice derives from the assumption that the displacement of surface points can be recovered more easily than the displacement of all points within the myocardium, given a sequence of images; thus learning from surface meshes may be more relevant for real applications. In this work we assume the trajectory of surface points to be entirely known, as opposed to the displacement in the direction normal to the contour only (aperture problem). Several variants to derive currents for 4D object representation can be discussed (e.g. [7]), but their relevance largely depends on the application and complete processing work flow from the original data.

In this work, we rely on the remark that the concatenation of smoothly deformed surface meshes can be visualized as a (3D) hyper-surface in 4D (Fig. 2). The ith simplex of this hyper-surface generates a current $\delta_{x_i}^{\eta_i}$, where x_i is its barycenter and η_i is the vector of $\mathbb{R}^4$ normal to its support and of length the volume of the simplex. The current associated to the series of meshes is the aggregation of such delta currents, $\sum_i \delta_{x_i}^{\eta_i}$. This construction captures both the geometry of the heart and its motion.

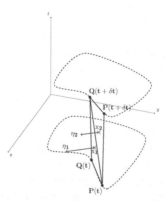

Fig. 2. Current generation from a mesh element, illustrated on an element of contour in 2D deformed in time. The simplex PQ is followed over two consecutive timesteps, which gives a quad embedded in 3D. The quad is divided into two triangles, from which we get two current deltas, applied at each triangle barycenter, orthogonal to the support of their corresponding triangles and of norm the area of the triangle. For a surface in 3D deformed over time, each element of the triangulation followed over two consecutive timesteps generates a hyper-prism embedded in 4D, which is in turn decomposed in three tetrahedra from which we obtain three momenta.

3.2 Shape Space Reduction

Since learning a direct mapping between the space of model parameters and the space of 3D+t currents is a cumbersome task, we introduce an intermediate step of dimensionality reduction via PCA. During the learning stage, we compute the mean current and principal modes of variation from the learning database of N currents $\{S_i\}_{1 \leq i \leq N}$ generated from the N training mesh sequences $\{M_i\}_{1 \leq i \leq N}$ as described in §3.1. This is achieved efficiently by computing the Gram matrix of the data $\mathbf{G}_{ij} = (S_i | S_j)$ column by column and using the "kernel trick"[17]. Each column of $\mathbf{G}$ is computed in $\mathcal{O}(N \cdot P)$, where P is the maximum number of momenta among all currents S_j (cf. §2.1). Finally, we compute an approximate compact representation at the scale Σ of the mean current $\bar{T}$ and of the K first modes of variation $\{T_k\}_{1 \leq k \leq K}$ to accelerate computations of inner products involving these currents[9].

At testing time and given a new current S, we derive its coordinates $v = (v_1, \cdots, v_K)$ in the reduced shape space by projection on the principal modes of variation, $v_k = (S - \bar{T} | T_k)$.

3.3   Regression Problem for Model Parameter Learning

It remains to link the physiological (model) parameters to the reduced shape space. Although we are ultimately interested in finding an optimal set of parameters $\mathrm{p} \in \mathbb{R}^d$ from an observation $v \in \mathbb{R}^K$ we will actually learn a mapping in the other direction, $f : \mathrm{p} \in \mathbb{R}^d \mapsto v \in \mathbb{R}^K$. We motivate this choice by three arguments. Firstly, the observation v is a deterministic output of the cardiac model given a parameter set p and thus the mapping f is well-defined; however there may be several parameter sets resulting in the same observable shape and deformation, as parameter identifiability is not *a priori* ensured. Secondly, the parameter space is expected to be of smaller dimensionality than the reduced shape space and therefore easier to sample for combinatorial reasons. Finally, we can also expect that the set of biologically admissible model parameters be relatively well-behaved; on the other hand few points in the shape space may actually relate to anatomically reasonable hearts: thus mapping every $v \in \mathbb{R}^k$ to a parameter set could be impractical.

The regression function f is learned by kernel ridge regression using a Gaussian kernel[12], and admits a straightforward close-form expression. During the testing phase, given a new observation v, we solve the optimization problem $\arg\min_{\mathrm{p}} \| f(\mathrm{p}) - v \|^2$ by Simulated Annealing[19]. This optimization problem involves an analytical mapping between low-dimensional spaces, as opposed to optimizing directly over the 4D meshes or currents. Thus it will not constitute a computational bottleneck regardless of the chosen optimization scheme. Naturally, if a prior on the likelihood of a given parameter set $\mathrm{p} \in \mathbb{R}^d$ were known (e.g. via a biophysical argument), it could be integrated in the cost function in the form of a prior energy term $\lambda \cdot R(\mathrm{p})$.

4   Experimental Results

In our first experiment we focus on the prediction of the maximum contractility parameter σ_0 of the BCS model, defined globally for the whole cardiac muscle. Building on the sensitivity analysis from [16], we consider that σ_0 covers the range of values from 10^6 to $2 \cdot 10^7$ in an anatomically plausible way. We form a training base of ten cases $\{\mathrm{p}_i, \mathcal{M}_i\}$ by sampling this range deterministically and launching simulations with the corresponding parameter sets, for a single heart geometry from the STACOM'2011

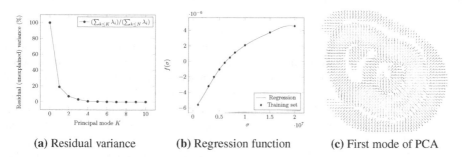

(a) Residual variance   (b) Regression function   (c) First mode of PCA

Fig. 3. PCA results for the first experiment. The projection of the first mode of variation on a plane orthogonal to the z-axis at a fixed time step is shown in (c), and can be interpreted as capturing the variability in the extent of the contraction of the muscle.

dataset. Following the PCA, the first principal mode of variation is found to explain 81% of the variance, thus we set the reduced shape space to be of dimension 1 ($K = 1$); the regression function ($\sigma = 0.3$, $\lambda = 10^{-5}$) bijectively maps the model parameter space and the reduced shape space. In all experiments, the model parameters are affinely mapped to $[-1, 1]$ for convenience, for the regression and optimization stages. We use an isotropic Gaussian kernel of width 1cm in space and 50ms in time.

In the spirit of cross-validation procedures, we evaluate the performance of our approach on an independent test set $\{p_j, \mathcal{M}_j\}_{0 \le j < N'}$ by randomly choosing parameter sets in the admissible range of parameters and launching the corresponding simulations. We thereafter refer to p_j as the *real* parameter (value) and to the output of our approach p_j^* as the *optimal* parameter (value). Our test set is of size $N' = 100$ samples. The whole personalization pipeline, from the current generation to the parameter optimization phase, takes roughly 2 minutes per sample on a regular laptop. We define the relative error on the parameter value for a given test sample j as $\epsilon_r p_j = |p_j^* - p_j|/p_j$. In addition to the relative error, we consider the absolute error over the range of admissible parameters, $\epsilon_a p_j = |p_j^* - p_j|/|p_{max} - p_{min}|$. We refer to $\epsilon_a p$ as an absolute error but express it for convenience as a percentage of the admissible parameter variation. Over the test set, we found a mean relative (resp. absolute) error of 9.2% (resp. 4.5%) and a median relative (resp. absolute) error of 6.8% (resp. 2.3%).

We are also interested in a preliminary evaluation of the robustness of our approach with respect to geometry changes. Ten samples are generated following the same procedure as before, but using another heart geometry of the STACOM dataset. The 10 mesh sequences are manually registered (*via* a similarity transform) to the training geometry based on the end-diastole mesh before applying the normal pipeline, as described in Section 3. The mean relative (resp. absolute) error on the contractility parameter over our sample is 25% (9.3%), with 15% (resp. 7.5%) median relative (absolute) error.

The second experiment proceeds similarly to the first one, but we simultaneously estimate the contractility σ_0, the relaxation rate k_{rs} and the viscosity μ. For the training phase, the parameter space is sampled on a $7 \times 7 \times 7$ grid with σ_0 in the range $[10^6, 2 \; 10^7]$, k_{rs} in $[5, 50]$ and μ in $[10^5, 8 \; 10^5]$. The explained variance with

1 eigenmode of the PCA (resp. 2 to 5) out of the $N = 343$ modes equals 63.2% of the total variance (resp. 80.3%, 89.5%, 94.1%, 96.7%). We set the dimension of the reduced shape space to $K = 3$. The performance is tested on $N' = 100$ random samples. Because we can no longer assume the parameter set to be identifiable *a priori*, we introduce another measure of the goodness of fit of our personalization by directly evaluating the error on the observations. Given two surface mesh sequences $\mathcal{M} = \{\mathcal{M}_i\}_{1 \leq i \leq T}$ and $\mathcal{M}' = \{\mathcal{M}'_i\}_{1 \leq i \leq T}$, we define the pseudo-distance $d_{\text{sur}}(\mathcal{M}, \mathcal{M}') = \max_i d_s(\mathcal{M}_i, \mathcal{M}'_i)$ where $d_s(\mathcal{M}_i, \mathcal{M}'_i)^2$ is the mean square distance of the points of the surface $\mathcal{M}_i$ to the surface $\mathcal{M}'_i$. Additionally given one-to-one correspondences between $\mathcal{M}$ and $\mathcal{M}'$, we can define the distance $d_{\text{nod}}(\mathcal{M}, \mathcal{M}') = \max_i d_p(\mathcal{M}_i, \mathcal{M}'_i)$, where $d_p(\mathcal{M}_i, \mathcal{M}'_i)$ is the mean distance between corresponding nodes of $\mathcal{M}_i$ and $\mathcal{M}'_i$. While d_{sur} intuitively relates to an upper bound for the matching between surface meshes at any time step, d_{nod} conveys more information about the quality of the matching of point trajectories. The results for this experiment are reported in Table 1. As a comparison, two mesh sequences corresponding to extreme values in the parameter set will yield a value for $d_{\text{sur}}(\mathcal{M}, \mathcal{M}')$ (resp. $d_{\text{nod}}(\mathcal{M}, \mathcal{M}')$) of the order of 6mm (resp. 8mm).

Table 1. Experiment 2 - results

	$\epsilon_r \sigma_0$ ($\epsilon_a \sigma_0$)	$\epsilon_r k_{rs}$ ($\epsilon_a k_{rs}$)	$\epsilon_r \mu$ ($\epsilon_a \mu$)	d_{sur} (mm)	d_{nod} (mm)
Mean	15.2% (8.0%)	48.8% (26.4%)	40.5% (20.0%)	0.92mm	1.42mm
Median	13.2% (6.3%)	44.7% (19.6%)	32.1% (17.5%)	0.80mm	1.32mm

In addition we compute the optimal parameters and performance indicators for a different choice of the reduced space dimension K, obtaining quasi-identical statistics for $K = 4$. Finally, we test here again the robustness with respect to changes of the heart geometry. Using the same procedure as before on 10 test samples on a different geometry, we find a mean error of 1.4mm and a median value at 1.3mm for d_{sur} (respectively, 1.8mm and 1.6mm for d_{nod}).

5   Discussion

Despite working around the bias and error introduced by the model and image processing in real applications, our synthetic experiments show promising performance for our framework in terms of accuracy, tolerance to non-linear effects of parameters, robustness and computational efficiency. The accuracy of our approach was found to be below the typical voxel dimension (1mm), while a priori optimizing among a very wide range of parameter values at test time, and using a reasonable number of training samples at learning time. Although a single geometry is used for the training phase, the accuracy was of the same order on similar (non-pathological) heart geometries. Naturally, further work should handle geometry variability in a proper way, taking it into account at the training stage, and adding "shape factors" to the model parameter space capturing 3D shape variability. Moreover the addition in the pipeline of a pre-clustering stage with respect to the heart geometry, so as to distinguish very different geometries and treat them separately, should reduce the number of samples required to cover the whole parameter space while achieving better model personalization.

The proposed framework also brings an interesting perspective on the issue of parameter identifiability. It should be noticed that we achieve good results in terms of spatial distance between the matched model and observations while significant differences in the parameter space may still be observed. Parameter identifiability encompasses two distinct aspects. Firstly, small variations of the parameter values may result in changes that are not noticeable at the scale of reference. This sensitivity to parameters partially explains the error on the retrieved set of parameters. In our approach, the kernel width for currents impacts the ability of the algorithm to discern shape differences. In the future we will experiment with smaller kernel widths and improve algorithms to handle increased computational cost. Secondly in joint parameter estimation, a whole subset in the parameter space may result in identical observations, which also affects parameter identifiability. Such considerations can be analyzed in depth at the regression or optimization steps: several parameter sets with similar costs along with a measure of local sensitivity around these values may be additionally output by the Simulated Annealing algorithm. Biophysical priors may also be introduced at the optimization step by penalizing unlikely parameter sets without adding significant computational cost.

Finally more efficient machine learning algorithms should be tested in lieu of PCA, so as to capture non-linear 4D shapes variation, and to obtain and exploit precise information about the manifold structure of 4D heart shapes. Not only will this be of help with parameter identifiability and to derive efficient representations in the reduced shape space, but it could also provide valuable feedback for "smart" sampling of the parameter space.

6   Conclusion

A machine-learning current-based method has been proposed in this paper for the personalization of electromechanical models of the heart from patient-specific kinematics. A framework to encapsulate information regarding shape and motion in a way that allows the efficient computation of statistics via 4D currents has been described. This approach has been evaluated on synthetic data using the BCS model, with the joint estimation of the maximum contraction, relaxation rate and viscosity. It is found that the proposed method is accurate, computationally efficient and robust.

Acknowledgments. This work was partly funded by Microsoft Research through its PhD Scholarship Programme and by the ERC Advanced Grant MedYMA.

References

1. Aronszajn, N.: Theory of reproducing kernels. Harvard University (1951)
2. Bestel, J., Clément, F., Sorine, M.: A Biomechanical Model of Muscle Contraction. In: Niessen, W.J., Viergever, M.A. (eds.) MICCAI 2001. LNCS, vol. 2208, pp. 1159–1161. Springer, Heidelberg (2001)

3. Chabiniok, R., Moireau, P., Lesault, P.F., Rahmouni, A., Deux, J.F., Chapelle, D.: Estimation of tissue contractility from cardiac cine-MRI using a biomechanical heart model. Biomechanics and Modeling in Mechanobiology 11(5), 609–630 (2012)
4. Chapelle, D., Le Tallec, P., Moireau, P., Sorine, M.: An energy-preserving muscle tissue model: formulation and compatible discretizations. IJMCE 10(2), 189–211 (2012)
5. Davis, G., Mallat, S., Avellaneda, M.: Adaptive greedy approximations. Constructive Approximation 13(1), 57–98 (1997)
6. Delingette, H., Billet, F., Wong, K., Sermesant, M., Rhode, K., Ginks, M., Rinaldi, C., Razavi, R., Ayache, N., et al.: Personalization of Cardiac Motion and Contractility from Images using Variational Data Assimilation. IEEE Trans. Biomed. Eng. 59(1), 20 (2012)
7. Durrleman, S.: Statistical models of currents for measuring the variability of anatomical curves, surfaces and their evolution. Ph.D. Thesis, INRIA (March 2010)
8. Durrleman, S., Pennec, X., Trouvé, A., Ayache, N.: Measuring Brain Variability Via Sulcal Lines Registration: A Diffeomorphic Approach. In: Ayache, N., Ourselin, S., Maeder, A. (eds.) MICCAI 2007, Part I. LNCS, vol. 4791, pp. 675–682. Springer, Heidelberg (2007)
9. Durrleman, S., Pennec, X., Trouvé, A., Ayache, N.: Sparse Approximation of Currents for Statistics on Curves and Surfaces. In: Metaxas, D., Axel, L., Fichtinger, G., Székely, G. (eds.) MICCAI 2008, Part II. LNCS, vol. 5242, pp. 390–398. Springer, Heidelberg (2008)
10. Gärtner, T., Flach, P., Kowalczyk, A., Smola, A.: Multi-instance kernels. In: Proceedings of the 19th International Conference on Machine Learning, pp. 179–186 (2002)
11. Haussler, D.: Convolution kernels on discrete structures. Tech. rep., Technical report, UC Santa Cruz (1999)
12. Hoerl, A., Kennard, R.: Ridge regression: Biased estimation for nonorthogonal problems. Technometrics pp. 55–67 (1970)
13. Imperiale, A., Chabiniok, R., Moireau, P., Chapelle, D.: Constitutive Parameter Estimation Methodology Using Tagged-MRI Data. In: Metaxas, D.N., Axel, L. (eds.) FIMH 2011. LNCS, vol. 6666, pp. 409–417. Springer, Heidelberg (2011)
14. Liu, H., Shi, P.: Maximum a posteriori strategy for the simultaneous motion and material property estimation of the heart. IEEE Trans. Biomed. Eng. 56(2), 378–389 (2009)
15. Mansi, T., Pennec, X., Sermesant, M., Delingette, H., Ayache, N.: ilogdemons: A demons-based registration algorithm for tracking incompressible elastic biological tissues. International Journal of Computer Vision 92(1), 92–111 (2011)
16. Marchesseau, S., Delingette, H., Sermesant, M., Rhode, K., Duckett, S.G., Rinaldi, C.A., Razavi, R., Ayache, N.: Cardiac Mechanical Parameter Calibration Based on the Unscented Transform. In: Ayache, N., Delingette, H., Golland, P., Mori, K. (eds.) MICCAI 2012, Part II. LNCS, vol. 7511, pp. 41–48. Springer, Heidelberg (2012)
17. Schölkopf, B., Smola, A.: Learning with kernels: Support vector machines, regularization, optimization, and beyond. The MIT Press (2002)
18. Vaillant, M., Glaunès, J.: Surface Matching via Currents. In: Christensen, G.E., Sonka, M. (eds.) IPMI 2005. LNCS, vol. 3565, pp. 381–392. Springer, Heidelberg (2005)
19. Xiang, Y., Gubian, S., Suomela, B., Hoeng, J.: Generalized simulated annealing for efficient global optimization: the GenSA package for R. The R Journal (2012) (forthcoming)

Author Index

CPSIA information can be obtained at www.ICGtesting.com
Printed in the USA
LVOW01s1321061013

355632LV00002B/73/P

9 783642 366192

THE HOMESTEADING HANDBOOK

A BACK TO BASICS GUIDE TO
GROWING YOUR OWN FOOD • CANNING
KEEPING CHICKENS • GENERATING YOUR OWN ENERGY
CRAFTING • HERBAL MEDICINE • AND MORE

ABIGAIL R. GEHRING

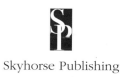

Skyhorse Publishing

THE HOMESTEADING HANDBOOK

www.skyhorsepublishing.com

20 19 18 17 16 15 14 13

Library of Congress Cataloging-in-Publication Data

Gehring, Abigail R.
  The homesteading handbook : back to basics guide to growing your own food, canning, keeping chickens, generating your own energy, crafting, herbal medicine, and more / Abigail R. Gehring.
      p. cm.
  ISBN 978-1-61608-265-9 (alk. paper)
 1. Agriculture--Handbooks, manuals, etc. 2. Family farms--Handbooks, manuals, etc. 3. Home economics, Rural--Handbooks, manuals, etc. 4. Sustainable living--Handbooks, manuals, etc. 5. Agriculture--United States--Handbooks, manuals, etc. I. Title.
  S501.2.G44 2011
  640--dc22
                                        2011017263

Printed in China

Contents

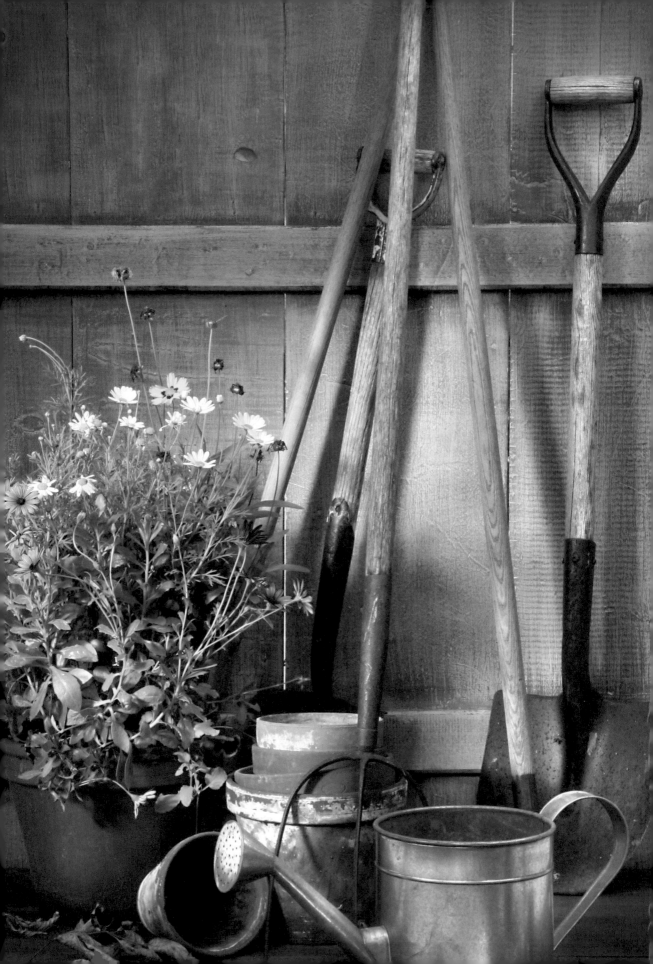

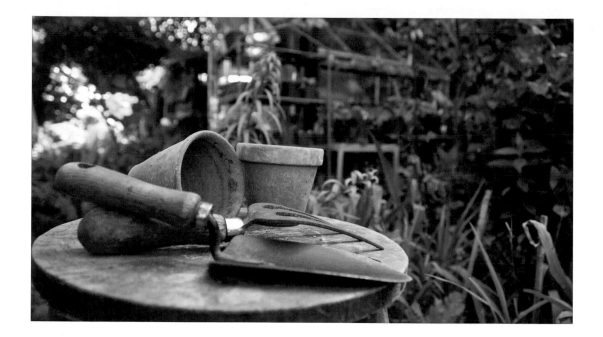

PART ONE

The Home Garden

"My green thumb came only as a result of the mistakes I made while learning to see things from the plant's point of view."

—*H. Fred Ale*

Creating a garden—whether it's a single tomato plant in a pot on your windowsill or a full acre chock-full of flowers and veggies—takes imagination, hard work, a bit of planning, patience, and a willingness to take risks. There are some factors you can control, like the condition of the soil you bury your seeds in, the time of year you start planting, and what plants you put where. But there will always be situations you can't predict; you might get a frost in June, an old discarded pumpkin seed might sprout up in the middle of your magnolias, or the cat could knock your basil plant off the counter to its demise on the kitchen floor. This element of surprise is one of the joys and challenges of gardening. If you can learn to skillfully navigate the factors in your control and accept the unpredictable circumstances with patience and a sense of humor, you'll have mastered a great life lesson. The following pages are meant to help you with that first part: gaining the knowledge and insight you need to give your garden the best chance of thriving. From understanding a plant's basic needs, to properly preparing soil, to protecting against weeds and harmful insects, this section covers all the gardening basics. Beyond that, you'll find information on growing plants without soil, tips for keeping your garden organic, and inspiration for gardening in urban environments. There is little in life as rewarding as enjoying a salad composed entirely of things you've picked from your own garden. But gardening is also about the process: If you can learn to love the feel of the dirt between your fingers, the burn in your muscles as you dig, and the quiet, slow way in which sprouts reach toward the sun, no moment of your labor will have been a waste, regardless of the end results.

Planning a Garden

Basic Plant Requirements

Before you start a garden, it's helpful to understand what plants need in order to thrive. Some plants, like dandelions, are tolerant of a wide variety of conditions, while others, such as orchids, have very specific requirements in order to grow successfully. Before spending time, effort, and money attempting to grow a new plant in a garden, to do some research to learn about the conditions that a particular plant needs in order to grow properly.

Environmental factors play a key role in the proper growth of plants. Some of the essential factors that influence this natural process are as follows:

1. Length of Day

The amount of time between sunrise and sunset is the most critical factor in regulating vegetative growth, blooming, flower development, and the initiation of dormancy. Plants utilize increasing day length as a cue to promote their growth in spring, while decreasing day length in fall prompts them to prepare for the impending cold weather. Many plants require specific day length conditions in order to bloom and flower.

2. Light

Light is the energy source for all plants. Cloudy, rainy days or any shade cast by nearby plants and structures can significantly reduce the amount of light available to the plant. In addition, plants adapted to thrive in shady spaces cannot tolerate full sunlight. In general, plants will only be able to survive where adequate sunlight reaches them at levels they are able to tolerate.

3. Temperature

Plants grow best within an optimal range of temperatures. This temperature range may vary drastically depending on the plant species. Some plants

Some gardens require more planning than others. Flower gardens can be carefully arranged to create patterns or to contain a specific range of colors, or they can be more casual, as this garden is. However, always keep in mind a plant's specific environmental needs before choosing a place for it.

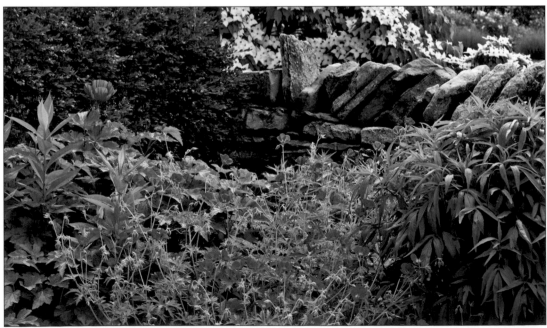

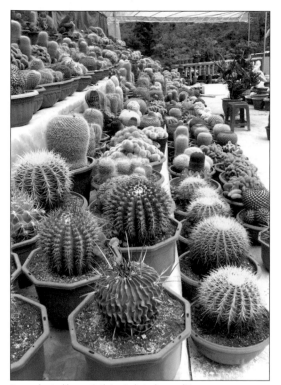

Some plants, like cacti, thrive in hot, dry conditions.

thrive in environments where the temperature range is quite wide; others can only survive within a very narrow temperature variance. Plants can only survive where temperatures allow them to carry on life-sustaining chemical reactions.

4. Cold

Plants differ by species in their ability to survive cold temperatures. Temperatures below 60°F injure some tropical plants. Conversely, arctic species can tolerate temperatures well below zero. The ability of a plant to withstand cold is a function of the degree of dormancy present in the plant, its water status, and its general health. Exposure to wind, bright sunlight, or rapidly changing temperatures can also compromise a plant's tolerance to the cold.

5. Heat

A plant's ability to tolerate heat also varies widely from species to species. Many plants that evolved to grow in arid, tropical regions are naturally very heat tolerant, while sub-arctic and alpine plants show very little tolerance for heat.

6. Water

Different types of plants have different water needs. Some plants can tolerate drought during the summer but need winter rains in order to flourish. Other plants need a consistent supply of moisture to grow well. Careful attention to a plant's need for supplemental water can help you to select plants that need a minimum of irrigation to perform well in your garden. If you have poorly drained, chronically wet soil, you can select lovely garden plants that naturally grow in bogs, marshlands, and other wet places.

7. Soil pH

A plant root's ability to take up certain nutrients depends on the pH—a measure of the acidity or alkalinity—of your soil. Most plants grow best in soils that have a pH between 6.0 and 7.0. Most ericaceous plants, such as azaleas and blueberries, need acidic soils with a pH below 6.0 to grow well. Lime can be used to raise the soil's pH, and materials containing sulfates, such as aluminum sulfate and iron sulfate, can be used to lower the pH. The solubility of many trace elements is controlled by pH, and plants can only use the soluble forms of these important micronutrients.

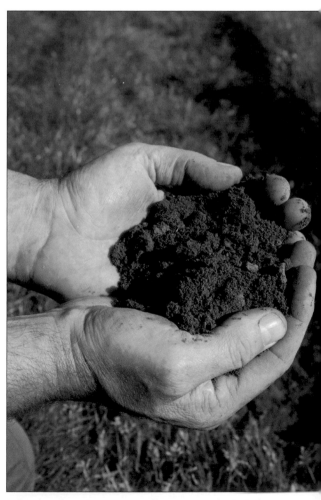

Feeling the soil can give you a sense of how nutrient-rich it is. Dark, crumbly, soft soil is usually full of nutrients. However, determining the pH requires a soil test (see page 9).

A Basic Plant Glossary

Here is some terminology commonly used in reference to plants and gardening:

annual—a plant that completes its life cycle in one year or season.

arboretum—a landscaped space where trees, shrubs, and herbaceous plants are cultivated for scientific study or educational purposes, and to foster appreciation of plants.

axil—the area between a leaf and the stem from which the leaf arises.

bract—a leaflike structure that grows below a flower or cluster of flowers and is often colorful. Colored bracts attract pollinators, and are often mistaken for petals. Poinsettia and flowering dogwood are examples of plants with prominent bracts.

cold hardy—capable of withstanding cold weather conditions.

conifers—plants that predate true, flowering plants in evolution; conifers lack true flowers and produce separate male and female strobili, or cones. Some conifers, such as yews, have fruits enclosed in a fleshy seed covering.

cultivar—a cultivated variety of a plant selected for a feature that distinguishes it from the species from which it was selected.

deciduous—having leaves that fall off or are shed seasonally to avoid adverse weather conditions, such as cold or drought.

herbaceous—having little or no woody tissue. Most perennials or annuals are herbaceous.

hybrid—a plant, or group of plants, that results from the interbreeding of two distinct cultivars, varieties, species, or genera.

inflorescence—a floral axis that contains many individual flowers in a specific arrangement; also known as a flower cluster.

native plant—a plant that lives or grows naturally in a particular region without direct or indirect human intervention.

panicle—a pyramidal, loosely branched flower cluster; a panicle is a type of inflorescence.

perennial—a plant that persists for several years, usually dying back to a perennial crown during the winter and initiating new growth each spring

shrub—a low-growing, woody plant, usually less than 15 feet tall, that often has multiple stems and may have a suckering growth habit (the tendency to sprout from the root system).

taxonomy—the study of the general principles of scientific classification, especially the orderly classification of plants and animals according to their presumed natural relationships.

tree—a woody perennial plant having a single, usually elongated main stem, or trunk, with few or no branches on its lower part.

wildflower—a herbaceous plant that is native to a given area and is representative of unselected forms of its species.

woody plant—a plant with persistent woody parts that do not die back in adverse conditions. Most woody plants are trees or shrubs.

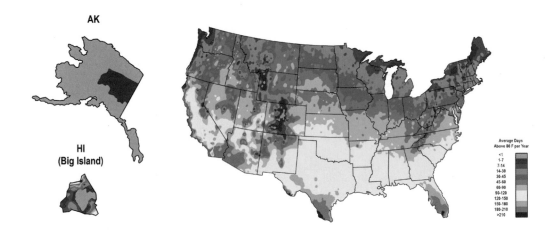

AK

HI
(Big Island)

Average Days
Above 86 F per Year

<1
1-7
7-14
14-30
30-45
45-60
60-90
90-120
120-150
150-180
180-210
>210

Parts of a Flower

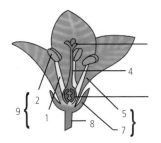

1—filament
2—anther
3—stigma
4—style
5—petal
6—ovary
7—sepal
8—pedicel
9—stamen
10—pistil
11—perianth

Selecting a Site for Your Garden

Selecting a site for your garden is the first step in growing the vegetables, fruits, and herbs that you want. You do not need a large space in order to grow a significant amount of vegetables, fruit, and herbs. Creating a garden that is about 25 feet square should be quite sufficient for a family. It is important that you don't start off with a space that is too large—it is better to start small and then work your way up if you find that gardening is something that you truly enjoy.

Five Factors to Consider When Choosing a Garden Site

1. Sunlight

Sunlight is crucial for the growth of vegetables and other plants. In order for your garden to grow, your plants will need at least six hours of direct sunlight per day. In order to make sure your garden receives an ample amount of sunlight, don't select a garden site that will be in the shade of trees, shrubs, houses, or other structures. Certain vegetables, such as broccoli and spinach, grow just fine in shadier spots, so if your garden does receive some shade, make sure to plant those types of vegetables in the shadier areas. However, on a whole, if your garden does not receive at least six hours of intense sunlight per day, it will not grow as efficiently or successfully.

2. Proximity

Another consideration is how close you place your garden to your home. If your garden is closer to your house and easy to reach, you will most likely use it more often—and to its fullest potential. Having a garden close to your home will help you to pick your vegetables and fruit at their peak ripeness, allowing you access to an abundance of fresh produce on a regular basis. Weeding, watering, and controlling pests are all more likely to be attended to if your garden is situated near your home. Overall, gardens placed closer to the home will receive more attention and thus be healthier and more productive.

3. Soil Quality

Contrary to some beliefs, you do not need high-quality soil to start and grow a productive garden. However, it is best to have soil that is fertile, is full of organic materials that provide nutrients to the plant roots, and is easy to dig and till. Loose, well-drained soil is ideal for

If you don't have enough space for a full garden, you can plant in flowerpots or other containers. Potted plants are especially convenient because you can move them around to get more light or to make watering easier.

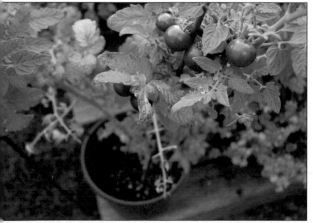

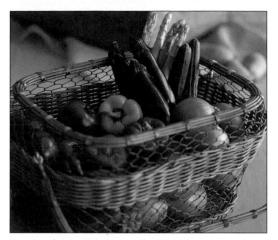

A garden of about 25 feet square should be adequate to produce enough vegetables for a family of four to six to enjoy.

growing a good garden. If there is a section of your yard where water does not easily drain after a good, soaking rain, it is best not to plant your garden in that area, as the excess water will most likely drown your garden plants. Furthermore, soils that are of a clay or sandy consistency are not as effective in growing plants. To make these types of soils more nutrient-rich and fertile, add in organic materials (such as compost or manure) to improve their quality.

4. Water Availability

Water is vital to keeping your garden green, healthy, and productive. A successful garden needs around 1 inch of water per week to thrive. Rain and irrigation systems are effective in maintaining this 1-inch-per-week quota. Situating your garden near a spigot or hose is ideal, allowing you to keep the soil moist and your plants happy.

5. Elevation

It is essential to make sure your garden is not located in an area where air cannot circulate and where frost quickly forms. Placing your garden in a low-lying area, such as at the base of a slope, should be avoided, as these lower areas do not warm as quickly in the spring, and frost forms quickly during the spring and fall since the cold air collects in these areas. Your garden should, if at all possible, be elevated slightly, on ground that is higher up. This way, your garden plants will be less likely to be affected by frost and you'll be able to start your garden growing earlier in the spring and harvest well into the fall.

Some Other Things to Consider

When planning out your garden, it is useful to sketch a diagram of what you want your garden to look like. What sorts of plants to you want to grow? Do you want a garden purely for growing vegetables or do you want to mix in some fruits, herbs, and wildflowers? Choosing the appropriate plants to grow next to each other will help your garden grow well and will provide you with

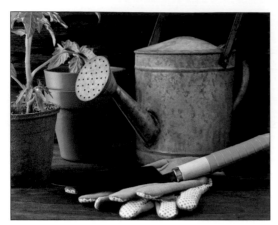

Gloves, a trowel, and a watering can are some of the most basic tools you should have on hand for gardening.

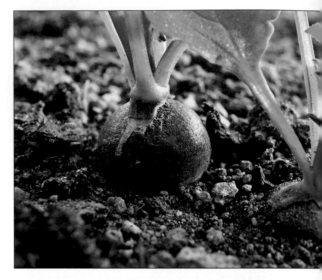

ample produce throughout the growing season (see the charts on this page).

When planting a garden, be sure to have access to many types of tools. You'll need a spade or digging fork for digging holes for seeds or seedlings (or, if the soil is loose enough, you can just use your hands). You'll also need a trowel, rake, or hoe to smooth over the garden surface. A measuring stick is helpful when spacing your plants or seeds (if you don't have a measuring stick, you can use a precut string to measure). If you are planting seedlings or established plants, you may need stakes and string to tie them up (so they don't fall over in inclement weather or when they start producing fruit or vegetables). Finally, if you are interested in installing an irrigation system for your garden, you will need to buy the appropriate materials for this purpose.

Companion Planting

Plants have natural substances built into their structures that repel or attract certain insects and can have an effect on the growth rate and even the flavor of the other plants around them. Thus, some plants aid each other's growth when planted in close proximity and others inhibit each other. Smart companion planting will help your garden remain healthy, beautiful, and in harmony, while deterring certain insect pests and other factors that could be potentially detrimental to your garden plants.

These charts list various types of garden vegetables, herbs, and flowers and their respective companion and "enemy" plants.

Vegetables

Type	Companion plant(s)	Avoid
Asparagus	Tomatoes, parsley, basil	Onion, garlic, potatoes
Beans	Eggplant	Tomatoes, onion, kales
Beets	Mint	Runner beans
Broccoli	Onion, garlic, leeks	Tomatoes, peppers, mustard

Type	Companion plant(s)	Avoid
Cabbage	Onion, garlic, leeks	Tomatoes, peppers, beans
Carrot	Leeks, beans	Radish
Celery	Daisies, snapdragons	Corn, aster flower
Corn	Legumes, squash, cucumber	Tomatoes, celery
Cucumber	Radishes, beets, carrots	Tomatoes
Eggplant	Marigolds, mint	Runner beans
Leeks	Carrots	Legumes
Lettuce	Radish, carrots	Celery, cabbage, parsley
Melon	Pumpkin, squash	None
Peppers	Tomatoes	Beans, cabbage, kales
Onion	Carrots	Peas, beans
Peas	Beans, corn	Onion, garlic
Potato	Horseradish	Tomatoes, cucumber
Tomatoes	Carrots, celery, parsley	Corn, peas, potato, kales

Herbs

Type	Companion Plant(s)	Avoid
Basil	Chamomile, anise	Sage
Chamomile	Basil, cabbage	Other herbs (it will become oily)
Cilantro	Beans, peas	None
Chives	Carrots	Peas, beans
Dill	Cabbage, cucumber	Tomatoes, carrots
Fennel	Dill	Everything else
Garlic	Cucumber, peas, lettuce	None
Oregano	Basil, peppers	None
Peppermint	Broccoli, cabbage	None
Rosemary	Sage, beans, carrots	None
Sage	Rosemary, beans	None
Summer savory	Onion, green beans	None

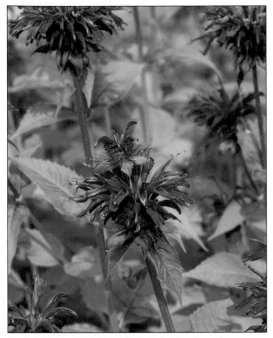

Bee balm does well in partial shade. Its bright color and sweet nectar have a tendency to attract bees and humming birds.

Flowering plants that do well in partial and full shade:

- Bee balm
- Bleeding heart
- Coleus
- Daylily
- Fern
- Globe daisy
- Impatiens
- Lily of the valley
- Pansy
- Persian violet
- Rue anemone
- Sweet alyssum
- Bellflower
- Cardinal flower
- Columbine
- Dichondra
- Forget-me-not
- Golden bleeding heart
- Leopardbane
- Meadow rue
- Periwinkle
- Primrose
- Snapdragon
- Thyme

Vegetable plants that can grow in partial shade:

- Arugula
- Beets
- Brussels sprouts
- Endive
- Leaf lettuce
- Radish
- Swiss chard
- Beans
- Broccoli
- Cauliflower
- Kale
- Peas
- Spinach

Flowers

Type	Companion Plant(s)	Avoid
Geraniums	Roses, tomatoes	None
Marigolds	Tomatoes, peppers, most plants	None
Petunias	Squash, asparagus	None
Sunflowers	Corn, tomatoes	None
Tansies	Roses, cucumber, squash	None

Plants for the Shade

It is best to situate your garden in an area that receives at least six hours of direct sunlight per day—especially if you want to grow vegetables or fruits. However, if the only part of your yard suitable for gardening is blocked by partial or full shade (or part of your sunlit garden receives partial shade during the day), you can still grow plenty of things in these areas—you just need to select plants that grow best in these types of environments. It is a good idea, either when buying seedlings from your local nursery or planting your own seeds, to read the accompanying label or packet or do a little research before planting to make sure your plants will thrive in a shadier environment.

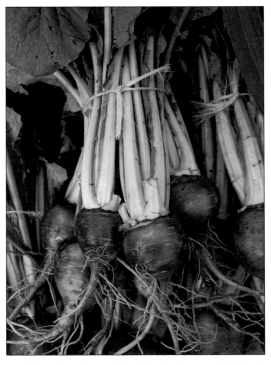

Beets like cool weather and do well in shady areas with rich soil. Plant beets at least 1 inch deep and 2 inches part. Weed regularly to ensure strong root development.

Improving Your Soil

When gardening, it is essential to have nutrient-rich, fertile soil in order to grow the best and healthiest plants—plants that will supply you with quality fruits, vegetables, and flowers. Sometimes, soil loses its fertility (or has minimum fertility based on the region in which you live), and so measures must be taken in order to improve your soil and, subsequently, your garden.

Soil Quality Indicators

Soil quality is an assessment of how well soil performs all of its functions now and how those functions are being preserved for future use. The quality of soil cannot just be determined by measuring row or garden yield, water quality, or any other single outcome, nor can it be measured directly. Thus, it is important to look at specific indicators to better understand the properties of soil. Plants can provide us with clues about how well the soil is functioning—whether a plant is growing and producing quality fruits and vegetables or failing to yield such things is a good indicator of the quality of the soil it's growing in.

Indicators are measurable properties of soil or plants that provide clues about how well the soil can function. Indicators can be physical, chemical, and biological properties, processes, or characteristics of soils. They can also be visual features of plants.

Useful indicators of soil quality:
- are easy to measure
- measure changes in soil functions
- encompass chemical, biological, and physical properties
- are accessible to many users
- are sensitive to variations in climate and management

Indicators can be assessed by qualitative or quantitative techniques, such as soil tests. After measurements are collected, they can be evaluated by looking for patterns and comparing results to measurements taken at a different time.

Good soil is usually dark, moist, and dense.

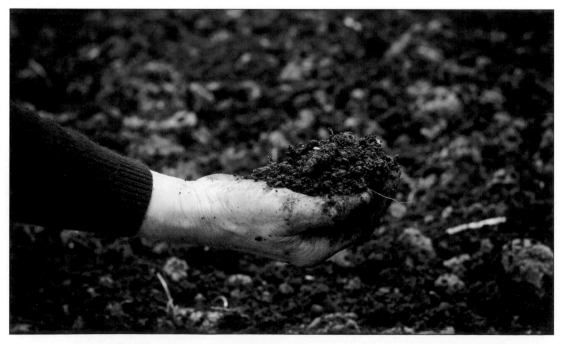

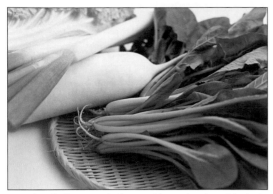

Spinach and other green, leafy vegetables tend to do well in shady areas. Just be sure they get enough water; trees or other shade-producing canopies can also block rainfall.

Examples of soil quality indicators:
1. Soil Organic Matter—promotes soil fertility, structure, stability, nutrient retention, and helps combat soil erosion.
2. Physical Indicators—these include soil structure, depth, infiltration and bulk density, and water hold capacity. Quality soil will retain and transport water and nutrients effectively; it will provide habitat for microbes; it will promote compaction and water movement; and, it will be porous and easy to work with.
3. Chemical Indicators—these include pH, electrical conductivity, and extractable nutrients. Quality soil will be at its threshold for plant, microbial, biological, and chemical activity; it will also have plant nutrients that are readily available.
4. Biological Indicators—these include microbial biomass, mineralizable nitrogen, and soil respiration. Quality soil is a good repository for nitrogen and other basic nutrients for prosperous plant growth; it has a high soil productivity and nitrogen supply; and there is a good amount of microbial activity.

Soil and Plant Nutrients

Nutrient Management

There are 20 nutrients that all plants require. Six of the most important nutrients, called macronutrients, are: calcium, magnesium, nitrogen, phosphorous, potassium, and sulfur. Of these, nitrogen, phosphorus, and potassium are essential to healthy plant growth and so are required in relatively large amounts. Nitrogen is associated with lush vegetative growth, phosphorus is required for flowering and fruiting, and potassium is necessary for durability and disease resistance. Calcium, sulfur, and magnesium are also required in comparatively large quantities and aid in the overall health of plants.

The other nutrients, referred to as micronutrients, are required in very small amounts. These include such elements as copper, zinc, iron, and boron. While both macro- and micronutrients are required for good plant growth, over-application of these nutrients can be as detrimental to the plant as a nutrient deficiency. Over-application of plant nutrients may not only impair plant growth, but may also contaminate groundwater by penetrating through the soil or may pollute surface waters.

Soil Testing

Testing your soil for nutrients and pH is important in order to provide your plants with the proper balance of nutrients (while avoiding over-application). If you are establishing a new lawn or garden, a soil test is strongly recommended. The cost of soil testing is minor in comparison to the cost of plant materials and labor. Correcting a problem before planting is much simpler and cheaper than afterwards.

Once your garden is established, continue to take periodic soil samples. While many people routinely lime their soil, this can raise the pH of the soil too high. Likewise, since many fertilizers tend to lower the soil's pH, it may drop below desirable levels after several years, depending on fertilization and other soil factors, so occasional testing is strongly encouraged.

Home tests for pH, nitrogen, phosphorus, and potassium are available from most garden centers. While these may give you a general idea of the nutrients in your soil, they are not as reliable as tests performed by the Cooperative Extension Service at land grant universities. University and other commercial testing services will provide more detail, and you can request special tests for micronutrients if you suspect a problem. In addition to the analysis of nutrients in your soil, these services often provide recommendations for the application of nutrients or how best to adjust the pH of your soil.

The test for soil pH is very simple. pH is a measure of how acidic or alkaline your soil is. A pH of 7 is considered neutral. Below 7 is acidic and above 7 is alkaline. Since pH greatly influences plant nutrients, adjusting the pH will often correct a nutrient problem. At a high pH, several of the micronutrients become less available for plant uptake. Iron deficiency is a common problem, even

This electronic soil tester runs on one AA battery and gives pH, nutrient, and moisture level readings within minutes.

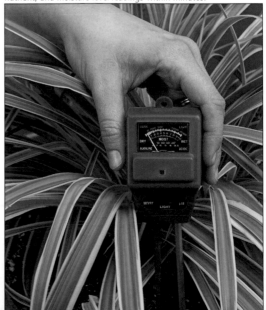

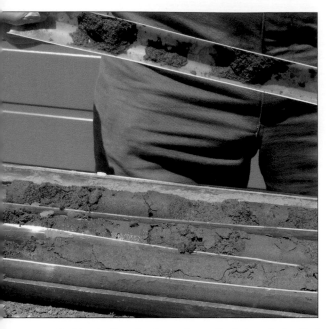

To determine the various layers of your soil, called your "soil profile," a core sample can be taken. This requires a boring machine, which will insert a hollow core rod, or "probe" like these shown here, deep into the ground to extract soil. The layers will be distinguishable by the change in soil color. Several core samples can be mixed together for a more accurate soil test.

Steps for Taking a Soil Test

1. If you intend to send your sample to the land grant university in your state, contact the local Cooperative Extension Service for information and sample bags. If you intend to send your sample to a private testing lab, contact them for specific details about submitting a sample.

2. Follow the directions carefully for submitting the sample. The following are general guidelines for taking a soil sample:

   - Sample when the soil is moist but not wet.
   - Obtain a clean pail or similar container.
   - Clear away the surface litter or grass.
   - With a spade or soil auger, dig a small amount of soil to a depth of 6 inches.
   - Place the soil in the clean pail.
   - Repeat steps 3 through 5 until the required number of samples has been collected.
   - Mix the samples together thoroughly.
   - From the mixture, take the sample that will be sent for analysis.
   - Send immediately. Do not dry before sending.

3. If you are using a home soil testing kit, follow the above steps for taking your sample. Follow the directions in the test kit carefully so you receive the most accurate reading possible.

at a neutral pH, for such plants as rhododendrons and blueberries. At a very low soil pH, other micronutrients may be too available to the plant, resulting in toxicity.

Phosphorus and potassium are tested regularly by commercial testing labs. While there are soil tests for nitrogen, these may be less reliable. Nitrogen is present in the soil in several forms that can change rapidly. Therefore, a precise analysis of nitrogen is more difficult to obtain. Most university soil test labs do not routinely test for nitrogen. Home testing kits often contain a test for nitrogen that may give you a general, though not necessarily completely accurate, idea of the presence of nitrogen in your garden soil.

Organic matter is often part of a soil test. Organic matter has a large influence on soil structure and so is highly desirable for your garden soil. Good soil structure improves aeration, water movement, and retention. This encourages increased microbial activity and root growth, both of which influence the availability of nutrients for plant growth. Soils high in organic matter tend to have a greater supply of plant nutrients compared to many soils low in organic matter. Organic matter tends to bind up some soil pesticides, reducing their effectiveness, and so this should be taken into consideration if you are planning to apply pesticides to your garden.

Tests for micronutrients are usually not performed unless there is reason to suspect a problem. Certain plants have greater requirements for specific micronutrients and may show deficiency symptoms if those nutrients are not readily available. (See the chart listing nutrient deficiency symptoms on page 57.)

Enriching Your Soil

Organic and Commercial Fertilizers and Returning Nutrients to Your Soil

Once you have the results of the soil test, you can add nutrients or soil amendments as needed to alter the pH. If you need to raise the soil's pH, use lime. Lime is most effective when it is mixed into the soil; therefore, it is best to apply before planting (if you apply lime in the fall, it has a better chance of correcting any soil acidity problems for the next growing season). For large areas, rototilling is most effective. For small areas or around plants, working the lime into the soil with a spade or cultivator is preferable. When working around plants, be careful not to dig too deeply or roughly so that you damage plant roots. Depending on the form of lime and the soil conditions, the change in pH may be gradual. It may take several months before a significant change is noted. Soils high in organic matter and clay tend to take larger amounts of lime to change the pH than do sandy soils.

If you need to lower the pH significantly, especially for plants such as rhododendrons, you can use aluminum sulfate. In all cases, follow the soil test or manufacturer's recommended rates of application. Again, mixing well into the soil is recommended.

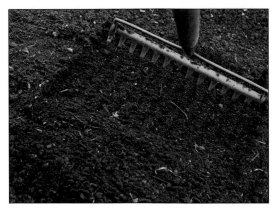

After rototilling or mixing in the fertilizer with a spade, you may wish to rake out the soil to make it smooth and well aerated.

There are numerous choices for providing nitrogen, phosphorus, and potassium, the nutrients your plants need to thrive. Nitrogen (N) is needed for healthy, green growth and regulation of other nutrients. Phosphorus (P) helps roots and seeds properly develop and resist disease. Potassium (K) is also important in root development and disease resistance. If your soil is of adequate fertility, applying compost may be the best method of introducing additional nutrients. While compost is relatively low in nutrients compared to commercial fertilizers, it is especially beneficial in improving the condition of the soil and is nontoxic. By keeping the soil loose, compost allows plant roots to grow well throughout the soil, helping them to extract nutrients from a larger area. A loose soil enriched with compost is also an excellent habitat for earthworms and other beneficial soil microorganisms that are essential for releasing nutrients for plant use. The nutrients from compost are also released slowly, so there is no concern about "burning" the plant with an over-application of synthetic fertilizer.

Manure is also an excellent source of plant nutrients and is an organic matter. Manure should be composted before applying, as fresh manure may be too strong and can injure plants. Be careful when composting manure. If left in the open, exposed to rain, nutrients may leach out of the manure and the runoff can contaminate nearby waterways. Make sure the manure is stored in a location away from wells and any waterways and that any runoff is confined or slowly released into a vegetated area. Improperly applied manure also can be a source of pollution. If you are not composting your own manure, you can purchase some at your local garden store. For best results, work composted manure into the soil around the plants or in your garden before planting.

If preparing a bed before planting, compost and manure may be worked into the soil to a depth of 8 to 12 inches. If adding to existing plants, work carefully around the plants so as not to harm the existing roots.

Green manures are another source of organic matter and plant nutrients. Green manures are crops that are grown and then tilled into the soil. As they break down, nitrogen and other plant nutrients become available. These manures may also provide additional benefits of reducing soil erosion. Green manures, such as rye and oats, are often planted in the fall after the crops have been harvested. In the spring, these are tilled under before planting.

With all organic sources of nitrogen, whether compost or manure, the nitrogen must be changed to an inorganic form before the plants can use it. Therefore, it is important to have well-drained, aerated soils that provide the favorable habitat for the soil microorganisms responsible for these conversions.

There are also numerous sources of commercial fertilizers that supply nitrogen, phosphorus, and potassium, though it is preferable to use organic fertilizers, such as compost and manures. However, if you choose to use a commercial fertilizer, it is important to know how to read the amount of nutrients contained in each bag. The first number on the fertilizer analysis is the percentage of nitrogen; the second number is phosphorus; and the third number is the potassium content. A fertilizer that has a 10-20-10 analysis contains twice as much of each of the nutrients as a 5-10-5. How much of each nutrient you need depends on your soil test results and the plants you are fertilizing.

As was mentioned before, nitrogen stimulates vegetative growth while phosphorus stimulates flowering.

Soil Test Reading	What to Do
High ph	Your soil is alkaline. To lower ph, add elemental sulfur, gypsum, or cottonseed meal. Sulfur can take several months to lower your soil's ph, as it must first convert to sulfuric acid with the help of the soil's bacteria.
Low ph	Your soil is too acidic. Add lime or wood ashes.
Low nitrogen	Add manure, horn or hoof meal, cottonseed meal, fish meal, or dried blood.
High nitrogen	Your soil may be over-fertilized. Water the soil frequently and don't add any fertilizer.
Low phosphorus	Add cottonseed meal, bonemeal, fish meal, rock phosphate, dried blood, or wood ashes.
High phosphorous	Your soil may be over-fertilized. Avoid adding phosphorous-rich materials and grow lots of plants to use up the excess.
Low potassium	Add potash, wood ashes, manure, dried seaweed, fish meal, or cottonseed meal.
High potassium	Continue to fertilize with nitrogen and phosphorous-rich soil additions, but avoid potassium-rich fertilizers for at least two years.
Poor drainage or too much drainage	If your soil is a heavy, clay-like consistency, it won't drain well. If it's too sandy, it won't absorb nutrients as it should. Mix in peat moss or compost to achieve a better texture.

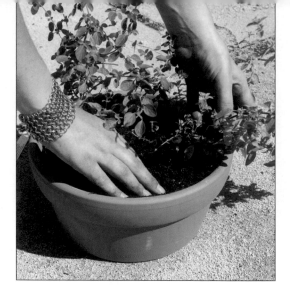

For potted plants, you can apply fertilizer around the edge of the pot if needed, but try to avoid direct contact between the plant's roots, leaves, or stem, and the fertilizer.

Too much nitrogen can inhibit flowering and fruit production. For many flowers and vegetables, a fertilizer higher in phosphorus than nitrogen is preferred, such as a 5-10-5. For lawns, nitrogen is usually required in greater amounts, so a fertilizer with a greater amount of nitrogen is more beneficial.

Fertilizer Application

Commercial fertilizers are normally applied as a dry, granular material or mixed with water and poured onto the garden. If using granular materials, avoid spilling on sidewalks and driveways because these materials are water soluble and can cause pollution problems if rinsed into storm sewers. Granular fertilizers are a type of salt, and if applied too heavily, they have the capability of burning the plants. If using a liquid fertilizer, apply directly to or around the base of each plant and try to contain it within the garden only.

In order to decrease the potential for pollution and to gain the greatest benefits from fertilizer, whether it's a commercial variety, compost, or other organic materials, apply it when the plants have the greatest need for the nutrients. Plants that are not actively growing do not have a high requirement for nutrients; thus, nutrients applied to dormant plants, or plants growing slowly due to cool temperatures, are more likely to be wasted. While light applications of nitrogen may be recommended for lawns in the fall, generally, nitrogen fertilizers should not be applied to most plants in the fall in regions of the country that experience cold winters. Since nitrogen encourages vegetative growth, if it is applied in the fall it may reduce the plant's ability to harden properly for winter.

In some gardens, you can reduce fertilizer use by applying it around the individual plants rather than broadcasting it across the entire garden. Much of the phosphorus in fertilizer becomes unavailable to the plants once spread on the soil. For better plant uptake, apply the fertilizer in a band near the plant. Do not apply directly to the plant or in contact with the roots, as it may burn and damage the plant and its root system.

A Cheap Way to Fertilize

If you are looking to save money while still providing your lawn and garden with extra nutrients, you can do so by simply mowing your lawn on a regular basis and leaving the grass clippings to decompose on the lawn, or spreading them around your garden to decompose into the soil. Annually, this will provide nutrients equivalent to one or two fertilizer applications and it is a completely organic means of boosting a soil's nutrient content.

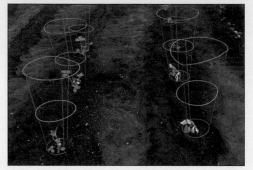

The fertilizer in this garden has only been applied to the garden rows.

Rules of Thumb for Proper Fertilizer Use

It is best to apply fertilizer before or at the time of planting. Fertilizers can either be spread over a large area or confined to garden rows, depending on the condition of your soil and the types of plants you will be growing. After spreading, till the fertilizer into the soil about 3 to 4 inches deep. Only spread about one half of the fertilizer this way and then dispatch the rest 3 inches to the sides of each row and also a little below each seed or established plant. This method, minus the spreader, is used when applying fertilizer to specific rows or plants by hand.

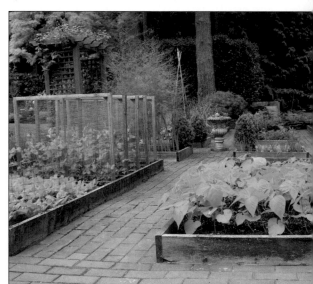

Composting in Your Backyard

Composting is nature's own way of recycling yard and household wastes by converting them into valuable fertilizer, soil organic matter, and a source of plant nutrients. The result of this controlled decomposition of organic matter—a dark, crumbly, earthy-smelling material—works wonders on all kinds of soil by providing vital nutrients and contributing to good aeration and moisture-holding capacity, to help plants grow and look better.

Composting can be as simple or as involved as you would like, depending on how much yard waste you have, how fast you want results, and the effort you are willing to invest. Since all organic matter eventually decomposes, composting speeds up the process by providing an ideal environment for bacteria and other decomposing microorganisms. The composting season coincides with the growing season, when conditions are favorable for plant growth, so those same conditions work well for biological activity in the compost pile. However, since compost generates heat, the process may continue later into the fall or winter. The final product—called humus or compost—looks and feels like fertile garden soil.

Compost Preparation

While a multitude of organisms, fungi, and bacteria is involved in the overall process, there are four basic ingredients for composting: nitrogen, carbon, water, and air.

A wide range of materials may be composted because anything that was once alive will naturally decompose. The starting materials for composting, commonly referred to as feed stocks, include leaves, grass clippings, straw, vegetable and fruit scraps, coffee grounds, livestock manure, sawdust, and shredded paper. However, some materials that should always be avoided include diseased plants, dead animals, noxious weeds, meat scraps that may attract animals, and dog or cat manure, which can carry disease. Since adding kitchen wastes to compost may attract flies and insects, make a hole in the center of your pile and bury the waste.

Most of your household food waste can be composted. Avoid composting meat scraps, dairy products, grains, or very greasy foods.

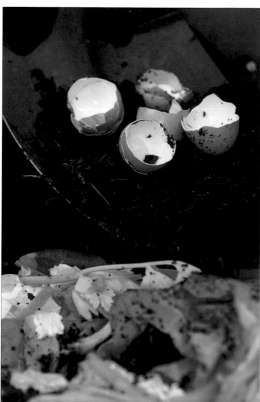

Common Composting Materials

Cardboard	Vegetable scraps
Coffee grounds	Weeds without seed heads
Corn cobs	Wood chips
Corn stalks	Woody brush
Food scraps	
Grass clippings	**Avoid using:**
Hedge trimmings	Bread and grains
Livestock manure	Cooking oil
Newspapers	Dairy products
Plant stalks	Dead animals
Pine needles	Diseased plant material
Old potting soil	Dog or cat manure
Sawdust	Grease or oily foods
Seaweed	Meat or fish scraps
Shredded paper	Noxious or invasive
Straw	weeds
Tea bags	Weeds with seed heads
Telephone books	
Tree leaves and twigs	

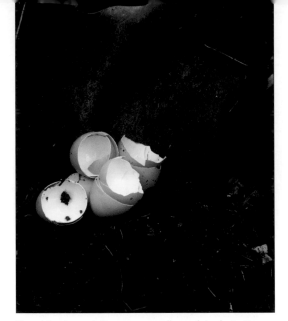

The calcium in eggshells encourages cell growth in plants. You can even mix crushed eggshells directly into the soil around tomatoes, zucchini, squash, and peppers to prevent blossom end rot. Eggshells also help deter slugs, snails, and cutworm.

For best results, you will want an even ratio of green, or wet, material, which is high in nitrogen, and brown, or dry, material, which is high in carbon. Simply layer or mix landscape trimmings and grass clippings, for example, with dried leaves and twigs in a pile or enclosure. If there is not a good supply of nitrogen-rich material, a handful of general lawn fertilizer or barnyard manure will help even out the ratio.

Though rain provides the moisture, you may need to water the pile in dry weather or cover it in extremely wet weather. The microorganisms in the compost pile function best when the materials are as damp as a wrung-out sponge—not saturated with water. A moisture content of 40 to 60 percent is preferable. To test for adequate moisture, reach into your compost pile, grab a handful of material, and squeeze it. If a few drops of water come out, it probably has enough moisture. If it doesn't, add water by putting a hose into the pile so that you aren't just wetting the top, or, better yet, water the pile as you turn it.

Air is the only part that cannot be added in excess. For proper aeration, you'll need to punch holes in the pile so it has many air passages. The air in the pile is usually used up faster than the moisture, and extremes of sun or rain can adversely affect this balance, so the materials must be turned or mixed up often with a pitchfork, rake, or other garden tool to add air that will sustain high temperatures, control odor, and yield faster decomposition.

Over time, you'll see that the microorganisms, which are small forms of plant and animal life, will break down the organic material. Bacteria are the first to break down plant tissue and are the most numerous and effective compost makers in your compost pile. Fungi and protozoans soon join the bacteria and, later in the cycle, centipedes, millipedes, beetles, sow bugs, nematodes, worms, and numerous others complete the composting process. With the right ingredients and favorable weather conditions, you can have a finished compost pile in a few weeks.

How to Make Your Own Backyard Composting Heap

1. Choose a level, well-drained site, preferably near your garden.
2. Decide whether you will be using a bin after checking on any local or state regulations for composting in urban areas, as some communities require rodent-proof bins. There are numerous styles of compost bins available, depending on your needs, ranging from a moveable bin formed by wire mesh to a more substantial wooden structure consisting of several compartments. You can also easily make your own bin using chicken wire or scrap wood. While a bin will help contain the pile, it is not absolutely necessary, as you can build your pile directly on the ground. To help with aeration, you may want to place some woody material on the ground where you will build your pile.
3. Ensure that your pile will have a minimum dimension of 3 feet all around, but is no taller than 5 feet, as not enough air will reach the microorganisms at the center if it is too tall. If you don't have this amount at one time, simply stockpile your materials until a sufficient quantity is available for proper mixing. When composting is completed, the total volume of the original materials is usually reduced by 30 to 50 percent.
4. Build your pile by using either alternating equal layers of high-carbon and high-nitrogen material or by mixing equal parts of both together and then heaping it into a pile. If you choose to alternate layers, make each layer 2 to 4 inches thick. Some composters find that mixing the two together is more effective than layering. Adding a few shovels of soil will also help get the pile off to a good start because soil adds commonly found, decomposing organisms to your compost.

As your compost begins to break down, you may notice gases escaping from the pile.

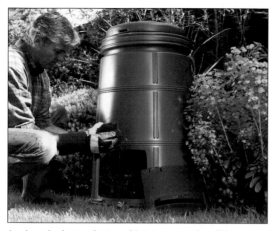

Any large bucket can be turned into a compost barrel. You can cut out a piece of the barrel for easy access to the compost, as shown here, or simply access the compost through the lid. Drilling holes in the sides and lids of the bucket will increase air circulation and speed up the process. Leave your bucket in the sun and shake it, roll it, or stir the contents regularly.

5. Keep the pile moist but not wet. Soggy piles encourage the growth of organisms that can live without oxygen and cause unpleasant odors.
6. Punch holes in the sides of the pile for aeration. The pile will heat up and then begin to cool. The most efficient decomposing bacteria thrive in temperatures between 110 and 160°F. You can track this with a compost thermometer, or you can simply reach into the pile to determine if it is uncomfortably hot to the touch. At these temperatures, the pile kills most weed seeds and plant diseases. However, studies have shown that compost produced at these temperatures has less ability to suppress diseases in the soil, since these temperatures may kill some of the beneficial bacteria necessary to suppress disease.
8. Check your bin regularly during the composting season to assure optimum moisture and aeration are present in the material being composted.
9. Move materials from the center to the outside of the pile and vice versa. Turn every day or two and you should get compost in less than four weeks. Turning every other week will make compost in one to three months. Finished compost will smell sweet and be cool and crumbly to the touch.

Other Types of Composting

Cold or Slow Composting

Cold composting allows you to just pile organic material on the ground or in a bin. This method requires no maintenance, but it will take several months to a year or more for the pile to decompose, though the process is faster in warmer climates than in cooler areas. Cold

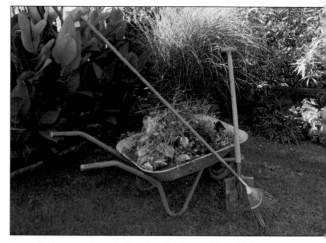

Grass clippings, weeds, and other plant debris can all be added to your compost pile.

composting works well if you are short on time needed to tend to the compost pile at least every other day, have little yard waste, and are not in a hurry to use the compost.

For this method, add yard waste as it accumulates. To speed up the process, shred or chop the materials by running over small piles of trimmings with your lawn mower, because the more surface area the microorganisms have to feed on, the faster the materials will break down.

Cold composting has been shown to be better at suppressing soil-borne diseases than hot composting and also leaves more non-decomposed bits of material, which can be screened out if desired. However, because of the low temperatures achieved during decomposition, weed seeds and disease-causing organisms may not be destroyed.

Vermicomposting

Vermicomposting uses worms to compost. This takes up very little space and can be done year-round in a basement or garage. It is an excellent way to dispose of kitchen wastes.

Here's how to make your own vermicomposting pile:
1. Obtain a plastic storage bin. One bin measuring 1 foot by 2 feet by 3½ feet will be enough to meet the needs of a family of six.
2. Drill 8 to 10 holes about ¼ inch in diameter in the bottom of the bin for drainage.
3. Line the bottom of the bin with a fine nylon mesh to keep the worms from escaping.
4. Put a tray underneath to catch the drainage.
5. Rip newspaper into pieces to use as bedding and pour water over the strips until they are thoroughly moist. Place these shredded bits on one side of your bin. Do not let them dry out.
6. Add worms to your bin. It's best to have about two pounds of worms (roughly 2,000 worms) per one pound of food waste. You may want to start with less food waste and increase the amount as your

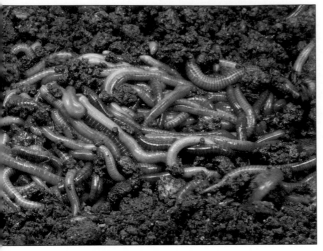

Worms will filter your organic waste through their systems and turn it into nutrient-rich humus.

worm population grows. Redworms are recommended for best composting, but other species can be used. Redworms are the common, small worms found in most gardens and lawns. You can collect them from under a pile of mulch or order them from a garden catalog.

7. Provide worms with food wastes such as vegetable peelings. Do not add fat or meat products. Limit their feed, as too much at once may cause the material to rot.

8. Keep the bin in a dark location away from extreme temperatures.

9. Wait about three months and you'll see that the worms have changed the bedding and food wastes into compost. At this time, open your bin in a bright light and the worms will burrow into the bedding. Add fresh bedding and more food to the other side of the bin. The worms should migrate to the new food supply.

10. Scoop out the finished compost and apply to your plants or save to use in the spring.

Uses for Compost

Compost contains nutrients, but it is not a substitute for fertilizers. Compost holds nutrients in the soil until plants can use them, loosens and aerates clay soils, and retains water in sandy soils.

To use as a soil amendment, mix 2 to 5 inches of compost into vegetable and flower gardens each year before planting. In a potting mixture, add one part compost to two parts commercial potting soil, or make your own mixture by using equal parts of compost and sand, or Perlite.

As a mulch, spread an inch or two of compost around annual flowers and vegetables, and up to 6 inches around trees and shrubs. Studies have shown that compost used as mulch, or mixed with the top 1-inch layer of soil, can help prevent some plant diseases, including some of those that cause damping of seedlings.

As a top dressing, mix finely sifted compost with sand and sprinkle evenly over lawns.

Common Problems

Composting is not an exact science. Experience will tell you what works best for you. If you notice that nothing is happening, you may need to add more nitrogen, water, or air, chip or grind the materials, or adjust the size of the pile.

If the pile is too hot, you probably have too much nitrogen and need to add additional carbon materials to reduce the heating.

A bad smell may indicate not enough air or too much moisture. Simply turn the pile or add dry materials to the wet pile to get rid of the odor.

Planting Your Garden

Once you've chosen a spot for your garden (as well as the size you want to make your garden bed), and prepared the soil with compost or other fertilizer, it's time to start planting. Seeds are very inexpensive at your local garden center, or you can browse through seed catalogs and order seeds that will do well in your area. Alternately, you can start with bedding plants (or seedlings) available at nurseries and garden centers.

Read the instructions on the back of the seed package or on the plastic tag in your plant pot. You may have to ask experts when to plant the seeds if this information is not stated on the back of the package. Some seeds (such as tomatoes) should be started indoors, in small pots or seed trays, before the last frost, and only transplanted outdoors when the weather warms up. For established plants or seedlings, be sure to plant as directed on the plant tag or consult your local nursery about the best planting times.

Some plugs are biodegradable so that you can insert them directly into the garden bed, rather than having to transplant them.

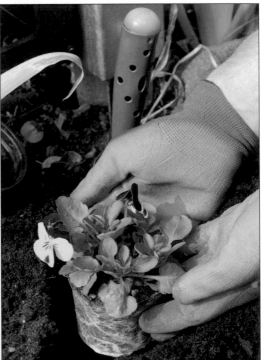

Seedlings

If you live in a cooler region with a shorter growing period, you will want to start some of your plants indoors. To do this, obtain plug flats (trays separated into many small cups or "cells") or make your own small planters by poking holes in the bottom of paper cups. Fill the cups two-thirds full with potting soil or composted soil. Bury the seed at the recommended depth, according to the instructions on the package. Tamp down the soil lightly and water. Keep the seedlings in a warm, well-lit place, such as the kitchen, to encourage germination.

Once the weather begins to warm up and you are fairly certain you won't be getting any more frosts (you can contact your local extension office to find out the last "frost free" date for your area) you can begin to acclimate your seedlings to the great outdoors. First place them in a partially shady spot outdoors that is protected from strong wind. After a couple of days, move them into direct sunlight, and then finally transplant them to the garden.

Recommended plants to start as seedlings

Crop [s] small seed [l] large seed (planting cell size)	Weeks before transplanting	Seed planting depth (inches)	Transplant spacing	
			Within row	between row
Broccoli [s]	(1)	4-6	1/4-1/2	8-10" 18-24"
Cabbage [s]	(1)	4-6	1/4-1/2	18-24" 30"
Cucumber [l]	(2)	4-5	1/2	2' 5-6'
Eggplant [s]	(2)	8	1/4	18" 18-24"
Herbs [s]	(1)	4	1/4	4-6" 12-18"
Lettuce [s]	(2)	4-5	1/4	12" 12"
Melon [l]	(3)	4-5	1/4	2-3' 6'
Onion [s]	(*)	8	1/4	4" 12"
Pepper [s]	(2)	8	1/4	12-18" 2-3'
Pumpkin [l]	(3)	2-4	1	5-6' 5-6'
Summer squash [l]	(3)	2-4	3/4-1	18" 2-3'
Tomato [s]	(3)	8	1/4	18"-24" 3'
Watermelon [l]	(3)	4-5	1/2-3/4	3-4' 3-4'
Winter squash [l]	(3)	2-4	1	3-4' 4-5'

Seeds can be sprouted and eaten on sandwiches, salads, or stirfries any time of the year. They are delicious and full of vitamins and proteins. Mung bean, soybean, alfalfa, wheat, corn, barley, mustard, clover, chickpeas, radish, and lentils all make good sprouts. Find seeds for sprouting from your local health food store or use dried peas, beans, or lentils from the grocery store. Never use seeds intended for planting unless you've harvested the seeds yourself—commercially available planting seeds are often treated with a poisonous chemical fungicide.

To grow sprouts, thoroughly rinse and strain the seeds, then soak overnight in cool water. You'll need about four times as much water as you have seeds. Drain the seeds and place them in a wide-mouthed bowl or on a cookie sheet with a lip. Sprinkle with water to keep the seeds slightly damp. You may wish to place the seeds on a damp paper towel to better hold in the moisture. Keep the seeds at 60 to 80°F and rinse twice a day, returning them to their bowl or tray after. Once sprouts are 1 to 1 ½ inches long (generally after 3 to 5 days), they are ready to eat.

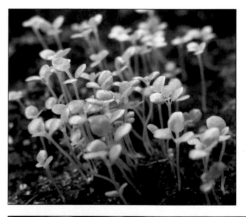

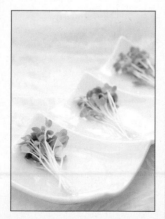

Radish sprouts are delicious on their own or in sandwiches or salads

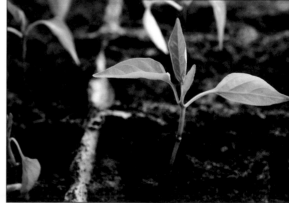

You can grow seedlings in any wood, metal, or plastic container that is at least 3 inches deep. Egg cartons work very well if you don't have access to regular plug flats. Just punch holes in the bottom for drainage.

How to Best Water Your Soil

After your seeds or seedlings are planted, the next step is to water your soil. Different soil types have different watering needs. You don't need to be a soil scientist to know how to water your soil properly. Here are some tips that can help to make your soil moist and primed for gardening:

1. Loosen the soil around plants so water and nutrients can be quickly absorbed.

2. Use a 1- to 2-inch protective layer of mulch on the soil surface above the root area. Cultivating and mulching help reduce evaporation and soil erosion.

3. Water your plants at the appropriate time of day. Early morning or night is the best time for watering, as evaporation is less likely to occur at these times. Do not water your plants when it is extremely windy outside. Wind will prevent the water from reaching the soil where you want it to go.

A gentle spray will soak into the soil without damaging the plants. The thin layer of mulch will help to keep the water from evaporating too quickly.

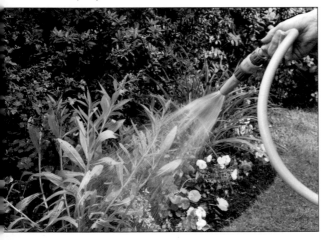

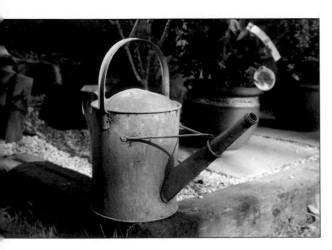

Types of Soil and Their Water Retention

Knowing the type of soil you are planting in will help you best understand how to properly water and grow your garden plants. Three common types of soil and their various abilities to absorb water are listed below:

Clay soil: In order to make this type of soil more loamy, add organic materials, such as compost, peat moss, and well-rotted leaves, in the spring before growing and also in the fall after harvesting your vegetables and fruits. Adding these organic materials allows this type of soil to hold more nutrients for healthy plant growth. Till or spade to help loosen the soil.

Since clay soil absorbs water very slowly, water only as fast as the soil can absorb the water.

Sandy soil: As with clay soil, adding organic materials in the spring and fall will help supplement the sandy soil and promote better plant growth and water absorption.

Left on its own (with no added organic matter) the water will run through sandy soil so quickly that plants won't be able to absorb it through their roots and will fail to grow and thrive.

Loam soil: This is the best kind of soil for gardening. It's a combination of sand, silt, and clay. Loamy soil is fertile, deep, easily crumbles, and is made up of organic matter. It will help promote the growth of quality fruits and vegetables, as well as flowers and other plants.

Loam absorbs water readily and stores it for plants to use. Water as frequently as the soil needs to maintain its moisture and to promote plant growth.

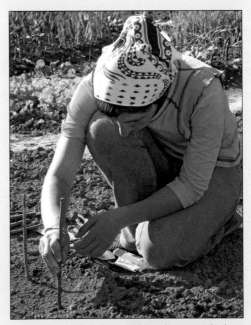

Sandy soil is usually lighter in color and won't easily clump together in your hands. It needs organic matter and plenty of water to be suitable for growing.

A good old-fashioned watering can is great for small gardens and potted plants.

Conserving Water

Wise use of water for hydrating your garden and lawn not only helps protect the environment, but saves money and also provides optimum growing
conditions for your plants. There are simple ways of reducing the amount of
water used for irrigation, such as growing xeriphytic species (plants that are
adapted to dry conditions), mulching, adding water-retaining organic matter
to the soil, and installing windbreaks and fences to slow winds and reduce
evapotranspiration.

You can conserve water by watering your plants and lawn in the early
morning, before the sun is too intense. This helps reduce the amount of water
lost due to evaporation. Furthermore, installing rain gutters and collecting
water from downspouts—in collection bins such as rain barrels—also helps
reduce water use.

How Plants Use Water

Water is a critical component of photosynthesis, the process by which plants
manufacture their own food from carbon dioxide and water in the presence
of light. Water is one of the many factors that can limit plant growth. Other
important factors include nutrients, temperature, and amount and duration
of sunlight.

Plants take in carbon dioxide through their stomata—microscopic openings
on the undersides of the leaves. The stomata are also the place where water
is lost, in a process called transpiration. Transpiration, along with evaporation
from the soil's surface, accounts for most of the moisture lost from the soil and
subsequently from the plants.

When there is a lack of water in the plant tissue, the stomata close to try
to limit excessive water loss. If the tissues lose too much water, the plant will
wilt. Plants adapted to dry conditions have developed certain characteristics
that support numerous mechanisms for reducing water loss—they typically
have narrow, hairy leaves and thick, fleshy stems and leaves. Pines, hemlocks,
and junipers are also well-adapted to survive extended periods of dry conditions—an environmental factor they encounter each winter when the frozen
soil prevents the uptake of water. Cacti, which have thick stems and leaves
reduced to spines, are the best example of plants well-adapted to extremely
dry environments.

Even very dry areas can be made
attractive with tasteful placement of
grasses, yarrow, and similar plants.

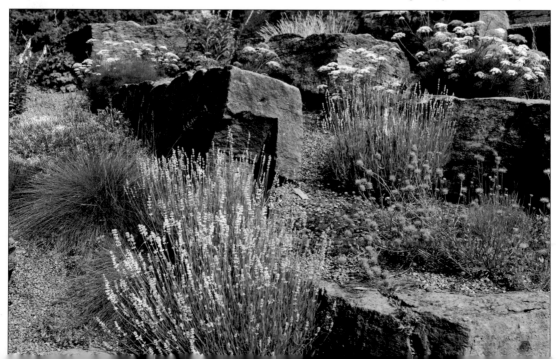

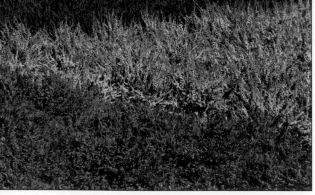

Heath flowers are well-adapted to dry environments and make a very attractive ground cover.

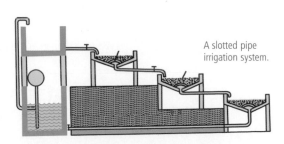

A slotted pipe irrigation system.

Choosing Plants for Low Water Use

You are not limited to cacti, succulents, or narrow-leafed evergreens when selecting plants adapted to low water requirements. Many plants growing in humid environments are well-adapted to low levels of soil moisture. Numerous plants found growing in coastal or mountainous regions have developed mechanisms for dealing with extremely sandy, excessively well-drained soils or rocky, cold soils in which moisture is limited for months at a time. Try alfalfa, aloe, artichokes, asparagus, blue hibiscus, chives, columbine, eucalyptus, garlic, germander, lamb's ear, lavender, ornamental grasses, prairie turnip, rosemary, sage, sedum, shrub roses, thyme, yarrow, yucca, and verbena.

Installing Irrigation Systems

An irrigation system can be easy to install, and there are many different products available for home irrigation systems. The simplest system consists of a soaker hose that is laid out around the plants and connected to an outdoor spigot. No installation is required, and the hose can be moved as needed to water the entire garden.

A slightly more sophisticated system is a slotted pipe system. Here are the steps needed in order to install this type of irrigation system in your garden:

1. Sketch the layout of your garden so you know what materials you will need. If you intend to water a vegetable garden, you may want one pipe next to every row or one pipe between every two rows.
2. Depending on the layout and type of garden, purchase the required lengths of pipe. You will need a length of solid pipe for the width of your garden, and perforated pipes that are the length of your lateral rows (and remember to buy one pipe for each row or two).
3. Measure the distances between rows and cut the solid pipe to the proper lengths.
4. Place T-connectors between the pieces of solid pipe.
5. In the approximate center of the solid pipe, place a T-connector to which a hose connector will be fitted.

Trickle Irrigation Systems

Trickle irrigation and drip irrigation systems help reduce water use and successfully meet the needs of most plants. With these systems, very small amounts of water are supplied to the bases of the plants. Since the water is applied directly to the soil—rather than onto the plant—evaporation from the leaf surfaces is reduced, thus allowing more water to effectively reach the roots. In these types of systems, the water is not wasted by being spread all over the garden; rather, it is applied directly to the appropriate source.

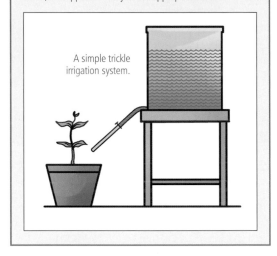

A simple trickle irrigation system.

6. Cut the perforated pipe to the length of the rows.
7. Attach the perforated pipes to the T-connectors so that the perforations are facing downward. Cap the end of the pipe.
8. Connect a garden hose to the hose connector on the solid pipe. Adjust the pressure of the water flowing from the spigot until the water slowly emerges from each of the perforated pipes.

Rain Barrels

Another very efficient and easy way to conserve water—and save money—is to buy or make your own rain barrel. A rain barrel is a large bin that is placed beneath a downspout and that collects rainwater runoff from a roof. The water collected in the rain barrel can then be routed through a garden hose and used to water your garden and lawn.

Rain barrels can be purchased from specialty home and garden stores, but a simple rain barrel is also quite easy to make. Here are simple instructions on how to make your own rain barrel.

Instructions

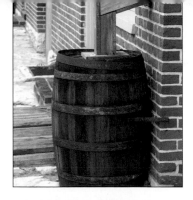

1. Obtain a suitable plastic barrel, a large plastic trashcan with a lid, or a wooden barrel (e.g., a wine barrel) that has not been stored dry for too many seasons, since it can start to leak. Good places to find plastic barrels include suppliers of dairy products, metal plating companies, and bulk food suppliers. Just be sure that nothing toxic or harmful to plants and animals (including you!) was stored in the barrel. A wine barrel can be obtained through a winery. Barrels that allow less light to penetrate through will eliminate the risk of algae growth and the establishment of other microorganisms.

2. Once you have your barrel, find a location for it under or near one of your home's downspouts. In order for the barrel to fit, you will probably need to shorten the downspout by a few feet. You can do this by removing the screws or rivets located at a joint of the downspout, or by simply cutting off the last few feet with a hacksaw or other cutter. If your barrel will not be able to fit underneath the downspout, you can purchase a flexible downspout at your local home improvement store. These flexible tubes will direct the water from the downspout into the barrel. An alternative, and aesthetically appealing, option is to use a rain chain—a large, metal chain that water can run down.

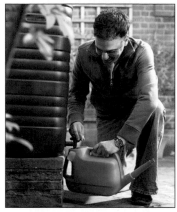

3. Create a level, stable platform for your rain barrel to sit on by raking the dirt under the spout, adding gravel to smooth out lawn bumps, or using bricks or concrete blocks to make a low platform. Keep in mind that a barrel full of water is very heavy, so if you decide to build a platform, make sure it is sturdy enough to hold such heavy weight.

4. If your barrel has a solid top, you'll need to make a good-sized hole in it for the downspout to pour into. You can do this using a hole-cutting attachment on a power drill or by drilling a series of smaller holes close together and then cutting out the remaining material with a hacksaw blade or a scroll saw.

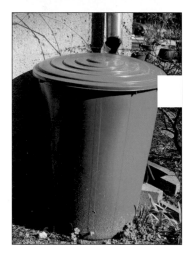

5. Mosquitoes are drawn to standing water, so to reduce the risk of breeding these insects, and to also keep debris from entering the barrel, fasten a piece of window screen to the underside of the top so it covers the entire hole.

6. Next, drill a hole so the hose bib you'll attach to the side of the barrel fits snugly. Place the hose bib as close to the bottom of the barrel as possible, so you'll be able to gain access to the maximum amount of water in the barrel. Attach the hose bib using screws driven into the barrel. You'll probably need to apply some caulking, plumber's putty, or silicon sealant around the joint between the barrel and the hose bib to prevent leaks, depending on the type of hardware you're using and how snug it fits in the hole you drilled.

7. Attach a second hose bib to the side of the barrel near the top, to act as an overflow drain. Attach a short piece of garden hose to this hose bib and route it to a flowerbed, lawn, or another nearby area that won't be damaged by some running water if your barrel gets too full (or, if you want to have a second rain barrel for excess water, you can attach it to another hose bib on a second barrel. If you are chaining multiple barrels together, one of them should have a hose attached to drain off the overflow.

8. Attach a garden hose to the lower hose bib and open the valve to allow collected rain water to flow to your plants. The lower bib can also be used to connect multiple rain barrels together for a larger water reservoir.

9. Consider using a drip irrigation system in conjunction with the rain barrels. Rain barrels don't achieve anything near the pressure of city water supplies, so you won't be able to use microsprinkler attachments, and you will need to use button attachments that are intended to deliver four times the amount of city-supplied water you need.

10. Now, wait for a heavy downpour and start enjoying your rain barrel!

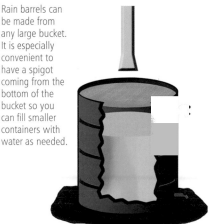

Rain barrels can be made from any large bucket. It is especially convenient to have a spigot coming from the bottom of the bucket so you can fill smaller containers with water as needed.

Mary Maddox and her husband and children maintain a full vegetable garden and raise chickens, ducks, turkeys, and a goose on less than half an acre of land. They describe their experiences and share tips on their blog, "The Yardstead," www.yardstead.com.

My husband, children, and I live in a small town in North Florida. Like most of our neighbors we live on a little less than ½ acre lot. We dream of becoming homesteaders on 10 to 15 acres but until that dream becomes reality, we do what we can on our small plot. We currently maintain a 30 ft. x 30 ft. vegetable garden, and keep chickens, ducks, turkeys, and a goose. These birds only require 3-4 sq. ft. per bird and are easy to care for in an appropriate size pen.

We keep between 10 and 20 chickens most of the time in a 72 sq. ft. pen, with an adjoining 200 sq. ft. pen for a few ducks, turkeys, and a goose. We supply our family, friends, and neighbors with fresh eggs year round and put a few chickens in the freezer as well. We recently were given a rooster by one of our neighbors and our hens have hatched their first babies this spring.

We try to keep something growing in the garden all year round. Each year we are able to grow enough squash and zucchini to eat fresh all spring and summer and put enough up in the freezer to last through the winter. We also grow enough onions and garlic most years to meet all our needs and share with our friends and family. We dabble in other vegetables and grow a variety of gourds on our fence line each year.

We have landscaped the yard with mostly edible plants and trees. Our backyard shade is provided by a pecan, mulberry, persimmon, and other trees. We have chosen some native shrubs, like the pineapple guava, that also produces edible flowers and fruit. We keep several dwarf citrus as potted plants that can be moved in and out of the house depending on our winter temperatures each year. Last fall we planted a few small canes of sugar cane. These clumps of sugar cane will be mostly for our children to enjoy in late summer each year.

We try to garden and care for our animals and yard with an emphasis on permaculture and we follow organic practices as much as possible. All of the yard waste and food waste we produce go first to the chickens and other birds who love to eat table scraps as well as grass

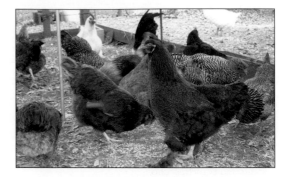

How to Make a Simple Rain Barrel

Things You'll Need

- A clean, plastic barrel, tall trash can with lid, or a wooden barrel that does not leak—a 55 gallon plastic drum or barrel does a very good job at holding rainwater
- Two hose bibs (a valve with a fitting for a garden hose on one end and a flange with a short pipe sticking out of it at the other end)
- Garden hose
- Plywood and paint (if your barrel doesn't already have a top)
- Window screen
- Wood screws
- Vegetable oil
- A drill
- A hacksaw
- A screwdriver

clippings and the like. They eat what they like and the leftovers along with the rich droppings are raked out occasionally and added to the compost pile. This provides us a constant supply of rich compost, which is the fertilizer we use in the garden. We also let some chickens roam the garden after the plants have grown to an 8-10 in. height. They do an excellent job of keeping the garden pest free by eating every bug they can find.

We love teaching our children about gardening and caring for animals and we all enjoy a healthy sense of self-reliance. We share our produce as much as possible and also try to share as much knowledge as possible with anyone who is interested.

Things to Consider

- Put some water in the barrel from a garden hose once everything is in place and any sealants have had time to thoroughly dry. The first good downpour is *not* the time to find out there's a leak in your barrel.
- If you don't own the property on which you are thinking of installing a rain barrel, be sure to get permission before altering the downspouts.
- If your barrel doesn't already have a solid top, cover it securely with a circle of painted plywood, an old trashcan lid screwed to the walls of the barrel, or a heavy tarp secured over the top of the barrel with bungee cords. This will protect children and small animals from falling into the barrel and drowning.
- As stated before, stagnant water is an excellent breeding ground for mosquitoes, so it would be a good idea to take additional steps to keep them out of your barrel by sealing all the openings into the barrel with caulk or putty. You might also consider adding enough non-toxic oil (such as vegetable cooking oil) to the barrel to form a film on top of the water that will prevent mosquito larvae from hatching.

  Always double check to make sure the barrel you're using (particularly if it is from a food distribution center or other recycled source) did not contain pesticides, industrial chemicals, weed killers, or other toxins or biological materials that could be harmful to you, your plants, or the environment. If you are concerned about this, it is best to purchase a new barrel or trashcan so there is no doubt about its safety.

Mulching in Your Garden and Yard

Mulching is one of the simplest and most beneficial practices you can use in your garden. Mulch is simply a protective layer of material that is spread on top of the soil to enrich the soil, prevent weed growth, and help provide a better growing environment for your garden plants and flowers.

Mulches can either be organic—such as grass clippings, bark chips, compost, ground corncobs, chopped cornstalks, leaves, manure, newspaper, peanut shells, peat moss, pine needles, sawdust, straw, and wood shavings—or inorganic—such as stones, brick chips, and plastic. Both organic and inorganic mulches have numerous benefits, including:

1. Protecting the soil from erosion
2. Reducing compaction from the impact of heavy rains
3. Conserving moisture, thus reducing the need for frequent watering
4. Maintaining a more even soil temperature
5. Preventing weed growth
6. Keeping fruits and vegetables clean
7. Keeping feet clean and allowing access to the garden even when it's damp
8. Providing a "finished" look to the garden

Organic mulches also have the benefit of improving the condition of the soil. As these mulches slowly decompose, they provide organic matter to help keep the soil loose. This improves root growth, increases the infiltration of water, improves the water-holding capacity of the soil, provides a source of plant nutrients, and establishes an ideal environment for earthworms and other beneficial soil organisms.

While inorganic mulches have their place in certain landscapes, they lack the soil-improving properties of organic mulches. Inorganic mulches, because of their permanence, may be difficult to remove if you decide to change your garden plans at a later date.

Wood chips or shavings are some of the most common forms of mulch.

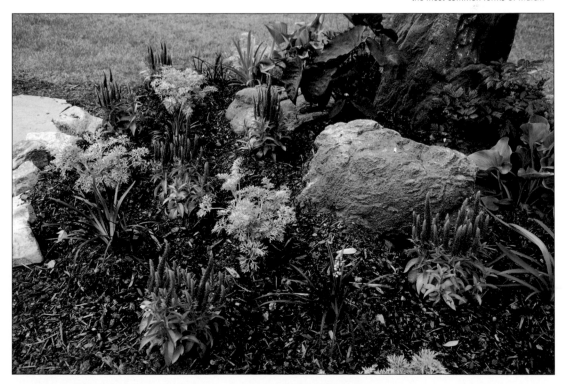

Where to Find Mulch Materials

You can find mulch materials right in your own backyard. They include:

1. Lawn clippings. They make an excellent mulch in the vegetable garden if spread immediately to avoid heating and rotting. The fine texture allows them to be spread easily, even around small plants.
2. Newspaper. As a mulch, newspaper works especially well to control weeds. Save your own newspapers and only use the text pages, or those with black ink, as color dyes may be harmful to soil microflora and fauna if composted and used. Use three or four sheets together, anchored with grass clippings or other mulch material to prevent them from blowing away.
3. Leaves. Leaf mold, or the decomposed remains of leaves, gives the forest floor its absorbent, spongy structure. Collect leaves in the fall and chop with a lawnmower or shredder. Compost leaves over winter, as some studies have indicated that freshly chopped leaves may inhibit the growth of certain crops.
4. Compost. The mixture makes wonderful mulch—if you have a large supply—as it not only improves the soil structure but also provides an excellent source of plant nutrients.
5. Bark chips and composted bark mulch. These materials are available at garden centers and are

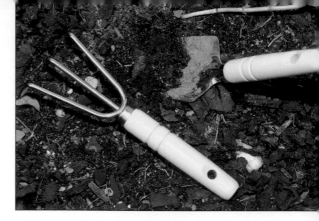

A trowel and hand fork are helpful for mulching small areas around and between plants.

sometimes used with landscape fabric or plastic that is spread atop the soil and beneath the mulch to provide additional protection against weeds. However, the barrier between the soil and the mulch also prevents any improvement in the soil condition and makes planting additional plants more difficult. Without the barrier, bark mulch makes a neat finish to the garden bed and will eventually improve the condition of the soil. It may last for one to three years or more, depending on the size of the chips or how well-composted the bark mulch is. Smaller chips are easier to spread, especially around small plants.

6. Hay and straw. These work well in the vegetable garden, although they may harbor weed seeds.
7. Seaweed mulch, ground corncobs, and pine needles. Depending on where you live, these materials may be readily available and can also be used as mulch. However, pine needles tend to increase the acidity of the soil, so they work best around acid-loving plants, such as rhododendrons and blueberries.

When choosing a mulch material, think of your primary objective. Newspaper and grass clippings are great for weed control, while bark mulch gives a perfect, finishing touch to a front-yard perennial garden. If you're looking for a cheap solution, consider using materials found in your own yard or see if your community offers chipped wood or compost to its residents.

If you want the mulch to stay in place for several years around shrubs, for example, you might want to consider using inorganic mulches. While they will not provide organic matter to the soil, they will be more or less permanent.

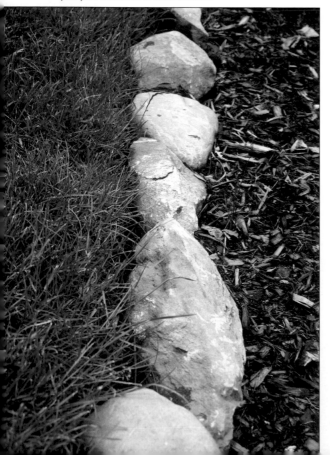

Mulch can be neat and attractive, especially if kept from spilling into your yard with a row or circle of stones.

Common Organic Mulching Materials

Bark chips	Chopped cornstalks
Compost	Grass clippings
Ground corncobs	Hay
Leaves	Manure
Newspaper	Peanut shells
Peat moss	Pine needles
Sawdust	Straw
Wood shavings	

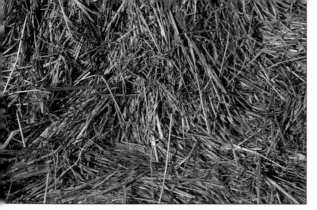

Hay and straw make excellent, inexpensive mulch.

When to Apply Mulch

Time of application depends on what you hope to achieve by mulching. Mulches, by providing an insulating barrier between the soil and the air, moderate the soil temperature. This means that a mulched soil in the summer will be cooler than an adjacent, unmulched soil; while in the winter, the mulched soil may not freeze as deeply. However, since mulch acts as an insulating layer, mulched soils tend to warm up more slowly in the spring and cool down more slowly in the fall than unmulched soils.

If you are using mulches in your vegetable or flower garden, it is best to apply or add additional mulch after the soil has warmed up in the spring. Organic mulches reduce the soil temperature by 8 to 10°F during the summer, so if they are applied to cold garden soils, the soil will warm up more slowly and plant maturity will be delayed.

Mulches used to help moderate winter temperatures can be applied late in the fall after the ground has frozen, but before the coldest temperatures arrive. Applying mulches before the ground has frozen may attract rodents looking for a warm over-wintering site. Delayed applications of mulch should prevent this problem.

Mulches used to protect plants over the winter should be composed of loose material, such as straw, hay, or pine boughs that will help insulate the plants without compacting under the weight of snow and ice. One of the benefits from winter applications of mulch is the reduction in the freezing and thawing of the soil in the late winter and early spring. These repeated cycles of freezing at night and then thawing in the warmth of the sun cause many small or shallow-rooted plants to be heaved out of the soil. This leaves their root systems exposed and results in injury, or death, of the plant. Mulching helps prevent these rapid fluctuations in soil temperature and reduces the chances of heaving.

How Much Do I Apply?

The amount of mulch to apply to your garden depends on the mulching material used. Spread bark mulch and wood chips 2 to 4 inches deep, keeping it an inch or two away from tree trunks.

Scatter chopped and composted leaves 3 to 4 inches deep. If using dry leaves, apply about 6 inches.

Grass clippings, if spread too thick, tend to compact and rot, becoming quite slimy and smelly. They should be applied 2 to 3 inches deep, and additional layers should be added as clippings decompose. Make sure not to use clippings from lawns treated with herbicides.

Sheets of newspaper should only be ¼ inch thick and covered lightly with grass clippings or other mulch material to anchor them. If other mulch materials are not available, cover the edges of the newspaper with soil.

If using compost, apply 3 to 4 inches deep, as it's an excellent material for enriching the soil.

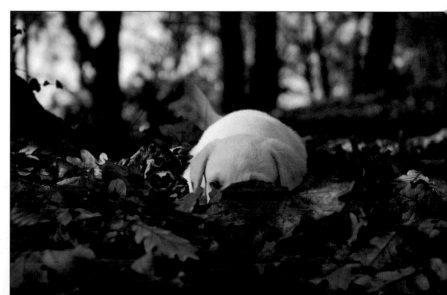

Gather fallen leaves in the fall and compost them or use them in large plastic bags as extra house insulation over the winter. Come spring, the decomposed leaves will be ready for mulch.

Organic Gardening

"Organically grown" food is food grown and processed using no synthetic fertilizers or pesticides. Pesticides derived from natural sources (such as biological pesticides—compost and manure) may be used in producing organically grown food.

Organic gardeners grow the healthiest, highest quality foods and flowers—all without the addition of chemical fertilizers, pesticides, or herbicides. Organic gardening methods are healthier, environmentally friendly, safe for animals and humans, and are typically less expensive, since you are working with natural materials. It is easy to grow and harvest organic foods in your backyard garden and typically, organic gardens are easier to maintain than gardens that rely on chemical and unnatural components to help them grow effectively.

Organic production is not simply the avoidance of conventional chemical inputs, nor is it the substitution of natural inputs for synthetic ones. Organic farmers apply techniques first used thousands of years ago, such as crop rotations and the use of composted animal manures and green manure crops, in ways that are economically sustainable in today's world.

Organic farming entails:

- Use of cover crops, green manures, animal manures, and crop rotations to fertilize the soil, maximize biological activity, and maintain long-term soil health.
- Use of biological control, crop rotations, and other techniques to manage weeds, insects, and diseases.
- An emphasis on biodiversity of the agricultural system and the surrounding environment.
- Reduction of external and off-farm inputs and elimination of synthetic pesticides and fertilizers and other materials, such as hormones and antibiotics.
- A focus on renewable resources, soil and water conservation, and management practices that restore, maintain, and enhance ecological balance.

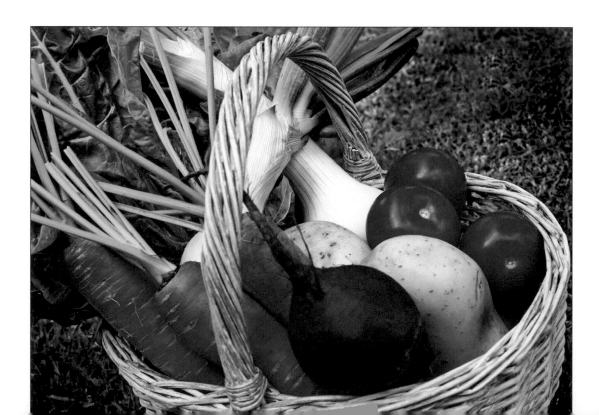

How to Start Your Own Organic Garden

Step One: Choose a Site for Your Garden

1. Think small, at least at first. A small garden takes less work and materials than a large one. If done well, a 4 x 4-foot garden will yield enough vegetables and fruit for you and your family to enjoy.

2. Be careful not to over-plant your garden. You do not want to end up with too many vegetables that will end up over-ripening or rotting in your garden.

3. You can even start a garden in a window box if you are unsure of your time and dedication to a larger bed.

Step Two: Make a Compost Pile

1. Compost is the main ingredient for creating and maintaining rich, fertile soil. You can use most organic materials to make compost that will provide your soil with essential nutrients. To start a compost pile, all you need are fallen leaves, weeds, grass clippings, and other vegetation that is in your yard. (See the Compost chapter for more details on how to make compost.)

Step Three: Add Soil

1. In order to have a thriving organic garden, you must have excellent soil. Adding organic material (such

as that in your compost pile) to your existing soil will only make it better. Soil containing copious amounts of organic material is very good for your garden. Organically rich soil:

- Nourishes your plants without any chemicals, keeping them natural
- Is easy to use when planting seeds or seedlings, and it also allows for weeds to be more easily picked
- Is softer than chemically treated soil, so the roots of your plants can spread and grow deeper
- Helps water and air find the roots

Step Four: Weed Control

1. Weeds are invasive to your garden plants and thus must be removed in order for your organic garden to grow efficiently. Common weeds that can invade your garden are ivy, mint, and dandelions.

2. Using a sharp hoe, go over each area of exposed soil frequently to keep weeds from sprouting. Also, plucking off the green portions of weeds will deprive them of the nutrients they need to survive.

3. Gently pull out weeds by hand to remove their root systems and to stop continued growth. Be careful when weeding around established plants so you don't uproot them as well.

4. Mulch unplanted areas of your garden so that weeds will be less likely to grow. You can find organic mulches, such as wood chips and grass clippings, at your local garden store. These mulches will not only discourage weed growth but will also eventually break down and help enrich the soil. Mulching also helps regulate soil

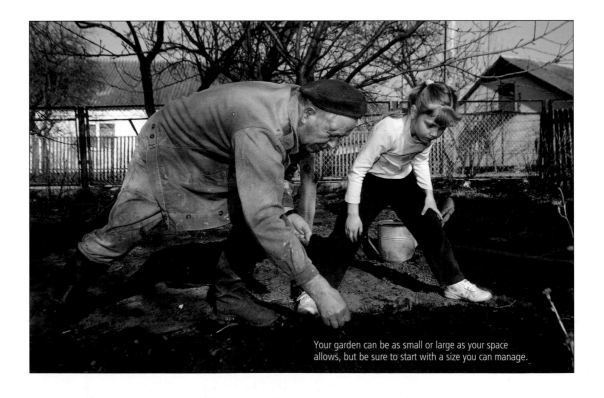

Your garden can be as small or large as your space allows, but be sure to start with a size you can manage.

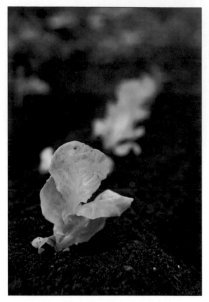

A row of lettuce thrives in the compost-fertilized soil.

temperatures and helps in conserving water by decreasing evaporation. (See the "Mulch" chapter for more on mulching.)

Step Five: Be Careful of Lawn Fertilizers

If you have a lawn and your organic garden is situated in it, be mindful that any chemicals you might place on your lawn may find their way into your organic garden. Therefore, refrain from fertilizing your lawn with chemicals and, if you wish to return nutrients to your grass, simply let your cut grass clippings remain in the yard to decompose naturally and enrich the soil beneath.

Things to Consider

- "Organic" means that you don't use any kinds of materials, such as paper or cardboard, that contain chemicals, and especially not fertilizer or pesticides. Make sure that these products do not find their way into your garden or compost pile.
- If you are adding grass clippings to your compost pile, make sure they don't come from a lawn that has been treated with chemical fertilizer.
- If you don't want to start a compost pile, simply add leaves and grass clippings directly to your garden bed. This will act like a mulch, deter weeds from growing, and will eventually break down to help return nutrients to your soil.
- If you find insects attacking your plants, the best way to control them is by picking them off by hand. Also practice crop rotation (planting different types of plants in a given area from year to year), which might reduce your pest problem. For some insects, just a strong stream of water is effective in removing them from your plants.
- Shy away from using bark mulch. It robs nitrogen from the soil as it decomposes and can also attract termites.

A hand fork can be useful in digging up tough roots of pesky weeds.

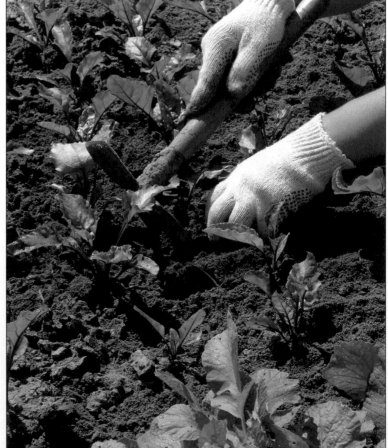

Terracing

Terraces can create several mini-gardens in your backyard. On steep slopes, terracing can make planting a garden possible. Terraces also prevent erosion by shortening a long slope into a series of shorter, more level steps. This allows heavy rains to soak into the soil rather than to run off and cause erosion and poor plant growth.

Materials Needed for Terraces

Numerous materials are available for building terraces. Treated wood is often used in terrace building and has several advantages: It is easy to work with, it blends well with plants and the surrounding environment, and it is often less expensive than other materials. There are many types of treated wood available for terracing—railroad ties and landscaping timbers are just two examples. These materials will last for years, which is crucial if you are hoping to keep your terraced garden intact for any length of time. There has been some concern about using these treated materials around plants, but studies by Texas A&M University and the Southwest Research Institute concluded that these materials are not harmful to gardens or people when used as recommended.

Other materials for terraces include bricks, rocks, concrete blocks, and similar masonry materials. Some masonry materials are made specifically for walls and terraces and can be more easily installed by a homeowner than other materials. These include fieldstone and brick. One drawback is that most stone or masonry products tend to be more expensive than wood, so if you are looking to save money, treated wood will make a sufficient terrace wall.

Terraces help prevent erosion and encourage vegetation on sloped ground.

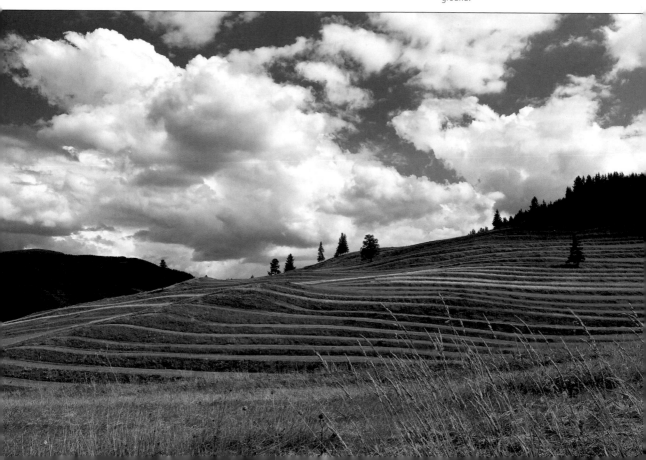

How High Should the Terrace Walls Be?

The steepness of the slope on which you wish to garden often dictates the appropriate height of the terrace wall. Make the terraces in your yard high enough so the land between them is fairly level. Be sure the terrace material is strong enough and anchored well to stay in place through freezing and thawing, and during heavy rainstorms. Do not underestimate the pressure of waterlogged soil behind a wall—it can be enormous and will cause improperly constructed walls to bulge or collapse.

Many communities have building codes for walls and terraces. Large projects will most likely need the expertise of a professional landscaper to make sure the walls can stand up to water pressure in the soil. Large terraces also need to be built with adequate drainage and tied back into the slope properly. Because of the expertise and equipment required to do this correctly, you will probably want to restrict terraces you build on your own to no more than a foot or two high.

Building Your Own Terrace

The safest way to build a terrace is by using the cut and fill method. With this method, little soil is disturbed, giving you protection from erosion should a sudden storm occur while the work is in progress. This method will also require little, if any, additional soil. Here are the steps needed to build your own terrace:

1. Contact your utility companies to identify the location of any buried utility lines and pipes before starting to dig.
2. Determine the rise and run of your slope. The rise is the vertical distance from the bottom of the slope to the top. The run is the horizontal distance between the top and the bottom. This will allow you to determine how many terraces you will need. For example, if your run is 20 feet and the rise is 8 feet, and you want each bed to be 5 feet wide, you will need four beds. The rise of each bed will be 2 feet.
3. Start building the beds at the bottom of your slope. You will need to dig a trench in which to place your first tier. The depth and width of the trench will vary depending on how tall the terrace will be and the specific building materials you are using. Follow the manufacturer's instructions carefully when using masonry products, as many of these have limits on the number of tiers or the height that can be safely built. If you are using landscape timbers and your terrace is low (less than 2 feet), you only need to bury the timber to about half its thickness or less. The width of the trench should be slightly wider than your timber. Make sure the bottom of the trench is firmly packed and completely level, and then place your timbers into the trench.
4. For the sides of your terrace, dig a trench into the slope. The bottom of this trench must be level with the bottom of the first trench. When the depth of the trench is one inch greater than the thickness of your timber, you have reached the back of the terrace and can stop digging.
5. Cut a piece of timber to the correct length and place it into the trench.
6. Drill holes through your timbers and pound long spikes, or pipes, through the holes and into the ground. A minimum of 18 inches of pipe length is recommended, and longer pipes may be needed in higher terraces for added stability.
7. Place the next tier of timbers on top of the first, overlapping the corners and joints. Pound a spike through both tiers to fuse them together.
8. Move the soil from the back of the bed to the front of the bed until the surface is level. Add another tier as needed.

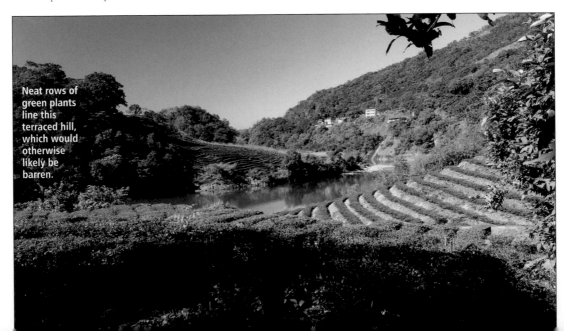

Neat rows of green plants line this terraced hill, which would otherwise likely be barren.

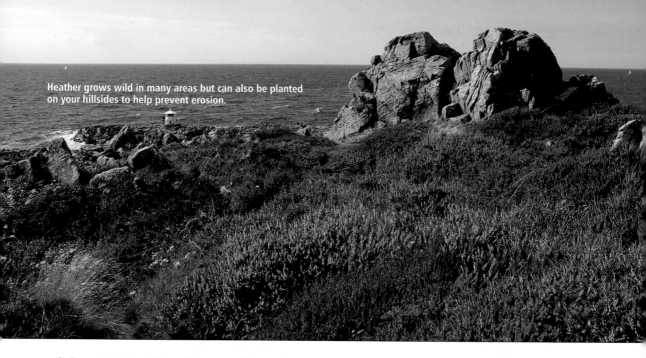

Heather grows wild in many areas but can also be planted on your hillsides to help prevent erosion.

9. Repeat, starting with step 2, to create the remaining terraces. In continuously connected terrace systems, the first timber of the second tier will also be the back wall of your first terrace.
10. The back wall of the last bed will be level with its front wall.
11. When finished, you can start to plant and mulch your terraced garden.

Other Ways to Make Use of Slopes in Your Yard

If terraces are beyond the limits of your time or money, you may want to consider other options for backyard slopes. If you have a slope that is hard to mow, consider using groundcovers on the slope rather than grass. There are many plants adapted to a wide range of light and moisture conditions that require little care (and do not need mowing) and provide soil erosion protection. These include:

- Juniper
- Wintercreeper
- Periwinkle
- Cotoneaster
- Potentilla
- Heathers and heaths

Strip-cropping is another way to deal with long slopes in your yard. Rather than terracing to make garden beds level, plant perennial beds and strips of grass across the slope. Once established, many perennials are effective in reducing erosion. Adding mulch also helps reduce erosion. If erosion does occur, it will be basically limited to the gardened area. The grass strips will act as filters to catch much of the soil that may run off the beds. Grass strips should be wide enough to mow easily, as well as wide enough to reduce erosion effectively.

Periwinkles require little maintenance, spread quickly, and will grow easily on a slope in your yard.

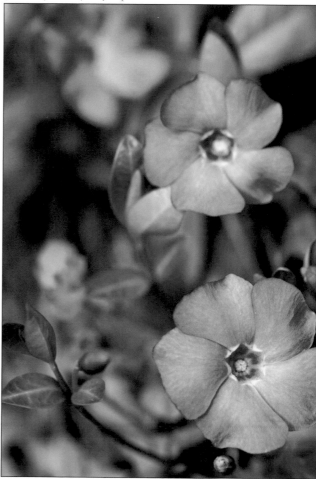

Start Your Own Vegetable Garden

If you want to start your own vegetable garden, just follow these simple steps and you'll be on your way to growing your own yummy vegetables—right in your own backyard.

Steps to Making Your Own Vegetable Garden

1. Select a site for your garden.
   - Vegetables grow best in well-drained, fertile soil (loamy soils are the best).
   - Some vegetables can cope with shady conditions, but most prefer a site with a good amount of sunshine—at least six hours a day of direct sunlight.
2. Remove all weeds in your selected spot and dispose of them. If you are using compost to supplement your garden soil, do not put the weeds on the compost heap, as they may germinate once again and cause more weed growth among your vegetable plants.
3. Prepare the soil by tilling it. This will break up large soil clumps and allow you to see and remove pesky weed roots. This would also be the appropriate time to add organic materials (such as compost) to the existing soil to help make it more fertile. The tools used for tilling will depend on the size of your garden. Some examples are:
   - Shovel and turning fork—using these tools is hard work, requiring strong upper body strength.
   - Rotary tiller—this will help cut up weed roots and mix the soil.
4. After the soil has been tilled, you are ready to begin planting. If you would like straight rows in your garden, a guide can be made from two wooden stakes and a bit of rope.

After soil is tilled it should be loose and free from weeds or root systems.

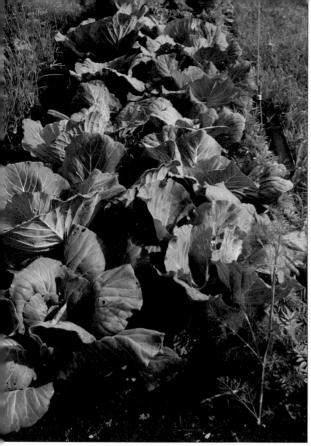

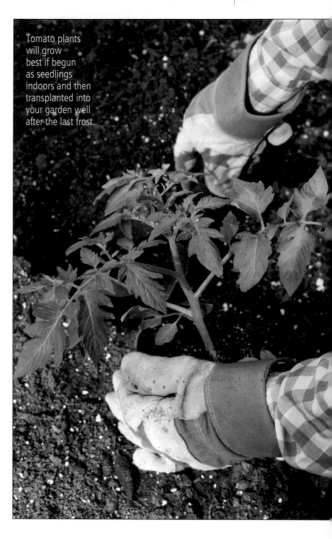

Tomato plants will grow best if begun as seedlings indoors and then transplanted into your garden well after the last frost.

You can often grow two crops of cabbage or other green leafy vegetables in one growing season if you start the garden early enough.

5. Vegetables can be grown from seeds or transplanted.
   • If your garden has problems with pests such as slugs, it's best to transplant older plants, as they are more likely to survive attacks from these organisms.
   • Transplanting works well for vegetables like tomatoes and onions, which usually need a head start to mature within a shorter growing season. These can be germinated indoors on seed trays on a windowsill before the growing season begins.
6. Follow these basic steps to grow vegetables from seeds:
   • Information on when and how deep to plant vegetable seeds is usually printed on seed packages or on various websites. You can also contact your local nursery or garden center to inquire after this information.
   • Measure the width of the seed to determine how deep it should be planted. Take the width and multiply by 2. That is how deep the seed should be placed in the hole. As a general rule, the larger the seed, the deeper it should be planted.
7. Water the plants and seeds well to ensure a good start. Make sure they receive water at least every other day, especially if there is no rain in the forecast.

A shovel is perfectly adequate for turning over soil in a small garden.

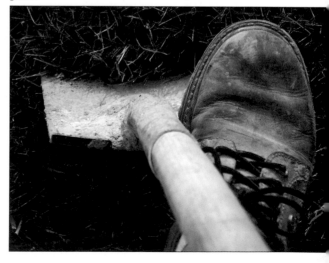

Things to Consider

- In the early days of a vegetable garden, all your plants are vulnerable to attack by insects and animals. It is best to plant multiples of the same plant to ensure that some survive. Placing netting and fences around your garden can help keep out certain animal pests. Coffee grains or slug traps filled with beer will also help protect your plants against insect pests.
- If sowing seed straight onto your bed, be sure to obtain a photograph of what your seedlings will look like so you don't mistake the growing plant for a weed.
- Weeding early on is very important to the overall success of your garden. Weeds steal water, nutrients, and light from your vegetables, which will stunt their growth and make it more difficult for them to thrive.

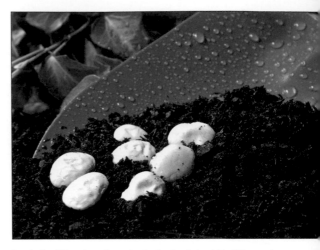

Seeds should be planted at a depth of twice their width. If the seed is ¼ inch wide, it should be planted ½ inch below the surface.

For very small seeds, such as carrot seeds, you can sprinkle 15 to 20 seeds per inch in a shallow channel. To make the row straight, tie a string to two small sticks and drive each stick into the ground on either side of your garden so that the string is taut. Use a hoe to dig a shallow channel in the string's shadow.

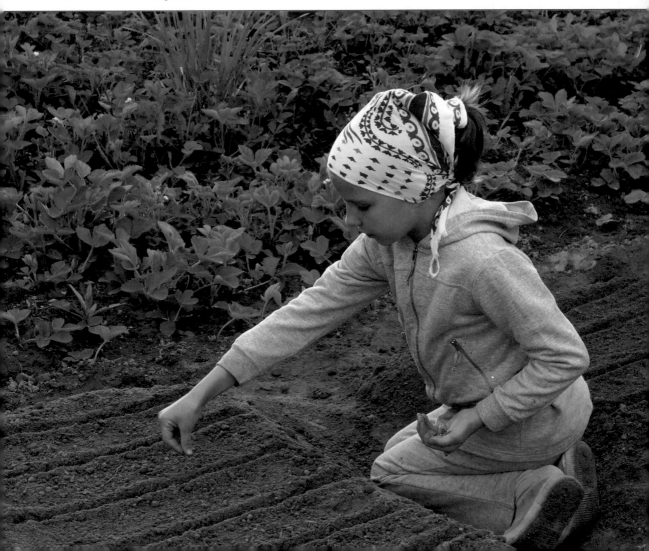

Start Your Own Flower Garden

If you are looking to grow a beautiful garden full of flowers, just follow these simple steps to achieve the perfect beginner's flower garden.

Step One: Start with a Small Garden

Gardening takes a lot of work, and so for the beginner gardener, tackling a large garden can be overwhelming. Start with a small flowerbed around 25 square feet. This will provide you with room for about 20 to 30 plants—enough room for three types of annuals and two types of perennials. As your gardening experience grows, so can the size of your garden!

If you are looking to start even smaller, you can always begin your first flower garden in a container, or create a border from treated wood or bricks and stones around your existing bed. That way, when you are ready to expand your garden, all you need to do is remove the temporary border and you'll be all set. Even a small container filled with a few different types of plants can be a wonderful addition to any yard.

Step Two: Plan Your Flower Garden

Draw up a plan of how you'd like your garden to look, and then dig a flowerbed to fit that plan. Planning your garden before gathering the seeds or plants and beginning the digging can give you a clearer sense of how your garden will be organized and can facilitate the planting process.

Step Three: Choose a Spot for Your Garden

It is important, when choosing where your flower garden will be located, that you consider an area that receives at least six hours of direct sunlight per day, as this will be adequate for a large variety of garden plants. Be careful that you will not be digging into utility lines or pipes, and that you place your garden at least a short distance away from fences or other structures.

If you live in a part of the country that is quite hot, it might be beneficial for your flowers to be placed in an area that gets some shade during the hot afternoon sun. Placing your garden on the east side of your home will help your flowers flourish. If your garden will get more than six hours of sunlight per day, it would be wise to choose flowers that thrive in hot, sunny spaces, and make sure to water them frequently.

It is also important to choose a spot that has good, fertile soil in which your flowers can grow. Try to avoid any areas with rocky, shallow soil or where water collects and pools. Make sure your garden is away from large trees and shrubs, as these plants will compete with your flowers for water and nutrients. If you are concerned that your soil may not contain enough nutrients for your flowers to grow properly, you can have a soil test done, which will tell you the pH of the soil. Depending on the results,

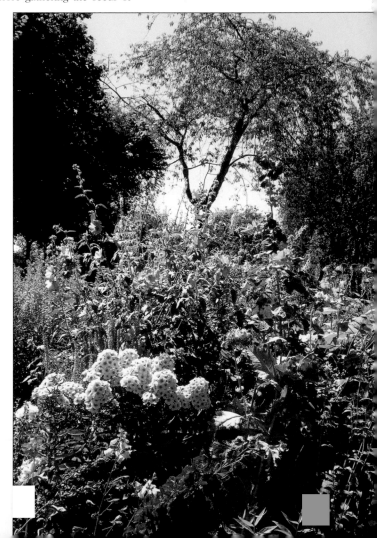

Flower gardens do not need to be as carefully organized as vegetable gardens. Experiment with different color combinations and flower varieties. In general, it's best to put taller plants toward the center or back of your garden so that the shorter flowers will still be visible.

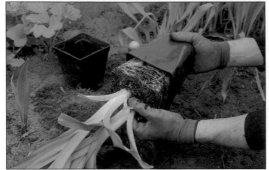

Some flowers, like lilies, do best if started in pots and then transplanted into your garden.

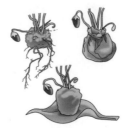

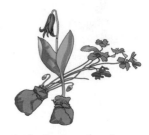

To transplant flowers from one growing location to another, dig up the plant, being careful not to damage the root system. Wrap the root ball in a large leaf or a cloth and tie at the top around the stems to keep the roots from drying out. Leaf wrappings do not need to be removed before replanting. Be sure to water the plant thoroughly after planting it in its new location.

you can then adjust the types of nutrients needed in your soil by adding organic materials or certain types of fertilizers.

Step Four: Start Digging

Now that you have a site picked out, mark out the boundaries with a hose or string. Remove the sod and any weed roots that may re-grow. Use your spade or garden fork to dig up the bed at least 8 to 12 inches deep, removing any rocks or debris you come across.

Once your bed is dug, level it and break up the soil with a rake. Add compost or manure if the soil is not fertile. If your soil is sandy, adding peat moss or grass clippings will help it hold more water. Work any additions into the top 6 inches of soil.

Step Five: Purchase Your Seeds or Plants

Once you've chosen which types of flowers you'd like to grow in your garden, visit your local garden store or nursery and pick out already-established plants or packaged seeds. Follow the planting instructions on the plant tabs or seed packets. The smaller plants should be situated in the front of the bed. Once your plants or seeds are in their holes, pack in the soil around them. Make sure to leave ample space between your seeds or plants for them to grow and spread out (most labels and packets will alert you to how large your flower should be expected to grow, so you can adjust the spacing as needed).

Step Six: Water Your Flower Garden

After your plants or seeds are first put into the ground, be sure they get a thorough watering. Continue to check your garden to see whether or not the soil is drying out. If so, give your garden a good soaking with the garden hose or watering can. The amount of water your garden needs is dependant on the climate you live in, the exposure to the sun, and how much rain your area has received.

Step Seven: Cutting Your Flowers

Once your flowers begin to bloom, feel free to cut them and display the beautiful blooms in your home. Pruning your flower garden (cutting the dead or dying blooms off the plant) will help certain plants to re-bloom. Also, if you have plants that are becoming top heavy, support them with a stake and some string so you can enjoy their blossoms to the fullest.

Things to Consider

- Annuals are plants that you need to replant every year. They are often inexpensive, and many have brightly colored flowers. Annuals can be rewarding for beginner gardeners, as they take little effort and provide lovely color to your garden. The following season, you'll need to replant or start over from seed.

Echinacea is beautiful as well as useful for medicinal purposes. It grows best in sunny areas. Plant in early spring for summer blooming, or about two months before the first frost for flowers the next year.

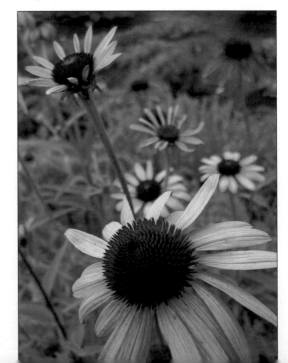

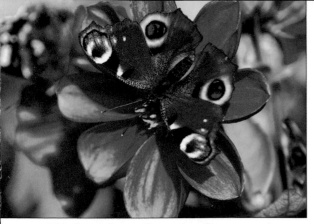

Bright, fragrant flowers will attract butterflies to your garden.

Barrel Plant Holder

If you have some perennials you want to display in your yard away from your flower garden, you can create a planter out of an old barrel. This plant holder is made by sawing an old barrel (wooden or metal) into two pieces and mounting it on short or tall legs—whichever design fits better in your yard. You can choose to either paint it or leave it natural. Filling the planter with good quality soil and compost and planting an array of multi-colored flowers into the barrel planter will brighten up your yard all summer long. If you do not want to mount the barrel on legs, it can be placed on the ground on a smooth and level surface where it won't easily tip over.

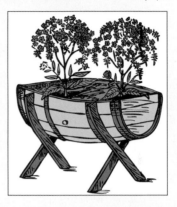

- Perennials last from one year to the next. They, too, will require annual maintenance but not yearly replanting. Perennials may require division, support, and extra care during winter months. Perennials may also need their old blooms and stems pruned and cut back every so often.

- Healthy, happy plants tend not to be as susceptible to pests and diseases. It is easier to practice prevention rather than curing existing problems. Do your best to give your plants good soil, nutrients, and appropriate moisture, and choose plants that are well-suited to your climate. This way, your garden will be more likely to grow to its maximum potential and your plants will be strong and healthy.

Garden centers or farm stands often sell flowers that are started in flats or plugs. Because the root systems are already established, they are easier to grow and create an instantly attractive garden.

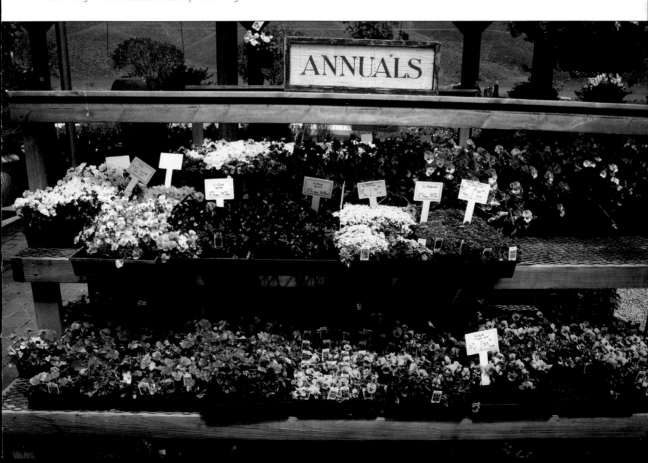

Rustic Plant Stand

If you'd like to incorporate a rustic, natural-looking plant stand in your garden or on your patio or deck, one can easily be made from a preexisting wooden box or by nailing boards together. This box should be mounted on legs (see picture below). To make the legs, saw the piece of wood meant for the leg in half to a length from the top equal to the depth of the box. Then, cross-cut and remove one half. The corner of the box can then be inserted in the middle of the crosscut and the leg nailed to the side of the box.

The plant stand can be decorated to suit your needs and preference. You can nail smaller, alternating twigs or cut branches around the stand to give it a more natural feel or you can simply paint it a soothing, natural color and place it in your yard.

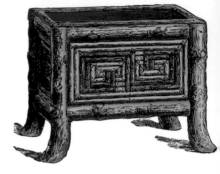

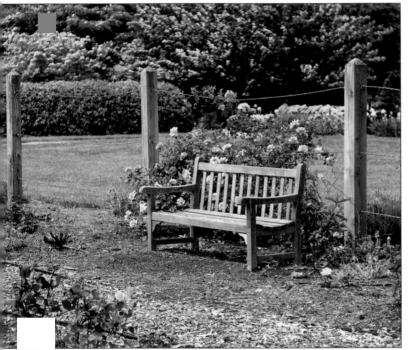

A fence can be set up around your garden to keep out deer and other wild animals. See page 181 for fence construction ideas.

Wooden Window Box

Planting perennial flowers and cascading plants in window boxes is the perfect way to brighten up the front exterior of your home. Making a simple wooden window box to hold your flowers and plants is quite easy. These boxes can be made from preexisting wooden boxes (such as fruit crates) or you can make your own out of simple boards. Whatever method you choose, make sure the boards are stout enough to hold the brads firmly.

The size of your window will ultimately determine the size of your box, but this plan calls for a box roughly 21 x 7 x 7 inches. You can decorate your boxes with waterproof paint or you can nail strips of wood or sticks to the panels. Make sure to cut a few holes in the bottom of the box to allow for water drainage.

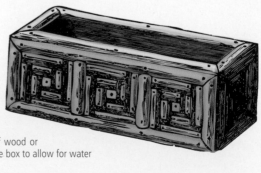

Planting Trees

Trees in your yard can become home to many different types of wildlife. Trees also reduce your cooling costs by providing shade, help clean the air, add beauty and color, provide shelter from the wind and the sun, and add value to your home.

Choosing a Tree

Choosing a tree should be a well-thought-out decision. Tree planting can be a significant investment, both in money and time. Selecting the proper tree for your yard can provide you with years of enjoyment, as well as significantly increase the value of your property. However, a tree that is inappropriate for your property can be a constant maintenance problem, or even a danger to your and others' safety. Before you decide to purchase a tree, take advantage of the many references on gardening at local libraries, universities, arboretums, native plant and gardening clubs, and nurseries. Some questions to consider in selecting a tree include:

1. What purpose will this tree serve?

Trees can serve numerous landscape functions, including beautification, screening of sights and sounds, shade and energy conservation, and wildlife habitat.

2. Is the species appropriate for your area?

Reliable nurseries will not sell plants that are not suitable for your area. However, some mass marketers have trees and shrubs that are not fitted for the environment in which they are sold. Even if a tree is hardy, it may not flower consistently from year to year if the environmental factors are not conducive for it to do so. If you are buying a tree for its spring flowers and fall fruits, consider climate when deciding which species of tree to plant.

- Be aware of microclimates. Microclimates are localized areas where weather conditions may vary from the norm. A very sheltered yard may support vegetation not normally adapted to the region. On the other hand, a north-facing slope may be significantly cooler or windier than surrounding areas, and survival of normally adapted plants may be limited.
- Select trees native to your area. These trees will be more tolerant of local weather and soil conditions, enhance natural biodiversity in your neighborhood, and be more beneficial to wildlife than many non-native trees. Avoid exotic trees that can invade other areas, crowd out native plants, and harm natural ecosystems.

3. How big will it get?

When planting a small tree, it is often difficult to imagine that in 20 years it will most likely be shading your entire yard. Unfortunately, many trees are planted and later removed when the tree grows beyond the dimensions of the property.

4. What is the average life expectancy of the tree?

Some trees can live for hundreds of years. Others are considered "short-lived" and may live for only 20 to 30 years. Many short-lived trees tend to be smaller, ornamental species. Short-lived species should not necessarily be ruled out when considering plantings, as they may have other desirable characteristics, such as size, shape, tolerance of

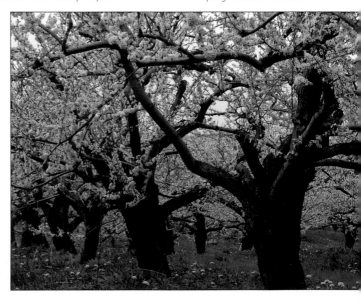

Fruit trees provide sweet-smelling flowers in the spring and fruit in the fall.

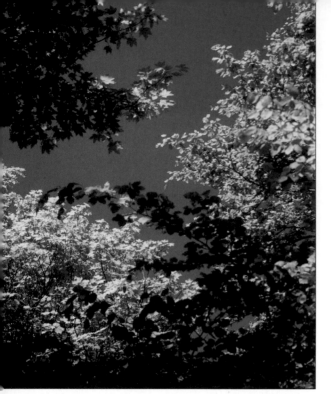

Full-grown trees create a shade-producing canopy of branches and leaves. Shade can be a good addition to your property, but be sure you don't plant trees in an area where you want a garden that requires full sun.

shade, or fruit, that would be useful in the landscape. These species may also fill a void in a young landscape and can be removed as other larger, longer-lived species mature.

5. Does it have any particular ornamental value, such as leaf color or flowers and fruits?

Some species provide beautiful displays of color for short periods in the spring or fall. Other species may have foliage that is reddish or variegated and can add color in your yard year-round. Trees bearing fruits or nuts can provide an excellent source of food for many species of wildlife.

6. Does it have any particular insect, disease, or other problem that may reduce its usefulness in the future?

Certain insects and diseases can cause serious problems for some desirable species in certain regions. Depending on the pest, control of the problem may be difficult and the pest may significantly reduce the attractiveness, if not the life expectancy, of the tree. Other species, such as the silver maple, are known to have weak wood that is susceptible to damage in ice storms or heavy winds. All these factors should be kept in mind, as controlling pests or dealing with tree limbs that have snapped in foul weather can be expensive and potentially damaging.

7. How common is this species in your neighborhood or town?

Some species are over-planted. Increasing the natural diversity in your area will provide habitat for wildlife and help limit the opportunity for a single pest to destroy large numbers of trees.

8. Is the tree evergreen or deciduous?

Evergreen trees will provide cover and shade year-round. They may also be more effective as wind and noise barriers. On the other hand, deciduous trees will give you summer shade but allow the winter sun to shine in. If planting a deciduous tree, keep these heating and cooling factors in mind when placing the tree in your yard.

Placement of Trees

Proper placement of trees is critical for your enjoyment and for their long-term survival. Check with local authorities about regulations pertaining to placement of trees in your area. Some communities have ordinances restricting placement of trees within a specified distance from a street, sidewalk, streetlight, or other city utilities.

Before planting your tree, consider the tree's potential maximum size. Ask yourself these simple questions:

1. When the tree nears maturity, will it be too close to your or a neighbor's house? An evergreen tree planted on your north side may block the winter sun from your next-door neighbor.
2. Will it provide too much shade for your vegetable and flower gardens? Most vegetables and many flowers require considerable amounts of sun. If you intend to grow these plants in your yard, consider how the placement of trees will affect these gardens.
3. Will the tree obstruct any driveways or sidewalks?
4. Will it cause problems for buried or overhead power lines and utility pipes?

Once you have taken these questions into consideration and have bought the perfect tree for your yard, it is time to start digging!

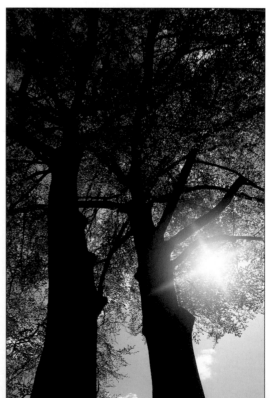

Planting a Tree

A properly planted and maintained tree will grow faster and live longer than one that is incorrectly planted. Trees can be planted almost any time of the year, as long as the ground is not frozen. Late summer or early fall is the optimum time to plant trees in many areas. By planting during these times, the tree has a chance to establish new roots before winter arrives and the ground freezes. When spring comes, the tree is then ready to grow. Another feasible time for planting trees is late winter or early spring. Planting in hot summer weather should be avoided if possible as the heat may cause the young tree to wilt. Planting in frozen soil during the winter is very difficult and is tough on tree roots. When the tree is dormant and the ground is frozen, there is no opportunity for the new roots to begin growing.

Trees can be purchased as container-grown, balled and burlapped (B&B), or bare root. Generally, container-grown are the easiest to plant and successfully establish in any season, including summer. With container-grown stock, the plant has been growing in a container for a period of time. When planting container-grown trees, little damage is done to the roots as the plant is transferred to the soil. Container-grown trees range in size from very small plants in gallon pots up to large trees in huge pots.

Bare root trees are usually extremely small plants. Because there is no soil around the roots, they must be planted when they are dormant to avoid drying out, and the roots must be kept moist until planted. Frequently, bare root trees are offered by seed and nursery mail order catalogs, or in the wholesale trade. Many state-operated nurseries and local conservation districts also sell bare root stock in bulk quantities for only a few cents per plant. Bare root plants are usually offered in the early spring and should be planted as soon as possible.

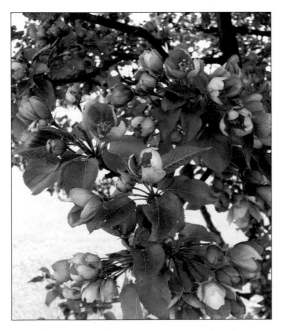

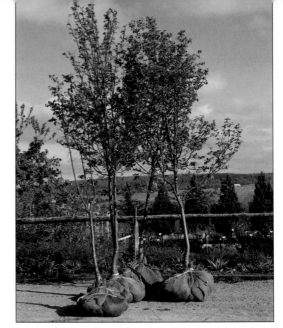

B&B trees are dug from a nursery, wrapped in burlap, and kept in the nursery for an additional period of time, giving the roots opportunity to regenerate. B&B plants can be quite large.

Be sure to carefully follow the planting instructions that come with your tree. If specific instructions are not available, here are some general tree-planting guidelines:

1. Before starting any digging, call your local utility companies to identify the location of any underground wires or lines. In the U.S., you can call 811 to have your utility lines marked for free.
2. Dig a hole twice as wide as, and slightly shallower than, the root ball. Roughen the sides and bottom of the hole with a pick or shovel so that the roots can easily penetrate the soil.
3. With a potted tree, gently remove the tree from the container. To do this, lay the tree on its side with the container end near the planting hole. Hit the bottom and sides of the container until the root ball is loosened. If roots are growing in a circular pattern around the root ball, slice through the roots on a couple of sides of the root ball. With trees wrapped in burlap, remove the string or wire that holds the burlap to the root crown; it is not necessary to remove the burlap completely. Plastic wraps must be completely removed. Gently separate circling roots on the root ball. Shorten exceptionally long roots and guide the shortened roots downward and outward. Root tips die quickly when exposed to light and air, so complete this step as quickly as possible.
4. Place the root ball in the hole. Leave the top of the root ball (where the roots end and the trunk begins) ½ to 1 inch above the surrounding soil, making sure not to cover it unless the roots are exposed. For bare root plants, make a mound of soil in the middle of the hole and spread plant roots out evenly over the mound. Do not set the tree too deep into the hole.
5. As you add soil to fill in around the tree, lightly tap the soil to collapse air pockets, or add water to help settle the soil. Form a temporary water basin

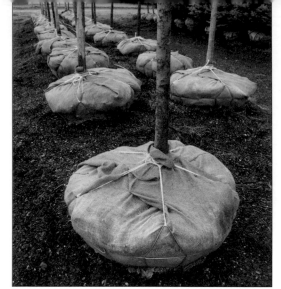

Burlap wraps do not need to be removed before planting your tree. They will decompose in the soil with time.

around the base of the tree to encourage water penetration, and be sure to water the tree thoroughly after planting. A tree with a dry root ball cannot absorb water; if the root ball is extremely dry, allow water to trickle into the soil by placing the hose at the trunk of the tree.

6. Place mulch around the tree. A circle of mulch, 3-foot in diameter, is common.

7. Depending on the size of the tree and the site condiions, staking the tree in place may be beneficial. Staking supports the tree until the roots are well established to properly anchor it. Staking should allow for some movement of the tree on windy days. After trees are established, remove all supporting wires. If these are not removed, they can girdle the tree, cut into the trunk, and eventually kill the tree.

Maintenance

For the first year or two, especially after a week or so of especially hot or dry weather, watch your tree closely for signs of moisture stress. If you see any leaf wilting or hard, caked soil, water the tree well and slowly enough to allow the water to soak in. This will encourage deep root growth. Keep the area under the tree mulched.

Some species of evergreen trees may need protection against winter sun and wind. A thorough watering in the fall before the ground freezes is recommended.

Fertilization is usually not needed for newly planted trees. Depending on the soil and growing conditions, fertilizer may be beneficial at a later time.

Things You'll Need

- Tree
- Shovel
- Watering can or garden hose
- Measuring stick
- Mulch
- Optional: scissors or knife to cut the burlap or container, stakes, and supporting wires

Pruning

Usually, pruning is not needed on newly planted trees. As the tree grows, lower branches may be pruned to provide clearance above the ground, or to remove dead or damaged limbs or suckers that sprout from the trunk. Sometimes larger trees need pruning to allow more light to enter the canopy. Small branches can be removed easily with pruners. Large branches should be removed with a pruning saw. All cuts should be vertical. This will allow the tree to heal quickly without the use of any artificial sealants. Major pruning should be done in late winter or early spring. At this time, the tree is more likely to "bleed," as sap is rising through the plant. This is actually healthy and will help prevent invasion by many disease-carrying organisms.

Under no circumstance should trees be topped (topping is chopping off large top tree branches). Not only does this practice ruin the natural shape of the tree, but it also increases its susceptibility to diseases and results in very narrow crotch angles (the angle between the trunk and the side branch). Narrow crotch angles are weaker than wide ones and more susceptible to damage from wind and ice. If a large tree requires major reduction in height or size, contact a professionally trained arborist.

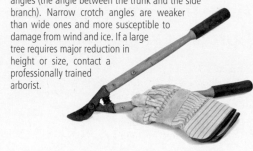

Young trees need protection against rodents, frost cracks, sunscald, lawn mowers, and weed whackers. In the winter months, mice and rabbits frequently girdle small trees by chewing away the bark at the snow level. Since the tissues that transport nutrients in the tree are located just under the bark, a girdled tree often dies in the spring when growth resumes. Weed whackers are also a common cause of girdling. In order to prevent girdling from occurring, use plastic guards, which are inexpensive and easy to control.

Frost cracking is caused by the sunny side of the tree expanding at a different rate than the colder, shaded side. This can cause large splits in the trunk. To prevent this, wrap young trees with paper tree wrap, starting from the base and wrapping up to the bottom branches. Sunscald can occur when a young tree is suddenly moved from a shady spot into direct sunlight. Light-colored tree wraps can be used to protect the trunk from sunscald.

Final Thoughts

Trees are natural windbreaks, slowing the wind and providing shelter and food for wildlife. Trees can help protect livestock, gardens, and larger crops. They also help prevent dust particles from adding to smog over urban areas. Tree plantings are key components of an effective conservation system and can provide your yard with beauty, shade, and rich, natural resources.

Container Gardening

An alternative to growing vegetables, flowers, and herbs in a traditional garden is to grow them in containers. While the amount that can be grown in a container is certainly limited, container gardens work well for tomatoes, peppers, cucumbers, herbs, salad greens, and many flowering annuals. Choose vegetable varieties that have been specifically bred for container growing. You can obtain this information online or at your garden center. Container gardening also brings birds and butterflies right to your doorstep. Hanging baskets of fuchsia or pots of snapdragons are frequently visited by hummingbirds, allowing for up-close observation.

Container gardening is an excellent method of growing vegetables, herbs, and flowers, especially if you do not have adequate outdoor space for a full garden bed. A container garden can be placed anywhere—on the patio, balcony, rooftop, or windowsill. Vegetables such as leaf lettuce, radishes, small tomatoes, and baby carrots can all be grown successfully in pots.

How to Grow Vegetables in a Container Garden

Here are some simple steps to follow for growing vegetables in containers.

1. Choose a sunny area for your container plants. Your plants will need at least five to six hours of sunlight a day. Some plants, such as cucumbers, may need more. Select plants that are suitable for container growing. Usually their name will have words such as "patio," "bush," "dwarf," "toy," or "miniature" in them. Peppers, onions, and carrots are also good choices.
2. Choose a planter that is at least 5 gallons, unless the plant is very small. Poke holes in the bottom if they don't already exist; the soil must be able to drain in order to prevent the roots from rotting. Avoid terracotta or dark colored pots as they tend to dry out quickly.

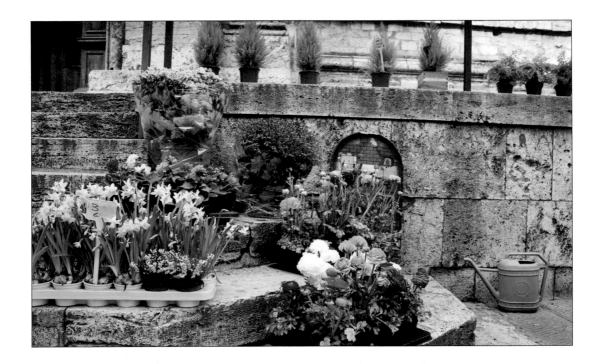

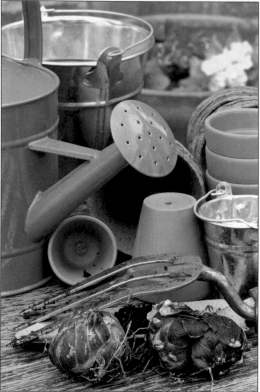

You only need a few simple tools for container gardening.

off pieces to use in cooking. Here's how to start your own herb container garden:

1. If your container doesn't already have holes in the bottom, poke several to allow the soil to drain. Pour gravel into the container until it is about a quarter of the way full. This will help the water drain and help to keep the soil from washing out.
2. Fill your container three-quarters of the way with potting soil or a soil-based compost.
3. It's best to use seedlings when planting herbs in containers. Tease the roots slightly, gently spreading them apart with your fingertips. This will encourage them to spread once planted. Place each herb into the pot and cover the root base with soil. Place herbs that will grow taller in the center of your container, and the smaller ones around the edges. Leave about four square inches of space between each seedling.
4. As you gently press in soil between the plants, leave an inch or so between the container's top and the soil. You don't want the container to overflow when you water the herbs.
5. Cut the tops off the taller herb plants to encourage them to grow faster and to produce more leaves.
6. Pour water into the container until it begins to leak out the bottom. Most herbs like to dry out between watering, and over-watering can cause some herbs to rot and die, so only water every few days unless the plants are in a very hot place.

3. Fill your container with potting soil. Good potting soil will have a mixture of peat moss and vermiculite. You can make your own potting soil using composted soil (see page 13). Read the directions on the seed packet or label to determine how deep to plant your seeds.
4. Check the moisture of the soil frequently. You don't want the soil to become muddy, but the soil should always feel damp to the touch. Do not wait until the plant is wilting to water it—at that point, it may be too late.

Things to Consider

- Follow normal planting schedules for your climate when determining when to plant your container garden.
- You may wish to line your container with porous materials such as shredded newspaper or rags to keep the soil from washing out. Be sure the water can still drain easily.

How to Grow Herbs in a Container

Herbs will thrive in containers if cared for properly. And if you keep them near your kitchen, you can easily snip

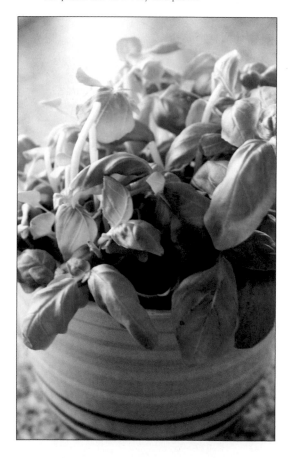

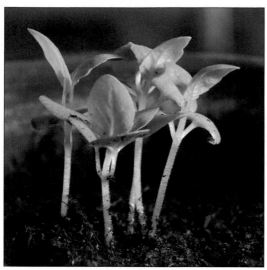

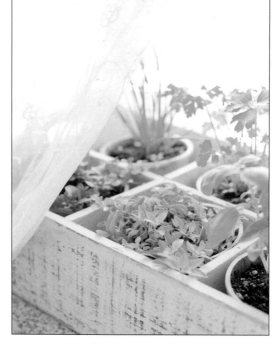

It's easiest to grow herbs from seedlings like these, though you can certainly grow them from seeds, too.

Things to Consider

- Growing several kinds of herbs together helps the plants to thrive. A few exceptions to this rule are oregano, lemon balm, and tea balm. These herbs should be planted on their own because they will overtake the other herbs in your container.
- You may wish to choose your herbs according to color to create attractive arrangements for your home. Any of the following herbs will grow well in containers:
- Silver herbs: artemsias, curry plans, santolinas
- Golden herbs: lemon thyme, calendula, nasturtium, sage, lemon balm
- Blue herbs: borage, hyssop, rosemary, catnip
- Green herbs: basil, mint, marjoram, thyme, parsley, chives, tarragon
- Pink and purple herbs: oregano (the flowers) are pink, lavender
- If you decide to transplant your herbs in the summer months, they will grow quite well outdoors and will give you a larger harvest.

How to Grow Flowers from Seeds in a Container

1. Cover the drainage hole in the bottom of the pot with a flat stone. This will keep the soil from trickling out when the plant is watered.
2. Fill the container with soil. The container should be filled almost to the top and for the best results, use potting soil from your local nursery or garden center

3. Make holes for the seeds. Refer to the seed packet to see how deep to make the holes. Always save the seed packet for future reference—it most likely has helpful directions about thinning young plants.
4. Place a seed in each hole. Pat the soil gently on top of each seed.
5. Use a light mist to water your seeds, making sure that the soil is only moist and not soaked.
6. Make sure your seeds get the correct amount of sunlight. Refer to the seed packet for the adequate amount of sunlight each seedling needs.
7. Watch your seeds grow. Most seeds take 3 to 17 days to sprout. Once the plants start sprouting, be sure to pull out plants that are too close together so the remaining plants will have enough space to establish good root systems.
8. Remember to water and feed your container plants. Keep the soil moist so your plants can grow. And in no time at all, you should have wonderful flowers growing in your container garden.

Preserving Your Container Plants

As fall approaches, frost will soon descend on your container plants and can ultimately destroy your garden. Container plants are particularly susceptible to frost damage, especially if you are growing tropical plants, perennials, and hardy woody plants in a single container garden. There are many ways that you can preserve and maintain your container garden plants throughout the winter season.

Preservation techniques will vary depending on the plants in your container garden. Tropical plants can be over-wintered using methods replicating a dry season, forcing the plant into dormancy; hardy perennials and woody shrubs need a cold dormancy to grow in the spring, so they must stay outside; cacti and succulents

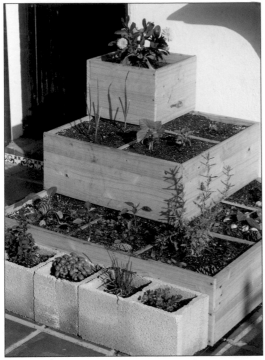

Cinder blocks or simple wooden planters made of scrap wood can make inexpensive container gardens.

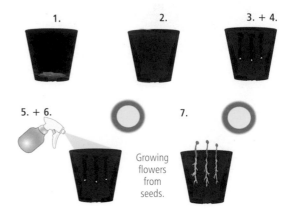

Growing flowers from seeds.

prefer their winters warm and dry and must be brought inside, while many annuals can be propagated by stem cuttings or can just be repotted and maintained inside.

Preserving Tropical Bulbs and Tubers

Many tropical plants, such as cannas, elephant ears, and angel's trumpets can be saved from an untimely death by over-wintering them in a dark corner or sunny window of your home, depending on the type of plant. A lot of bulbous and tuberous tropical plants have a natural dry season (analogous to our winter) when their leafy parts die off, leaving the bulb behind. Don't throw the bulbs away. After heavy frosts turn the aboveground plant parts to mush, cut the damaged foliage off about 4 inches above the thickened bulb. Then, dig them up and remove all excess soil from the roots. At this point, you can determine if the clump needs dividing. If it needs dividing, be sure to dust all cut surfaces with a sulfur-based fungicide made for bulbs to prevent the wounds from rotting. Cut the roots back to 1 inch from the bulb and leave to dry out evenly. Rotten bulbs or roots need to be thrown away so infection doesn't spread to the healthy bulbs.

A bulb's or tuber's drying time can last up to two weeks if it is sitting on something absorbent like newspaper and located somewhere shaded and dry—preferably around 50°F—such as a garage or basement. Once clean and dry, bulbs should be stored all winter in damp (not soggy) milled peat moss. This prevents the bulbs from drying out any further, which could cause

them to die. Many gardeners don't have a perfectly cool basement or garage to keep bulbs dormant. Alternative methods for dry storage include a dark closet with the door cracked for circulation, a cabinet, or underneath a bed in a cardboard box with a few holes punched for airflow. The important thing to keep in mind is that the bulb needs to be kept on the dry side, in the dark, and moderately warm.

If a bulb was grown as a single specimen in its own pot, the entire pot can be placed in a garage that stays above 50°F or a cool basement and allowed to dry out completely. Cut all aboveground plant parts flush with the soil and don't water until the outside temperatures stabilize above 60°F. Often, bulbs break dormancy unexpectedly in this dry pot method. If this happens, pots can be moved to a sunny location near a window and watered sparingly until they can be placed outside. The emerging leaves will be stunted, but once outside, the plant will replace any spindly leaves with lush, new ones.

Annuals

Many herbaceous annuals can also be saved for the following year. By rooting stem cuttings in water on a sunny windowsill, plants like impatiens, coleus, sweet potato vine cultivars, and purple heart can be held over winter until needed in the spring. Otherwise, the plants can be cut back by half, potted in a peat-based, soilless mix, and placed on a sunny windowsill. With a wide assortment of "annuals" available on the market, some research is required to determine which annuals can be over-wintered successfully. True annuals (such as basils, cockscomb, and zinnias)—regardless of any treatment given—will go to seed and die when brought inside.

Cacti and Succulents

If you planted a mixed dry container this year and want to retain any of the plants for next year, they should be removed from the main container and repotted into a high-sand-content soil mix for cacti and succulents. Keep them near a sunny window and water when dry. Many succulents and cacti do well indoors, either in a heated garage or a moderately sunny corner of a living room.

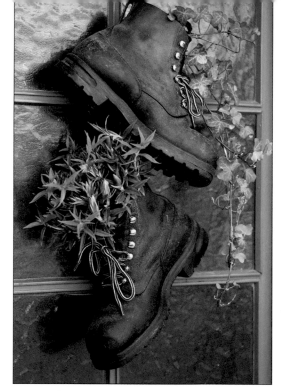

You can make container gardens out of almost anything.

ers. Crack-resistant, four-season containers can house perennials and woody shrubs year-round. Below is a list of specific perennials and woody plants that do well in both hot and cold weather, indoors and out:

- Shade perennials, like coral bells, lenten rose, assorted hardy ferns, and Japanese forest grass are great for all weather containers.
- Sun-loving perennials, such as sedges, some salvias, purple coneflower, daylily, spiderwort, and bee blossom are also very hardy and do well in year-round containers. Interplant them with cool growing plants, like kale, pansies, and Swiss chard, for fall and spring interest.
- Woody shrubs and vines—many of which have great foliage interest with four-season appeal—are ideal for container gardens. Red-twigged dogwood cultivars, clematis vine cultivars, and dwarf crape myrtle cultivars are great container additions that can stay outdoors year-round.

If the container has to be removed, hardy perennials and woody shrubs can be temporarily planted in the ground and mulched. Dig them from the garden in the spring, if you wish, and replant into a container. Or, leave them in their garden spot and start over with fresh ideas and new plant material for your container garden.

Sustainable Plants and Money in Your Pocket

Over-wintering is a great form of sustainable plant conservation achieved simply and effectively by adhering to each plant's cultural and environmental needs. With careful planning and storage techniques, you'll save money as well as plant material. The beauty and interest you've created in this season's well-grown container garden can also provide enjoyment for years to come.

As with other tropical plants, succulents also need time to adjust to sunnier conditions in the spring. Move them to a shady spot outside when temperatures have stabilized above 60°F and then gradually introduce them to brighter conditions.

Hardy Perennials, Shrubs, and Vines

Hardy perennials, woody shrubs, and vines needn't be thrown away when it's time to get rid of accent contain-

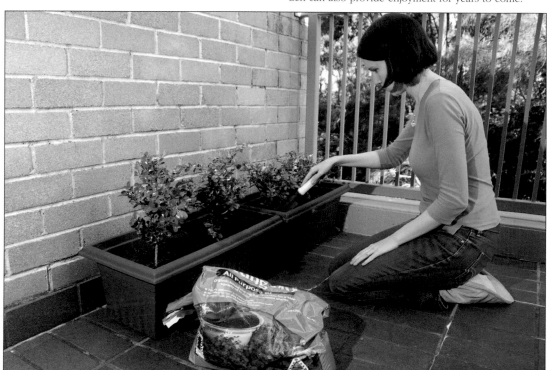

Rooftop Gardens

If you live in an urban area and don't have a lawn, that does not mean that you cannot have a garden. Whether you live in an apartment building or own your own home without yard space, you can grow your very own garden, right on your roof!

Is Your Roof Suitable for a Rooftop Garden?

Theoretically, any roof surface can be greened—even sloped or curved roofs can support a layer of sod or wildflowers. However, if the angle of your roof is over 30 degrees you should consult with a specialist. Very slanted roofs make it difficult to keep the soil in place until the plant's roots take hold. Certainly, a flat roof, approximating level ground conditions is the easiest on which to grow a garden, though a slight slant can be helpful in allowing drainage.

Also consider how much weight your roof can bear. A simple, lightweight rooftop garden will weigh between 13 and 30 pounds per square foot. Add to this your own weight—or that of anyone who will be tending or enjoying the garden—gardening tools, and, if you live in a colder climate, the additional weight of snow in the winter.

Will a Rooftop Garden Cause Water Leakage or Other Damage?

No. In fact, planting beds or surfaces are often used to protect and insulate roofs. However, you should take some precautions to protect your roof:

1. Cover your roof with a layer of waterproof material, such as a heavy-duty pond liner. You may want to place an old rug on top of the waterproof material to help it stay in place and to give additional support to the materials on top.

Rooftop gardens are becoming more popular in urban areas around the world.

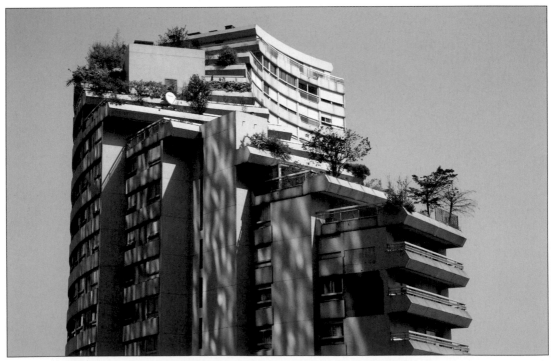

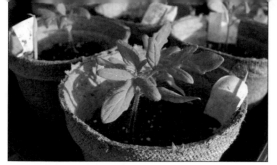

You can use container plants on your rooftop rather than laying a garden directly on the roof. However, still be sure that your roof is sturdy enough to hold the pots and the people who will be tending them.

Benefits of Rooftop Gardening

- Create more outdoor green space within your urban environment.
- Grow your own fresh vegetables—even in the city.
- Improve air quality and reduce CO_2 emissions.
- Help delay storm water runoff.
- Give additional insulation to building roofs.
- Reduce noise.

---

2. Place a protective drainage layer on top of the waterproof material. Otherwise, shovels, shoe heels, or dropped tools could puncture the roof. Use a coarse material such as gravel, pumice, or expanded shale.
3. Place a filter layer on top of the drainage layer to keep soil in place so that it won't clog up your drainage. A lightweight polyester geotextile (an inexpensive, non-woven fabric found at most home improvement stores) is ideal for this. Note that if your roof has an angle of over 10 degrees, only install the filter layer around the edges of the roof as it can increase slippage.
4. Using moveable planters or containers, modular walkways and surfacing treatment, and compartmentalized planting beds will make it easier to fix leaks should they appear.

Things to Consider

1. If you live in a very hot area, you may want to build small wooden platforms to elevate your plants above the hot rooftop. This will help increase the ventilation around the plants.
2. When determining whether or not your roof is strong enough to support a garden, remember that large pots full of water and soil will be very heavy, and if the roof is not strong enough, your garden could cause structural damage.
3. You can use pots or other containers on your rooftop rather than making a full garden bed. You should still first find out how much weight your roof can hold and choose lightweight containers.
4. Consider adding a fence or railing around your roof, especially if children will be helping in the garden.

How to Make a Rooftop Garden

Preparation

1. Before you begin, find out if it is possible and legal to create a garden on your roof. You don't want to spend lots of time and money preparing for a garden and then find out that it is prohibited.
2. Make sure that the roof is able to hold the weight of a rooftop garden. If so, figure out how much weight it can hold. Remember this when making the garden and use lighter containers and soil as needed.

Setting Up the Garden

1. Install your waterproof, protective drainage, and filter layers, as described earlier. If your roof is angled, you may want to place a wooden frame around the edges of the roof to keep the layers from sliding off. Be sure to use rot-resistant wood and cut outlets into the frame to allow excess water to drain away. Layer pebbles around the outlets to aid drainage and to keep vegetation from clogging them.
2. Add soil to your garden. It should be 1–4 inches thick and will be best if it's a mix of ¾ inorganic soil (crushed brick or a similar granular material) and ¼ organic compost.

Planting and Maintaining the Garden

1. Start planting. You can plant seeds, seedlings, or transplant mature plants. Choose plants that are wind-resistant and won't need a great deal of maintenance. Sedums make excellent rooftop plants as they require very little attention once planted, are hardy, and are attractive throughout most of the year. Most vegetables can be grown in-season on rooftops, though the wind will make taller vegetables (like corn or beans) difficult to grow. If your roof is slanted, plant drought-resistant plant varieties near the peak, as they'll get less water.
2. Water your garden immediately after planting, and then regularly throughout the growing season, unless rain does the work for you.

Raised Beds

If you live in an area where the soil is wet (preventing a good vegetable garden from growing in the spring), find it difficult to bend over to plant and cultivate your vegetables or flowers, or if you just want a different look to your backyard garden, consider building a raised bed.

A raised bed is an interesting and affordable way to garden. It creates an ideal environment for growing vegetables, since the soil concentration can be closely monitored and, as it is raised above the ground, it reduces the compaction of plants from people walking on the soil.

Raised beds are typically 2 to 6 feet wide and as long as needed. In most cases, a raised bed consists of a "frame" that is filled in with nutrient-rich soil (including compost or organic fertilizers) and is then planted with a variety of vegetables or flowers, depending on the gardener's preference. By controlling the bed's construction and the soil mixture that goes into the bed, a gardener can effectively reduce the amount of weeds that will grow in the garden.

When planting seeds or young sprouts in a raised bed, it is best to space the plants equally from each other on all sides. This will ensure that the leaves will be touching once the plant is mature, thus saving space and reducing the soil's moisture loss.

How to Make a Raised Bed

Step One: Plan Out Your Raised Bed

1. Think about how you'd like your raised bed to look, and then design the shape. A raised bed is not extremely complicated, and all you need to do is build an open-top and open-bottom box (if you are ambitious, you can create a raised bed in the shape of a circle, hexagon, or star). The main purpose of this box is to hold soil.
2. Make a drawing of your raised bed, measure your available garden space, and add those measurements to your drawing. This will allow you to determine how much material is needed. Generally, your bed should be at least 24 inches in height.

Raised beds make neat, attractive gardens and make it easy to monitor the condition of the soil.

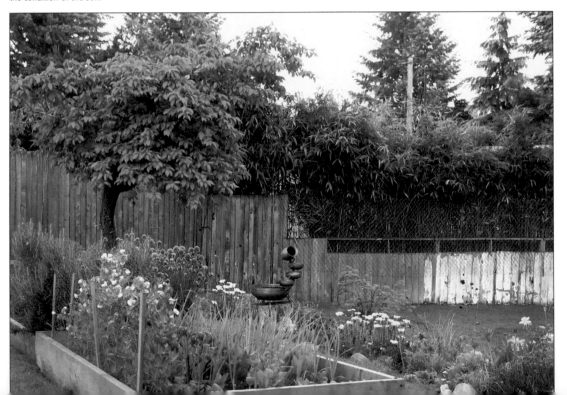

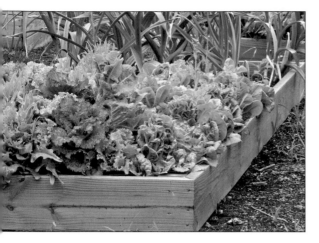

Follow the package instructions for how best to mix it in.
3. Decide what you want to plant. Some people like to grow flowers in their raised beds; others prefer to grow vegetables. If you do want to grow food, raised beds are excellent choices for salad greens, carrots, onions, radishes, beets, and other root crops.

Things to Consider

1. To save money, try to dig up and use soil from your yard. Potting soil can be expensive, and yard soil is just as effective when mixed with compost.
2. Be creative when building your raised planting bed. You can construct a great raised bed out of recycled goods or old lumber.
3. You can convert your raised bed into a greenhouse. Just add hoops to your bed by bending and connecting PVC pipe over the bed. Then clip greenhouse plastic to the PVC pipes, and you have your own greenhouse.
4. Make sure to water your raised bed often. Because it is above ground, your raised bed will not retain water as well as the soil in the ground. If you keep your bed narrow, it will help conserve water.
5. Decorate or illuminate your raised bed to make it a focal point in your yard.
6. If you use lumber to construct your raised bed, keep a watch out for termites.
7. Beware of old, pressure-treated lumber, as it may contain arsenic and could potentially leak into the root systems of any vegetables you might grow in your raised bed. Newer pressure-treated lumber should not contain these toxic chemicals.

3. Decide what kind of material you want to use for your raised bed. You can use lumber, plastic, synthetic wood, railroad ties, bricks, rocks, or a number of other items to hold the dirt. Using lumber is the easiest and most efficient method.
4. Gather your supplies.

Step Two: Build Your Raised Bed

1. Make sure your bed will be situated in a place that gets plenty of sunlight. Carefully assess your placement, as your raised bed will be fairly permanent.
2. Connect the sides of your bed together (with either screws or nails) to form the desired shape of your bed. If you are using lumber, you can use 4 x 4-inch posts to serve as the corners of your bed, and then nail or screw the sides to these corner posts. By doing so, you will increase the strength of the structure and ensure that the dirt will stay inside.
3. Cut a piece of gardening plastic to fit inside your raised bed, and lay it out in the appropriate location. This will significantly reduce the amount of weeds growing in your garden.
4. Place your frame over the gardening plastic (this might take two people).

Step Three: Start Planting

1. Add some compost into the bottom of the bed and then layer potting soil on top of the compost. If you have soil from other parts of your yard, feel free to use that in addition to the compost and potting soil. Plan on filling at least ⅓ of your raised bed with compost or composted manure (available from nurseries or garden centers in 40-pound bags).
2. Mix in dry organic fertilizers (like wood ash, bone meal, and blood meal) while building your bed.

Things You'll Need

- Forms for your raised bed (consider using 4 x 4-inch posts cut to 24 inches in height for corners, and 2 x 12-inch boards for the sides)
- Nails or screws
- Hammer or screwdriver
- Plastic liner (to act as a weed barrier at the bottom of your bed)
- Shovel
- Compost, or composting manure
- Soil (either potting soil or soil from another part of your yard)
- Rake (to smooth out the soil once in the bed)
- Seeds or young plants
- Optional: PVC piping and greenhouse plastic (to convert your raised bed to a greenhouse)

Growing Plants without Soil

Plants grown in soilless cultures still need the basic requirements of plant growth, such as temperature, light (if indoors, use a heat-lamp and set the container near or on a windowsill), water, oxygen (you can produce good airflow by using a small, rotating fan indoors), carbon dioxide, and mineral nutrients (derived from solutions). But palnts grown without soil have their roots either free-floating in a nutrient-rich solution or bedded in a soil-like medium, such as sand, gravel, brick shards, Perlite, or rockwool. These plants do not have to exert as much energy to gather nutrients from the soil and thus they grow more quickly and, usually, more productively.

Types of Soilless Systems

There are two main types of soilless cultures that can be used in order to grow plants and vegetables. The first is a water culture, in which plants are supplied with mineral nutrients directly from the water solution. The second, called aggregate culture or "sand culture," uses an aggregate (such as sand, gravel, or Perlite) as soil to provide an anchoring support for the plant roots. Both types of hydroponics are effective in growing soilless plants and in providing essential nutrients for healthy and productive plant growth.

The Benefits and Drawbacks of Growing Plants in a Hydroponics System

Hydroponics is the method of growing plants in a container filled with a nutrient-rich bath (water with special fertilizer) and no soil.

Lettuce is especially well-suited to hydroponics systems.

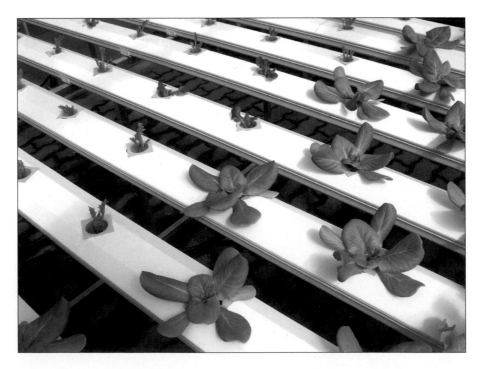

Water Culture

The main advantage of using a water culture system is that a significant part of the nutrient solution is always in contact with the plants' roots. This provides an adequate amount of water and nutrients. The main challenges of this system are providing sufficient air supply for the roots and providing the roots with proper support and anchorage.

Water culture systems are not extremely expensive, though the cost does depend on the price of the chemicals and water used in the preparation of the nutrient solutions, the size of your container, and whether or not your are using mechanized objects, such as pumps and filters. You can decrease the cost by starting small and using readily available materials.

Materials Needed to Make Your Own Water Culture

A large water culture system will need either a wood or concrete tank 6 to 18 inches deep and 2 to 3 feet wide. If you use a wooden container, be sure there are no knots in the wood and seal the tank with non-creosote or tar asphalt.

For small water culture systems, which are recommended for beginners, glass jars, earthenware crocks, or plastic buckets will suffice as your holding tanks. If your container is transparent, be sure to paint the outside of the container with black paint to keep the light out (and to keep algae from growing inside your system). Keep a narrow, vertical strip unpainted in order to see the level of the nutrient solution inside your container.

The plant bed should be 3 or more inches deep and large enough to cover the container or tank. In order to support the weight of the litter (where your seeds or seedlings are placed), cover the bottom of the bed with chicken wire and then fill the bed with litter (wood shavings, sphagnum moss, peat, or other organic materials that do not easily decay). If you are starting your plants from seeds, germinate the seeds in a bed of sand and then transplant to the water culture bed, keeping the bed moist until the plants get their roots down into the nutrient solution.

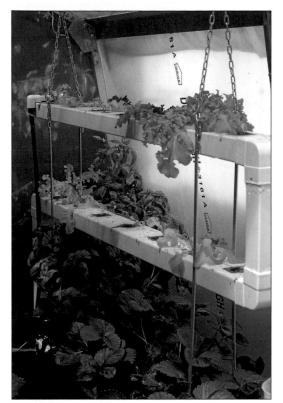

In this type of hydroponics system, a dripper releases the nutrient solution into the top layer of piping. It then flows in a steady stream down through the other layers of piping.

Benefits:

- Plants can be grown in areas where normal plant agriculture is difficult (such as deserts and other arid places, or cities).
- Most terrestrial plants will grow in a hydroponics system.
- There is minimal weed growth.
- The system takes up less space than soil system.
- It conserves water.
- No fear of contaminated runoff from garden fertilizers.
- There is less labor and cost involved.
- Certain seasonal plants can be raised during any season.
- The quality of produce is generally consistent.
- Old nutrient solution can be used to water houseplants.

Drawbacks:

- Can cause salmonella to grow due to the wet and confined conditions.
- More difficult to grow root vegetables, such as carrots and potatoes.
- If nutrient solution is not regularly changed, plants can become nutrient deficient and thus not grow or produce.

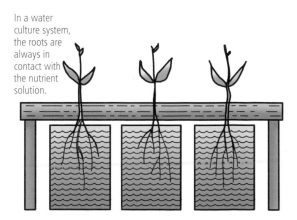

In a water culture system, the roots are always in contact with the nutrient solution.

Aeration

A difficulty in using water culture is keeping the solution properly aerated. It is important to keep enough space between the seed bed and the nutrient solution so the plant's roots can receive proper oxygen. In order to make sure that air can easily flow into the container, either prop up the seed bed slightly to allow air flow or drill a hole in your container just above the highest solution level.

To make sure there is sufficient oxygen reaching the plant roots, you can install an aquarium pump in your water culture system. Just make sure that the water is not agitated too much or the roots may be damaged. You can also use an air stone or perforated pipe to gently introduce air flow into your container.

Water Supply

Your hydroponics system needs an adequate supply of fresh water to maintain healthy plant life. Make sure that the natural minerals in your water are not going to adversely affect your hydroponics plants. If there is too much sodium in your water (usually an effect of softened water), it could become toxic to your plants. In general, the minerals in water are not harmful to the growth of your plants.

Nutrient Solution

You may add nutrient solution by hand, by a gravity-feed system, or mechanically. In smaller water culture systems, mixing the nutrient solution in a small container and adding it by hand, as needed, is typically adequate.

If you are using a larger setup, a gravity-feed system will work quite well. In this type of system, the nutrient solution is mixed in a vat and then tapped from the vat into your container as needed. You can use a plastic container or larger earthenware jar as the vat.

A pump can also be used to supply your system with adequate nutrient solution. You can insert the pump into the vat and then transfer the solution to your hydroponics system.

When your plants are young, it is important to keep the space between your seed bed and the nutrient solution small (that way, the young plant roots can reach the nutrients). As your plants grow, the amount of space between the bed and solution should increase (but do this slowly and keep the level rather consistent).

If the temperature is rather high and there is increased evaporation, it is important to keep the roots at the correct level in the water and change the nutrient solution every day, if needed.

Drain your container every two weeks and then renew the nutrient solution from your vat or by hand. This must be done in a short amount of time so the roots do not dry out.

Transplanting

When transplanting your seedlings, it's important that you are careful with the tiny root systems. Gently work

Things You'll Need

- External pump
- Air line or tubing
- Air stones
- Waterproof bin, bucket, or fish tank to use as a reserve
- Styrofoam
- Net pots
- Type of growing medium, such as rockwool or grow rocks
- Hydroponics nutrients, such as grow formula, bloom formula, supplements, and pH
- Black spray paint (this is only required if the reservoir is transparent)
- Knife, box cutter, or scissors
- Tape measure

the roots through the support netting and down into the nutrient solution. Then fill in the support netting with litter to help the plant remain upright.

How to Build a Simple, Homemade Hydroponics System

Steps to Building Your Hydroponics System:

1. Find a container to use as a reservoir, such as a fish tank, a bin, or a bucket of some sort. The reservoir should be painted black if it is not lightproof (or covered with a thick, black trash bag if you want to reuse the tank at some point), and allowed to dry before moving on to the next step. Allowing light to enter the reservoir will promote the growth of algae. It is a good idea to use a reservoir that is the same dimensions (length and width) from top to bottom.

2. Using a knife or sharp object, score a line on the tank (scratch off some paint in a straight line from top to bottom). This will be your water level meter, which will allow you to see how much water is in the reservoir and will give you a more accurate and convenient view of the nutrient solution level in your tank.

3. Use a tape measure to determine the length and width of your reservoir. Measure the inside of the reservoir from one end to the other. Once you have the dimensions, cut the Styrofoam ¼ inch smaller than the size of the reservoir. For example, if your dimensions are 36 x 20 inches, you should cut the Styrofoam to 35¾ x 19¾ inches. The Styrofoam should fit nicely in the reservoir, with just enough room to adjust to any water level changes. If the reservoir tapers off at the bottom (the bottom is smaller in dimension than the top) the floater (Styrofoam) should be 2 to 4 inches smaller than the reservoir, or more if necessary.

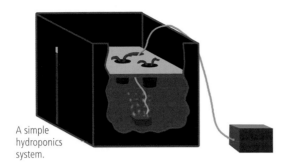

A simple hydroponics system.

4. Do not place the Styrofoam in the reservoir yet. First, you need to cut holes for the net pots. Put the net pots on the Styrofoam where you want to place each plant. Using a pen or pencil, trace around the bottom of each net pot. Use a knife or box cutter to follow the trace lines and cut the holes for pots. On one end of the Styrofoam, cut a small hole for the air line to run into the reservoir.

5. The number of plants you can grow will depend on the size of the garden you build and the types of crops you want to grow. Remember to space plants appropriately so that each receives ample amounts of light.

6. The pump you choose must be strong enough to provide enough oxygen to sustain plant life. Ask for advice choosing a pump at your local hydroponics supply store or garden center.

7. Connect the air line to the pump and attach the air stone to the free end. The air line should be long enough to travel from the pump into the bottom of the reservoir, or at least float in the middle of the tank so the oxygen bubbles can get to the plant roots. It also must be the right size for the pump you choose. Most pumps will come with the correct size air line. To determine the tank's capacity, use a one-gallon bucket or bottle and fill the reservoir. Remember to count how many gallons it takes to fill the reservoir and you will know the correct capacity of your tank.

Setting Up Your Hydroponics System

1. Fill the reservoir with the nutrient solution.
2. Place the Styrofoam into the reservoir.
3. Run the air line through the designated hole or notch.

Things to Consider

- A homemade hydroponics system like this is not ideal for large-scale production of plants or for commercial usage. This particular system does not offer a way to conveniently change the nutrient solution. An extra container would be required to hold the floater while you change the solution.
- Lettuce, watercress, tomatoes, cucumbers, and herbs grow especially well hydroponically.

4. Fill the net pots with growing medium and place one plant in each pot.

5. Put the net pots into the designated holes in the Styrofoam.

6. Plug in the pump, turn it on, and start growing with your fully functional, homemade hydroponics system.

Aggregate Culture

Aggregate culture systems utilize different mediums that act in place of soil to stabilize the plant and its roots. The aggregate in the container is flooded with the nutrient solution. The advantage of this type of system is that there is not as much trouble with aerating the roots. Also, aggregate culture systems allow for the easy transplantation of seedlings into the aggregate medium and it is less expensive.

Materials Needed for an Aggregate Culture System

The container should be watertight to help conserve the nutrient solution. Large tanks can be made of concrete or wood, and smaller operations can effectively be done in glass jars, earthenware containers, or plastic buckets. Make sure to paint transparent containers black.

Aggregate materials may differ greatly, depending on what type you choose to use. Silica sand (well washed) is one of the best materials that can be used. Any other type of coarse-textured sand is also effective, but make sure it does not contain lime. Sand holds moisture quite well and it allows for easy transplantation. A mixture of sand and gravel together is also an effective aggregate. Other materials, such as peat moss, vermiculite, wood shavings, and coco peat, are also good aggregates. You can find aggregate materials at your local garden center, home center, or garden-supply house.

Aeration

Aggregate culture systems allow much easier aeration than water culture systems. Draining and refilling the container with nutrient solution helps the air to move in and out of the aggregate material. This brings a fresh supply of oxygen to the plant roots.

Water Supply

The same water requirements are needed for this type of hydroponics system as for a water culture system. Minerals in the water tend to collect in the aggregate material, so it's a good idea to flush the material with fresh water every few weeks.

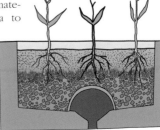

Nutrient Solution

The simplest way of adding the nutrient solution to aggregate cultures is to pour it over the aggregates by hand. You may also use a manual gravity-feed system with buckets or vats. Attach the vat to the bottom of the container with a flexible hose, raise the vat to flood the container, and lower it to drain it. Cover the vat to prevent evaporation and replenish it with new nutrient solution once every two weeks.

A gravity drip-feed system also works well and helps reduce the amount of work you do. Place the vat higher than the container, and then control the solution drip so it is just fast enough to keep the aggregate moist.

It is important that the nutrient solution is added and drained or raised and lowered at least once a day. In hotter weather, the aggregate material may need more wetting with the solution. Make sure that the material is not drying out the roots. Drenching the aggregate with solution often will not harm the plants but letting the roots dry out could have detrimental effects.

Always replace your nutrient solution after two weeks. Not replacing the solution will cause salts and harmful fertilizer residues to build up, which may ultimately damage your plants.

Planting

You may use either seedlings or rooted cuttings in an aggregate culture system. The aggregate should be flooded and solution drained before planting to create a moist, compacted seed bed. Seeds may also be planted directly into the aggregate material. Do not plant the seeds too deep, and flood the container frequently with water to keep the aggregate moist. Once the seedlings have germinated, you may start using the nutrient solution.

If you are transplanting seedlings from a germination bed, make sure they have germinated in soilless material, as any soil left on the roots may cause them to rot and may hamper them in obtaining nutrients from the solution.

Pre-mixed Chemicals

Many of the essential nutrients needed for hydroponic plant growth are now available already mixed in their correct proportions. You may find these solutions in catalogs or from garden-supply stores. They are typically inexpensive and only small quantities are needed to help your plants grow strong and healthy. Always follow the directions on the container when using pre-mixed chemicals.

Making Your Own Solution

In the event that you want to make your own nutrient solution, here is a formula for a solution that will provide all the major elements required for your plants to grow.

You can obtain all of these chemicals from garden-supply stores or drugstores.

Making Nutrient Solutions

For plants to grow properly, they must receive nitrogen, phosphorous, potassium, calcium, magnesium, sulfur, iron, manganese, boron, zinc, copper, molybdenum, and chlorine. There is a wide range of nutrient solutions that can be used. If your plants are receiving inadequate amounts of nutrients, they will show this in different ways. This means that you must proceed with caution when selecting and adding the minerals that will be present in your nutrient solution.

It is important to have pure nutrient materials when preparing the solution. Using fertilizer-grade chemicals is always the best route to go, as it is cheapest. Make sure the containers are closed and not exposed to air. Evaporated solutions increase the amount of salt which could harm your plants.

Salt	Grade	Nutrients	Amt. for 25 gallons of solution
Potassium phosphate	Technical	Potassium, phosphorus	½ ounce (1 Tbsp)
Potassium nitrate	Fertilizer	Potassium, nitrogen	2 ounces (4 Tbsp of powdered salt)
Calcium nitrate	Fertilizer	Calcium, nitrogen	3 ounces (7 Tbsp)
Magnesium sulfate	Fertilizer	Magnesium, sulfur	1½ ounces (4 Tbsp)

After all the chemicals have been mixed into the solution, check the pH of the solution. A pH of 7.0 is neutral; anything below 7.0 is acidic and anything above is alkaline. Certain plants grow best in certain pHs. Plants that grow well at a lower pH (between 4.5 and 5.5) are azaleas, buttercups, gardenias, and roses; plants that grow well at a neutral pH are potatoes, zinnias, and pumpkins; most plants grow best in a slightly acidic pH (between 5.5 and 6.5).

To determine the pH of your solution, use a pH indicator (these are usually paper strips). The strip will change color when placed in different levels of pH. If you find your pH level to be above your desired range, you can bring it down by adding dilute sulfuric acid in small quantities using an eyedropper. Keep retesting until you reach your desired pH level.

Plant Nutrient Deficiencies

When plants are lacking nutrients, they typically display these deficiencies outwardly. Following is a list of symptoms that might occur if a plant is lacking a certain type of nutrient. If your plants display any of these symptoms, it is imperative that the level of that particular nutrient be increased.

Deficient Nutrient	Symptoms
Boron	Tip of the shoot dies; stems and petioles are brittle
Calcium	Tip of the shoot dies; tips of the young leaves die; tips of the leaves are hooked
Iron	New upper leaves turn yellow between the veins; edges and tips of leaves may die
Magnesium	Lower leaves are yellow between the veins; leaf margins curl up or down; leaves die
Manganese	New upper leaves have dead spots; leaf might appear netted
Nitrogen	Leaves are small and light green; lower leaves are lighter than upper leaves; weak stalks
Phosphorous	Dark-green foliage; lower leaves are yellow between the veins; purplish color on leaves
Potassium	Lower leaves might be mottled; dead areas near tips of leaves; yellowing at leaf margins and toward the center
Sulfur	Light-green upper leaves; leaf veins are lighter than surrounding area

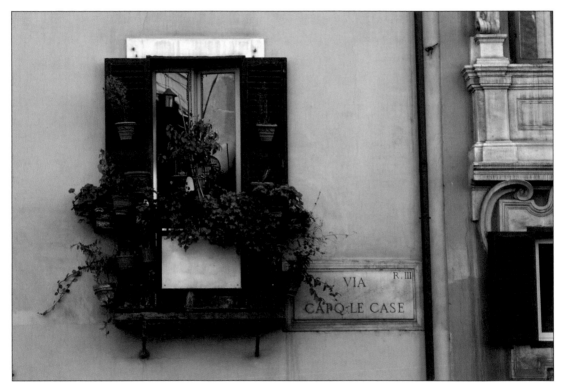

Aggregate culture is especially useful in urban areas where quality soil is not readily available. If the only spot you have for a garden is outside your window, you should still be able to grow a variety of flowers, vegetables, or herbs.

Pest and Disease Management

Pest management can be one of the greatest challenges to the home gardener. Yard pests include weeds, insects, diseases, and some species of wildlife. Weeds are plants that are growing out of place. Insect pests include an enormous number of species, from tiny thrips that are nearly invisible to the naked eye, to the large larvae of the tomato hornworm. Plant diseases are caused by fungi, bacteria, viruses, and other organisms—some of which are only now being classified. Poor plant nutrition and misuse of pesticides also can cause injury to plants. Slugs, mites, and many species of wildlife, such as rabbits, deer, and crows can be extremely destructive as well.

Identify the Problem

Careful identification of the problem is essential before taking measures to control the issue in your garden. Some insect damage may at first appear to be a disease, especially if no visible insects are present. Nutrient problems may also mimic diseases. Herbicide damage, resulting from misapplication of chemicals, can also be mistaken for other problems. Learning about different types of garden pests is the first step in keeping your plants healthy and productive.

Insects and Mites

All insects have six legs, but other than that they are extremely different depending on the species. Some insects include such organisms as beetles, flies, bees, ants, moths, and butterflies. Mites and spiders have eight legs—they are not, in fact, insects but will be treated as such for the purposes of this section.

Insects damage plants in several ways. The most visible damage caused by insects is chewed plant leaves and flowers. Many pests are visible and

Leaf damage from Japanese beetles

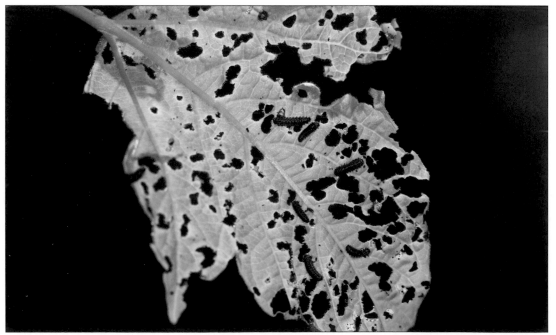

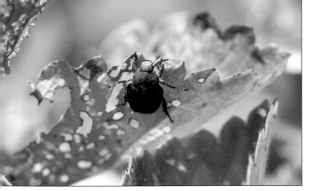

A Japanese beetles eats holes in a leaf

Other insects cause damage to plants by boring into stems, fruits, and leaves, possibly disrupting the plant's ability to transport water. They also create opportunities for disease organisms to attack the plants. You may suspect the presence of boring insects if you see small accumulations of sawdust-like material on plant stems or fruits. Common examples of boring insects include squash vine borers and corn borers.

Integrated Pest Management (IPM)

It is difficult, if not impossible, to prevent all pest problems in your garden every year. If your best prevention efforts have not been entirely successful, you may need to use some control methods. Integrated pest management (IPM) relies on several techniques to keep pests at acceptable population levels without excessive use of chemical controls. The basic principles of IPM include monitoring (scouting), determining tolerable injury levels (thresholds), and applying appropriate strategies and tactics to solve the pest issue. Unlike other methods of pest control where pesticides are applied on a rigid schedule, IPM applies only those controls that are needed, when they are needed, to control pests that will cause more than a tolerable level of damage to the plant.

Monitoring

Monitoring is essential for a successful IPM program. Check your plants regularly. Look for signs of damage from insects and diseases as well as indications of ade-

can be readily identified, including the Japanese beetle, Colorado potato beetle, and numerous species of caterpillars such as tent caterpillars and tomato hornworms. Other chewing insects, however, such as cutworms (which are caterpillars), come out at night to eat, and burrow into the soil during the day. These are much harder to identify but should be considered likely culprits if young plants seem to disappear overnight or are found cut off at ground level.

Sucking insects are extremely common in gardens and can be very damaging to your vegetable plants and flowers. The most known of these insects are leafhoppers, aphids, mealy bugs, thrips, and mites. These insects insert their mouthparts into the plant tissues and suck out the plant juices. They also may carry diseases that they spread from plant to plant as they move about the yard. You may suspect that these insects are present if you notice misshapen plant leaves or flower petals. Often the younger leaves will appear curled or puckered. Flowers developing from the buds may only partially develop if they've been sucked by these bugs. Look on the undersides of the leaves—that is where many insects tend to gather.

Certain kinds of worms and beetles will leave damaging holes in your plants.

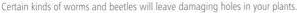

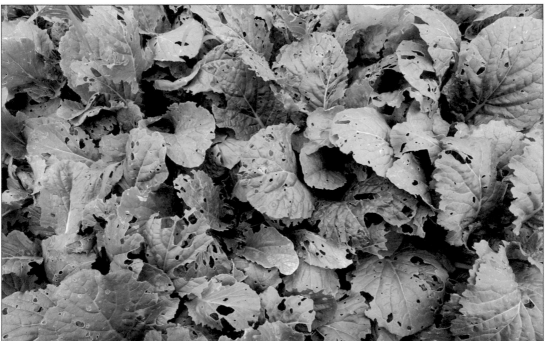

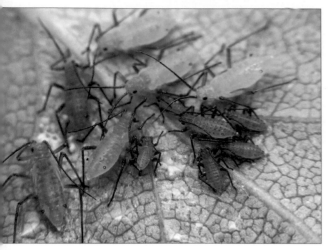

Aphids

quate fertility and moisture. Early identification of potential problems is essential.

There are thousands of insects in a garden, many of which are harmless or even beneficial to the plants. Proper identification is needed before control strategies can be adopted. It is important to recognize the different stages of insect development for several reasons. The caterpillar eating your plants may be the larvae of the butterfly you were trying to attract. Any small larvae with six spots on its back is probably a young ladybug, a very beneficial insect.

Thresholds

It is not necessary to kill every insect, weed, or disease organism invading your garden in order to maintain the plants' health. When dealing with garden pests, an economic threshold comes into play and is the point where the damage caused by the pest exceeds the cost of control. In a home garden, this can be difficult to determine. What you are growing and how you intend to use it will determine how much damage you are willing to tolerate. Remember that larger plants, especially those close to harvest, can tolerate more damage than a tiny seedling. A few flea beetles on a radish seedling may warrant control, whereas numerous Japanese beetles eating the leaves of beans close to harvest may not.

If the threshold level for control has been exceeded, you may need to employ control strategies. Effective and safe strategies can be discussed with your local Cooperative Extension Service, garden centers, or nurseries.

Mechanical/Physical Control Strategies

Many insects can simply be removed by hand. This method is definitely preferable if only a few, large insects are causing the problem. Simply remove the insect from the plant and drop it into a container of soapy water or vegetable oil. Be aware that some insects have prickly

Beneficial Insects that Help Control Pest Populations

Insect	Pest Controlled
Green lacewings	Aphids, mealy bugs, thrips, and spider mites
Ladybugs	Aphids and Colorado potato beetles
Praying mantises	Almost any insect
Ground beetles	Caterpillars that attack trees and shrubs
Seedhead weevils and other beetles	Weeds

spines or excrete oily substances that can cause injury to humans. Use caution when handling unfamiliar insects. Wear gloves or remove insects with tweezers.

Many insects can be removed from plants by spraying water from a hose or sprayer. Small vacuums can also be used to suck up insects. Traps can be used effectively for some insects as well. These come in a variety of styles depending on the insect to be caught. Many traps rely on the use of pheromones—naturally occurring chemicals produced by the insects and used to attract the opposite sex during mating. They are extremely specific for each species and, therefore, will not harm beneficial species. One caution with traps is that they may actually draw more insects into your yard, so don't place them directly into your garden. Other traps (such as yellow and blue sticky cards) are more generic and will attract numerous species. Different insects are attracted to different colors of these traps. Sticky cards also can be used effectively to monitor insect pests.

Other Pest Controls

Diatomaceous earth, a powder-like dust made of tiny marine organisms called diatoms, can be used to reduce damage from soft-bodied insects and slugs. Spread this material on the soil—it is sharp and cuts or irritates these soft organisms. It is harmless to other organisms. In order to trap slugs, put out shallow dishes of beer.

Biological Controls

Biological controls are nature's way of regulating pest populations. Biological controls rely on predators and parasites to keep organisms under control. Many of our present pest problems result from the loss of predator species and other biological control factors.

Some biological controls include birds and bats that eat insects. A single bat can eat up to 600 mosquitoes an hour. Many bird species eat insect pests on trees and in the garden.

Chemical Controls

When using biological controls, be very careful with pesticides. Most common pesticides are broad spectrum,

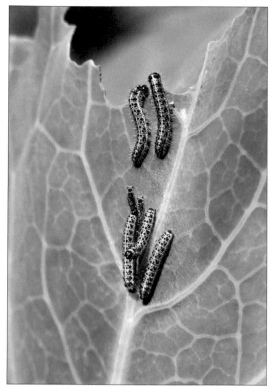

Cutworms

stream of water from a hose all work to dislodge insects from your garden plants.

Another solution is to also consider using plants that naturally repel insects. These plants have their own chemical defense systems, and when planted among flowers and vegetables, they help keep unwanted insects away.

Plant Diseases

Plant disease identification is extremely difficult. In some cases, only laboratory analysis can conclusively identify some diseases. Disease organisms injure plants in several ways: Some attack leaf surfaces and limit the plant's ability to carry on photosynthesis; others produce substances that clog plant tissues that transport water and nutrients; still other disease organisms produce toxins that kill the plant or replace plant tissue with their own.

which means that they kill a wide variety of organisms. Spray applications of insecticides are likely to kill numerous beneficial insects as well as the pests. Herbicides applied to weed species may drift in the wind or vaporize in the heat of the day and injure non-targeted plants. Runoff of pesticides can pollute water. Many pesticides are toxic to humans as well as pets and small animals that may enter your yard. Try to avoid using these types of pesticides at all costs—and if you do use them, read the labels carefully and avoid spraying them on windy days.

Some common, non-toxic household substances are as effective as many toxic pesticides. A few drops of dishwashing detergent mixed with water and sprayed on plants is extremely effective in controlling many soft-bodied insects, such as aphids and whiteflies. Crushed garlic mixed with water may control certain insects. A baking soda solution has been shown to help control some fungal diseases on roses.

Alternatives to Pesticides and Chemicals

When used incorrectly, pesticides can pollute water. They also kill beneficial as well as harmful insects. Natural alternatives prevent both of these events from occurring and save you money. Consider using natural alternatives for chemical pesticides: Non-detergent insecticidal soaps, garlic, hot pepper spray, 1 teaspoon of liquid soap in a gallon of water, used dishwater, or a forceful

Natural Pest Repellants

Pest	Repellant
Ant	Mint, tansy, or pennyroyal
Aphids	Mint, garlic, chives, coriander, or anise
Bean leaf beetle	Potato, onion, or turnip
Codling moth	Common oleander
Colorado potato bug	Green beans, coriander, or nasturtium
Cucumber beetle	Radish or tansy
Flea beetle	Garlic, onion, or mint
Imported cabbage worm	Mint, sage, rosemary, or hyssop
Japanese beetle	Garlic, larkspur, tansy, rue, or geranium
Leaf hopper	Geranium or petunia
Mice	Onion
Root knot nematodes	French marigolds
Slugs	Prostrate rosemary or wormwood
Spider mites	Onion, garlic, cloves, or chives
Squash bug	Radish, marigolds, tansy, or nasturtium
Stink bug	Radish
Thrips	Marigolds
Tomato hornworm	Marigolds, sage, or borage
Whitefly	Marigolds or nasturtium

Symptoms that are associated with plant diseases may include the presence of mushroom-like growths on trunks of trees; leaves with a grayish, mildewed appearance; spots on leaves, flowers, and fruits; sudden wilting or death of a plant or branch; sap exuding from branches or trunks of trees; and stunted growth.

Misapplication of pesticides and nutrients, air pollutants, and other environmental conditions—such as flooding and freezing—can also mimic some disease problems. Yellowing or reddening of leaves and stunted growth may indicate a nutritional problem. Leaf curling or misshapen growth may be a result of herbicide application.

Pest and Disease Management Practices

Preventing pests should be your first goal when growing a garden, although it is unlikely that you will be able to avoid all pest problems because some plant seeds and disease organisms may lay dormant in the soil for years.

Diseases need three elements to become established in plants: the disease organism, a susceptible species, and the proper environmental conditions. Some disease organisms can live in the soil for years; other organisms are carried in infected plant material that falls to the ground. Some disease organisms are carried by insects. Good sanitation will help limit some problems with disease. Choosing resistant varieties of plants also prevents many diseases from occurring. Rotating annual plants in a garden can also prevent some diseases.

Plants that have adequate, but not excessive, nutrients are better able to resist attacks from both diseases and insects. Excessive rates of nitrogen often result in extremely succulent vegetative growth and can make plants more susceptible to insect and disease problems, as well as decreasing their winter hardiness. Proper watering and spacing of plants limits the spread of some diseases and provides good aeration around plants, so diseases that fester in standing water cannot multiply. Trickle irrigation, where water is applied to the soil and not the plant leaves, may be helpful.

Removal of diseased material certainly limits the spread of some diseases. It is important to clean up litter

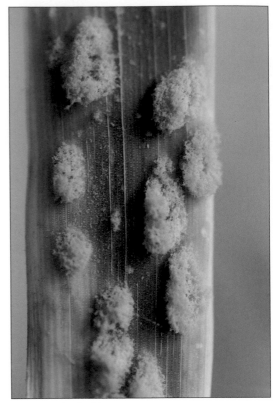

Powdery mildew leaf disease

dropped from diseased plants. Prune diseased branches on trees and shrubs to allow for more air circulation. When pruning diseased trees and shrubs, disinfect your pruners between cuts with a solution of chlorine bleach to avoid spreading the disease from plant to plant. Also try to control insects that may carry diseases to your plants.

You can make your own natural fungicide by combining 5 teaspoons each of baking soda and hydrogen peroxide with a gallon of water. Spray on your infected plants. Milk diluted with water is also an effective fungicide, due to the potassium phosphate in it, which boosts a plant's immune system. The more diluted the solution, the more frequently you'll need to spray the plant.

Harvesting Your Garden

It is essential, in order to get the best freshness, flavor, and nutritional benefits from your garden vegetables and fruits, to harvest them at the appropriate time. The vegetable's stage of maturity and the time of day at which it is harvested are essential for good-tasting and nutritious produce. Overripe vegetables and fruits will be stringy and coarse. When possible, harvest your vegetables during the cool part of the morning. If you are going to can and preserve your vegetables and fruits, do so as soon as possible. Or, if this process must be delayed, cool the vegetables in ice water or crushed ice and store them in the refrigerator. Here are some brief guidelines for harvesting various types of common garden produce:

Asparagus—Harvest the spears when they are at least 6 to 8 inches tall by snapping or cutting them at ground level. A few spears may be harvested the second year after crowns are set out. A full harvest season will last four to six weeks during the third growing season.

Beans, snap—Harvest before the seeds develop in the pod. Beans are ready to pick if they snap easily when bent in half.

Beans, lima—Harvest when the pods first start to bulge with the enlarged seeds. Pods must still be green, not yellowish.

Broccoli—Harvest the dark green, compact cluster, or head, while the buds are shut tight, before any yellow flowers appear. Smaller side shoots will develop later, providing a continuous harvest.

Brussels sprouts—Harvest the lower sprouts (small heads) when they are about 1 to 1 ½ inches in diameter by twisting them off. Removing the lower leaves along the stem will help to hasten the plant's maturity.

Cabbage—Harvest when the heads feel hard and solid.

Cantaloupe—Harvest when the stem slips easily from the fruit with a gentle tug. Another indicator of ripeness is when the netting on the skin becomes rounded and the flesh between the netting turns from a green to a tan color.

Carrots—Harvest when the roots are ¾ to 1 inch in diameter. The largest roots generally have darker tops.

Cauliflower—When preparing to harvest, exclude sunlight when the curds (heads) are 1 to 2 inches in diameter by loosely tying the outer leaves

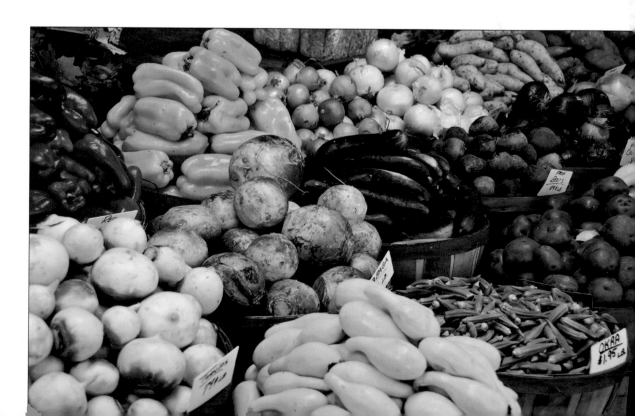

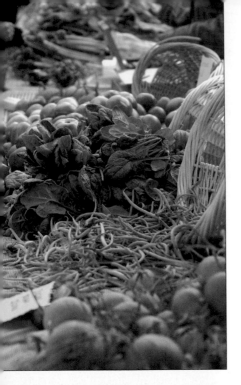

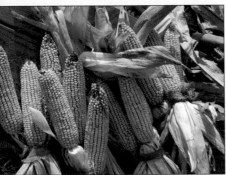

Dried corn can be made into cornmeal by removing the kernels from the husk and grinding them in a food processor.

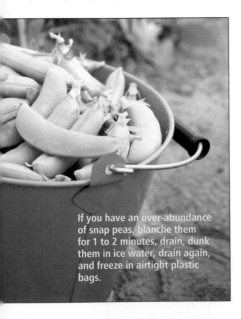

If you have an over-abundance of snap peas, blanche them for 1 to 2 minutes, drain, dunk them in ice water, drain again, and freeze in airtight plastic bags.

together above the curd with a string or rubber band. This process is known as blanching. Harvest the curds when they are 4 to 6 inches in diameter but still compact, white, and smooth. The head should be ready 10 to 15 days after tying the leaves.

Collards—Harvest older, lower leaves when they reach a length of 8 to 12 inches. New leaves will grow as long as the central growing point remains, providing a continuous harvest. Whole plants may be harvested and cooked if desired.

Corn, sweet—The silks begin to turn brown and dry out as the ears mature. Check a few ears for maturity by opening the top of the ear and pressing a few kernels with your thumbnail. If the exuded liquid is milky rather than clear, the ear is ready for harvesting. Cooking a few ears is also a good way to test for maturity.

Cucumbers—Harvest when the fruits are 6 to 8 inches in length. Harvest when the color is deep green and before yellow color appears. Pick four to five times per week to encourage continuous production. Leaving mature cucumbers on the vine will stop the production of the entire plant.

Eggplant—Harvest when the fruits are 4 to 5 inches in diameter and their color is a glossy, purplish black. The fruit is getting too ripe when the color starts to dull or become bronzed. Because the stem is woody, cut—do not pull—the fruit from the plant. A short stem should remain on each fruit.

Kale—Harvest by twisting off the outer, older leaves when they reach a length of 8 to 10 inches and are medium green in color. Heavy, dark green leaves are overripe and are likely to be tough and bitter. New leaves will grow, providing a continuous harvest.

Lettuce—Harvest the older, outer leaves from leaf lettuce as soon as they are 4 to 6 inches long. Harvest heading types when the heads are moderately firm and before seed stalks form.

Mustard—Harvest the leaves and leaf stems when they are 6 to 8 inches long; new leaves will provide a continuous harvest until they become too strong in flavor and tough in texture, due to temperature extremes.

Okra—Harvest young, tender pods when they are 2 to 3 inches long. Pick the okra at least every other day during the peak growing season. Overripe pods become woody and are too tough to eat.

Onions—Harvest when the tops fall over and begin to turn yellow. Dig up the onions and allow them to dry out in the open sun for a few days to toughen the skin. Then remove the dried soil by brushing the onions lightly. Cut the stem, leaving 2 to 3 inches attached, and store in a net-type bag in a cool, dry place.

Peas—Harvest regular peas when the pods are well rounded; edible-pod varieties should be harvested when the seeds are fully developed but still fresh and bright green. Pods are getting too old when they lose their brightness and turn light or yellowish green.

Peppers—Harvest sweet peppers with a sharp knife when the fruits are firm, crisp, and full size. Green peppers will turn red if left on the plant. Allow hot peppers to attain their bright red color and full flavor while attached to the vine; then cut them and hang them to dry.

Potatoes (Irish)—Harvest the tubers when the plants begin to dry and die down. Store the tubers in a cool, high-humidity location with good ventilation, such as the basement or crawl space of your house. Avoid exposing the tubers to light, as greening, which denotes the presence of dangerous alkaloids, will occur even with small amounts of light.

Pumpkins—Harvest pumpkins and winter squash before the first frost. After the vines dry up, the fruit color darkens and the skin surface resists puncture from your thumbnail. Avoid bruising or scratching the fruit while handling it. Leave a 3- to 4-inch portion of the stem

Don't cut asparagus below the soil as it could damage other buds on the crown that would otherwise send up new spears.

attached to the fruit and store it in a cool, dry location with good ventilation.

Radishes—Harvest when the roots are ½ to 1½ inches in diameter. The shoulders of radish roots often appear through the soil surface when they are mature. If left in the ground too long, the radishes will become tough and woody.

Rutabagas—Harvest when the roots are about 3 inches in diameter. The roots may be stored in the ground and used as needed, if properly mulched.

Spinach—Harvest by cutting all the leaves off at the base of the plant when they are 4 to 6 inches long. New leaves will grow, providing additional harvests.

Squash, summer—Harvest when the fruit is soft, tender, and 6 to 8 inches long. The skin color often changes to a dark, glossy green or yellow, depending on the variety. Pick every two to three days to encourage continued production.

Sweet potatoes—Harvest the roots when they are large enough for use before the first frost. Avoid bruising or scratching the potatoes during handling. Ideal storage conditions are at a temperature of 55°F and a relative humidity of 85 percent. The basement or crawl space of a house may suffice.

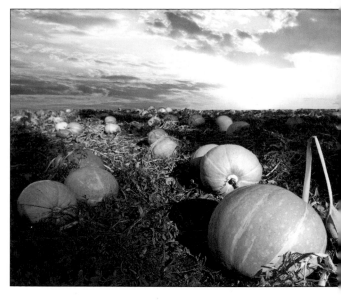

Swiss chard—Harvest by breaking off the developed outer leaves 1 inch above the soil. New leaves will grow, providing a continuous harvest.

Tomatoes—Harvest the fruits at the most appealing stage of ripeness, when they are bright red. The flavor is best at room temperature, but ripe fruit may be held in the refrigerator at 45 to 50°F for 7 to 10 days.

Turnips—Harvest the roots when they are 2 to 3 inches in diameter but before heavy fall frosts occur. The tops may be used as salad greens when the leaves are 3 to 5 inches long.

Watermelons—Harvest when the watermelon produces a dull thud rather than a sharp, metallic sound when thumped—this means the fruit is ripe. Other ripeness indicators are a deep yellow rather than a white color where the melon touches the ground, brown tendrils on the stem near the fruit, and a rough, slightly ridged feel to the skin surface.

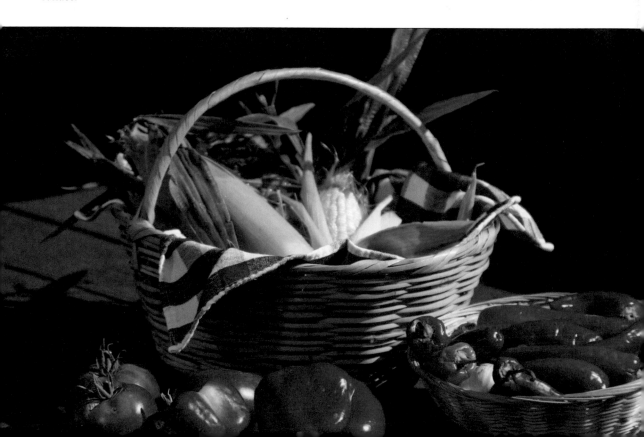

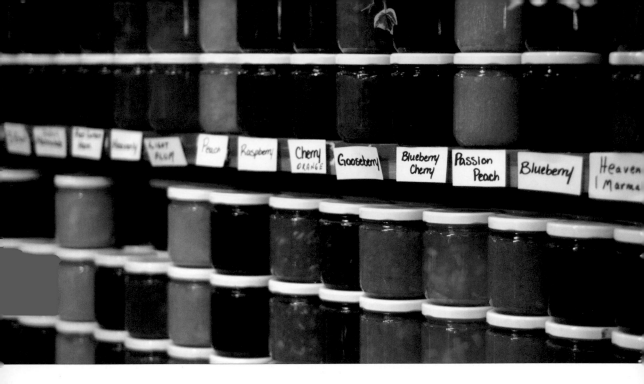

PART TWO   The Pantry

One of the greatest pleasures of self-sufficiency is preparing, preserving, and eating your own food. After the hard work of planting and tending your gardens, or raising animals for eggs, milk, or meat, your kitchen will become a joyful laboratory where you can create wonderful foods from the fruits of your labor to enjoy or to share. With a little preparation, your pantry can become a treasure trove of canned and dried foods, ready to draw from all winter long. There is something distinctly rewarding about running out to the garden to pick salad makings in the summer, or reaching into the cupboard for a new jar of strawberry jam in the middle of the winter. It's a gift more and more people are finding time to accept, as the quality of supermarket offerings seems to plummet and a new awareness of the benefits of locally grown food sweeps across rural and urban areas alike. If you don't have the space or time to grow or produce your own food, there are farmers' markets springing up all over where you can find fresh, delicious produce, meats, baked goods, and dairy products to enjoy on your own or to inspire a festive dinner party. Whether you go to the garden, the pantry, or the market for your food, remember the work that went into its growth and preparation and you will begin to see food not only as a necessity and a pleasure, but as a great gift.

Canning

Introduction to Canning

On the next few pages, you will find descriptions of proper canning methods, with details on how canning works and why it is both safe and economical. Much of the information here is from the USDA, which has done extensive research on home canning and preserving. If you are new to home canning, read this section carefully as it will help to ensure success with the recipes that follow

Whether you are a seasoned home canner or this is your first foray into food preservation, it is important to follow directions carefully. With some recipes it is okay to experiment with varied proportions or added ingredients, and with others it is important to stick to what's written. In many instances it is noted whether creative liberty is a good idea for a particular recipe, but if you are not sure, play it safe—otherwise you may end up with a jam that is too runny, a vegetable that is mushy, or a product that is spoiled. Take time to read the directions and prepare your foods and equipment adequately, and you will find that home canning is safe, economical, tremendously satisfying, and a great deal of fun!

Why Can Foods?

Canning is fun and a good way to preserve your precious produce. As more and more farmers' markets make their way into urban centers, city dwellers are also discovering how rewarding it is to make seasonal treats last all year round. Besides the value of your labor, canning home-grown or locally grown food may save you half the cost of buying commercially canned food. And what makes a nicer, more thoughtful gift than a jar of homemade jam, tailored to match the recipient's favorite fruits and flavors?

The nutritional value of home canning is an added benefit. Many vegetables begin to lose their vitamins as soon as they are harvested. Nearly half

Canned jams and nut butters.

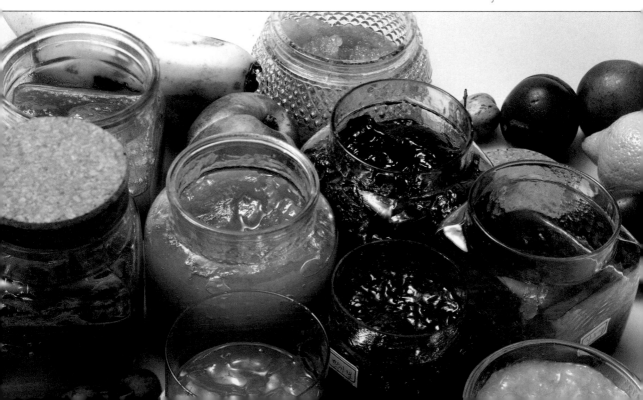

the vitamins may be lost within a few days unless the fresh produce is kept cool or preserved. Within one to two weeks, even refrigerated produce loses half or more of certain vitamins. The heating process during canning destroys from one-third to one-half of vitamins A and C, thiamin, and riboflavin. Once canned, foods may lose from 5 percent to 20 percent of these sensitive vitamins each year. The amounts of other vitamins, however, are only slightly lower in canned compared with fresh food. If vegetables are handled properly and canned promptly after harvest, they can be more nutritious than fresh produce sold in local stores.

The advantages of home canning are lost when you start with poor quality foods; when jars fail to seal properly; when food spoils; and when flavors, texture, color, and nutrients deteriorate during prolonged storage. The tips that follow explain many of these problems and recommend ways to minimize them.

How Canning Preserves Foods

The high percentage of water in most fresh foods makes them very perishable. They spoil or lose their quality for several reasons:

- Growth of undesirable microorganisms—bacteria, molds, and yeasts
- Activity of food enzymes
- Reactions with oxygen
- Moisture loss

Microorganisms live and multiply quickly on the surfaces of fresh food and on the inside of bruised, insect-damaged, and diseased food. Oxygen and enzymes are present throughout fresh food tissues.

Proper canning practices include:

- Carefully selecting and washing fresh food
- Peeling some fresh foods
- Hot packing many foods
- Adding acids (lemon juice, citric acid, or vinegar) to some foods
- Using acceptable jars and self-sealing lids
- Processing jars in a boiling-water or pressure canner for the correct amount of time

Collectively, these practices remove oxygen; destroy enzymes; prevent the growth of undesirable bacteria, yeasts, and molds; and help form a high vacuum in jars. High vacuums form tight seals, which keep liquid in and air and microorganisms out.

CANNING began in France, at the turn of the nineteenth century, when Napoleon Bonaparte was desperate for a way to keep his troops well-fed while on the march. In 1800, he decided to hold a contest, offering 12,000 francs to anyone who could devise a suitable method of food preservation. Nicolas François Appert, a French confectioner, rose to the challenge, considering that if wine could be preserved in bottles, perhaps food could be as well. He experimented until he was able to prove that heating food to boiling after it had been sealed in airtight glass bottles prevented the food from deteriorating. Interestingly, this all took place about 100 years before Louis Pasteur found that heat could destroy bacteria. Nearly ten years after the contest began, Napoleon personally presented Nicolas with the cash reward.

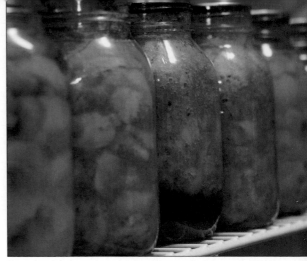

Canned applesauce and peaches line this pantry's shelves.

Canning Glossary

Acid foods—Foods that contain enough acid to result in a pH of 4.6 or lower. Includes most tomatoes; fermented and pickled vegetables; relishes; jams, jellies, and marmalades; and all fruits except figs. Acid foods may be processed in boiling water.

Ascorbic acid—The chemical name for vitamin C. Commonly used to prevent browning of peeled, light-colored fruits and vegetables.

Blancher—A 6- to 8-quart lidded pot designed with a fitted, perforated basket to hold food in boiling water or with a fitted rack to steam foods. Useful for loosening skins on fruits to be peeled or for heating foods to be hot packed.

Boiling-water canner—A large, standard-sized, lidded kettle with jar rack designed for heat-processing seven quarts or eight to nine pints in boiling water.

Botulism—An illness caused by eating a toxin produced by growth of *Clostridium botulinum* bacteria in moist, low-acid food containing less than 2 percent oxygen and stored between 40°F and 120°F. Proper heat processing destroys this bacterium in canned food. Freezer temperatures inhibit its growth in frozen food. Low moisture controls its growth in dried food. High oxygen controls its growth in fresh foods.

Canning—A method of preserving food that employs heat processing in airtight, vacuum-sealed containers so that food can be safely stored at normal home temperatures.

Canning salt—Also called pickling salt. It is regular table salt without the anti-caking or iodine additives.

Citric acid—A form of acid that can be added to canned foods. It increases the acidity of low-acid foods and may improve their flavor.

Cold pack—Canning procedure in which jars are filled with raw food. "Raw pack" is the preferred term for describing this practice. "Cold pack" is often used incorrectly to refer to foods that are open-kettle canned or jars that are heat-processed in boiling water.

Enzymes—Proteins in food that accelerate many flavor, color, texture, and nutritional changes, especially when food is cut, sliced, crushed, bruised, or exposed

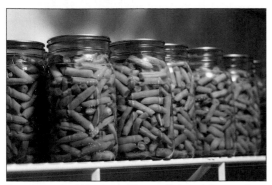
Green beans should be chopped into small pieces before canning.

to air. Proper blanching or hot-packing practices destroy enzymes and improve food quality.

Exhausting—Removing air from within and around food and from jars and canners. Exhausting or venting of pressure canners is necessary to prevent botulism in low-acid canned foods.

Headspace—The unfilled space above food or liquid in jars that allows for food expansion as jars are heated and for forming vacuums as jars cool.

Heat processing—Treatment of jars with sufficient heat to enable storing food at normal home temperatures.

Hermetic seal—An absolutely airtight container seal that prevents reentry of air or microorganisms into packaged foods.

Hot pack—Heating of raw food in boiling water or steam and filling it hot into jars.

Low-acid foods—Foods that contain very little acid and have a pH above 4.6. The acidity in these foods is insufficient to prevent the growth of botulism bacteria. Vegetables, some varieties of tomatoes, figs, all meats, fish, seafood, and some dairy products are low-acid foods. To control all risks of botulism, jars of these foods must be either heat processed in a pressure canner or acidified to a pH of 4.6 or lower before being processed in boiling water.

Microorganisms—Independent organisms of microscopic size, including bacteria, yeast, and mold. In a suitable environment, they grow rapidly and may divide or reproduce every 10 to 30 minutes. Therefore, they reach high populations very quickly. Microorganisms are sometimes intentionally added to ferment foods, make antibiotics, and for other reasons. Undesirable microorganisms cause disease and food spoilage.

Mold—A fungus-type microorganism whose growth on food is usually visible and colorful. Molds may grow on many foods, including acid foods like jams and jellies and canned fruits. Recommended heat processing and sealing practices prevent their growth on these foods.

A large stockpot with a lid can be used in place of a boiling-water canner for high-acid foods like tomatoes, pickles, apples, peaches, and jams. Simply place a rack inside the pot so that the jars do not rest directly on the bottom of the pot.

Mycotoxins—Toxins produced by the growth of some molds on foods.

Open-kettle canning—A non-recommended canning method. Food is heat-processed in a covered kettle, filled while hot into sterile jars, and then sealed. Foods canned this way have low vacuums or too much air, which permits rapid loss of quality in foods. Also, these foods often spoil because they become recontaminated while the jars are being filled.

Pasteurization—Heating food to temperatures high enough to destroy disease-causing microorganisms.

pH—A measure of acidity or alkalinity. Values range from 0 to 14. A food is neutral when its pH is 7.0. Lower values are increasingly more acidic; higher values are increasingly more alkaline.

PSIG—Pounds per square inch of pressure as measured by a gauge.

Pressure canner—A specifically designed metal kettle with a lockable lid used for heat-processing low-acid food. These canners have jar racks, one or more safety devices, systems for exhausting air, and a way to measure or control pressure. Canners with 20- to 21-quart capacity are common. The minimum size of canner that should be used has a 16-quart capacity and can hold seven one-quart jars. Use of pressure saucepans with a capacity of less than 16 quarts is not recommended.

Raw pack—The practice of filling jars with raw, unheated food. Acceptable for canning low-acid foods, but allows more rapid quality losses in acid foods that are heat-processed in boiling water. Also called "cold pack."

Style of pack—Form of canned food, such as whole, sliced, piece, juice, or sauce. The term may also be used to specify whether food is filled raw or hot into jars.

Vacuum—A state of negative pressure that reflects how thoroughly air is removed from within a jar of processed food; the higher the vacuum, the less air left in the jar.

Peel potatoes before canning them.
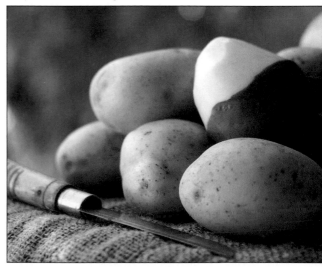

Proper Canning Practices

Growth of the bacterium *Clostridium botulinum* in canned food may cause botulism—a deadly form of food poisoning. These bacteria exist either as spores or as vegetative cells. The spores, which are comparable to plant seeds, can survive harmlessly in soil and water for many years. When ideal conditions exist for growth, the spores produce vegetative cells, which multiply rapidly and may produce a deadly toxin within three to four days in an environment consisting of:

* A moist, low-acid food
* A temperature between 40°F and 120°F, and
* Less than 2 percent oxygen.

Botulinum spores are on most fresh food surfaces. Because they grow only in the absence of air, they are harmless on fresh foods. Most bacteria, yeasts, and molds are difficult to remove from food surfaces. Washing fresh food reduces their numbers only slightly. Peeling root crops, underground stem crops, and tomatoes reduces their numbers greatly. Blanching also helps, but the vital controls are the method of canning and use of the recommended research-based processing times. These processing times ensure destruction of the largest expected number of heat-resistant microorganisms in home-canned foods.

Properly sterilized canned food will be free of spoilage if lids seal and jars are stored below 95°F. Storing jars at 50 to 70°F enhances retention of quality.

Food Acidity and Processing Methods

Whether food should be processed in a pressure canner or boiling-water canner to control botulism bacteria depends on the acidity in the food. Acidity may be natural, as in most fruits, or added, as in pickled food. Low-acid canned foods contain too little acidity

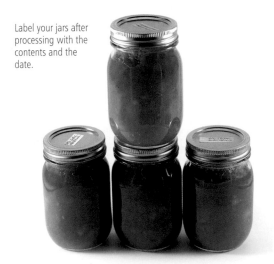

Label your jars after processing with the contents and the date.

to prevent the growth of these bacteria. Other foods may contain enough acidity to block their growth or to destroy them rapidly when heated. The term "pH" is a measure of acidity: the lower its value, the more acidic the food. The acidity level in foods can be increased by adding lemon juice, citric acid, or vinegar.

Low-acid foods have pH values higher than 4.6. They include red meats, seafood, poultry, milk, and all fresh vegetables except for most tomatoes. Most products that are mixtures of low-acid and acid foods also have pH values above 4.6 unless their ingredients include enough lemon juice, citric acid, or vinegar to make them acid foods. Acid foods have a pH of 4.6 or lower. They include fruits, pickles, sauerkraut, jams, jellies, marmalade, and fruit butters.

Although tomatoes usually are considered an acid food, some are now known to have pH values slightly above 4.6. Figs also have pH values slightly above 4.6. Therefore, if they are to be canned as acid foods, these products must be acidified to a pH of 4.6 or lower with lemon juice or citric acid. Properly acidified tomatoes and figs are acid foods and can be safely processed in a boiling-water canner.

Botulinum spores are very hard to destroy at boiling-water temperatures; the higher the canner temperature, the more easily they are destroyed. Therefore, all low-acid foods should be sterilized at temperatures of 240 to 250°F, attainable with pressure canners operated at 10 to 15 PSIG. (PSIG means pounds per square inch of pressure as measured by a gauge.) At these temperatures, the time needed to destroy bacteria in low-acid canned foods ranges from 20 to 100 minutes. The exact time depends on the kind of food being canned, the way it is packed into jars, and the size of jars. The time needed to safely process low-acid foods in boiling water ranges from 7 to 11 hours; the time needed to process acid foods in boiling water varies from 5 to 85 minutes.

Know Your Altitude

It is important to know your approximate elevation or altitude above sea level in order to determine a safe processing time for canned foods. Since the boiling temperature of liquid is lower at higher elevations, it is critical that additional time be given for the safe processing of foods at altitudes above sea level.

What Not to Do

Open-kettle canning and the processing of freshly filled jars in conventional ovens, microwave ovens, and dishwashers are not recommended because these practices do not prevent all risks of spoilage. Steam canners are not recommended because processing times for use with current models have not been adequately researched. Because steam canners may not heat foods in the same manner as boiling-water canners, their use with boiling-water processing times may result in spoilage. So-called canning powders are useless as preservatives and do not replace the need for proper heat processing.

It is not recommended that pressures in excess of 15 PSIG be applied when using new pressure-canning equipment.

Ensuring High-Quality Canned Foods

Examine food carefully for freshness and wholesomeness. Discard diseased and moldy food. Trim small diseased lesions or spots from food.

Can fruits and vegetables picked from your garden or purchased from nearby producers when the products are at their peak of quality—within 6 to 12 hours after harvest for most vegetables. However, apricots, nectarines, peaches, pears, and plums should be ripened one or more days between harvest and canning. If you must delay the canning of other fresh produce, keep it in a shady, cool place.

Fresh, home-slaughtered red meats and poultry should be chilled and canned without delay. Do not can meat from sickly or diseased animals. Put fish and seafood on ice after harvest, eviscerate immediately, and can them within two days.

Maintaining Color and Flavor in Canned Food

To maintain good natural color and flavor in stored canned food, you must:
- Remove oxygen from food tissues and jars,
- Quickly destroy the food enzymes, and
- Obtain high jar vacuums and airtight jar seals.

Follow these guidelines to ensure that your canned foods retain optimal colors and flavors during processing and storage:
- Use only high-quality foods that are at the proper maturity and are free of diseases and bruises.
- Use the hot-pack method, especially with acid foods to be processed in boiling water.
- Don't unnecessarily expose prepared foods to air; can them as soon as possible.
- While preparing a canner load of jars, keep peeled, halved, quartered, sliced or diced apples, apricots, nectarines, peaches, and pears in a solution of 3 grams (3,000 milligrams) ascorbic acid to 1 gallon of cold water. This procedure is also useful in maintaining the natural color of mushrooms and potatoes and for preventing stem-end discoloration in cherries and grapes. You can get ascorbic acid in several forms:

Pure powdered form—Seasonally available among canning supplies in supermarkets. One level teaspoon of pure powder weighs about 3 grams. Use 1 teaspoon per gallon of water as a treatment solution.

Vitamin C tablets—Economical and available year-round in many stores. Buy 500-milligram tablets; crush and dissolve six tablets per gallon of water as a treatment solution.

Commercially prepared mixes of ascorbic and citric acid—Seasonally available among canning supplies in supermarkets. Sometimes citric acid powder is sold

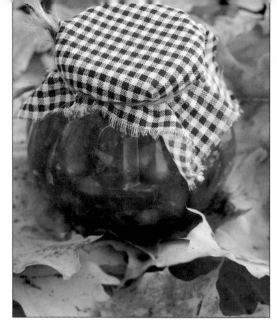

in supermarkets, but it is less effective in controlling discoloration. If you choose to use these products, follow the manufacturer's directions.
- Fill hot foods into jars and adjust headspace as specified in recipes.
- Tighten screw bands securely, but if you are especially strong, not as tightly as possible.
- Process and cool jars.
- Store the jars in a relatively cool, dark place, preferably between 50 and 70°F.
- Can no more food than you will use within a year.

Advantages of Hot Packing

Many fresh foods contain from 10 percent to more than 30 percent air. The length of time that food will last at premium quality depends on how much air is removed from the food before jars are sealed. The more air that is removed, the higher the quality of the canned product.

Raw packing is the practice of filling jars tightly with freshly prepared but unheated food. Such foods, especially fruit, will float in the jars. The entrapped air in and around the food may cause discoloration within two to three months of storage. Raw packing is more suitable for vegetables processed in a pressure canner.

Hot packing is the practice of heating freshly prepared food to boiling, simmering it three to five minutes, and promptly filling jars loosely with the boiled food.

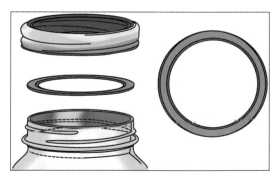

Hot packing is the best way to remove air and is the preferred pack style for foods processed in a boiling-water canner. At first, the color of hot-packed foods may appear no better than that of raw-packed foods, but within a short storage period, both color and flavor of hot-packed foods will be superior.

Whether food has been hot packed or raw packed, the juice, syrup, or water to be added to the foods should be heated to boiling before it is added to the jars. This practice helps to remove air from food tissues, shrinks food, helps keep the food from floating in the jars, increases vacuum in sealed jars, and improves shelf life. Preshrinking food allows you to add more food to each jar.

Controlling Headspace

The unfilled space above the food in a jar and below its lid is termed headspace. It is best to leave a ¼-inch headspace for jams and jellies, ½-inch for fruits and tomatoes to be processed in boiling water, and from 1 to 1¼ inches in low-acid foods to be processed in a pressure canner.

This space is needed for expansion of food as jars are processed and for forming vacuums in cooled jars. The extent of expansion is determined by the air content in the food and by the processing temperature. Air expands greatly when heated to high temperatures—the higher the temperature, the greater the expansion. Foods expand less than air when heated.

Jars and Lids

Food may be canned in glass jars or metal containers. Metal containers can be used only once. They require special sealing equipment and are much more costly than jars.

Mason-type jars designed for home canning are ideal for preserving food by pressure or boiling-water canning. Regular and wide-mouthed threaded mason jars with self-sealing lids are the best choices. They are available in half-pint, pint, 1½-pint, and quart sizes. The standard jar mouth opening is about 2⅜ inches. Wide-mouthed jars have openings of about 3 inches, making them more easily filled and emptied. Regular-mouthed decorative jelly jars are available in 8-ounce and 12-ounce sizes.

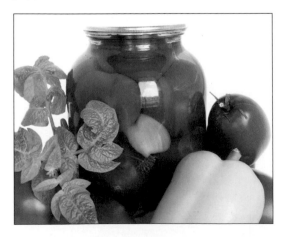

With careful use and handling, mason jars may be reused many times, requiring only new lids each time. When lids are used properly, jar seals and vacuums are excellent.

Jar Cleaning

Before reuse, wash empty jars in hot water with detergent and rinse well by hand, or wash in a dishwasher. Rinse thoroughly, as detergent residue may cause unnatural flavors and colors. Scale or hard-water films on jars are easily removed by soaking jars for several hours in a solution containing 1 cup of vinegar (5 percent acid) per gallon of water.

Sterilization of Empty Jars

Use sterile jars for all jams, jellies, and pickled products processed less than 10 minutes. To sterilize empty jars, put them right side up on the rack in a boiling-water canner. Fill the canner and jars with hot (not boiling) water to 1 inch above the tops of the jars. Boil for 10 minutes. Remove and drain hot, sterilized jars one at a time. Save the hot water for processing filled jars. Fill jars with food, add lids, and tighten screw bands.

Empty jars used for vegetables, meats, and fruits to be processed in a pressure canner need not be sterilized beforehand. It is also unnecessary to sterilize jars for fruits, tomatoes, and pickled or fermented foods that will be processed 10 minutes or longer in a boiling-water canner.

Lid Selection, Preparation, and Use

The common self-sealing lid consists of a flat metal lid held in place by a metal screw band during processing. The flat lid is crimped around its bottom edge to form a trough, which is filled with a colored gasket material. When jars are processed, the lid gasket softens and flows slightly to cover the jar-sealing surface, yet allows air to escape from the jar. The gasket then forms an airtight seal as the jar cools. Gaskets in unused lids work well for at least five years from date of manufacture. The gasket material in older, unused lids may fail to seal on jars.

It is best to buy only the quantity of lids you will use in a year. To ensure a good seal, carefully follow the manufacturer's directions in preparing lids for use. Examine all metal lids carefully. Do not use old, dented, or deformed lids or lids with gaps or other defects in the sealing gasket.

After filling jars with food, release air bubbles by inserting a flat, plastic (not metal) spatula between the food and the jar. Slowly turn the jar and move the spatula up and down to allow air bubbles to escape. Adjust the headspace and then clean the jar rim (sealing surface) with a dampened paper towel. Place the lid, gasket down, onto the cleaned jar-sealing surface. Uncleaned jar-sealing surfaces may cause seal failures.

Then fit the metal screw band over the flat lid. Follow the manufacturer's guidelines enclosed with or on the box for tightening the jar lids properly.

- If screw bands are too tight, air cannot vent during processing, and food will discolor during storage. Overtightening also may cause lids to buckle and jars to break, especially with raw-packed, pressure-processed food.
- If screw bands are too loose, liquid may escape from jars during processing, seals may fail, and the food will need to be reprocessed.

Do not retighten lids after processing jars. As jars cool, the contents in the jar contract, pulling the self-sealing lid firmly against the jar to form a high vacuum. Screw bands are not needed on stored jars. They can be removed easily after jars are cooled. When removed, washed, dried, and stored in a dry area, screw bands may be used many times. If left on stored jars, they become difficult to remove, often rust, and may not work properly again.

Selecting the Correct Processing Time

When food is canned in boiling water, more processing time is needed for most raw-packed foods and for quart jars than is needed for hot-packed foods and pint jars.

To destroy microorganisms in acid foods processed in a boiling-water canner, you must:
- Process jars for the correct number of minutes in boiling water.
- Cool the jars at room temperature.

To destroy microorganisms in low-acid foods processed with a pressure canner, you must:
- Process the jars for the correct number of minutes at 240°F (10 PSIG) or 250°F (15 PSIG).
- Allow canner to cool at room temperature until it is completely depressurized.

The food may spoil if you fail to use the proper processing times, fail to vent steam from canners properly, process at lower pressure than specified, process for fewer minutes than specified, or cool the canner with water.

Processing times for haft-pint and pint jars are the same, as are times for 1½-pint and quart jars. For some products, you have a choice of processing at 5, 10, or 15 PSIG. In these cases, choose the canner pressure (PSIG) you wish to use and match it with your pack style (raw or hot) and jar size to find the correct processing time.

Recommended Canners

There are two main types of canners for heat-processing home-canned food: boiling-water canners and pressure canners. Most are designed to hold seven one-quart jars or eight to nine one-pint jars. Small pressure canners hold four one-quart jars; some large pressure canners hold eighteen one-pint jars in two layers but hold only seven quart jars. Pressure saucepans with smaller volume capacities are not recommended for use in canning. Treat small pressure canners the same as standard larger canners; they should be vented using the typical venting procedures.

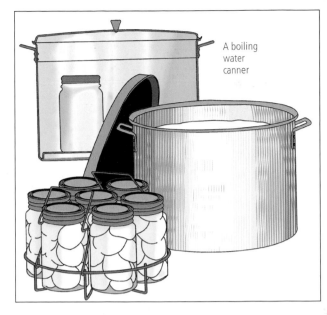

A boiling water canner

Low-acid foods must be processed in a pressure canner to be free of botulism risks. Although pressure canners also may be used for processing acid foods, boiling-water canners are recommended because they are faster. A pressure canner would require from 55 to 100 minutes to can a load of jars; the total time for canning most acid foods in boiling water varies from 25 to 60 minutes.

A boiling-water canner loaded with filled jars requires about 20 to 30 minutes of heating before its water begins to boil. A loaded pressure canner requires about 12 to 15 minutes of heating before it begins to vent, another 10 minutes to vent the canner, another 5 minutes to pressurize the canner, another 8 to 10 minutes to process the acid food, and, finally, another 20 to 60 minutes to cool the canner before removing jars.

Boiling-Water Canners

These canners are made of aluminum or porcelain-covered steel. They have removable perforated racks and fitted lids. The canner must be deep enough so that at least 1 inch of briskly boiling water will cover the tops of jars during processing. Some boiling-water canners do not have flat bottoms. A flat bottom must be used on an electric range. Either a flat or ridged bottom can be used on a gas burner. To ensure uniform processing of all jars with an electric range, the canner should be no more than 4 inches wider in diameter than the element on which it is heated.

Using a Boiling-Water Canner

Follow these steps for successful boiling-water canning:
1. Fill the canner halfway with water.
2. Preheat water to 140°F for raw-packed foods and to 180°F for hot-packed foods.
3. Load filled jars, fitted with lids, into the canner rack and use the handles to lower the rack into

the water; or fill the canner, one jar at a time, with a jar lifter.

4. Add more boiling water, if needed, so the water level is at least 1 inch above jar tops.
5. Turn heat to its highest position until water boils vigorously.
6. Set a timer for the minutes required for processing the food.
7. Cover with the canner lid and lower the heat setting to maintain a gentle boil throughout the processing time.
8. Add more boiling water, if needed, to keep the water level above the jars.
9. When jars have been boiled for the recommended time, turn off the heat and remove the canner lid.
10. Using a jar lifter, remove the jars and place them on a towel, leaving at least 1 inch of space between the jars during cooling.

Pressure Canners

Pressure canners for use in the home have been extensively redesigned in recent years. Models made before the 1970s were heavy-walled kettles with clamp-on lids. They were fitted with a dial gauge, a vent port in the form of a petcock or counterweight, and a safety fuse. Modern pressure canners are lightweight, thin-walled kettles; most have turn-on lids. They have a jar rack, gasket, dial or weighted gauge, an automatic vent or cover lock, a vent port (steam vent) that is closed with a counterweight or weighted gauge, and a safety fuse.

Pressure does not destroy microorganisms, but high temperatures applied for a certain period of time do. The success of destroying all microorganisms capable of growing in canned food is based on the temperature obtained in pure steam, free of air, at sea level. At sea level, a canner operated at a gauge pressure of 10 pounds provides an internal temperature of 240°F.

Air trapped in a canner lowers the inside temperature and results in under-processing. The highest volume of

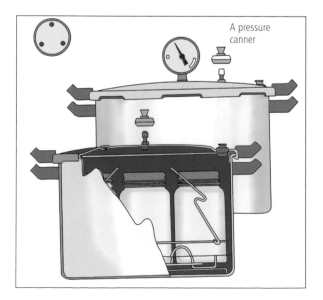

A pressure canner

air trapped in a canner occurs in processing raw-packed foods in dial-gauge canners. These canners do not vent air during processing. To be safe, all types of pressure canners must be vented 10 minutes before they are pressurized.

To vent a canner, leave the vent port uncovered on newer models or manually open petcocks on some older models. Heating the filled canner with its lid locked into place boils water and generates steam that escapes through the petcock or vent port. When steam first escapes, set a timer for 10 minutes. After venting 10 minutes, close the petcock or place the counterweight or weighted gauge over the vent port to pressurize the canner.

Weighted-gauge models exhaust tiny amounts of air and steam each time their gauge rocks or jiggles during processing. The sound of the weight rocking or jiggling indicates that the canner is maintaining the recommended pressure and needs no further attention until the load has been processed for the set time. Weighted-gauge canners cannot correct precisely for higher altitudes, and at altitudes above 1,000 feet must be operated at a pressure of 15.

Check dial gauges for accuracy before use each year and replace if they read high by more than 1 pound at 5, 10, or 15 pounds of pressure. Low readings cause over-processing and may indicate that the accuracy of the gauge is unpredictable. If a gauge is consistently low, you may adjust the processing pressure. For example, if the directions call for 12 pounds of pressure and your dial gauge has tested 1 pound low, you can safely process at 11 pounds of pressure. If the gauge is more than 2 pounds low, it is unpredictable, and it is best to replace it. Gauges may be checked at most USDA county extension offices, which are located in every state across the country. To find one near you, visit www.csrees.usda.gov.

Handle gaskets of canner lids carefully and clean them according to the manufacturer's directions. Nicked or dried gaskets will allow steam leaks during pressurization of canners. Gaskets of older canners may need to be lightly coated with vegetable oil once per year, but newer models are pre-lubricated. Check your canner's instructions.

Lid safety fuses are thin, metal inserts or rubber plugs designed to relieve excessive pressure from the canner. Do not pick at or scratch fuses while cleaning lids. Use only canners that have Underwriter's Laboratory (UL) approval to ensure their safety.

Replacement gauges and other parts for canners are often available at stores offering canner equipment or from canner manufacturers. To order parts, list canner model number and describe the parts needed.

Using a Pressure Canner

Follow these steps for successful pressure canning:
1. Put 2 to 3 inches of hot water in the canner. Place filled jars on the rack, using a jar lifter. Fasten canner lid securely.
2. Open petcock or leave weight off vent port. Heat at the highest setting until steam flows from the petcock or vent port.

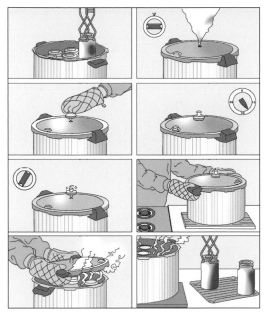

Using a pressure canner

3. Maintain high heat setting, exhaust steam 10 minutes, and then place weight on vent port or close petcock. The canner will pressurize during the next three to five minutes.

4. Start timing the process when the pressure reading on the dial gauge indicates that the recommended pressure has been reached or when the weighted gauge begins to jiggle or rock.

5. Regulate heat under the canner to maintain a steady pressure at or slightly above the correct gauge pressure. Quick and large pressure variations during processing may cause unnecessary liquid losses from jars. Weighted gauges on Mirro canners should jiggle about two or three times per minute. On Presto canners, they should rock slowly throughout the process.

When processing time is completed, turn off the heat, remove the canner from heat if possible, and let the canner depressurize. Do not force-cool the canner. If you cool it with cold running water in a sink or open the vent port before the canner depressurizes by itself, liquid will spurt from the jars, causing low liquid levels and jar seal failures. Force-cooling also may warp the canner lid of older model canners, causing steam leaks.

Depressurization of older models should be timed. Standard size heavy-walled canners require about 30 minutes when loaded with pints and 45 minutes with quarts. Newer thin-walled canners cool more rapidly and are equipped with vent locks. These canners are depressurized when their vent lock piston drops to a normal position.

1. After the vent port or petcock has been open for two minutes, unfasten the lid and carefully remove it. Lift the lid away from you so that the steam does not burn your face.

2. Remove jars with a lifter, and place on towel or cooling rack, if desired.

Cooling Jars

Cool the jars at room temperature for 12 to 24 hours. Jars may be cooled on racks or towels to minimize heat damage to counters. The food level and liquid volume of raw-packed jars will be noticeably lower after cooling because air is exhausted during processing, and food shrinks. If a jar loses excessive liquid during processing, do not open it to add more liquid. As long as the seal is good, the product is still usable.

Testing Jar Seals

After cooling jars for 12 to 24 hours, remove the screw bands and test seals with one of the following methods:

Method 1: Press the middle of the lid with a finger or thumb. If the lid springs up when you release your finger, the lid is unsealed and reprocessing will be necessary.

Method 2: Tap the lid with the bottom of a teaspoon. If it makes a dull sound, the lid is not sealed. If food is in contact with the underside of the lid, it will also cause a dull sound. If the jar lid is sealed correctly, it will make a ringing, high-pitched sound.

Method 3: Hold the jar at eye level and look across the lid. The lid should be concave (curved down slightly in the center). If center of the lid is either flat or bulging, it may not be sealed.

Reprocessing Unsealed Jars

If a jar fails to seal, remove the lid and check the jar-sealing surface for tiny nicks. If necessary, change the jar, add a new, properly prepared lid, and reprocess within 24 hours using the same processing time.

Another option is to adjust headspace in unsealed jars to 1½ inches and freeze jars and contents instead of reprocessing. However, make sure jars have straight sides. Freezing may crack jars with "shoulders."

Foods in single, unsealed jars could be stored in the refrigerator and consumed within several days.

Storing Canned Foods

If lids are tightly vacuum-sealed on cooled jars, remove screw bands, wash the lid and jar to remove food residue, then rinse and dry jars. Label and date the jars and store them in a clean, cool, dark, dry place. Do not store jars at temperatures above 95°F or near hot pipes, a range, a furnace, in an uninsulated attic, or in direct sunlight. Under these conditions, food will lose quality

Testing jar seals

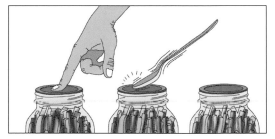

in a few weeks or months and may spoil. Dampness may corrode metal lids, break seals, and allow recontamination and spoilage.

Accidental freezing of canned foods will not cause spoilage unless jars become unsealed and re-contaminated. However, freezing and thawing may soften food. If jars must be stored where they may freeze, wrap them in newspapers, place them in heavy cartons, and cover them with more newspapers and blankets.

Identifying and Handling Spoiled Canned Food

Growth of spoilage bacteria and yeast produces gas, which pressurizes the food, swells lids, and breaks jar seals. As each stored jar is selected for use, examine its lid for tightness and vacuum. Lids with concave centers have good seals.

Next, while holding the jar upright at eye level, rotate the jar and examine its outside surface for streaks of dried food originating at the top of the jar. Look at the contents for rising air bubbles and unnatural color.

While opening the jar, smell for unnatural odors and look for spurting liquid and cotton-like mold growth (white, blue, black, or green) on the top food surface and underside of lid. Do not taste food from a stored jar you discover to have an unsealed lid or that otherwise shows signs of spoilage.

All suspect containers of spoiled, low-acid foods should be treated as having produced botulinum toxin and should be handled carefully as follows:
- If the suspect glass jars are unsealed, open, or leaking, they should be detoxified before disposal.
- If the suspect glass jars are sealed, remove lids and detoxify the entire jar, contents, and lids.

Detoxification Process

Carefully place the suspect containers and lids on their sides in an eight-quart-volume or larger stockpot, pan, or boiling-water canner. Wash your hands thoroughly. Carefully add water to the pot. The water should completely cover the containers with a minimum of 1 inch of water above the containers. Avoid splashing the water. Place a lid on the pot and heat the water to boiling. Boil 30 minutes to ensure detoxifying the food and all container components. Cool and discard lids and food in the trash or bury in soil.

Thoroughly clean all counters, containers, and equipment including can opener, clothing, and hands that may have come in contact with the food or the containers. Discard any sponges or washcloths that were used in the cleanup. Place them in a plastic bag and discard in the trash.

Canned Foods for Special Diets

The cost of commercially canned, special diet food often prompts interest in preparing these products at home. Some low-sugar and low-salt foods may be easily and safely canned at home. However, it may take some experimentation to create a product with the desired color, flavor, and texture. Start with a small batch and then make appropriate adjustments before producing large quantities.

Canning without Sugar

In canning regular fruits without sugar, it is very important to select fully ripe but firm fruits of the best quality. It is generally best to can fruit in its own juice, but blends of unsweetened apple, pineapple, and white grape juice are also good for pouring over solid fruit pieces. Adjust headspaces and lids and use the processing recommendations for regular fruits. Add sugar substitutes, if desired, when serving.

Fruit

There's nothing quite like opening a jar of home-preserved strawberries in the middle of a winter snowstorm. It takes you right back to the warm, early-summer sunshine, the smell of the strawberry patch's damp earth, and the feel of the firm berries as you snipped them from the vines. Best of all, you get to indulge in the sweet, summery flavor even as the snow swirls outside the windows.

Preserving fruit is simple, safe, and it allows you to enjoy the fruits of your summer's labor all year-round. On the next pages, you will find reference charts for processing various fruits and fruit products in a dial-gauge pressure canner or a weighted-gauge pressure canner. The same information is also included with each recipe's directions. In some cases, a boiling-water canner will serve better; for these instances, directions for its use are offered instead.

Adding syrup to canned fruit helps to retain its flavor, color, and shape, although it does not prevent spoilage. To maintain the most natural flavor, use the Very Light Syrup listed in the table found on page 78. Many fruits that are typically packed in heavy syrup are just as good—and a lot better for you—when packed in lighter syrups. However, if you're preserving fruit that's on the sour side, like cherries or tart apples, you might want to splurge on one of the sweeter versions.

Syrups

Adding syrup to canned fruit helps to retain its flavor, color, and shape, although jars still need to be processed to prevent spoilage. Follow the chart into the right for syrups of varying sweetness. Light corn syrups or mild-flavored honey may be used to replace up to half the table sugar called for in syrups.

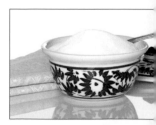

Directions
1. Bring water and sugar to a boil in a medium saucepan.
2. Pour over raw fruits in jars.

Process Times for Fruits and Fruit Products in a Dial-Gauge Pressure Canner*

Type of Fruit	Style of Pack	Jar Size	Process Time	Canner Pressure (PSI) at Altitudes of:			
				0–2,000 ft	2,001–4,000 ft	4,001–6,000 ft	6,001–8,000 ft
Applesauce	Hot	Pints	8 minutes	6 lbs	7 lbs	8 lbs	9 lbs
	Hot	Quarts	10 minutes	6 lbs	7 lbs	8 lbs	9 lbs
Apples, sliced	Hot	Pints or Quarts	8 minutes	6 lbs	7 lbs	8 lbs	9 lbs
Berries, whole	Hot	Pints or Quarts	8 minutes	6 lbs	7 lbs	8 lbs	9 lbs
	Raw	Pints	8 minutes	6 lbs	7 lbs	8 lbs	9 lbs
	Raw	Quarts	10 minutes	6 lbs	7 lbs	8 lbs	9 lbs
Cherries, sour or sweet	Hot	Pints	8 minutes	6 lbs	7 lbs	8 lbs	9 lbs
	Hot	Quarts	10 minutes	6 lbs	7 lbs	8 lbs	9 lbs
	Raw	Pints or Quarts	10 minutes	6 lbs	7 lbs	8 lbs	9 lbs
Fruit purées	Hot	Pints or Quarts	8 minutes	6 lbs	7 lbs	8 lbs	9 lbs
Grapefruit or orange sections	Hot	Pints or Quarts	8 minutes	6 lbs	7 lbs	8 lbs	9 lbs
	Raw	Pints	8 minutes	6 lbs	7 lbs	8 lbs	9 lbs
	Raw	Quarts	10 minutes	6 lbs	7 lbs	8 lbs	9 lbs
Peaches, apricots, or nectarines	Hot or Raw	Pints or Quarts	10 minutes	6 lbs	7 lbs	8 lbs	9 lbs
Pears	Hot	Pints or Quarts	10 minutes	6 lbs	7 lbs	8 lbs	9 lbs
Plums	Hot or Raw	Pints or Quarts	10 minutes	6 lbs	7 lbs	8 lbs	9 lbs
Rhubarb	Hot	Pints or Quarts	8 minutes	6 lbs	7 lbs	8 lbs	9 lbs

*After the process is complete, turn off the heat and remove the canner lid. Wait 5 to 10 minutes before removing jars.

Process Times for Fruits and Fruit Products in a Weighted-Gauge Pressure Canner*

Type of Fruit	Style of Pack	Jar Size	Process Time	Canner Pressure (PSI) at Altitudes of:	
				0–1,000 ft	Above 1,000 ft
Applesauce	Hot	Pints	8 minutes	5 lbs	10 lbs
	Hot	Quarts	10 minutes	5 lbs	10 lbs
Apples, sliced	Hot	Pints or Quarts	8 minutes	5 lbs	10 lbs
Berries, whole	Hot	Pints or Quarts	8 minutes	5 lbs	10 lbs
	Raw	Pints	8 minutes	5 lbs	10 lbs
	Raw	Quarts	10 minutes	5 lbs	10 lbs
Cherries, sour or sweet	Hot	Pints	8 minutes	5 lbs	10 lbs
	Hot	Quarts	10 minutes	5 lbs	10 lbs
	Raw	Pints or Quarts	10 minutes	5 lbs	10 lbs
Fruit purées	Hot	Pints or Quarts	8 minutes	5 lbs	10 lbs
Grapefruit or orange sections	Hot	Pints or Quarts	8 minutes	5 lbs	10 lbs
	Raw	Pints	8 minutes	5 lbs	10 lbs
	Raw	Quarts	10 minutes	5 lbs	10 lbs
Peaches, apricots, or nectarines	Hot or Raw	Pints or Quarts	10 minutes	5 lbs	10 lbs
Pears	Hot	Pints or Quarts	10 minutes	5 lbs	10 lbs
Plums	Hot or Raw	Pints or Quarts	10 minutes	5 lbs	10 lbs
Rhubarb	Hot	Pints or Quarts	8 minutes	5 lbs	10 lbs

*After the process is complete, turn off the heat and remove the canner lid. Wait 5 to 10 minutes before removing jars.

Sugar and Water in Syrup

Syrup Type	Approx. % Sugar	Measures of Water and Sugar				Fruits Commonly Packed in Syrup
		For 9-Pt Load*		For 7-Qt Load		
		Cups Water	Cups Sugar	Cups Water	Cups Sugar	
Very Light	10	6½	¾	10½	1¼	Approximates natural sugar levels in most fruits and adds the fewest calories.
Light	20	5¾	1½	9	2¼	Very sweet fruit. Try a small amount the first time to see if your family likes it.
Medium	30	5¼	2¼	8¼	3¾	Sweet apples, sweet cherries, berries, grapes.
Heavy	40	5	3¼	7¾	5¼	Tart apples, apricots, sour cherries, gooseberries, nectarines, peaches, pears, plums.
Very Heavy	50	4¼	4¼	6½	6¾	Very sour fruit. Try a small amount the first time to see if your family likes it.

*This amount is also adequate for a four-quart load.

Apple Juice

The best apple juice is made from a blend of varieties. If you don't have your own apple press, try to buy fresh juice from a local cider maker within 24 hours after it has been pressed.

Directions
1. Refrigerate juice for 24 to 48 hours.
2. Without mixing, carefully pour off clear liquid and discard sediment. Strain the clear liquid through a paper coffee filter or double layers of damp cheesecloth.
3. Heat quickly in a saucepan, stirring occasionally, until juice begins to boil.
4. Fill immediately into sterile pint or quart jars or into clean, half-gallon jars, leaving ¼-inch headspace.
5. Adjust lids and process. See below for recommended times for a boiling-water canner.

Process Times for Apple Juice in a Boiling-Water Canner*

Style of Pack	Jar Size	Process Time at Altitudes of:		
		0– 1,000 ft	1,001– 6,000 ft	Above 6,000 ft
Hot	Pints or Quarts	5 min	10	15
	Half-gallons	10	15	20

*After the process is complete, turn off the heat and remove the canner lid. Wait five minutes before removing jars.

Apple Butter

The best apple varieties to use for apple butter include Jonathan, Winesap, Stayman, Golden Delicious, and Macintosh apples, but any of your favorite varieties will work. Don't bother to peel the apples, as you will strain the fruit before cooking it anyway. This recipe will yield eight to nine pints.

Ingredients
8 lbs apples
2 cups vinegar
2¼ cups packed brown sugar
2 cups cider
2¼ cups white sugar
2 tbsp ground cinnamon
1 tbsp ground cloves

Directions
1. Wash, stem, quarter, and core apples.
2. Cook slowly in cider and vinegar until soft. Press fruit through a colander, food mill, or strainer.
3. Cook fruit pulp with sugar and spices, stirring frequently. To test for doneness, remove a spoonful and hold it away from steam for 2 minutes. If the butter remains mounded on the spoon, it is done. If you're still not sure, spoon a small quantity onto a plate. When a rim of liquid does not separate around the edge of the butter, it is ready for canning.
4. Fill while hot into sterile half-pint or pint jars, leaving ¼-inch headspace. Quart jars need not be presterilized.

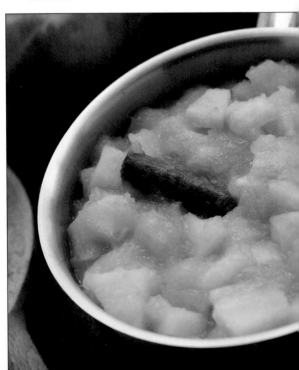

Process Times for Apple Butter in a Boiling-Water Canner*

		Process Time at Altitudes of:		
Style of Pack	Jar Size	0–1,000 ft	1,001–6,000 ft	Above 6,000 ft
Hot	Half-pints or Pints	5 minutes	10 minutes	15 minutes
	Quarts	10 minutes	15 minutes	20 minutes

*After the process is complete, turn off the heat and remove the canner lid. Wait five minutes before removing jars.

Applesauce

Besides being delicious on its own or paired with dishes like pork chops or latkes, applesauce can be used as a butter substitute in many baked goods. Select apples that are sweet, juicy, and crisp. For a tart flavor, add one to two pounds of tart apples to each three pounds of sweeter fruit.

Quantity

1. An average of 21 pounds of apples is needed per canner load of seven quarts.
2. An average of 13½ pounds of apples is needed per canner load of nine pints.
3. A bushel weighs 48 pounds and yields 14 to 19 quarts of sauce—an average of three pounds per quart.

Directions

1. Wash, peel, and core apples. Slice apples into water containing a little lemon juice to prevent browning.
2. Place drained slices in an 8- to 10-quart pot. Add ½ cup water. Stirring occasionally to prevent burning, heat quickly until tender (5 to 20 minutes, depending on maturity and variety).
3. Press through a sieve or food mill, or skip the pressing step if you prefer chunky-style sauce. Sauce may be packed without sugar, but if desired, sweeten to taste (start with ⅛ cup sugar per quart of sauce).
4. Reheat sauce to boiling. Fill jars with hot sauce, leaving ½-inch headspace. Adjust lids and process.

Process Times for Applesauce in a Boiling-Water Canner*

		Process Time at Altitudes of:			
Style of Pack	Jar Size	0–1,000 ft	1,001–3,000 ft	3,001–6,000 ft	Above 6,000 ft
Hot	Pints	15 minutes	20 minutes	20 minutes	25 minutes
	Quarts	20 minutes	25 minutes	30 minutes	35 minutes

*After the process is complete, turn off the heat and remove the canner lid. Wait five minutes before removing jars.

Process Times for Applesauce in a Dial-Gauge Pressure Canner*

			Canner Pressure (PSI) at Altitudes of:			
Style of Pack	Jar Size	Process Time	0–2,000 ft	2,001–4,000 ft	4,001–6,000 ft	6,001–8,000 ft
Hot	Pints	8 minutes	6 lbs	7 lbs	8 lbs	9 lbs
	Quarts	10 minutes	6 lbs	7 lbs	8 lbs	9 lbs

*After the canner is completely depressurized, remove the weight from the vent port or open the petcock. Wait 10 minutes; then unfasten the lid and remove it carefully. Lift the lid with the underside away from you so that the steam coming out of the canner does not burn your face.

Process Times for Applesauce in a Weighted-Gauge Pressure Canner*

			Canner Pressure (PSI) at Altitudes of:	
Style of Pack	Jar Size	Process Time	0–1,000 ft	Above 1,000 ft
Hot	Pints	8 minutes	5 lbs	10 lbs
	Quarts	10 minutes	5 lbs	10 lbs

*After the canner is completely depressurized, remove the weight from the vent port or open the petcock. Wait 10 minutes, then unfasten the lid and remove it carefully. Lift the lid with the underside away from you so that the steam coming out of the canner does not burn your face.

Apricots, Halved or Sliced

Apricots are excellent in baked goods, stuffing, chutney, or on their own. Choose firm, well-colored, mature fruit for best results.

Quantity

- An average of 16 pounds is needed per canner load of seven quarts.
- An average of 10 pounds is needed per canner load of nine pints.

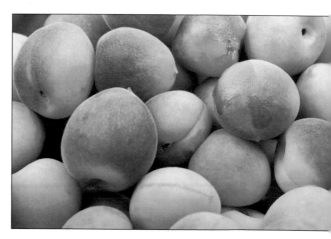

- A bushel weighs 50 pounds and yields 20 to 25 quarts—an average of 2¼ pounds per quart.

Directions

1. Dip fruit in boiling water for 30 to 60 seconds until skins loosen. Dip quickly in cold water and slip off skins.
2. Cut in half, remove pits, and slice if desired. To prevent darkening, keep peeled fruit in water with a little lemon juice.
3. Prepare and boil a very light, light, or medium syrup (see page 78) or pack apricots in water, apple juice, or white grape juice.

Process Times for Halved or Sliced Apricots in a Dial-Gauge Pressure Canner*

Style of Pack	Jar Size	Process Time	Canner Pressure (PSI) at Altitudes of:			
			0–2,000 ft	2,001–4,000 ft	4,001–6,000 ft	6,001–8,000 ft
Hot or Raw	Pints or Quarts	10 minutes	6 lbs	7 lbs	8 lbs	9 lbs

*After the process is complete, turn off the heat and remove the canner lid. Wait five minutes before removing jars.

Process Times for Halved or Sliced Apricots in a Weighted-Gauge Pressure Canner*

Style of Pack	Jar Size	Process Time	Canner Pressure (PSI) at Altitudes of:	
			0–1,000 ft	Above 1,000 ft
Hot or Raw	Pints or Quarts	10 minutes	5 lbs	10 lbs

*After the process is complete, turn off the heat and remove the canner lid. Wait five minutes before removing jars.

Berries, Whole

Preserved berries are perfect for use in pies, muffins, pancakes, or in poultry or pork dressings. Nearly every berry preserves well, including blackberries, blueberries, currants, dewberries, elderberries, gooseberries, huckleberries, loganberries, mulberries, and raspberries. Choose ripe, sweet berries with uniform color.

Quantity

- An average of 12 pounds is needed per canner load of seven quarts.
- An average of 8 pounds is needed per canner load of nine pints.
- A 24-quart crate weighs 36 pounds and yields 18 to 24 quarts—an average of 1¾ pounds per quart.

Directions

1. Wash 1 or 2 quarts of berries at a time. Drain, cap, and stem if necessary. For gooseberries, snip off heads and tails with scissors.
2. Prepare and boil preferred syrup, if desired (see page 78). Add ½ cup syrup, juice, or water to each clean jar.

Hot pack—(Best for blueberries, currants, elderberries, gooseberries, and huckleberries) Heat berries in boiling water for 30 seconds and drain. Fill jars and cover with hot juice, leaving ½-inch headspace.

Raw pack—Fill jars with any of the raw berries, shaking down gently while filling. Cover with hot syrup, juice, or water, leaving ½-inch headspace.

Recommended Process Times for Whole Berries in a Boiling-Water Canner*

Style of Pack	Jar Size	Process Time at Altitudes of:			
		0–1,000 ft	1,001–3,000 ft	3,001–6,000 ft	Above 6,000 ft
Hot	Pints or Quarts	15 minutes	20 minutes	20 minutes	25 minutes
Raw	Pints	15 minutes	20 minutes	20 minutes	25 minutes
Raw	Quarts	20 minutes	25 minutes	30 minutes	35 minutes

*After the process is complete, turn off the heat and remove the canner lid. Wait five minutes before removing jars.

Process Times for Whole Berries in a Dial-Gauge Pressure Canner*

Style of Pack	Jar Size	Process Time	Canner Pressure (PSI) at Altitudes of:			
			0–2,000 ft	2,001–4,000 ft	4,001–6,000 ft	6,001–8,000 ft
Hot	Pints or Quarts	8 minutes	6 lbs	7 lbs	8 lbs	9 lbs
Raw	Pints	8 minutes	6 lbs	7 lbs	8 lbs	9 lbs
Raw	Quarts	10 minutes	6 lbs	7 lbs	8 lbs	9 lbs

*After the process is complete, turn off the heat and remove the canner lid. Wait five minutes before removing jars.

Process Times for Whole Berries in a Weighted-Gauge Pressure Canner*

Style of Pack	Jar Size	Process Time	Canner Pressure (PSI) at Altitudes of:	
			0–1,000 ft	Above 1,000 ft
Hot	Pints or Quarts	8 minutes	5 lbs	10 lbs
Raw	Pints	8 minutes	5 lbs	10 lbs
Raw	Quarts	10 minutes	5 lbs	10 lbs

*After the process is complete, turn off the heat and remove the canner lid. Wait five minutes before removing jars.

Berry Syrup

Juices from fresh or frozen blueberries, cherries, grapes, raspberries (black or red), and strawberries are easily made into toppings for use on ice cream and pastries. For an elegant finish to cheesecakes or pound cakes, drizzle a thin stream in a zigzag across the top just before serving. Berry syrups are also great additions to smoothies or milkshakes. This recipe makes about nine half-pints.

Directions
1. Select 6½ cups of fresh or frozen berries of your choice. Wash, cap, and stem berries and crush in a saucepan.
2. Heat to boiling and simmer until soft (5 to 10 minutes). Strain hot through a colander placed in a large pan and drain until cool enough to handle.

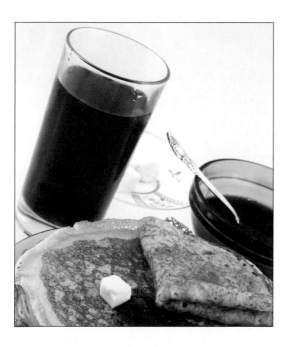

3. Strain the collected juice through a double layer of cheesecloth or jelly bag. Discard the dry pulp. The yield of the pressed juice should be about 4½ to 5 cups.
4. Combine the juice with 6¾ cups of sugar in a large saucepan, bring to a boil, and simmer 1 minute.
5. Fill into clean half-pint or pint jars, leaving ½-inch headspace. Adjust lids and process.

> To make syrup with whole berries, rather than crushed, save 1 or 2 cups of the fresh or frozen fruit, combine these with the sugar, and simmer until soft. Remove from heat, skim off foam, and fill into clean jars, following processing directions for regular berry syrup.

Process Times for Berry Syrup in a Boiling-Water Canner*

Style of Pack	Jar Size	Process Time at Altitudes of:		
		0–1,000 ft	1,001–6,000 ft	Above 6,000 ft
Hot	Half-pints or Pints	10 minutes	15 minutes	20 minutes

*After the process is complete, turn off the heat and remove the canner lid. Wait five minutes before removing jars.

Fruit Purées

Almost any fruit can be puréed for use as baby food, in sauces, or just as a nutritious snack. Puréed prunes and apples can be used as a butter replacement in many baked goods. Use this recipe for any fruit except figs and tomatoes.

Directions
1. Stem, wash, drain, peel, and remove pits if necessary. Measure fruit into large saucepan, crushing slightly if desired.
2. Add 1 cup hot water for each quart of fruit. Cook slowly until fruit is soft, stirring frequently. Press through sieve or food mill. If desired, add sugar to taste.
3. Reheat pulp to boil, or until sugar dissolves (if added). Fill hot into clean jars, leaving ¼-inch headspace. Adjust lids and process.

Process Times for Fruit Purées in a Boiling-Water Canner*

Style of Pack	Jar Size	Process Time at Altitudes of:		
		0–1,000 ft	1,001–6,000 ft	Above 6,000 ft
Hot	Pints or Quarts	15 minutes	20 minutes	25 minutes

*After the process is complete, turn off the heat and remove the canner lid. Wait five minutes before removing jars.

Process Times for Fruit Purées in a Dial-Gauge Pressure Canner*

Style of Pack	Jar Size	Process Time	Canner Pressure (PSI) at Altitudes of:			
			0–2,000 ft	2,001–4,000 ft	4,001–6,000 ft	6,001–8,000 ft
Hot	Pints or Quarts	8 minutes	6 lbs	7 lbs	8 lbs	9 lbs

*After the canner is completely depressurized, remove the weight from the vent port or open the petcock. Wait 10 minutes, then unfasten the lid and remove it carefully. Lift the lid with the underside away from you so that the steam coming out of the canner does not burn your face.

Process Times for Fruit Purées in a Weighted-Gauge Pressure Canner*

Style of Pack	Jar Size	Process Time (Min)	Canner Pressure (PSI) at Altitudes of:	
			0–1,000 ft	Above 1,000 ft
Hot	Pints or Quarts	8 minutes	5 lbs	10 lbs

*After the canner is completely depressurized, remove the weight from the vent port or open the petcock. Wait 10 minutes; then unfasten the lid and remove it carefully. Lift the lid with the underside away from you so that the steam coming out of the canner does not burn your face.

Grape Juice

Purple grapes are full of antioxidants and help to reduce the risk of heart disease, cancer, and Alzheimer's disease. For juice, select sweet, well-colored, firm, mature fruit.

Quantity

- An average of 24½ pounds is needed per canner load of seven quarts.
- An average of 16 pounds per canner load of nine pints.
- A lug weighs 26 pounds and yields seven to nine quarts of juice—an average of 3½ pounds per quart.

Directions

1. Wash and stem grapes. Place grapes in a saucepan and add boiling water to cover. Heat and simmer slowly until skin is soft.
2. Strain through a damp jelly bag or double layers of cheesecloth, and discard solids. Refrigerate juice for 24 to 48 hours.
3. Without mixing, carefully pour off clear liquid and save; discard sediment. If desired, strain through a paper coffee filter for a clearer juice.

4. Add juice to a saucepan and sweeten to taste. Heat and stir until sugar is dissolved. Continue heating with occasional stirring until juice begins to boil. Fill into jars immediately, leaving ¼-inch headspace. Adjust lids and process.

Process Times for Grape Juice in a Boiling-Water Canner*

Style of Pack	Jar Size	Process Time at Altitudes of:		
		0–1,000 ft	1,001–6,000 ft	Above 6,000 ft
Hot	Pints or Quarts	5 minutes	10 minutes	15 minutes
	Half-gallons	10 minutes	15 minutes	20 minutes

*After the process is complete, turn off the heat and remove the canner lid. Wait five minutes before removing jars.

Peaches, Halved or Sliced

Peaches are delicious in cobblers, crisps, and muffins, or grilled for a unique cake topping. Choose ripe, mature fruit with minimal bruising.

Quantity

- An average of 17½ pounds is needed per canner load of seven quarts.
- An average of 11 pounds is needed per canner load of nine pints.
- A bushel weighs 48 pounds and yields 16 to 24 quarts—an average of 2½ pounds per quart.

Directions

1. Dip fruit in boiling water for 30 to 60 seconds until skins loosen. Dip quickly in cold water and slip off skins. Cut in half, remove pits, and slice if desired. To prevent darkening, keep peeled fruit in ascorbic acid solution.
2. Prepare and boil a very light, light, or medium syrup or pack peaches in water, apple juice, or white grape juice. Raw packs make poor-quality peaches.

   Hot pack—In a large saucepan, place drained fruit in syrup, water, or juice and bring to boil. Fill jars with hot fruit and cooking liquid, leaving ½-inch headspace. Place halves in layers, cut side down.

   Raw pack—Fill jars with raw fruit, cut side down, and add hot water, juice, or syrup, leaving ½-inch headspace.
3. Adjust lids and process.

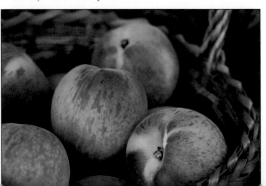

Process Times for Halved or Sliced Peaches in a Boiling-Water Canner*

Style of Pack	Jar Size	Process Time at Altitudes of:			
		0–1,000 ft	1,001–3,000 ft	3,001–6,000 ft	Above 6,000 ft
Hot	Pints	20 minutes	25 minutes	30 minutes	35 minutes
	Quarts	25 minutes	30 minutes	35 minutes	40 minutes
Raw	Pints	25 minutes	30 minutes	35 minutes	40 minutes
	Quarts	30 minutes	35 minutes	40 minutes	45 minutes

*After the process is complete, turn off the heat and remove the canner lid. Wait five minutes before removing jars.

Process Times for Halved or Sliced Peaches in a Dial-Gauge Pressure Canner*

Style of Pack	Jar Size	Process Time	Canner Pressure (PSI) at Altitudes of:			
			0–2,000 ft	2,001–4,000 ft	4,001–6,000 ft	6,001–8,000 ft
Hot or Raw	Pints or Quarts	10 minutes	6 lbs	7 lbs	8 lbs	9 lbs

*After the canner is completely depressurized, remove the weight from the vent port or open the petcock. Wait 10 minutes; then unfasten the lid and remove it carefully. Lift the lid with the underside away from you so that the steam coming out of the canner does not burn your face.

Process Times for Halved or Sliced Peaches in a Weighted-Gauge Pressure Canner*

Style of Pack	Jar Size	Process Time	Canner Pressure (PSI) at Altitudes of:	
			0–1,000 ft	Above 1,000 ft
Hot or Raw	Pints or Quarts	10 minutes	5 lbs	10 lbs

*After the canner is completely depressurized, remove the weight from the vent port or open the petcock. Wait 10 minutes; then unfasten the lid and remove it carefully. Lift the lid with the underside away from you so that the steam coming out of the canner does not burn your face.

Pears, Halved

Choose ripe, mature fruit for best results. For a special treat, filled halved pears with a mixture of chopped dried apricots, pecans, brown sugar, and butter; bake or microwave until warm and serve with vanilla ice cream.

Quantity

- An average of 17½ pounds is needed per canner load of seven quarts.
- An average of 11 pounds is needed per canner load of nine pints.
- A bushel weighs 50 pounds and yields 16 to 25 quarts—an average of 2½ pounds per quart.

Directions

1. Wash and peel pears. Cut lengthwise in halves and remove core. A melon baller or metal measuring spoon works well for coring pears. To prevent discoloration, keep pears in water with a little lemon juice.
2. Prepare a very light, light, or medium syrup (see page 78) or use apple juice, white grape juice, or water. Raw packs make poor quality pears. Boil drained pears for 5 minutes in syrup, juice, or water. Fill jars with hot fruit and cooking liquid, leaving ½-inch headspace. Adjust lids and process.

Process Times for Halved Pears in a Boiling-Water Canner*

Style of Pack	Jar Size	Process Time at Altitudes of:			
		0–1,000 ft	1,001–3,000 ft	3,001–6,000 ft	Above 6,000 ft
Hot	Pints	20 minutes	25 minutes	30 minutes	35 minutes
	Quarts	25 minutes	30 minutes	35 minutes	40 minutes

*After the process is complete, turn off the heat and remove the canner lid. Wait five minutes before removing jars.

Process Times for Halved Pears in a Dial-Gauge Pressure Canner*

Style of Pack	Jar Size	Process Time	Canner Pressure (PSI) at Altitudes of:			
			0–2,000 ft	2,001–4,000 ft	4,001–6,000 ft	6,001–8,000 ft
Hot	Pints or Quarts	10 minutes	6 lbs	7 lbs	8 lbs	9 lbs

*After the canner is completely depressurized, remove the weight from the vent port or open the petcock. Wait 10 minutes; then unfasten the lid and remove it carefully. Lift the lid with the underside away from you so that the steam coming out of the canner does not burn your face.

Process Times for Halved Pears in a Weighted-Gauge Pressure Canner*

Style of Pack	Jar Size	Process Time	Canner Pressure (PSI) at Altitudes of:	
			0– 1,000 ft	Above 1,000 ft
Hot	Pints or Quarts	10 minutes	5 lbs	10 lbs

*After the canner is completely depressurized, remove the weight from the vent port or open the petcock. Wait 10 minutes; then unfasten the lid and remove it carefully. Lift the lid with the underside away from you so that the steam coming out of the canner does not burn your face.

Rhubarb, Stewed

Rhubarb in the garden is a sure sign that spring has sprung and summer is well on its way. But why not enjoy rhubarb all year-round? The brilliant red stalks make it as appropriate for a holiday table as for an early summer feast. Rhubarb is also delicious in crisps, cobblers, or served hot over ice cream. Select young, tender, well-colored stalks from the spring or, if available, late fall crop.

Quantity

- An average of 10½ pounds is needed per canner load of seven quarts.
- An average of 7 pounds is needed per canner load of nine pints.
- A lug weighs 28 pounds and yields 14 to 28 quarts—an average of 1½ pounds per quart.

Directions

1. Trim off leaves. Wash stalks and cut into ½-inch to 1-inch pieces.
2. Place rhubarb in a large saucepan, and add ½ cup sugar for each quart of fruit. Let stand until juice appears. Heat gently to boiling. Fill jars without delay, leaving ½-inch headspace. Adjust lids and process.

Process Times for Stewed Rhubarb in a Boiling-Water Canner*

Style of Pack	Jar Size	Process Time at Altitudes of:		
		0– 1,000 ft	1,001– 6,000 ft	Above 6,000 ft
Hot	Pints or Quarts	15 minutes	20 minutes	25 minutes

*After the process is complete, turn off the heat and remove the canner lid. Wait five minutes before removing jars.

Process Times for Stewed Rhubarb in a Dial-Gauge Pressure Canner*

Style of Pack	Jar Size	Process Time	Canner Pressure (PSI) at Altitudes of			
			0– 2,000 ft	2,001– 4,000 ft	4,001– 6,000 ft	6,001– 8,000 ft
Hot	Pints or Quarts	8 minutes	6 lbs	7 lbs	8 lbs	9 lbs

*After the canner is completely depressurized, remove the weight from the vent port or open the petcock. Wait 10 minutes; then unfasten the lid and remove it carefully. Lift the lid with the underside away from you so that the steam coming out of the canner does not burn your face.

Process Times for Stewed Rhubarb in a Weighted-Gauge Pressure Canner*

Style of Pack	Jar Size	Process Time	Canner Pressure (PSI) at Altitudes of:	
			0–1,000 ft	Above 1,000 ft
Hot	Pints or Quarts	8 minutes	5 lbs	10 lbs

*After the canner is completely depressurized, remove the weight from the vent port or open the petcock. Wait 10 minutes; then unfasten the lid and remove it carefully. Lift the lid with the underside away from you so that the steam coming out of the canner does not burn your face.

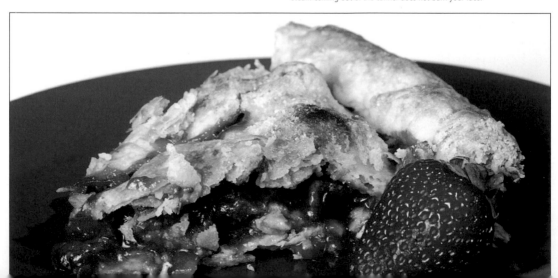

Canned Pie Fillings

Using a pre-made pie filling will cut your pie preparation time by more than half, but most commercially produced fillings are oozing with high fructose corn syrup and all manner of artificial coloring and flavoring. (Food coloring is not at all necessary, but if you're really concerned about how the inside of your pie will look, appropriate amounts are added to each recipe as an optional ingredient.) Making and preserving your own pie fillings means that you can use your own fresh ingredients and adjust the sweetness to your taste. Because some folks like their pies rich and sweet and others prefer a natural tart flavor, you might want to first make a single quart, make a pie with it, and see how you like it. Then you can adjust the sugar and spices in the recipe to suit your personal preferences before making a large batch. Experiment with combining fruits or adding different spices, but the amount of lemon juice should not be altered, as it aids in controlling the safety and storage stability of the fillings.

These recipes use Clear Jel (sometimes sold as Clear Jel A), a chemically modified cornstarch that produces excellent sauce consistency even after fillings are canned and baked. By using Clear Jel, you can lower the sugar content of your fillings without sacrificing safety, flavor, or texture. (Note: Instant Clear Jel is not meant to be cooked and should not be used for these recipes. Sure-Gel is a natural fruit pectin and is not a suitable substitute for Clear Jel. Cornstarch, tapioca starch, or arrowroot starch can be used in place of Clear Jel, but the finished product is likely to be runny.) One pound of Clear Jel costs less than five dollars and is enough to make fillings for about 14 pies. It will keep for at least a year if stored in a cool, dry place. Clear Jel is increasingly available among canning and freezing supplies in some stores. Alternately, you can order it by the pound at any of the following online stores:
- www.barryfarm.com
- www.kitchenkrafts.com
- www.theingredientstore.com

When using frozen cherries and blueberries, select unsweetened fruit. If sugar has been added, rinse it off while fruit is frozen. Thaw fruit, then collect, measure, and use juice from fruit to partially replace the water specified in the recipe.

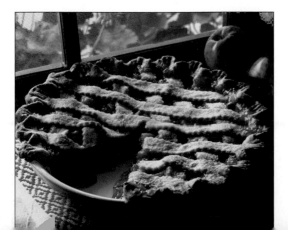

Apple Pie Filling

Use firm, crisp apples, such as Stayman, Golden Delicious, or Rome varieties for the best results. If apples lack tartness, use an additional ¼ cup of lemon juice for each six quarts of slices. Ingredients are included for a one-quart (enough for one 8-inch pie) or a seven-quart recipe.

Ingredients

	1 Quart	7 Quarts
Blanched, sliced fresh apples	3½ cups	6 quarts
Granulated sugar	¾ cup + 2 tbsp	5½ cups
Clear Jel®	¼ cup	1½ cup
Cinnamon	¼ tsp	1 tbsp
Cold water	½ cup	2½ cups
Apple juice	¾ cup	5 cups
Bottled lemon juice	2 tbsp	¾ cup
Nutmeg (optional)	⅛ tsp	1 tsp

Directions
1. Wash, peel, and core apples. Prepare slices ½ inch wide and place in water containing a little lemon juice to prevent browning.
2. For fresh fruit, place 6 cups at a time in 1 gallon of boiling water. Boil each batch 1 minute after the water returns to a boil. Drain, but keep heated fruit in a covered bowl or pot.
3. Combine sugar, Clear Jel, and cinnamon in a large kettle with water and apple juice. Add nutmeg, if desired. Stir and cook on medium-high heat until mixture thickens and begins to bubble.
4. Add lemon juice and boil 1 minute, stirring constantly. Fold in drained apple slices immediately and fill jars with mixture without delay, leaving 1-inch headspace. Adjust lids and process immediately.

Process Times for Apple Pie Filling in a Boiling-Water Canner*

Style of Pack	Jar Size	0–1,000 ft	1,001–3,000 ft	3,001–6,000 ft	Above 6,000 ft
Hot	Pints or Quarts	25 minutes	30 minutes	35 minutes	40 minutes

*After the process is complete, turn off the heat and remove the canner lid. Wait five minutes before removing jars.

Blueberry Pie Filling

Select fresh, ripe, and firm blueberries. Unsweetened frozen blueberries may be used. If sugar has been added, rinse it off while fruit is still frozen. Thaw fruit, then collect, measure, and use juice from fruit to partially replace the water specified in the recipe. Ingredients are included for a one-quart (enough for one 8-inch pie) or seven-quart recipe.

Ingredients

	1 Quart	7 Quarts
Fresh or thawed blueberries	3½ cups	6 quarts
Granulated sugar	¾ cup + 2 tbsp	6 cups
Clear Jel®	¼ cup + 1 tbsp	2¼ cup
Cold water	1 cup	7 cups
Bottled lemon juice	3½ cups	½ cup
Blue food coloring (optional)	3 drops	20 drops
Red food coloring (optional)	1 drop	7 drops

Directions

1. Wash and drain blueberries. Place 6 cups at a time in 1 gallon boiling water. Allow water to return to a boil and cook each batch for 1 minute. Drain but keep heated fruit in a covered bowl or pot.
2. Combine sugar and Clear Jel in a large kettle. Stir. Add water and food coloring if desired. Cook on medium-high heat until mixture thickens and begins to bubble.
3. Add lemon juice and boil 1 minute, stirring constantly. Fold in drained berries immediately and fill jars with mixture without delay, leaving 1-inch headspace. Adjust lids and process immediately.

Process Times for Blueberry Pie Filling in a Boiling-Water Canner*

Style of Pack	Jar Size	Process Time at Altitudes of:			
		0– 1,000 ft	1,001– 3,000 ft	3,001– 6,000 ft	Above 6,000 ft
Hot	Pints or Quarts	30 minutes	35 minutes	40 minutes	45 minutes

*After the process is complete, turn off the heat and remove the canner lid. Wait five minutes before removing jars.

Cherry Pie Filling

Select fresh, very ripe, and firm cherries. Unsweetened frozen cherries may be used. If sugar has been added, rinse it off while the fruit is still frozen. Thaw fruit, then collect, measure, and use juice from fruit to partially replace the water specified in the recipe. Ingredients are included for a one-quart (enough for one 8-inch pie) or seven-quart recipe.

Ingredients

	1 Quart	7 Quarts
Fresh or thawed sour cherries	3⅓ cups	6 quarts
Granulated sugar	1 cup	7 cups
Clear Jel®	¼ cup + 1 tbsp	1-¾ cups
Cold water	1⅓ cups	9⅓ cups
Bottled lemon juice	1 tbsp + 1 tsp	½ cup
Cinnamon (optional)	⅛ tsp	1 tsp
Almond extract (optional)	¼ tsp	2 tsp
Red food coloring (optional)	6 drops	¼ tsp

Directions

1. Rinse and pit fresh cherries, and hold in cold water. To prevent stem end from browning, use water with a little lemon juice. Place 6 cups at a time in 1 gallon boiling water. Boil each batch 1 minute after the water returns to a boil. Drain but keep heated fruit in a covered bowl or pot.
2. Combine sugar and Clear Jel in a large saucepan and add water. If desired, add cinnamon, almond extract, and food coloring. Stir mixture and cook over medium-high heat until mixture thickens and begins to bubble.
3. Add lemon juice and boil 1 minute, stirring constantly. Fold in drained cherries immediately and fill jars with mixture without delay, leaving 1-inch headspace. Adjust lids and process immediately.

Process Times for Cherry Pie Filling in a Boiling-Water Canner*

Style of Pack	Jar Size	Process Time at Altitudes of:			
		0– 1,000 ft	1,001– 3,000 ft	3,001– 6,000 ft	Above 6,000 ft
Hot	Pints or Quarts	30 minutes	35 minutes	40 minutes	45 minutes

*After the process is complete, turn off the heat and remove the canner lid. Wait five minutes before removing jars.

Festive Mincemeat Pie Filling

Mincemeat pie originated as "Christmas Pie" in the eleventh century, when the English crusaders returned from the Holy Land bearing oriental spices. They added three of these spices—cinnamon, cloves, and nutmeg—to their meat pies to represent the three gifts that the magi brought to the Christ child. Mincemeat pies are traditionally small and are perfect paired with a mug of hot buttered rum. Walnuts or pecans can be used in place of meat if preferred. This recipe yields about seven quarts.

Ingredients

2 cups finely chopped suet

4 lbs ground beef or 4 lbs ground venison and 1 lb sausage

5 qts chopped apples

2 lbs dark, seedless raisins

1 lb white raisins

2 qts apple cider

2 tbsp ground cinnamon

2 tsp ground nutmeg

½ tsp cloves

5 cups sugar

2 tbsp salt

Directions

1. Cook suet and meat in water to avoid browning. Peel, core, and quarter apples. Put suet, meat, and apples through food grinder using a medium blade.
2. Combine all ingredients in a large saucepan and simmer 1 hour or until slightly thickened. Stir often.
3. Fill jars with mixture without delay, leaving 1-inch headspace. Adjust lids and process.

Process Times for Festive Mincemeat Pie Filling in a Dial-Gauge Pressure Canner*

Style of Pack	Jar Size	Process Time	Canner Pressure (PSI) at Altitudes of:			
			0–2,000 ft	2,001–4,000 ft	4,001–6,000 ft	6,000–8,000 ft
Hot	Quarts	90 minutes	11 lbs	12 lbs	13 lbs	14 lbs

*After the canner is completely depressurized, remove the weight from the vent port or open the petcock. Wait 10 minutes, then unfasten the lid and remove it carefully. Lift the lid with the underside away from you so that the steam coming out of the canner does not burn your face.

Making Jams and Jellies without Added Pectin

If you are not sure if a fruit has enough of its own pectin, combine 1 tablespoon of rubbing alcohol with 1 tablespoon of extracted fruit juice in a small glass. Let stand 2 minutes. If the mixture forms into one solid mass, there's plenty of pectin. If you see several weak blobs, you need to add pectin or combine with another high-pectin fruit.

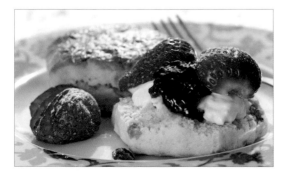

Process Times for Festive Mincemeat Pie Filling in a Weighted-Gauge Pressure Canner*

Style of Pack	Jar Size	Process Time	Canner Pressure (PSI) at Altitudes of:	
			0–1,000 ft	Above 1,000 ft
Hot	Quarts	90 minutes	10 lbs	15 lbs

*After the canner is completely depressurized, remove the weight from the vent port or open the petcock. Wait 10 minutes, then unfasten the lid and remove it carefully. Lift the lid with the underside away from you so that the steam coming out of the canner does not burn your face.

Jams, Jellies, and Other Fruit Spreads

Homemade jams and jellies have lots more flavor than store-bought, over-processed varieties. The combinations of fruits and spices are limitless, so have fun experimenting with these recipes. If you can bear to part with your creations when you're all done, they make wonderful gifts for any occasion.

Pectin is what makes jams and jellies thicken and gel. Many fruits, such as crab apples, citrus fruits, sour plums, currants, quinces, green apples, or Concord grapes, have plenty of their own natural pectin, so there's no need to add more pectin to your recipes. You can use less sugar when you don't add pectin, but you will have to boil the fruit for longer. Still, the process is relatively simple and you don't have to worry about having store-bought pectin on hand.

To use fresh fruits with a low-pectin content or canned or frozen fruit juice, powdered or liquid pectin must be added for your jams and jellies to thicken and set properly. Jelly or jam made with added pectin requires less cooking and generally gives a larger yield. These products have more natural fruit flavors, too. In addition, using added pectin eliminates the need to test hot jellies and jams for proper gelling.

Beginning this section are descriptions of the differences between methods, and tips for success with whichever you use.

Jelly Without Added Pectin

Making jelly without added pectin is not an exact science. You can add a little more or less sugar according to your taste, substitute honey for up to ½ of the sugar, or experiment with combining small amounts of low-pectin fruits with other high-pectin fruits. The Ingredients table below shows you the basics for common high-pectin fruits. Use it as a guideline as you experiment with other fruits.

As fruit ripens, its pectin content decreases, so use fruit that has recently been picked, and mix ¾ ripe fruit with ¼ under-ripe. Cooking cores and peels along with the fruit will also increase the pectin level. Avoid using canned or frozen fruit as they contain very little pectin.

Be sure to wash all fruit thoroughly before cooking. One pound of fruit should yield at least 1 cup of clear juice.

Ingredients

Fruit	Water to be Added per Pound of Fruit	Minutes to Simmer Fruit before Extracting Juice	Ingredients Added to Each Cup of Strained Juice		Yield from 4 Cups of Juice (Half-pints)
			Sugar (Cups)	Lemon Juice (Tsp)	
Apples	1 cup	20 to 25	¾	1½ (opt)	4 to 5
Blackberries	None or ¼ cup	5 to 10	¾ to 1	None	7 to 8
Crab apples	1 cup	20 to 25	1	None	4 to 5
Grapes	None or ¼ cup	5 to 10	¾ to 1	None	8 to 9
Plums	½ cup	15 to 20	¾	None	8 to 9

Directions

1. Crush soft fruits or berries; cut firmer fruits into small pieces (there is no need to peel or core the fruits, as cooking all the parts adds pectin).
2. Add water to fruits that require it, as listed in the Ingredients table above. Put fruit and water in large saucepan and bring to a boil. Then simmer according to the times in the chart until fruit is soft, while stirring to prevent scorching.
3. When fruit is tender, strain through a colander, then strain through a double layer of cheesecloth or a jelly bag. Allow juice to drip through, using a stand or colander to hold the bag. Avoid pressing or squeezing the bag or cloth as it will cause cloudy jelly.
4. Using no more than 6 to 8 cups of extracted fruit juice at a time, measure fruit juice, sugar, and lemon juice according to the Ingredients table, and heat to boiling.
5. Stir until the sugar is dissolved. Boil over high heat to the jellying point. To test jelly for doneness, use one of the following methods:

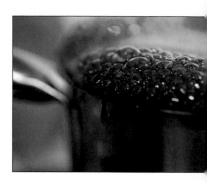

Temperature test—Use a jelly or candy thermometer and boil until mixture reaches the following temperatures:

Sea Level	1,000 ft	2,000 ft	3,000 ft	4,000 ft	5,000 ft	6,000 ft	7,000 ft	8,000 ft
220°F	218°F	216°F	214°F	212°F	211°F	209°F	207°F	205°F

Sheet or spoon test—Dip a cool, metal spoon into the boiling jelly mixture. Raise the spoon about 12 inches above the pan (out of steam). Turn the spoon so the liquid runs off the side. The jelly is done when the syrup forms two drops that flow together and sheet or hang off the edge of the spoon.

6. Remove from heat and quickly skim off foam. Fill sterile jars with jelly. Use a measuring cup or ladle the jelly through a wide-mouthed funnel, leaving ¼-inch headspace. Adjust lids and process.

Process Times for Jelly without Added Pectin in a Boiling Water Canner*

Style of Pack	Jar Size	Process Time at Altitudes of:		
		0–1,000 ft	1,001–6,000 ft	Above 6,000 ft
Hot	Half-pints or pints	5 minutes	10 minutes	15 minutes

*After the process is complete, turn off the heat and remove the canner lid. Wait five minutes before removing jars.

Lemon Curd

Lemon curd is a rich, creamy spread that can be used on (or in) a variety of teatime treats—crumpets, scones, cake fillings, tartlets, or meringues are all enhanced by its tangy-sweet flavor. Follow the recipe carefully, as variances in ingredients, order, and temperatures may lead to a poor texture or flavor. For Lime Curd, use the same recipe but substitute 1 cup bottled lime juice and ¼ cup fresh lime zest for the lemon juice and zest. This recipe yields about three to four half-pints.

Ingredients

2½ cups superfine sugar*

---

* If superfine sugar is not available, run granulated sugar through a grinder or food processor for 1 minute, let settle, and use in place of superfine sugar. Do not use powdered sugar.

½ cup lemon zest (freshly zested), optional
1 cup bottled lemon juice**
¾ cup unsalted butter, chilled, cut into approximately
¾-inch pieces
7 large egg yolks
4 large whole eggs

Directions

1. Wash 4 half-pint canning jars with warm, soapy water. Rinse well; keep hot until ready to fill. Prepare canning lids according to manufacturer's directions.

2. Fill boiling water canner with enough water to cover the filled jars by 1 to 2 inches. Use a thermometer to preheat the water to 180°F by the time filled jars are ready to be added. **Caution:** Do not heat the water in the canner to more than 180°F before jars are added. If the water in the canner is too hot when jars are added, the process time will not be long enough. The time it takes for the canner to reach boiling after the jars are added is expected to be 25 to 30 minutes for this product. Process time starts after the water in the canner comes to a full boil over the tops of the jars.

3. Combine the sugar and lemon zest in a small bowl, stir to mix, and set aside about 30 minutes. Pre-measure the lemon juice and prepare the chilled butter pieces.

4. Heat water in the bottom pan of a double boiler*** until it boils gently. The water should not boil vigorously or touch the bottom of the top double boiler pan or bowl in which the curd is to be cooked. Steam produced will be sufficient for the cooking process to occur.

5. In the top of the double boiler, on the countertop or table, whisk the egg yolks and whole eggs together until thoroughly mixed. Slowly whisk in the sugar and zest, blending until well-mixed and smooth. Blend in the lemon juice and then add the butter pieces to the mixture.

6. Place the top of the double boiler over boiling water in the bottom pan. Stir gently but continuously with a silicone spatula or cooking spoon, to prevent the mixture from sticking to the bottom of the pan. Continue cooking until the mixture reaches a temperature of 170°F. Use a food thermometer to monitor the temperature.

7. Remove the double boiler pan from the stove and place on a protected surface, such as a dishcloth or towel on the countertop. Continue to stir gently until the curd thickens (about 5 minutes). Strain

** Bottled lemon juice is used to standardize acidity. Fresh lemon juice can vary in acidity and is not recommended.

*** If a double boiler is not available, a substitute can be made with a large bowl or saucepan that can fit partway down into a saucepan of a smaller diameter. If the bottom pan has a larger diameter, the top bowl or pan should have a handle or handles that can rest on the rim of the lower pan.

curd through a mesh strainer into a glass or stainless steel bowl; discard collected zest.

8. Fill hot, strained curd into the clean, hot half-pint jars, leaving ½-inch headspace. Remove air bubbles and adjust headspace if needed. Wipe rims of jars with a dampened, clean paper towel; apply two-piece metal canning lids. Process. Let cool, undisturbed, for 12 to 24 hours and check for seals.

Process Times for Lemon Curd in a Boiling-Water Canner*

Style of Pack	Jar Size	Process Time at Altitudes of:		
		0–1,000 ft	1,001–6,000 ft	Above 6,000 ft
Hot	Half-pints	15 minutes	20 minutes	25 minutes

*After the process is complete, turn off the heat and remove the canner lid. Wait five minutes before removing jars.

Jam Without Added Pectin

Making jam is even easier than making jelly, as you don't have to strain the fruit. However, you'll want to be sure to remove all stems, skins, and pits. Be sure to wash and rinse all fruits thoroughly before cooking, but don't let them soak. For best flavor, use fully ripe fruit. Use the Ingredients table below as a guideline as you experiment with less common fruits.

Ingredients

Fruit	Quantity (Crushed)	Sugar	Lemon Juice	Yield (Half-pints)
Apricots	4 to 4 ½ cups	4 cups	2 tbsp	5 to 6
Berries*	4 cups	4 cups	None	3 to 4
Peaches	5 ½ to 6 cups	4 to 5 cups	2 tbsp	6 to 7

*Includes blackberries, boysenberries, dewberries, gooseberries, loganberries, raspberries, and strawberries.

1. Remove stems, skins, seeds, and pits; cut into pieces and crush. For berries, remove stems and blossoms and crush. Seedy berries may be put through a sieve or food mill. Measure crushed fruit into large saucepan using the ingredient quantities specified above.

2. Add sugar and bring to a boil while stirring rapidly and constantly. Continue to boil until mixture thickens. Use one of the following tests to determine when jams and jellies are ready to fill. Remember that the jam will thicken as it cools.

Temperature test—Use a jelly or candy thermometer and boil until mixture reaches the temperature for your altitude.								
Sea Level	**1,000 ft**	**2,000 ft**	**3,000 ft**	**4,000 ft**	**5,000 ft**	**6,000 ft**	**7,000 ft**	**8,000 ft**
220°F	218°F	216°F	214°F	212°F	211°F	209°F	207°F	205°F

Refrigerator test—Remove the jam mixture from the heat. Pour a small amount of boiling jam on a cold plate and put it in the freezer compartment of a refrigerator for a few minutes. If the mixture gels, it is ready to fill.

3. Remove from heat and skim off foam quickly. Fill sterile jars with jam. Use a measuring cup or ladle the jam through a wide-mouthed funnel, leaving ¼-inch headspace. Adjust lids and process.

Process Times for Jams without Added Pectin in a Boiling-Water Canner*

Style of Pack	Jar Size	**Process Time at Altitudes of:**		
		0–1,000 ft	1,001–6,000 ft	Above 6,000 ft
Hot	Half-pints	5 minutes	10 minutes	15 minutes

*After the process is complete, turn off the heat and remove the canner lid. Wait five minutes before removing jars.

Jams and Jellies With Added Pectin

To use fresh fruits with a low-pectin content or canned or frozen fruit juice, powdered or liquid pectin must be added for your jams and jellies to thicken and set properly. Jelly or jam made with added pectin requires less cooking and generally gives a larger yield. These products have more natural fruit flavors, too. In addition, using added pectin eliminates the need to test hot jellies and jams for proper gelling.

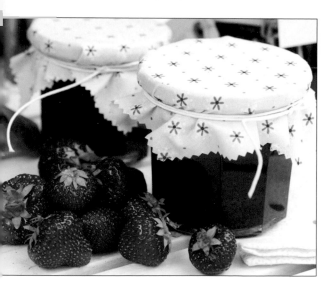

Commercially produced pectin is a natural ingredient, usually made from apples and available at most grocery stores. There are several types of pectin now commonly available; liquid, powder, low-sugar, and no-sugar pectins each have their own advantages and downsides. Pomona's Universal Pectin® is a citrus pectin that allows you to make jams and jellies with little or no sugar. Because the order of combining ingredients depends on the type of pectin used, it is best to follow the common jam and jelly recipes that are included right on most pectin packages. However, if you want to try something a little different, follow one of the following recipes for mixed fruit and spiced fruit jams and jellies.

Tips
- Adding ½ teaspoon of butter or margarine with the juice and pectin will reduce foaming. However, these may cause off-flavor in a long-term storage of jellies and jams.
- Purchase fresh fruit pectin each year. Old pectin may result in poor gels.
- Be sure to use mason canning jars, self-sealing two-piece lids, and a five-minute process (corrected for altitude, as necessary) in boiling water.

Process Times for Jams and Jellies with Added Pectin in a Boiling-Water Canner*

Style of Pack	Jar Size	**Process Time at Altitudes of:**		
		0–1,000 ft	1,001–6,000 ft	Above 6,000 ft
Hot	Half-pints	5 minutes	10 minutes	15 minutes

*After the process is complete, turn off the heat and remove the canner lid. Wait five minutes before removing jars.

Pear-Apple Jam

This is a delicious jam perfect for making at the end of autumn, just before the frost gets the last apples. For a warming, spicy twist, add a teaspoon of fresh, grated ginger along with the cinnamon. This recipe yields seven to eight half-pints.

Ingredients

2 cups peeled, cored, and finely chopped pears (about 2 lbs)

1 cup peeled, cored, and finely chopped apples

¼ tsp ground cinnamon

6½ cups sugar

⅓ cup bottled lemon juice

6 oz liquid pectin

Directions

1. Peel, core, and slice apples and pears into a large saucepan and stir in cinnamon. Thoroughly mix sugar and lemon juice with fruits and bring to a boil over high heat, stirring constantly and crushing fruit with a potato masher as it softens.
2. Once boiling, immediately stir in pectin. Bring to a full rolling boil and boil hard 1 minute, stirring constantly.
3. Remove from heat, quickly skim off foam, and fill sterile jars, leaving ¼-inch headspace. Adjust lids and process.

Process Times for Pear-Apple Jam in a Boiling Water Canner*

Style of Pack	Jar Size	Process Time at Altitudes of:		
		0–1,000 ft	1,001–6,000 ft	Above 6,000 ft
Hot	Half-pints	5 minutes	10 minutes	15 minutes

*After the process is complete, turn off the heat and remove the canner lid. Wait five minutes before removing jars.

Strawberry-Rhubarb Jelly

Strawberry-rhubarb jelly will turn any ordinary piece of bread into a delightful treat. You can also spread it on shortcake or pound cake for a simple and unique dessert. This recipe yields about seven half-pints.

Ingredients

1½ lbs red stalks of rhubarb

1½ qts ripe strawberries

½ tsp butter or margarine to reduce foaming (optional)

6 cups sugar

6 oz liquid pectin

Directions

1. Wash and cut rhubarb into 1-inch pieces and blend or grind. Wash, stem, and crush strawberries, one layer at a time, in a saucepan. Place both fruits in a jelly bag or double layer of cheesecloth and gently squeeze juice into a large measuring cup or bowl.
2. Measure 3½ cups of juice into a large saucepan. Add butter and sugar, thoroughly mixing into juice. Bring to a boil over high heat, stirring constantly.
3. As soon as mixture begins to boil, stir in pectin. Bring to a full, rolling boil and boil hard 1 minute, stirring constantly. Remove from heat, quickly skim off foam, and fill sterile jars, leaving ¼-inch headspace. Adjust lids and process.

Process Times for Strawberry-Rhubarb Jelly in a Boiling-Water Canner*

Style of Pack	Jar Size	Process Time at Altitudes of:		
		0–1,000 ft	1,001–6,000 ft	Above 6,000 ft
Hot	Half-pints or pints	5 minutes	10 minutes	15 minutes

*After the process is complete, turn off the heat and remove the canner lid. Wait five minutes before removing jars.

Blueberry-Spice Jam

This is a summery treat that is delicious spread over waffles with a little butter. Using wild blueberries results in a stronger flavor, but cultivated blueberries also work well. This recipe yields about five half-pints.

Ingredients

2½ pints ripe blueberries

1 tbsp lemon juice

½ tsp ground nutmeg or cinnamon

¾ cup water

5½ cups sugar

1 box (1¾ oz) powdered pectin

Directions

1. Wash and thoroughly crush blueberries, adding one layer at a time, in a saucepan. Add lemon juice, spice, and water. Stir pectin and bring to a full, rolling boil over high heat, stirring frequently.
2. Add the sugar and return to a full, rolling boil. Boil hard for 1 minute, stirring constantly. Remove from heat, quickly skim off foam, and fill sterile jars, leaving ¼-inch headspace. Adjust lids and process.

Process Times for Blueberry-Spice Jam in a Boiling-Water Canner*

Style of Pack	Jar Size	Process Time at Altitudes of:		
		0–1,000 ft	1,001–6,000 ft	Above 6,000 ft
Hot	Half-pints or pints	5 minutes	10 minutes	15 minutes

*After the process is complete, turn off the heat and remove the canner lid. Wait five minutes before removing jars.

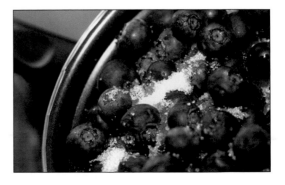

Grape-Plum Jelly

If you think peanut butter and jelly sandwiches are only for kids, try grape-plum jelly spread with a natural nut butter over a thick slice of whole wheat bread. You'll change your mind. This recipe yields about 10 half-pints.

Ingredients
3½ lbs ripe plums
3 lbs ripe Concord grapes
8½ cups sugar
1 cup water
½ tsp butter or margarine to reduce foaming (optional)
1 box (1¾ oz) powdered pectin

Directions
1. Wash and pit plums; do not peel. Thoroughly crush the plums and grapes, adding one layer at a time, in a saucepan with water. Bring to a boil, cover, and simmer 10 minutes.
2. Strain juice through a jelly bag or double layer of cheesecloth. Measure sugar and set aside. Combine 6½ cups of juice with butter and pectin in large saucepan. Bring to a hard boil over high heat, stirring constantly.
3. Add the sugar and return to a full, rolling boil. Boil hard for 1 minute, stirring constantly. Remove from heat, quickly skim off foam, and fill sterile jars, leaving ¼-inch headspace. Adjust lids and process.

Process Times for Grape-Plum Jelly in a Boiling-Water Canner*

Style of Pack	Jar Size	Process Time at Altitudes of:		
		0–1,000 ft	1,001–6,000 ft	Above 6,000 ft
Hot	Half-pints or pints	5 minutes	10 minutes	15 minutes

*After the process is complete, turn off the heat and remove the canner lid. Wait five minutes before removing jars.

Making Reduced-Sugar Fruit Spreads

A variety of fruit spreads may be made that are tasteful, yet lower in sugars and calories than regular jams and jellies. The most straightforward method is probably to buy low-sugar pectin and follow the directions on the package, but the following recipes show alternate methods of using gelatin or fruit pulp as thickening agents. Gelatin recipes should not be processed and should be refrigerated and used within four weeks.

Peach-Pineapple Spread

This recipe may be made with any combination of peaches, nectarines, apricots, and plums. You can use no sugar, up to two cups of sugar, or a combination of sugar and another sweetener (such as honey, Splenda, or agave nectar). Note that if you use aspartame, the spread may lose its sweetness within three to four weeks. Add cinnamon or star anise if desired. This recipe yields five to six half-pints.

Ingredients
4 cups drained peach pulp (follow directions below)
2 cups drained unsweetened crushed pineapple
¼ cup bottled lemon juice
2 cups sugar (optional)

Directions
1. Thoroughly wash 4 to 6 pounds of firm, ripe peaches. Drain well. Peel and remove pits. Grind fruit flesh with a medium or coarse blade, or crush with a fork (do not use a blender).
2. Place ground or crushed peach pulp in a 2-quart saucepan. Heat slowly to release juice, stirring constantly, until fruit is tender. Place cooked fruit in a jelly bag or strainer lined with four layers of cheesecloth. Allow juice to drip about 15 minutes. Save the juice for jelly or other uses.
3. Measure 4 cups of drained peach pulp for making spread. Combine the 4 cups of pulp, pineapple, and lemon juice in a 4-quart saucepan. Add up to 2 cups of sugar or other sweetener, if desired, and mix well.
4. Heat and boil gently for 10 to 15 minutes, stirring enough to prevent sticking. Fill jars quickly, leaving ¼-inch headspace. Adjust lids and process.

Process Times for Peach-Pineapple Spread in a Boiling-Water Canner*

Style of Pack	Jar Size	Process Time at Altitudes of:			
		0–1,000 ft	1,001–3,000 ft	3,001–6,000 ft	Above 6,000 ft
Hot	Half-pints	15 minutes	20 minutes	20 minutes	25 minutes
	Pints	20 minutes	25 minutes	30 minutes	35 minutes

*After the process is complete, turn off the heat and remove the canner lid. Wait five minutes before removing jars.

Refrigerated Apple Spread

This recipe uses gelatin as a thickener, so it does not require processing but it should be refrigerated and used within four weeks. For spiced apple jelly, add two sticks of cinnamon and four whole cloves to mixture before boiling. Remove both spices before adding the sweetener and food coloring (if desired). This recipe yields four half-pints.

Ingredients
2 tbsp unflavored gelatin powder
1 qt bottle unsweetened apple juice
2 tbsp bottled lemon juice
2 tbsp liquid low-calorie sweetener (e.g., sucralose, honey, or 1–2 tsp liquid stevia)

Directions
1. In a saucepan, soften the gelatin in the apple and lemon juices. To dissolve gelatin, bring to a full,

rolling boil and boil 2 minutes. Remove from heat.

2. Stir in sweetener and food coloring (if desired). Fill jars, leaving ¼-inch headspace. Adjust lids. Refrigerate (do not process or freeze).

Refrigerated Grape Spread

This is a simple, tasty recipe that doesn't require processing. Be sure to refrigerate and use within four weeks. This recipe makes three half-pints.

Ingredients

2 tbsp unflavored gelatin powder
1 bottle (24 oz) unsweetened grape juice
2 tbsp bottled lemon juice
2 tbsp liquid low-calorie sweetener (e.g., sucralose, honey, or 1–2 tsp liquid stevia)

Directions

1. In a saucepan, heat the gelatin in the grape and lemon juices until mixture is soft. Bring to a full, rolling boil to dissolve gelatin. Boil 1 minute and remove from heat. Stir in sweetener.
2. Fill jars quickly, leaving ¼-inch headspace. Adjust lids. Refrigerate (do not process or freeze).

Remaking Soft Jellies

Sometimes jelly just doesn't turn out right the first time. Jelly that is too soft can be used as a sweet sauce to drizzle over ice cream, cheesecake, or angel food cake, but it can also be re-cooked into the proper consistency.

To Remake with Powdered Pectin

1. Measure jelly to be re-cooked. Work with no more than 4 to 6 cups at a time. For each quart (4 cups) of jelly, mix ¼ cup sugar, ½ cup water, 2 tablespoons bottled lemon juice, and 4 teaspoons powdered pectin. Bring to a boil while stirring.
2. Add jelly and bring to a rolling boil over high heat, stirring constantly. Boil hard for ½ minute. Remove from heat, quickly skim foam off jelly, and fill sterile

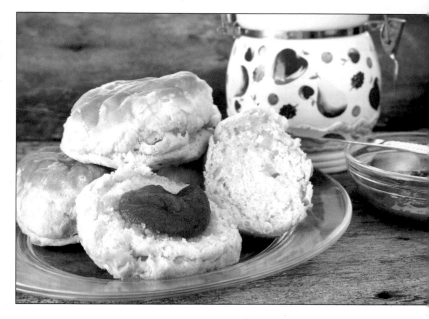

jars, leaving ¼-inch headspace. Adjust new lids and process as recommended.

To Remake With Liquid Pectin

1. Measure jelly to be re-cooked. Work with no more than 4 to 6 cups at a time. For each quart (4 cups) of jelly, measure into a bowl ¾ cup sugar, 2 tablespoons bottled lemon juice, and 2 tablespoons liquid pectin.
2. Bring jelly only to boil over high heat, while stirring. Remove from heat and quickly add the sugar, lemon juice, and pectin. Bring to a full, rolling boil, stirring constantly. Boil hard for 1 minute. Quickly skim off foam and fill sterile jars, leaving ¼-inch headspace. Adjust new lids and process as recommended.

To Remake without Added Pectin

1. For each quart of jelly, add 2 tablespoons bottled lemon juice. Heat to boiling and continue to boil for 3 to 4 minutes.
2. To test jelly for doneness, use one of the following methods:

Temperature test—Use a jelly or candy thermometer and boil until mixture reaches the following temperatures at the altitudes below:

Sea Level	1,000 ft	2,000 ft	3,000 ft	4,000 ft	5,000 ft	6,000 ft	7,000 ft	8,000 ft
220°F	218°F	216°F	214°F	212°F	211°F	209°F	207°F	205°F

Sheet or spoon test—Dip a cool metal spoon into the boiling jelly mixture. Raise the spoon about 12 inches above the pan (out of steam). Turn the spoon so the liquid runs off the side. The jelly is done when the syrup forms two drops that flow together and sheet or hang off the edge of the spoon.

3. Remove from heat, quickly skim off foam, and fill sterile jars, leaving ¼-inch headspace. Adjust new lids and process.

Process Times for Remade Soft Jellies in a Boiling-Water Canner

Style of Pack	Jar Size	Process Time at Altitudes of:		
		0–1,000 ft	1,001–6,000 ft	Above 6,000 ft
Hot	Half-pints or pints	5 minutes	10 minutes	15 minutes

*After the process is complete, turn off the heat and remove the canner lid. Wait five minutes before removing jars.

Vegetables, Pickles, and Tomatoes

Beans or Peas, Shelled or Dried (All Varieties)

Shelled or dried beans and peas are inexpensive and easy to buy or store in bulk, but they are not very convenient when it comes to preparing them to eat. Hydrating and canning beans or peas enable you to simply open a can and use them rather than waiting for them to soak. Sort and discard discolored seeds before rehydrating.

Quantity

- An average of five pounds is needed per canner load of seven quarts.
- An average of 3¼ pounds is needed per canner load of nine pints—an average of ¾ pounds per quart.

Directions

1. Place dried beans or peas in a large pot and cover with water. Soak 12 to 18 hours in a cool place. Drain water. To quickly hydrate beans, you may cover sorted and washed beans with boiling water in a saucepan. Boil 2 minutes, remove from heat, soak 1 hour, and drain.

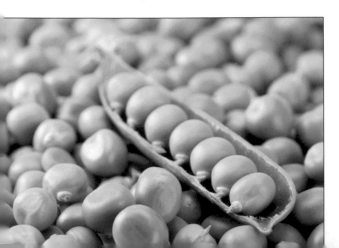

2. Cover beans soaked by either method with fresh water and boil 30 minutes. Add ½ teaspoon of salt per pint or 1 teaspoon per quart to each jar, if desired. Fill jars with beans or peas and cooking water, leaving 1-inch headspace. Adjust lids and process.

Process Times for Beans or Peas in a Dial-Gauge Pressure Canner*

Style of Pack	Jar Size	Process Time	Canner Pressure (PSI) at Altitudes of:			
			0–2,000 ft	2,001–4,000 ft	4,001–6,000 ft	6,001–8,000 ft
Hot	Pints	75 minutes	11 lbs	12 lbs	13 lbs	14 lbs
	Quarts	90 minutes	11 lbs	12 lbs	13 lbs	14 lbs

*After the canner is completely depressurized, remove the weight from the vent port or open the petcock. Wait 10 minutes; then unfasten the lid and remove it carefully. Lift the lid with the underside away from you so that the steam coming out of the canner does not burn your face.

Process Times for Beans or Peas in a Weighted-Gauge Pressure Canner*

Style of pack	Jar Size	Process Time	Canner Pressure (PSI) at Altitudes of:	
			0–1,000 ft	Above 1,000 ft
Hot	Pints	75 minutes	10 lbs	15 lbs
	Quarts	90 minutes	10 lbs	15 lbs

*After the canner is completely depressurized, remove the weight from the vent port or open the petcock. Wait 10 minutes, then unfasten the lid and remove it carefully. Lift the lid with the underside away from you so that the steam coming out of the canner does not burn your face.

Baked Beans

Baked beans are an old New England favorite, but every cook has his or her favorite variation. Two recipes are included here, but feel free to alter them to your own taste.

Quantity

- An average of five pounds of beans is needed per canner load of seven quarts.
- An average of 3¼ pounds is needed per canner load of nine pints—an average of ¾ pounds per quart.

Directions

1. Sort and wash dry beans. Add 3 cups of water for each cup of dried beans. Boil 2 minutes, remove from heat, soak 1 hour, and drain.

2. Heat to boiling in fresh water, and save liquid for making sauce. Make your choice of the following sauces:

Tomato Sauce—Mix 1 quart tomato juice, 3 tablespoons sugar, 2 teaspoons salt, 1 tablespoon chopped onion, and ¼ teaspoon each of ground cloves, allspice, mace, and cayenne pepper. Heat to boiling. Add 3 quarts cooking liquid from beans and bring back to boiling.

Molasses Sauce—Mix 4 cups water or cooking liquid from beans, 3 tablespoons dark molasses, 1 tablespoon vinegar, 2 teaspoons salt, and ¾ teaspoon powdered dry mustard. Heat to boiling.

3. Place seven ¾-inch pieces of pork, ham, or bacon in an earthenware crock, a large casserole, or a pan. Add beans and enough molasses sauce to cover beans.

4. Cover and bake 4 to 5 hours at 350°F. Add water as needed—about every hour. Fill jars, leaving 1-inch headspace. Adjust lids and process.

Process Times for Baked Beans in a Dial-Gauge Pressure Canner*

Style of Pack	Jar Size	Process Time	Canner Pressure (PSI) at Altitudes of:			
			0–2,000 ft	2,001–4,000 ft	4,001–6,000 ft	6,001–8,000 ft
Hot	Pints	65 minutes	11 lbs	12 lbs	13 lbs	14 lbs
	Quarts	75 minutes	11 lbs	12 lbs	13 lbs	14 lbs

*After the canner is completely depressurized, remove the weight from the vent port or open the petcock. Wait 10 minutes, then unfasten the lid and remove it carefully. Lift the lid with the underside away from you so that the steam coming out of the canner does not burn your face.

Process Times for Baked Beans in a Weighted-Gauge Pressure Canner*

Style of pack	Jar Size	Process Time	Canner Pressure (PSI) at Altitudes of:	
			0–1,000 ft	Above 1,000 ft
Hot	Pints	65 minutes	10 lbs	15 lbs
	Quarts	75 minutes	10 lbs	15 lbs

*After the canner is completely depressurized, remove the weight from the vent port or open the petcock. Wait 10 minutes, then unfasten the lid and remove it carefully. Lift the lid with the underside away from you so that the steam coming out of the canner does not burn your face.

Green Beans

This process will work equally well for snap, Italian, or wax beans. Select filled but tender, crisp pods, removing any diseased or rusty pods.

Quantity

- An average of 14 pounds is needed per canner load of seven quarts.
- An average of nine pounds is needed per canner load of nine pints.
- A bushel weighs 30 pounds and yields 12 to 20 quarts—an average of 2 pounds per quart.

Directions

1. Wash beans and trim ends. Leave whole, or cut or break into 1-inch pieces.

Hot pack—Cover with boiling water; boil 5 minutes. Fill jars loosely, leaving 1-inch headspace.

Raw pack—Fill jars tightly with raw beans, leaving 1-inch headspace. Add 1 teaspoon of salt per quart to each jar, if desired. Add boiling water, leaving 1-inch headspace.

2. Adjust lids and process.

Process Times for Green Beans in a Dial-Gauge Pressure Canner*

Style of Pack	Jar Size	Process Time	Canner Pressure (PSI) at Altitudes of:			
			0–2,000 ft	2,001–4,000 ft	4,001–6,000 ft	6,001–8,000 ft
Hot or Raw	Pints	20 minutes	11 lb	12 lb	13 lb	14 lb
	Quarts	25 minutes	11 lb	12 lb	13 lb	14 lb

*After the canner is completely depressurized, remove the weight from the vent port or open the petcock. Wait 10 minutes, then unfasten the lid and remove it carefully. Lift the lid with the underside away from you so that the steam coming out of the canner does not burn your face.

Process Times for Green Beans in a Weighted-Gauge Pressure Canner*

| Style of Pack | Jar Size | Process Time | Canner Pressure (PSI) at Altitudes of: | |
			0–1,000 ft	Above 1,000 ft
Hot or Raw	Pints	20 minutes	10 lbs	15 lbs
	Quarts	25 minutes	10 lbs	15 lbs

*After the canner is completely depressurized, remove the weight from the vent port or open the petcock. Wait 10 minutes; then unfasten the lid and remove it carefully. Lift the lid with the underside away from you so that the steam coming out of the canner does not burn your face.

Beets

You can preserve beets whole, cubed, or sliced, according to your preference. Beets that are 1 to 2 inches in diameter are the best, as larger ones tend to be too fibrous.

Quantity

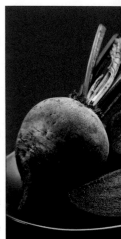

- An average of 21 pounds (without tops) is needed per canner load of seven quarts.
- An average of 13½ pounds is needed per canner load of nine pints.
- A bushel (without tops) weighs 52 pounds and yields 15 to 20 quarts—an average of three pounds per quart.

Directions
1. Trim off beet tops, leaving an inch of stem and roots to reduce bleeding of color. Scrub well. Cover with boiling water. Boil until skins slip off easily, about 15 to 25 minutes depending on size.
2. Cool, remove skins, and trim off stems and roots. Leave baby beets whole. Cut medium or large beets into ½-inch cubes or slices. Halve or quarter very large slices. Add 1 teaspoon of salt per quart to each jar, if desired.
3. Fill jars with hot beets and fresh hot water, leaving 1-inch headspace. Adjust lids and process.

Process Times for Beets in a Dial-Gauge Pressure Canner*

| Style of Pack | Jar Size | Process Time | Canner Pressure (PSI) at Altitudes of: | | | |
			0–2,000 ft	2,001–4,000 ft	4,001–6,000 ft	6,001–8,000 ft
Hot	Pints	30 minutes	11 lbs	12 lbs	13 lbs	14 lbs
	Quarts	35 minutes	11 lbs	12 lbs	13 lbs	14 lbs

*After the canner is completely depressurized, remove the weight from the vent port or open the petcock. Wait 10 minutes, then unfasten the lid and remove it carefully. Lift the lid with the underside away from you so that the steam coming out of the canner does not burn your face.

Process Times for Beets in a Weighted-Gauge Pressure Canner*

| Style of Pack | Jar Size | Process Time | Canner Pressure (PSI) at Altitudes of: | |
			0–1,000 ft	Above 1,000 ft
Hot or Raw	Pints	30 minutes	10 lbs	15 lbs
	Quarts	35 minutes	10 lbs	15 lbs

*After the canner is completely depressurized, remove the weight from the vent port or open the petcock. Wait 10 minutes; then unfasten the lid and remove it carefully. Lift the lid with the underside away from you so that the steam coming out of the canner does not burn your face.

Carrots

Carrots can be preserved sliced or diced according to your preference. Choose small carrots, preferably 1 to 1¼ inches in diameter, as larger ones are often too fibrous.

Quantity

- An average of 17½ pounds (without tops) is needed per canner load of seven quarts.
- An average of 11 pounds is needed per canner load of nine pints.
- A bushel (without tops) weighs 50 pounds and yields 17 to 25 quarts—an average of 2½ pounds per quart.

Directions

1. Wash, peel, and rewash carrots. Slice or dice.

Hot pack—Cover with boiling water; bring to boil and simmer for 5 minutes. Fill jars with carrots, leaving 1-inch headspace.

Raw pack—Fill jars tightly with raw carrots, leaving 1-inch headspace.

2. Add 1 teaspoon of salt per quart to the jar, if desired. Add hot cooking liquid or water, leaving 1-inch headspace. Adjust lids and process.

Process Times for Carrots in a Dial-Gauge pressure Canner*

Style of Pack	Jar Size	Process Time	Canner Pressure (PSI) at Altitudes of:			
			0–2,000 ft	2,001– 4,000 ft	4,001– 6,000 ft	6,001– 8,000 ft
Hot or Raw	Pints	25 minutes	11 lbs	12 lbs	13 lbs	14 lbs
	Quarts	30 minutes	11 lbs	12 lbs	13 lbs	14 lbs

*After the canner is completely depressurized, remove the weight from the vent port or open the petcock. Wait 10 minutes; then unfasten the lid and remove it carefully. Lift the lid with the underside away from you so that the steam coming out of the canner does not burn your face.

Process Times for Carrots in a Weighted-Gauge Pressure Canner*

Style of Pack	Jar Size	Process Time	Canner Pressure (PSI) at Altitudes of:	
			0–1,000 ft	Above 1,000 ft
Hot or Raw	Pints	25 minutes	10 lb	15 lb
	Quarts	30 minutes	10 lb	15 lb

*After the canner is completely depressurized, remove the weight from the vent port or open the petcock. Wait 10 minutes; then unfasten the lid and remove it carefully. Lift the lid with the underside away from you so that the steam coming out of the canner does not burn your face.

Corn, Cream Style

The creamy texture comes from scraping the corncobs thoroughly and including the juices and corn pieces with the kernels. If you want to add milk or cream, butter, or other ingredients, do so just before serving (do not add dairy products before canning). Select ears containing slightly immature kernels for this recipe.

Quantity

- An average of 20 pounds (in husks) of sweet corn is needed per canner load of nine pints.
- A bushel weighs 35 pounds and yields 12 to 20 pints—an average of 2¼ pounds per pint.

Directions

1. Husk corn, remove silk, and wash ears. Cut corn from cob at about the center of kernel. Scrape remaining corn from cobs with a table knife.

Hot pack—To each quart of corn and scrapings in a saucepan, add 2 cups of boiling water. Heat to boiling. Add ½ teaspoon salt to each jar, if desired. Fill pint jars with hot corn mixture, leaving 1-inch headspace.

Raw pack—Fill pint jars with raw corn, leaving 1-inch headspace. Do not shake or press down. Add ½ teaspoon salt to each jar, if desired. Add fresh boiling water, leaving 1-inch headspace.

2. Adjust lids and process.

Process Times for Cream-Style Corn in a Dial-Gauge Pressure Canner

Style of pack	Jar Size	Process Time	Canner Pressure (PSI) at Altitudes of:			
			0–2,000 ft	2,001–4,000 ft	4,001–6,000 ft	6,001–8,000 ft
Hot	Pints	85 minutes	11 lbs	12 lbs	13 lbs	14 lbs
Raw	Pints	95 minutes	11 lbs	12 lbs	13 lbs	14 lbs

*After the canner is completely depressurized, remove the weight from the vent port or open the petcock. Wait 10 minutes; then unfasten the lid and remove it carefully. Lift the lid with the underside away from you so that the steam coming out of the canner does not burn your face.

Process Times for Cream-Style Corn in a Weighted-Gauge Pressure Canner*

Style of Pack	Jar Size	Process Time	Canner Pressure (PSI) at Altitudes of:	
			0–1,000 ft	Above 1,000 ft
Hot	Pints	85 minutes	10 lb	15 lb
Raw	Pints	95 minutes	10 lb	15 lb

*After the canner is completely depressurized, remove the weight from the vent port or open the petcock. Wait 10 minutes; then unfasten the lid and remove it carefully. Lift the lid with the underside away from you so that the steam coming out of the canner does not burn your face.

Corn, Whole Kernel

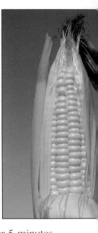

Select ears containing slightly immature kernels. Canning of some sweeter varieties or kernels that are too immature may cause browning. Try canning a small amount to test color and flavor before canning large quantities.

Quantity

- An average of 31½ pounds (in husks) of sweet corn is needed per canner load of seven quarts.
- An average of 20 pounds is needed per canner load of nine pints.
- A bushel weighs 35 pounds and yields 6 to 11 quarts—an average of 4½ pounds per quart.

Directions

1. Husk corn, remove silk, and wash. Blanch 3 minutes in boiling water. Cut corn from cob at about three-fourths the depth of kernel. Do not scrape cob, as it will create a creamy texture.

Hot pack—To each quart of kernels in a saucepan, add 1 cup of hot water, heat to boiling, and simmer 5 minutes. Add 1 teaspoon of salt per quart to each jar, if desired. Fill jars with corn and cooking liquid, leaving 1-inch headspace.

Raw pack—Fill jars with raw kernels, leaving 1-inch headspace. Do not shake or press down. Add 1 teaspoon of salt per quart to the jar, if desired.

2. Add fresh boiling water, leaving 1-inch headspace. Adjust lids and process.

Process Times for Whole Kernel Corn in a Dial-Gauge Pressure Canner*

Style of Pack	Jar Size	Process Time	Canner Pressure (PSI) at Altitudes of:			
			0–2,000 ft	2,001–4,000 ft	4,001–6,000 ft	6,001–8,000 ft
Hot or Raw	Pints	55 minutes	11 lbs	12 lbs	13 lbs	14 lbs
	Quarts	85 minutes	11 lbs	12 lbs	13 lbs	14 lbs

*After the canner is completely depressurized, remove the weight from the vent port or open the petcock. Wait 10 minutes; then unfasten the lid and remove it carefully. Lift the lid with the underside away from you so that the steam coming out of the canner does not burn your face.

Process Times for Whole Kernel Corn in a Weighted-Gauge Pressure Canner*

Style of Pack	Jar Size	Process Time	Canner Pressure (PSI) at Altitudes of:	
			0–1,000 ft	Above 1,000 ft
Hot or Raw	Pints	55 minutes	10 lbs	15 lbs
	Quarts	85 minutes	10 lbs	15 lbs

*After the canner is completely depressurized, remove the weight from the vent port or open the petcock. Wait 10 minutes; then unfasten the lid and remove it carefully. Lift the lid with the underside away from you so that the steam coming out of the canner does not burn your face.

Mixed Vegetables

Use mixed vegetables in soups, casseroles, pot pies, or as a quick side dish. You can change the suggested proportions or substitute other favorite vegetables, but avoid leafy greens, dried beans, cream-style corn, winter squash, and sweet potatoes as they will ruin the consistency of the other vegetables. This recipe yields about seven quarts.

Ingredients
6 cups sliced carrots
6 cups cut, whole-kernel sweet corn
6 cups cut green beans
6 cups shelled lima beans
4 cups diced or crushed tomatoes
4 cups diced zucchini

Directions

1. Carefully wash, peel, de-shell, and cut vegetables as necessary. Combine all vegetables in a large pot or kettle, and add enough water to cover pieces.

2. Add 1 teaspoon salt per quart to each jar, if desired. Boil 5 minutes and fill jars with hot pieces and liquid, leaving 1-inch headspace. Adjust lids and process.

Process Times for Mixed Vegetables in a Dial-Gauge Pressure Canner*

Style of Pack	Jar Size	Process Time	Canner Pressure (PSI) at Altitudes of:			
			0–2,000 ft	2,001–4,000 ft	4,001–6,000 ft	6,001–8,000 ft
Hot	Pints	75 minutes	11 lbs	12 lbs	13 lbs	14 lbs
	Quarts	90 minutes	11 lbs	12 lbs	13 lbs	14 lbs

*After the canner is completely depressurized, remove the weight from the vent port or open the petcock. Wait 10 minutes; then unfasten the lid and remove it carefully. Lift the lid with the underside away from you so that the steam coming out of the canner does not burn your face.

Process Times for Mixed Vegetables in a Weighted-Gauge Pressure Canner*

Style of Pack	Jar Size	Process Time	Canner Pressure (PSI) at Altitudes of:	
			0–1,000 ft	Above 1,000 ft
Hot	Pints	75 minutes	10 lbs	15 lbs
	Quarts	90 minutes	10 lbs	15 lbs

*After the canner is completely depressurized, remove the weight from the vent port or open the petcock. Wait 10 minutes; then unfasten the lid and remove it carefully. Lift the lid with the underside away from you so that the steam coming out of the canner does not burn your face.

Peas, Green or English, Shelled

Green and English peas preserve well when canned, but sugar snap and Chinese edible pods are better frozen. Select filled pods containing young, tender, sweet seeds, and discard any diseased pods.

Quantity

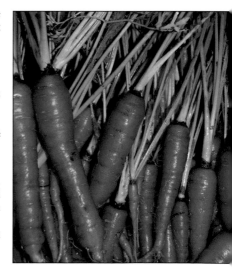

- An average of 31½ pounds (in pods) is needed per canner load of seven quarts.
- An average of 20 pounds is needed per canner load of nine pints.
- A bushel weighs 30 pounds and yields 5 to 10 quarts—an average of 4½ pounds per quart.

Directions

1. Shell and wash peas. Add 1 teaspoon of salt per quart to each jar, if desired.

Hot pack—Cover with boiling water. Bring to a boil in a saucepan, and boil 2 minutes. Fill jars loosely with hot peas, and add cooking liquid, leaving 1-inch headspace.

Raw pack—Fill jars with raw peas, and add boiling water, leaving 1-inch headspace. Do not shake or press down on peas.

2. Adjust lids and process.

Process Times for Peas in a Dial-Gauge Pressure Canner*

Style of Pack	Jar Size	Process Time	Canner Pressure (PSI) at Altitudes of:			
			0–2,000 ft	2,001–4,000 ft	4,001–6,000 ft	6,001–8,000 ft
Hot or Raw	Pints or Quarts	40 minutes	11 lbs	12 lbs	13 lbs	14 lbs

*After the canner is completely depressurized, remove the weight from the vent port or open the petcock. Wait 10 minutes; then unfasten the lid and remove it carefully. Lift the lid with the underside away from you so that the steam coming out of the canner does not burn your face.

Process Times for Peas in a Weighted-Gauge Pressure Canner*

Style of Pack	Jar Size	Process Time	Canner Pressure (PSI) at Altitudes of:	
			0–1,000 ft	Above 1,000 ft
Hot or Raw	Pints or Quarts	40 minutes	10 lbs	15 lbs

*After the canner is completely depressurized, remove the weight from the vent port or open the petcock. Wait 10 minutes; then unfasten the lid and remove it carefully. Lift the lid with the underside away from you so that the steam coming out of the canner does not burn your face.

Potatoes, Sweet

Sweet potatoes can be preserved whole, in chunks, or in slices, according to your preference. Choose small to medium-sized potatoes that are mature and not too fibrous. Can within one to two months after harvest.

Quantity

- An average of 17½ pounds is needed per canner load of seven quarts.
- An average of 11 pounds is needed per canner load of nine pints.
- A bushel weighs 50 pounds and yields 17 to 25 quarts—an average of 2½ pounds per quart.

Directions
1. Wash potatoes and boil or steam until partially soft (15 to 20 minutes). Remove skins. Cut medium potatoes, if needed, so that pieces are uniform in size. Do not mash or purée pieces.
2. Fill jars, leaving 1-inch headspace. Add 1 teaspoon salt per quart to each jar, if desired. Cover with your choice of fresh boiling water or syrup, leaving 1-inch headspace. Adjust lids and process.

Process Times for Sweet Potatoes in a Dial-Gauge Pressure Canner*

Style of Pack	Jar Size	Process Time	Canner Pressure (PSI) at Altitudes of:			
			0–2,000 ft	2,001–4,000 ft	4,001–6,000 ft	6,001–8,000 ft
Hot	Pints	65 minutes	11 lbs	12 lbs	13 lbs	14 lbs
	Quarts	90 minutes	11 lbs	12 lbs	13 lbs	14 lbs

*After the canner is completely depressurized, remove the weight from the vent port or open the petcock. Wait 10 minutes; then unfasten the lid and remove it carefully. Lift the lid with the underside away from you so that the steam coming out of the canner does not burn your face.

Process Times for Sweet Potatoes in a Weighted-Gauge Pressure Canner*

Style of Pack	Jar Size	Process Time	Canner Pressure (PSI) at Altitudes of:	
			0–1,000 ft	Above 1,000 ft
Hot	Pints	65 minutes	10 lbs	15 lbs
	Quarts	90 minutes	10 lbs	15 lbs

*After the canner is completely depressurized, remove the weight from the vent port or open the petcock. Wait 10 minutes; then unfasten the lid and remove it carefully. Lift the lid with the underside away from you so that the steam coming out of the canner does not burn your face.

Pumpkin and Winter Squash

Pumpkin and squash are great to have on hand for use in pies, soups, quick breads, or as side dishes. They should have a hard rind and stringless, mature pulp. Small pumpkins (sugar or pie varieties) are best. Before using for pies, drain jars and strain or sieve pumpkin or squash cubes.

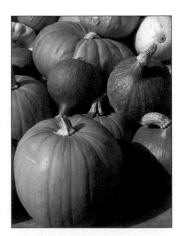

Quantity

- An average of 16 pounds is needed per canner load of seven quarts.
- An average of 10 pounds is needed per canner load of nine pints—an average of 2¼ pounds per quart.

Directions
1. Wash, remove seeds, cut into 1-inch-wide slices, and peel. Cut flesh into 1-inch cubes. Boil 2 minutes in water. Do not mash or purée.
2. Fill jars with cubes and cooking liquid, leaving 1-inch headspace. Adjust lids and process.

Process Times for Pumpkin and Winter Squash in a Dial-Gauge Pressure Canner*

Style of Pack	Jar Size	Process Time	Canner Pressure (PSI) at Altitudes of:			
			0–2,000 ft	2,001–4,000 ft	4,001–6,000 ft	6,001–8,000 ft
Hot	Pints	55 minutes	11 lbs	12 lbs	13 lbs	14 lbs
	Quarts	90 minutes	11 lbs	12 lbs	13 lbs	14 lbs

*After the canner is completely depressurized, remove the weight from the vent port or open the petcock. Wait 10 minutes; then unfasten the lid and remove it carefully. Lift the lid with the underside away from you so that the steam coming out of the canner does not burn your face.

Process Times for Pumpkin and Winter Squash in a Weighted-Gauge Pressure Canner*

Style of Pack	Jar Size	Process Time	Canner Pressure (PSI) at Altitudes of:	
			0–1,000 ft	Above 1,000 ft
Hot	Pints	55 minutes	10 lbs	15 lbs
	Quarts	90 minutes	10 lbs	15 lbs

*After the canner is completely depressurized, remove the weight from the vent port or open the petcock. Wait 10 minutes; then unfasten the lid and remove it carefully. Lift the lid with the underside away from you so that the steam coming out of the canner does not burn your face.

Succotash

To spice up this simple, satisfying dish, add a little paprika and celery salt before serving. It is also delicious made into a pot pie, with or without added chicken, turkey, or beef. This recipe yields seven quarts.

Ingredients
1 lb unhusked sweet corn or 3 qts cut whole kernels
14 lbs mature green podded lima beans or 4 qts shelled lima beans
2 qts crushed or whole tomatoes (optional)

Directions
1. Husk corn, remove silk, and wash. Blanch 3 minutes in boiling water. Cut corn from cob at about three-fourths the depth of kernel. Do not scrape cob, as it will create a creamy texture. Shell lima beans and wash thoroughly.

Hot pack—Combine all prepared vegetables in a large kettle with enough water to cover the pieces. Add 1 teaspoon salt to each quart jar, if desired. Boil gently 5 minutes and fill jars with pieces and cooking liquid, leaving 1-inch headspace.

Raw pack—Fill jars with equal parts of all prepared vegetables, leaving 1-inch headspace. Do not shake or press down pieces. Add 1 teaspoon salt to each quart jar, if desired. Add fresh boiling water, leaving 1-inch headspace.

2. Adjust lids and process.

Process Times for Succotash in a Dial-Gauge Pressure Canner*

Style of Pack	Jar Size	Process Time	Canner Pressure (PSI) at Altitudes of:			
			0–2,000 ft	2,001–4,000 ft	4,001–6,000 ft	6,001–8,000 ft
Hot or Raw	Pints	60 minutes	11 lbs	12 lbs	13 lbs	14 lbs
	Quarts	85 minutes	11 lbs	12 lbs	13 lbs	14 lbs

*After the canner is completely depressurized, remove the weight from the vent port or open the petcock. Wait 10 minutes; then unfasten the lid and remove it carefully. Lift the lid with the underside away from you so that the steam coming out of the canner does not burn your face.

Process Times for Succotash in a Weighted-Gauge Pressure Canner*

Style of Pack	Jar Size	Process Time	Canner Pressure (PSI) at Altitudes of:	
			0–1,000 ft	Above 1,000 ft
Hot or Raw	Pints	60 minutes	10 lbs	15 lbs
	Quarts	85 minutes	10 lbs	15 lbs

*After the canner is completely depressurized, remove the weight from the vent port or open the petcock. Wait 10 minutes; then unfasten the lid and remove it carefully. Lift the lid with the underside away from you so that the steam coming out of the canner does not burn your face.

Soups

Vegetable, dried bean or pea, meat, poultry, or seafood soups can all be canned. Add pasta, rice, or other grains to soup just prior to serving, as grains tend to get soggy when canned. If dried beans or peas are used, they *must* be fully rehydrated first. Dairy products should also be avoided in the canning process.

Directions
1. Select, wash, and prepare vegetables.
2. Cook vegetables. For each cup of dried beans or peas, add 3 cups of water, boil 2 minutes, remove from heat, soak 1 hour, and heat to boil. Drain and combine with meat broth, tomatoes, or water to cover. Boil 5 minutes.
3. Salt to taste, if desired. Fill jars halfway with solid mixture. Add remaining liquid, leaving 1-inch headspace. Adjust lids and process.

Process Times for Soups in a Dial-Gauge Pressure Canner*

			Canner Pressure (PSI) at Altitudes of:			
Style of Pack	Jar Size	Process Time	0– 2,000 ft	2,001–4,000 ft	4,001–6,000 ft	6,001– 8,000 ft
Hot	Pints	60** minutes	11 lbs	12 lbs	13 lbs	14 lbs
	Quarts	75** minutes	11 lbs	12 lbs	13 lbs	14 lbs

**Caution: Process 100 minutes if soup contains seafood.

*After the canner is completely depressurized, remove the weight from the vent port or open the petcock. Wait 10 minutes; then unfasten the lid and remove it carefully. Lift the lid with the underside away from you so that the steam coming out of the canner does not burn your face.

Process Times for Soups in a Weighted-Gauge Pressure Canner*

			Canner Pressure (PSI) at Altitudes of:	
Style of Pack	Jar Size	Process Time	0–1,000 ft	Above 1,000 ft
Hot	Pints	60** minutes	10 lbs	15 lbs
	Quarts	75** minutes	10 lbs	15 lbs

**Caution: Process 100 minutes if soup contains seafood.

*After the canner is completely depressurized, remove the weight from the vent port or open the petcock. Wait 10 minutes; then unfasten the lid and remove it carefully. Lift the lid with the underside away from you so that the steam coming out of the canner does not burn your face.

Meat Stock (Broth)

"Good broth will resurrect the dead," says a South American proverb. Bones contain calcium, magnesium, phosphorus, and other trace minerals, while cartilage and tendons hold glucosamine, which is important for joints and muscle health. When simmered for extended periods, these nutrients are released into the water and broken down into a form that our bodies can absorb. Not to mention that good broth is the secret to delicious risotto, reduction sauces, gravies, and dozens of other gourmet dishes.

Beef
1. Saw or crack fresh, trimmed beef bones to enhance extraction of flavor. Rinse bones and place in a large stockpot or kettle, cover bones with water, add pot cover, and simmer 3 to 4 hours.
2. Remove bones, cool broth, and pick off meat. Skim off fat, add meat removed from bones to broth, and reheat to boiling. Fill jars, leaving 1-inch headspace. Adjust lids and process.

Chicken or Turkey
1. Place large carcass bones in a large stockpot, add enough water to cover bones, cover pot, and simmer 30 to 45 minutes or until meat can be easily stripped from bones.
2. Remove bones and pieces, cool broth, strip meat, discard excess fat, and return meat to broth. Reheat to boiling and fill jars, leaving 1-inch headspace. Adjust lids and process.

Process Times for Meat Stock in a Dial-Gauge Pressure Canner*

			Canner Pressure (PSI) at Altitudes of:			
Style of Pack	Jar Size	Process Time	0–2,000 ft	2,001–4,000 ft	4,001–6,000 ft	6,001–8,000 ft
Hot	Pints	20 minutes	11 lbs	12 lbs	13 lbs	14 lbs
	Quarts	25 minutes	11 lbs	12 lbs	13 lbs	14 lbs

*After the canner is completely depressurized, remove the weight from the vent port or open the petcock. Wait 10 minutes; then unfasten the lid and remove it carefully. Lift the lid with the underside away from you so that the steam coming out of the canner does not burn your face.

Process Times for Meat Stock in a Weighted-Gauge Pressure Canner*

| Style of Pack | Jar Size | Process Time | Canner Pressure (PSI) at Altitudes of: | |
			0–1,000 ft	Above 1,000 ft
Hot	Pints	20 minutes	10 lbs	15 lbs
	Quarts	25 minutes	10 lbs	15 lbs

*After the canner is completely depressurized, remove the weight from the vent port or open the petcock. Wait 10 minutes; then unfasten the lid and remove it carefully. Lift the lid with the underside away from you so that the steam coming out of the canner does not burn your face.

Fermented Foods and Pickled Vegetables

Pickled vegetables play a vital role in Italian antipasto dishes, Chinese stir-fries, British piccalilli, and much of Russian and Finnish cuisine. And, of course, the Germans love their sauerkraut, kimchee is found on nearly every Korean dinner table, and many an American won't eat a sandwich without a good, strong dill pickle on the side.

Fermenting vegetables is not complicated, but you'll want to have the proper containers, covers, and weights ready before you begin. For containers, keep the following in mind:

- A once-gallon container is needed for each five pounds of fresh vegetables. Therefore, a five-gallon stone crock is of ideal size for fermenting about 25 pounds of fresh cabbage or cucumbers.
- Food-grade plastic and glass containers are excellent substitutes for stone crocks. Other one- to three-gallon non-food-grade plastic containers may be used if lined inside with a clean food-grade plastic bag. **Caution: Be certain that foods contact only food-grade plastics. Do not use garbage bags or trash liners.**
- Fermenting sauerkraut in quart and half-gallon mason jars is an acceptable practice, but may result in more spoilage losses.

Some vegetables, like cabbage and cucumbers, need to be kept 1 to 2 inches under brine while fermenting. If you find them floating to top of the container, here are some suggestions:

- After adding prepared vegetables and brine, insert a suitably sized dinner plate or glass pie plate inside the fermentation container. The plate must be slightly smaller than the container opening, yet large enough to cover most of the shredded cabbage or cucumbers.
- To keep the plate under the brine, weight it down with two to three sealed quart jars filled with water. Covering the container opening with a clean, heavy bath towel helps to prevent contamination from insects and molds while the vegetables are fermenting.
- Fine quality fermented vegetables are also obtained when the plate is weighted down with a very large, clean, plastic bag filled with three quarts of water containing 4½ tablespoons of salt. Be sure to seal the plastic bag. Freezer bags sold

for packaging turkeys are suitable for use with five-gallon containers.

Be sure to wash the fermentation container, plate, and jars in hot, sudsy water, and rinse well with very hot water before use.

Dill Pickles

Feel free to alter the spices in this recipe, but stick to the same proportion of cucumbers, vinegar, and water. Check the label of your vinegar to be sure it contains 5 percent acetic acid. Fully fermented pickles may be stored in the original container for about four to six months, provided they are refrigerated and surface scum and molds are removed regularly, but canning is a better way to store fully fermented pickles.

Ingredients

Use the following quantities for each gallon capacity of your container:

4 lbs of 4-inch pickling cucumbers
2 tbsp dill seed or 4 to 5 heads fresh or dry dill weed
½ cup salt
¼ cup vinegar (5 percent acetic acid)
8 cups water and one or more of the following ingredients:
2 cloves garlic (optional)
2 dried red peppers (optional)
2 tsp whole mixed pickling spices (optional)

Directions

1. Wash cucumbers. Cut 1⁄16-inch slice off blossom end and discard. Leave ¼ inch of stem attached. Place half of dill and spices on bottom of a clean, suitable container.

2. Add cucumbers, remaining dill, and spices. Dissolve salt in vinegar and water and pour over cucumbers. Add suitable cover and weight. Store where temperature is between 70°F and 75°F for about 3 to 4 weeks while fermenting. Temperatures of 55°F to 65°F are acceptable, but the fermentation will take 5 to 6 weeks. Avoid temperatures above 80°F, or pickles will become too soft during fermentation. Fermenting pickles cure slowly. Check the container several times a week and promptly remove surface scum or mold. **Caution: If the pickles become soft, slimy, or develop a disagreeable odor, discard them.**

3. Once fully fermented, pour the brine into a pan, heat slowly to a boil, and simmer 5 minutes. Filter brine through paper coffee filters to reduce cloudi-

ness, if desired. Fill jars with pickles and hot brine, leaving ½-inch headspace. Adjust lids and process in a boiling water canner, or use the low-temperature pasteurization treatment described here:

Low-Temperature Pasteurization Treatment

The following treatment results in a better product texture but must be carefully managed to avoid possible spoilage.

1. Place jars in a canner filled halfway with warm (120°F to 140°F) water. Then, add hot water to a level 1 inch above jars.
2. Heat the water enough to maintain 180°F to 185°F water temperature for 30 minutes. Check with a candy or jelly thermometer to be certain that the water temperature is at least 180°F during the entire 30 minutes. Temperatures higher than 185°F may cause unnecessary softening of pickles.

Process Times for Dill Pickles in a Boiling-Water Canner*

Style of Pack	Jar Size	Process Time at Altitudes of:		
		0–1,000 ft	1,001–6,000 ft	Above 6,000 ft
Raw	Pints	10 minutes	15 minutes	20 minutes
	Quarts	15 minutes	20 minutes	25 minutes

*After the process is complete, turn off the heat and remove the canner lid. Wait five minutes before removing jars.

Sauerkraut

For the best sauerkraut, use firm heads of fresh cabbage. Shred cabbage and start kraut between 24 and 48 hours after harvest. This recipe yields about nine quarts.

Ingredients

25 lbs cabbage
¾ cup canning or pickling salt

Directions

1. Work with about 5 pounds of cabbage at a time. Discard outer leaves. Rinse heads under cold running water and drain. Cut heads in quarters and remove cores. Shred or slice to the thickness of a quarter.
2. Put cabbage in a suitable fermentation container (see page 103 for suggestions on containers, lids, and weights), and add 3 tablespoons of salt. Mix thoroughly, using clean hands. Pack firmly until salt draws juices from cabbage.
3. Repeat shredding, salting, and packing until all cabbage is in the container. Be sure it is deep enough so that its rim is at least 4 or 5 inches above the cabbage. If juice does not cover cabbage, add boiled and cooled brine (1½ tablespoons of salt per quart of water).
4. Add plate and weights; cover container with a clean bath towel. Store at 70°F to 75°F while fermenting. At temperatures between 70°F and 75°F, kraut will be fully fermented in about 3 to 4 weeks; at 60°F to 65°F, fermentation may take 5 to 6 weeks. At tem-

peratures lower than 60°F, kraut may not ferment. Above 75°F, kraut may become soft.

Note: If you weigh the cabbage down with a brine-filled bag, do not disturb the crock until normal fermentation is completed (when bubbling ceases). If you use jars as weight, you will have to check the kraut 2 to 3 times each week and remove scum if it forms. Fully fermented kraut may be kept tightly covered in the refrigerator for several months or it may be canned as follows:

Hot pack—Bring kraut and liquid slowly to a boil in a large kettle, stirring frequently. Remove from heat and fill jars rather firmly with kraut and juices, leaving ½-inch headspace.

Raw pack—Fill jars firmly with kraut and cover with juices, leaving ½-inch headspace.

5. Adjust lids and process.

Process Times for Sauerkraut in a Boiling-Water Canner*

Style of Pack	Jar Size	Process Time at Altitudes of:			
		0–1,000 ft	1,001–3,000 ft	3,001–6,000 ft	Above 6,000 ft
Hot	Pints	10 minutes	15 minutes	15 minutes	20 minutes
	Quarts	15 minutes	20 minutes	20 minutes	25 minutes
Raw	Pints	20 minutes	25 minutes	30 minutes	35 minutes
	Quarts	25 minutes	30 minutes	35 minutes	40 minutes

*After the process is complete, turn off the heat and remove the canner lid. Wait five minutes before removing jars.

Pickled Three-Bean Salad

This is a great side dish to bring to a summer picnic or potluck. Feel free to add or adjust spices to your taste. This recipe yields about five to six half-pints.

Ingredients

1½ cups cut and blanched green or yellow beans (prepared as below)
1½ cups canned, drained red kidney beans
1 cup canned, drained garbanzo beans
½ cup peeled and thinly sliced onion (about 1 medium onion)
½ cup trimmed and thinly sliced celery (1½ medium stalks)
½ cup sliced green peppers (½ medium pepper)
½ cup white vinegar (5 percent acetic acid)
¼ cup bottled lemon juice
¾ cup sugar
1¼ cups water
¼ cup oil
½ tsp canning or pickling salt

Directions

1. Wash and snap off ends of fresh beans. Cut or snap into 1- to 2-inch pieces. Blanch 3 minutes and cool immediately. Rinse kidney beans with tap water and drain again. Prepare and measure all other vegetables.
2. Combine vinegar, lemon juice, sugar, and water and bring to a boil. Remove from heat. Add oil and salt and mix well. Add beans, onions, celery, and green pepper to solution and bring to a simmer.
3. Marinate 12 to 14 hours in refrigerator, then heat entire mixture to a boil. Fill clean jars with solids. Add hot liquid, leaving ½-inch headspace. Adjust lids and process.

Process Times for Pickled Three-Bean Salad in a Boiling Water Canner*

Style of Pack	Jar Size	Process Time at Altitudes of:		
		0–1,000 ft	1,001–6,000 ft	Above 6,000 ft
Hot	Half-pints or Pints	15 minutes	20 minutes	25 minutes

Pickled Horseradish Sauce

Select horseradish roots that are firm and have no mold, soft spots, or green spots. Avoid roots that have begun to sprout. The pungency of fresh horseradish fades within one to two months, even when refrigerated, so make only small quantities at a time. This recipe yields about two half-pints.

Ingredients

2 cups (¾ lb) freshly grated horseradish
1 cup white vinegar (5 percent acetic acid)
½ tsp canning or pickling salt
¼ tsp powdered ascorbic acid

Directions

1. Wash horseradish roots thoroughly and peel off brown outer skin. Grate the peeled roots in a food processor or cut them into small cubes and put through a food grinder.
2. Combine ingredients and fill into sterile jars, leaving ¼-inch headspace. Seal jars tightly and store in a refrigerator.

Marinated Peppers

Any combination of bell, Hungarian, banana, or jalapeño peppers can be used in this recipe. Use more jalapeño peppers if you want your mix to be hot, but remember to wear rubber or plastic gloves while handling them or wash hands thoroughly with soap and water before touching your face. This recipe yields about nine half-pints.

Ingredients

4 lbs firm peppers
1 cup bottled lemon juice
2 cups white vinegar (5 percent acetic acid)
1 tbsp oregano leaves

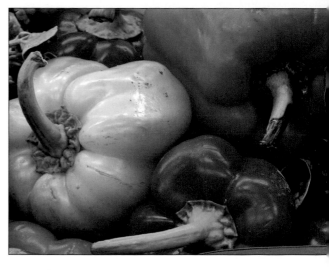

1 cup olive or salad oil
½ cup chopped onions
2 tbsp prepared horseradish (optional)
2 cloves garlic, quartered (optional)
2¼ tsp salt (optional)

Directions

1. Select your favorite pepper. Peppers may be left whole or quartered. Wash, slash two to four slits in each pepper, and blanch in boiling water or blister to peel tough-skinned hot peppers. Blister peppers using one of the following methods:
   Oven or broiler method—Place peppers in a hot oven (400°F) or broiler for 6 to 8 minutes or until skins blister.
   Range-top method—Cover hot burner, either gas or electric, with heavy wire mesh. Place peppers on burner for several minutes until skins blister.
2. Allow peppers to cool. Place in pan and cover with a damp cloth. This will make peeling the peppers easier. After several minutes of cooling, peel each pepper. Flatten whole peppers.
3. Mix all remaining ingredients except garlic and salt in a saucepan and heat to boiling. Place ¼ garlic clove (optional) and ¼ teaspoon salt in each half-pint or ½ teaspoon per pint. Fill jars with peppers, and add hot, well-mixed oil/pickling solution over peppers, leaving ½-inch headspace. Adjust lids and process.

Process Times for Marinated Peppers in a Boiling-Water Canner*

Style of Pack	Jar Size	Process Time at Altitudes of:			
		0–1,000 ft	1,001–3,000 ft	3,001–6,000 ft	Above 6,000 ft
Raw	Half-pints and Pints	15 minutes	20 minutes	20 minutes	25 minutes

*After the process is complete, turn off the heat and remove the canner lid. Wait five minutes before removing jars.

Piccalilli

Piccalilli is a nice accompaniment to roasted or braised meats and is common in British and Indian meals. It can also be mixed with mayonnaise or crème fraîche as the basis of a French remoulade. This recipe yields nine half-pints.

Ingredients
6 cups chopped green tomatoes
1½ cups chopped sweet red peppers
1½ cups chopped green peppers
2¼ cups chopped onions
7½ cups chopped cabbage
½ cup canning or pickling salt
3 tbsp whole mixed pickling spice
4½ cups vinegar (5 percent acetic acid)
3 cups brown sugar

Directions
1. Wash, chop, and combine vegetables with salt. Cover with hot water and let stand 12 hours. Drain and press in a clean, white cloth to remove all possible liquid.
2. Tie spices loosely in a spice bag and add to combined vinegar and brown sugar and heat to a boil in a saucepan. Add vegetables and boil gently 30 minutes or until the volume of the mixture is reduced by one-half. Remove spice bag.
3. Fill hot sterile jars with hot mixture, leaving ½-inch headspace. Adjust lids and process.

Process Times for Piccalilli in a Boiling-Water Canner

Style of Pack	Jar Size	Process Time at Altitudes of:		
		0–1,000 ft	1,001–6,000 ft	Above 6,000 ft
Hot	Half-pints or Pints	5 minutes	10 minutes	15 minutes

*After the process is complete, turn off the heat and remove the canner lid. Wait five minutes before removing jars.

Bread-and-Butter Pickles

These slightly sweet, spiced pickles will add flavor and crunch to any sandwich. If desired, slender (1 to 1½ inches in diameter) zucchini or yellow summer squash can be substituted for cucumbers. After processing and cooling, jars should be stored four to five weeks to develop ideal flavor. This recipe yields about eight pints.

Ingredients
6 lbs of 4- to 5-inch pickling cucumbers
8 cups thinly sliced onions (about 3 pounds)
½ cup canning or pickling salt
4 cups vinegar (5 percent acetic acid)
4½ cups sugar
2 tbsp mustard seed
1½ tbsp celery seed
1 tbsp ground turmeric
1 cup pickling lime (optional—for use in variation below for making firmer pickles)

Directions
1. Wash cucumbers. Cut ⅟₁₆ inch off blossom end and discard. Cut into ³⁄₁₆-inch slices. Combine cucumbers and onions in a large bowl. Add salt. Cover with 2 inches crushed or cubed ice. Refrigerate 3 to 4 hours, adding more ice as needed.
2. Combine remaining ingredients in a large pot. Boil 10 minutes. Drain cucumbers and onions, add to pot, and slowly reheat to boiling. Fill jars with slices and cooking syrup, leaving ½-inch headspace.
3. Adjust lids and process in boiling-water canner, or use the low-temperature pasteurization treatment described below.

Low-Temperature Pasteurization Treatment
The following treatment results in a better product texture but must be carefully managed to avoid possible spoilage.
1. Place jars in a canner filled halfway with warm (120°F to 140°F) water. Then, add hot water to a level 1 inch above jars.
2. Heat the water enough to maintain 180°F to 185°F water temperature for 30 minutes. Check with a candy or jelly thermometer to be certain that the water temperature is at least 180°F during the entire 30 minutes. Temperatures higher than 185°F may cause unnecessary softening of pickles.

Variation for firmer pickles: Wash cucumbers. Cut ⅟₁₆ inch off blossom end and discard. Cut into ³⁄₁₆-inch slices. Mix 1 cup pickling lime and ½ cup salt to 1 gallon water in a 2- to 3-gallon crock or enamelware container. Avoid inhaling lime dust while mixing the lime-water solution. Soak cucumber slices in lime water for 12 to 24 hours, stirring occasionally. Remove from lime solution, rinse, and resoak 1 hour in fresh cold water. Repeat the rinsing and soaking steps two more times. Handle carefully, as slices will be brittle. Drain well.

Process Times for Bread-and-Butter Pickles in a Boiling-Water Canner*

Style of Pack	Jar Size	Process Time at Altitudes of:		
		0–1,000 ft	1,001–6,000 ft	Above 6,000 ft
Hot	Pints or Quarts	10 minutes	15 minutes	20 minutes

*After the process is complete, turn off the heat and remove the canner lid. Wait five minutes before removing jars.

Quick Fresh-Pack Dill Pickles

For best results, pickle cucumbers within twenty-four hours of harvesting, or immediately after purchasing. This recipe yields seven to nine pints.

Ingredients
8 lbs of 3- to 5-inch pickling cucumbers
2 gallons water
1¼ to 1½ cups canning or pickling salt
1½ qts vinegar (5 percent acetic acid)

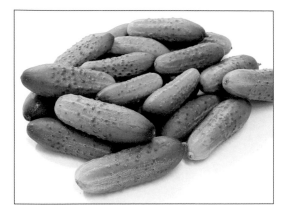
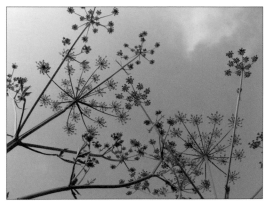

¼ cup sugar

2 to 2¼ quarts water

2 tbsp whole mixed pickling spice

3 to 5 tbsp whole mustard seed (2 tsp to 1 tsp per pint jar)

14 to 21 heads of fresh dill (1½ to 3 heads per pint jar) *or*

4½ to 7 tbsp dill seed (1-½ tsp to 1 tbsp per pint jar)

Directions

1. Wash cucumbers. Cut ¹⁄₁₆-inch slice off blossom end and discard, but leave ¼-inch of stem attached. Dissolve ¾ cup salt in 2 gallons water. Pour over cucumbers and let stand 12 hours. Drain.

2. Combine vinegar, ½ cup salt, sugar and 2 quarts water. Add mixed pickling spices tied in a clean white cloth. Heat to boiling. Fill jars with cucumbers. Add 1 tsp mustard seed and 1½ heads fresh dill per pint.

3. Cover with boiling pickling solution, leaving ½-inch headspace. Adjust lids and process.

Process Times for Quick Fresh-Pack Dill Pickles in a Boiling-Water Canner*

Style of Pack	Jar Size	Process Time at Altitudes of:		
		0–1,000 ft	1,001–6,000 ft	Above 6,000 ft
Raw	Pints	10 minutes	15 minutes	20 minutes
	Quarts	15 minutes	20 minutes	25 minutes

*After the process is complete, turn off the heat and remove the canner lid. Wait five minutes before removing jars.

Pickle Relish

A food processor will make quick work of chopping the vegetables in this recipe. Yields about nine pints.

Ingredients

3 qts chopped cucumbers

3 cups each of chopped sweet green and red peppers

1 cup chopped onions

¾ cup canning or pickling salt

4 cups ice

8 cups water

4 tsp each of mustard seed, turmeric, whole allspice, and whole cloves

2 cups sugar

6 cups white vinegar (5 percent acetic acid)

Directions

1. Add cucumbers, peppers, onions, salt, and ice to water and let stand 4 hours. Drain and re-cover vegetables with fresh ice water for another hour. Drain again.

2. Combine spices in a spice or cheesecloth bag. Add spices to sugar and vinegar. Heat to boiling and pour mixture over vegetables. Cover and refrigerate 24 hours.

3. Heat mixture to boiling and fill hot into clean jars, leaving ½-inch headspace. Adjust lids and process.

Process Times for Pickle Relish in a Boiling-Water Canner*

Style of Pack	Jar Size	Process Time at Altitudes of:		
		0–1,000 ft	1,001–6,000 ft	Above 6,000 ft
Hot	Half-pints or Pints	10 minutes	15 minutes	20 minutes

*After the process is complete, turn off the heat and remove the canner lid. Wait five minutes before removing jars.

Quick Sweet Pickles

Quick and simple to prepare, these are the sweet pickles to make when you're short on time. After processing and cooling, jars should be stored four to five weeks to develop ideal flavor. If desired, add two slices of raw whole onion to each jar before filling with cucumbers. This recipe yields about seven to nine pints.

Ingredients

8 lbs of 3- to 4-inch pickling cucumbers

⅓ cup canning or pickling salt

4½ cups sugar

3½ cups vinegar (5 percent acetic acid)

2 tsp celery seed

1 tbsp whole allspice
2 tbsp mustard seed
1 cup pickling lime (optional)

Directions
1. Wash cucumbers. Cut ⅟16 inch off blossom end and discard, but leave ¼ inch of stem attached. Slice or cut in strips, if desired.
2. Place in bowl and sprinkle with salt. Cover with 2 inches of crushed or cubed ice. Refrigerate 3 to 4 hours. Add more ice as needed. Drain well.
3. Combine sugar, vinegar, celery seed, allspice, and mustard seed in 6-quart kettle. Heat to boiling.

Hot pack—Add cucumbers and heat slowly until vinegar solution returns to boil. Stir occasionally to make sure mixture heats evenly. Fill sterile jars, leaving ½-inch headspace.

Raw pack—Fill jars, leaving ½-inch headspace.
4. Add hot pickling syrup, leaving ½-inch headspace. Adjust lids and process.

Variation for firmer pickles: Wash cucumbers. Cut ⅟16 inch off blossom end and discard, but leave ¼ inch of stem attached. Slice or strip cucumbers. Mix 1 cup pickling lime and ⅓ cup salt with 1 gallon water in a 2- to 3-gallon crock or enamelware container. **Caution: Avoid inhaling lime dust while mixing the lime-water solution.** Soak cucumber slices or strips in lime-water solution for 12 to 24 hours, stirring occasionally. Remove from lime solution, rinse, and soak 1 hour in fresh cold water. Repeat the rinsing and soaking two more times. Handle carefully, because slices or strips will be brittle. Drain well.

Process Times for Quick Sweet Pickles in a Boiling-Water Canner*

Style of Pack	Jar Size	Process Time at Altitudes of:		
		0–1,000 ft	1,001–6,000 ft	Above 6,000 ft
Hot	Pints or Quarts	5 minutes	10 minutes	15 minutes
Raw	Pints	10 minutes	15 minutes	20 minutes
	Quarts	15 minutes	20 minutes	25 minutes

*After the process is complete, turn off the heat and remove the canner lid. Wait five minutes before removing jars.

Reduced-Sodium Sliced Sweet Pickles

Whole allspice can be tricky to find. If it's not available at your local grocery store, it can be ordered at www.spicebarn.com or at www.gourmetsleuth .com. This recipe yields about four to five pints.

Ingredients
4 lbs (3- to 4-inch) pickling cucumbers
Canning syrup: 1⅔ cups distilled white vinegar (5 percent acetic acid)
3 cups sugar
1 tbsp whole allspice
2¼ tsp celery seed
Brining solution: 1 qt distilled white vinegar (5 percent acetic acid)
1 tbsp canning or pickling salt
1 tbsp mustard seed
½ cup sugar

Directions
1. Wash cucumbers and cut ⅟16-inch off blossom end, and discard. Cut cucumbers into ¼-inch slices. Combine all ingredients for canning syrup in a saucepan and bring to boiling. Keep syrup hot until used.
2. In a large kettle, mix the ingredients for the brining solution. Add the cut cucumbers, cover, and simmer until the cucumbers change color from bright to dull green (about 5 to 7 minutes). Drain the cucumber slices.
3. Fill jars, and cover with hot canning syrup leaving ½-inch headspace. Adjust lids and process.

Process Times for Reduced-Sodium Sliced Sweet Pickles in a Boiling-Water Canner*

Style of Pack	Jar Size	Process Time at Altitudes of:		
		0–1,000 ft	1,001–6,000 ft	Above 6,000 ft
Hot	Pints	10 minutes	15 minutes	20 minutes

*After the process is complete, turn off the heat and remove the canner lid. Wait five minutes before removing jars.

Tomatoes

Canned tomatoes should be a staple in every cook's pantry. They are easy to prepare and, when made with garden-fresh produce, make ordinary soups, pizza, or pastas into five-star meals. Be sure to select only dis-

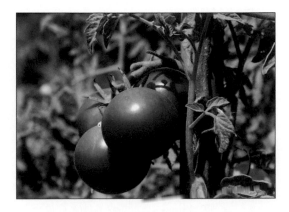

ease-free, preferably vine-ripened, firm fruit. Do not can tomatoes from dead or frost-killed vines.

Green tomatoes are more acidic than ripened fruit and can be canned safely with the following recommendations.

- To ensure safe acidity in whole, crushed, or juiced tomatoes, add two tablespoons of bottled lemon juice or ½ teaspoon of citric acid per quart of tomatoes. For pints, use one tablespoon bottled lemon juice or ¼ teaspoon citric acid.
- Acid can be added directly to the jars before filling with product. Add sugar to offset acid taste, if desired. Four tablespoons of 5 percent acidity vinegar per quart may be used instead of lemon juice or citric acid. However, vinegar may cause undesirable flavor changes.
- Using a pressure canner will result in higher quality and more nutritious canned tomato products. If your pressure canner cannot be operated above 15 PSI, select a process time at a lower pressure.

Tomato Juice

Tomato juice is a good source of vitamin A and C and is tasty on its own or in a cocktail. It's also the secret ingredient in some very delicious cakes. If desired, add carrots, celery, and onions, or toss in a few jalapeños for a little kick.

Quantity

- An average of 23 pounds is needed per canner load of seven quarts, or an average of 14 pounds per canner load of nine pints.

- A bushel weighs 53 pounds and yields 15 to 18 quarts of juice—an average of 3¼ pounds per quart.

Directions

1. Wash tomatoes, remove stems, and trim off bruised or discolored portions. To prevent juice from separating, quickly cut about 1 pound of fruit into quarters and put directly into saucepan. Heat immediately to boiling while crushing.
2. Continue to slowly add and crush freshly cut tomato quarters to the boiling mixture. Make sure the mixture boils constantly and vigorously while you add the remaining tomatoes. Simmer 5 minutes after you add all pieces.
3. Press heated juice through a sieve or food mill to remove skins and seeds. Add bottled lemon juice or citric acid to jars. Heat juice again to boiling.
4. Add 1 teaspoon of salt per quart to the jars, if desired. Fill jars with hot tomato juice, leaving ½-inch headspace. Adjust lids and process.

Process Times for Tomato Juice in a Boiling-Water Canner*

Style of Pack	Jar Size	Process Time at Altitudes of:			
		0–1,000 ft	1,001–3,000 ft	3,001–6,000 ft	Above 6,000 ft
Hot	Pints	35 minutes	40 minutes	45 minutes	50 minutes
	Quarts	40 minutes	45 minutes	50 minutes	55 minutes

*After the process is complete, turn off the heat and remove the canner lid. Wait five minutes before removing jars.

Process Times for Tomato Juice in a Dial-Gauge Pressure Canner*

Style of Pack	Jar Size	Process Time	Canner Gauge Pressure (PSI) at Altitudes of:			
			0–2,000 ft	2,001–4,000 ft	4,001–6,000 ft	6,001–8,000 ft
Hot	Pints or Quarts	20 minutes	6 lbs	7 lbs	8 lbs	9 lbs
		15 minutes	11 lbs	12 lbs	13 lbs	14 lbs

*After the canner is completely depressurized, remove the weight from the vent port or open the petcock. Wait 10 minutes; then unfasten the lid and remove it carefully. Lift the lid with the underside away from you so that the steam coming out of the canner does not burn your face.

Process Times for Tomato Juice in a Weighted-Gauge Pressure Canner*

Style of Pack	Jar Size	Process Time	Canner Gauge Pressure (PSI) at Altitudes of:	
			0–1,000 ft	Above 1,000 ft
Hot	Pints or Quarts	20 minutes	5 lbs	10 lbs
		15 minutes	10 lbs	15 lbs

Crushed Tomatoes with No Added Liquid

Crushed tomatoes are great for use in soups, stews, thick sauces, and casseroles. Simmer crushed tomatoes with kidney beans, chili powder, sautéed onions, and garlic to make an easy pot of chili.

Quantity

- An average of 22 pounds is needed per canner load of seven quarts.

- An average of 14 fresh pounds is needed per canner load of nine pints.
- A bushel weighs 53 pounds and yields 17 to 20 quarts of crushed tomatoes—an average of 2¾ pounds per quart.

Directions

1. Wash tomatoes and dip in boiling water for 30 to 60 seconds or until skins split. Then dip in cold water, slip off skins, and remove cores. Trim off any bruised or discolored portions and quarter.
2. Heat ⅙ of the quarters quickly in a large pot, crushing them with a wooden mallet or spoon as they are added to the pot. This will exude juice. Continue heating the tomatoes, stirring to prevent burning.
3. Once the tomatoes are boiling, gradually add remaining quartered tomatoes, stirring constantly. These remaining tomatoes do not need to be crushed; they will soften with heating and stirring. Continue until all tomatoes are added. Then boil gently 5 minutes.
4. Add bottled lemon juice or citric acid to jars. Add 1 teaspoon of salt per quart to the jars, if desired. Fill jars immediately with hot tomatoes, leaving ½-inch headspace. Adjust lids and process.

Process Times for Crushed Tomatoes in a Dial-Gauge Pressure Canner*

Style of Pack	Jar Size	Process Time	Canner Gauge Pressure (PSI) at Altitudes of:			
			0–2,000 ft	2,001–4,000 ft	4,001–6,000 ft	6,001–8,000 ft
Hot	Pints or Quarts	20 minutes	6 lbs	7 lbs	8 lbs	9 lbs
		15 minutes	11 lbs	12 lbs	13 lbs	14 lbs

*After the canner is completely depressurized, remove the weight from the vent port or open the petcock. Wait 10 minutes; then unfasten the lid and remove it carefully. Lift the lid with the underside away from you so that the steam coming out of the canner does not burn your face.

Process Times for Crushed Tomatoes in a Weighted-Gauge Pressure Canner*

Style of Pack	Jar Size	Process Time	Canner Gauge Pressure (PSI) at Altitudes of:	
			0–1,000 ft	Above 1,000 ft
Hot	Pints or Quarts	20 minutes	5 lbs	10 lbs
		15 minutes	10 lbs	15 lbs

*After the canner is completely depressurized, remove the weight from the vent port or open the petcock. Wait 10 minutes; then unfasten the lid and remove it carefully. Lift the lid with the underside away from you so that the steam coming out of the canner does not burn your face.

Process Times for Crushed Tomatoes in a Boiling-Water Canner*

Style of Pack	Jar Size	Process Time at Altitudes of:			
		0–1,000 ft	1,001–3,000 ft	3,001–6,000 ft	Above 6,000 ft
Hot	Pints	35 minutes	40 minutes	45 minutes	50 minutes
	Quarts	45 minutes	50 minutes	55 minutes	60 minutes

*After the process is complete, turn off the heat and remove the canner lid. Wait five minutes before removing jars.

Tomato Sauce

This plain tomato sauce can be spiced up before using in soups or in pink or red sauces. The thicker you want your sauce, the more tomatoes you'll need.

Quantity

For thin sauce:
- An average of 35 pounds is needed per canner load of seven quarts.
- An average of 21 pounds is needed per canner load of nine pints.
- A bushel weighs 53 pounds and yields 10 to 12 quarts of sauce—an average of five pounds per quart.

For thick sauce:
- An average of 46 pounds is needed per canner load of seven quarts.
- An average of 28 pounds is needed per canner load of nine pints.
- A bushel weighs 53 pounds and yields seven to nine quarts of sauce—an average of 6½ pounds per quart.

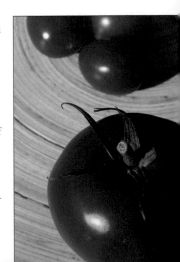

Directions

1. Prepare and press as for making tomato juice (see page 109). Simmer in a large saucepan until sauce reaches desired consistency. Boil until volume is reduced by about one-third for thin sauce, or by one-half for thick sauce.
2. Add bottled lemon juice or citric acid to jars. Add 1 teaspoon of salt per quart to the jars, if desired. Fill jars, leaving ¼-inch headspace. Adjust lids and process.

Process Times for Tomato Sauce in a Boiling-Water Canner*

Style of Pack	Jar Size	Process Time at Altitudes of:			
		0–1,000 ft	1,001–3,000 ft	3,001–6,000 ft	Above 6,000 ft
Hot	Pints	35 minutes	40 minutes	45 minutes	50 minutes
	Quarts	40 minutes	45 minutes	50 minutes	55 minutes

*After the process is complete, turn off the heat and remove the canner lid. Wait five minutes before removing jars.

Process Times for Tomato Sauce in a Dial-Gauge Pressure Canner*

Style of Pack	Jar Size	Process Time	Canner Gauge Pressure (PSI) at Altitudes of:			
			0–2,000 ft	2,001–4,000 ft	4,001–6,000 ft	6,001–8,000 ft
Hot	Pints or Quarts	20 minutes	6 lbs	7 lbs	8 lbs	9 lbs
		15 minutes	11 lbs	12 lbs	13 lbs	14 lbs

*After the canner is completely depressurized, remove the weight from the vent port or open the petcock. Wait 10 minutes; then unfasten the lid and remove it carefully. Lift the lid with the underside away from you so that the steam coming out of the canner does not burn your face.

Process Times for Tomato Sauce in a Weighted-Gauge Pressure Canner*

Style of Pack	Jar Size	Process Time	Canner Gauge Pressure (PSI) at Altitudes of:	
			0–1,000 ft	Above 1,000 ft
Hot	Pints or Quarts	20 minutes	5 lbs	10 lbs
		15 minutes	10 lbs	15 lbs

*After the canner is completely depressurized, remove the weight from the vent port or open the petcock. Wait 10 minutes; then unfasten the lid and remove it carefully. Lift the lid with the underside away from you so that the steam coming out of the canner does not burn your face.

Tomatoes, Whole or Halved, Packed in Water

Whole or halved tomatoes are used for scalloped tomatoes, savory pies (baked in a pastry crust with parmesan cheese, mayonnaise, and seasonings), or stewed tomatoes.

Quantity

- An average of 21 pounds is needed per canner load of seven quarts.
- An average of 13 pounds is needed per canner load of nine pints.
- A bushel weighs 53 pounds and yields 15 to 21 quarts—an average of three pounds per quart.

Directions

1. Wash tomatoes. Dip in boiling water for 30 to 60 seconds or until skins split; then dip in cold water. Slip off skins and remove cores. Leave whole or halve.
2. Add bottled lemon juice or citric acid to jars. Add 1 teaspoon of salt per quart to the jars, if desired. For hot pack products, add enough water to cover the tomatoes and boil them gently for 5 minutes.
3. Fill jars with hot tomatoes or with raw peeled tomatoes. Add the hot cooking liquid to the hot pack, or hot water for raw pack to cover, leaving ½-inch headspace. Adjust lids and process.

Process Times for Water-Packed Whole Tomatoes in a Boiling-Water Canner*

Style of Pack	Jar Size	Process Time at Altitudes of:			
		0–1,000 ft	1,001–3,000 ft	3,001–6,000 ft	Above 6,000 ft
Hot or Raw	Pints	40 minutes	45 minutes	50 minutes	55 minutes
	Quarts	45 minutes	50 minutes	55 minutes	60 minutes

*After the process is complete, turn off the heat and remove the canner lid. Wait five minutes before removing jars.

Process Times for Water-Packed Whole Tomatoes in a Dial-Gauge Pressure Canner*

Style of Pack	Jar Size	Process Time	Canner Gauge Pressure (PSI) at Altitudes of:			
			0–2,000 ft	2,001–4,000 ft	4,001–6,000 ft	6,001–8,000 ft
Hot or Raw	Pints or Quarts	15 minutes	6 lbs	7 lbs	8 lbs	9 lbs
		10 minutes	11 lbs	12 lbs	13 lbs	14 lbs

*After the canner is completely depressurized, remove the weight from the vent port or open the petcock. Wait 10 minutes; then unfasten the lid and remove it carefully. Lift the lid with the underside away from you so that the steam coming out of the canner does not burn your face.

Process Times for Water-Packed Whole Tomatoes in a Weighted-Gauge Pressure Canner*

Style of Pack	Jar Size	Process Time	Canner Gauge Pressure (PSI) at Altitudes of:	
			0–1,000 ft	Above 1,000 ft
Hot or Raw	Pints or Quarts	15 minutes	5 lbs	10 lbs
		10 minutes	10 lbs	15 lbs

*After the canner is completely depressurized, remove the weight from the vent port or open the petcock. Wait 10 minutes; then unfasten the lid and remove it carefully. Lift the lid with the underside away from you so that the steam coming out of the canner does not burn your face.

Spaghetti Sauce without Meat

Homemade spaghetti sauce is like a completely different food than store-bought varieties—it tastes fresher, is more flavorful, and is far more nutritious. Adjust spices to taste, but do not increase proportions of onions, peppers, or mushrooms. This recipe yields about nine pints.

Ingredients
30 lbs tomatoes
1 cup chopped onions
5 cloves garlic, minced
1 cup chopped celery or green pepper
1 lb fresh mushrooms, sliced (optional)
4½ tsp salt
2 tbsp oregano
4 tbsp minced parsley
2 tsp black pepper
¼ cup brown sugar
¼ cup vegetable oil

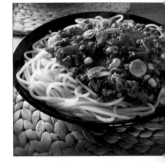

Directions
1. Wash tomatoes and dip in boiling water for 30 to 60 seconds or until skins split. Dip in cold water and slip off skins. Remove cores and quarter tomatoes. Boil 20 minutes, uncovered, in large saucepan. Put through food mill or sieve.
2. Sauté onions, garlic, celery, or peppers, and mushrooms (if desired) in vegetable oil until tender. Combine sautéed vegetables and tomatoes and add spices, salt, and sugar. Bring to a boil.
3. Simmer uncovered, until thick enough for serving. Stir frequently to avoid burning. Fill jars, leaving 1-inch headspace. Adjust lids and process.

Process Times for Spaghetti Sauce without Meat in a Dial-Gauge Pressure Canner*

Style of Pack	Jar Size	Process Time	Canner Gauge Pressure (PSI) at Altitudes of:			
			0–2,000 ft	2,001–4,000 ft	4,001–6,000 ft	6,001–8,000 ft
Hot	Pints	20 minutes	11 lbs	12 lbs	13 lbs	14 lbs
	Quarts	25 minutes	11 lbs	12 lbs	13 lbs	14 lbs

*After the canner is completely depressurized, remove the weight from the vent port or open the petcock. Wait 10 minutes; then unfasten the lid and remove it carefully. Lift the lid with the underside away from you so that the steam coming out of the canner does not burn your face.

Process Times for Spaghetti Sauce without Meat in a Weighted-Gauge Pressure Canner*

Style of Pack	Jar Size	Process Time	Canner Gauge Pressure (PSI) at Altitudes of:	
			0–1,000 ft	Above 1,000 ft
Hot	Pints	20 minutes	10 lbs	15 lbs
	Quarts	25 minutes	10 lbs	15 lbs

*After the canner is completely depressurized, remove the weight from the vent port or open the petcock. Wait 10 minutes; then unfasten the lid and remove it carefully. Lift the lid with the underside away from you so that the steam coming out of the canner does not burn your face.

Tomato Ketchup

Ketchup forms the base of several condiments, including Thousand Island dressing, fry sauce, and barbecue sauce. And, of course, it's an American favorite in its own right. This recipe yields six to seven pints.

Ingredients
24 lbs ripe tomatoes
3 cups chopped onions
¾ tsp ground red pepper (cayenne)
4 tsp whole cloves
3 sticks cinnamon, crushed
1-½ tsp whole allspice
3 tbsp celery seeds
3 cups cider vinegar (5 percent acetic acid)
1-½ cups sugar
¼ cup salt

Directions
1. Wash tomatoes. Dip in boiling water for 30 to 60 seconds or until skins split. Dip in cold water. Slip off skins and remove cores. Quarter tomatoes into 4-gallon stockpot or a large kettle. Add onions and red pepper. Bring to boil and simmer 20 minutes, uncovered.
2. Combine remaining spices in a spice bag and add to vinegar in a 2-quart saucepan. Bring to boil. Turn off heat and let stand until tomato mixture has been cooked 20 minutes. Then, remove spice bag and combine vinegar and tomato mixture. Boil about 30 minutes.
3. Put boiled mixture through a food mill or sieve. Return to pot. Add sugar and salt, boil gently, and stir frequently until volume is reduced by one-half or until mixture rounds up on spoon without separation. Fill pint jars, leaving ⅛-inch headspace. Adjust lids and process.

Process Times for Tomato Ketchup in a Boiling-Water Canner*

Style of Pack	Jar Size	Process Time at Altitudes of:		
		0–1,000 ft	1,001–6,000 ft	Above 6,000 ft
Hot	Pints	15 minutes	20 minutes	25 minutes

*After the process is complete, turn off the heat and remove the canner lid. Wait five minutes before removing jars.

Chile Salsa (Hot Tomato-Pepper Sauce)

For fantastic nachos, cover corn chips with chile salsa, add shredded Monterey jack or cheddar cheese, bake under broiler for about five minutes, and serve with guacamole and sour cream. Be sure to wear rubber gloves while handling chiles or wash hands thoroughly with soap and water before touching your face. This recipe yields six to eight pints.

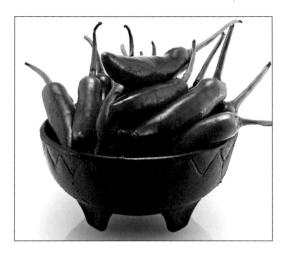

Ingredients
5 lbs tomatoes
2 lbs chile peppers
1 lb onions
1 cup vinegar (5 percent)
3 tsp salt
½ tsp pepper

Directions
1. Wash and dry chiles. Slit each pepper on its side to allow steam to escape. Peel peppers using one of the following methods:

Oven or broiler method:
Place chiles in oven (400°F) or broiler for 6 to 8 minutes until skins blister. Cool and slip off skins.

Range-top method:
Cover hot burner, either gas or electric, with heavy wire mesh. Place chiles on burner for several minutes until skins blister. Allow peppers to cool. Place in a pan and cover with a damp cloth. This will make peeling the peppers easier. After several minutes, peel each pepper.

2. Discard seeds and chop peppers. Wash tomatoes and dip in boiling water for 30 to 60 seconds or until skins split. Dip in cold water, slip off skins, and remove cores.
3. Coarsely chop tomatoes and combine chopped peppers, onions, and remaining ingredients in a large saucepan. Heat to boil, and simmer 10 minutes. Fill jars, leaving ½-inch headspace. Adjust lids and process.

Process Times for Chile Salsa in a Boiling-Water Canner*

Style of Pack	Jar Size	Process Time at Altitudes of:		
		0–1,000 ft	1,001–6,000 ft	Above 6,000 ft
Hot	Pints	15 minutes	20 minutes	25 minutes

*After the process is complete, turn off the heat and remove the canner lid. Wait five minutes before removing jars.

Drying and Freezing

Drying

Drying fruits, vegetables, herbs, and even meat is a great way to preserve foods for longer-term storage, especially if your pantry or freezer space is limited. Dried foods take up much less space than their fresh, frozen, or canned counterparts. Drying requires relatively little preparation time and is simple enough that kids will enjoy helping. Drying with a food dehydrator will ensure the fastest, safest, and best-quality results. However, you can also dry produce in the sunshine, in your oven, or strung up over a woodstove.

For more information on food drying, check out *So Easy to Preserve, 5th ed.* from the Cooperative Extension Service, the University of Georgia. Much of the information that follows is adapted from this excellent source.

Drying with a Food Dehydrator

Food dehydrators use electricity to produce heat and have a fan and vents for air circulation. Dehydrators are efficiently designed to dry foods fast at around 140°F. Look for food dehydrators in discount department stores, mail-order catalogs, the small appliance section of a department store, natural food stores, and seed or garden supply catalogs. Costs vary depending on features. Some models are expandable and additional trays can be purchased later. Twelve square feet of drying space dries about a half-bushel of produce.

Dehydrator Features to Look For

- Double-wall construction of metal or high-grade plastic. Wood is not recommended, because it is a fire hazard and is difficult to clean.
- Enclosed heating elements
- Countertop design
- An enclosed thermostat from 85 to 160°F
- Fan or blower

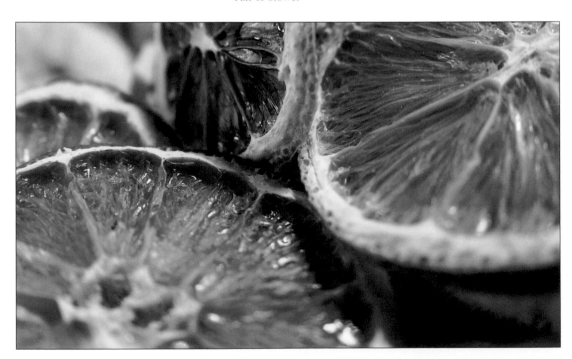

- Four to 10 open mesh trays made of sturdy, light-weight plastic for easy washing
- Underwriters Laboratory (UL) seal of approval
- A one-year guarantee
- Convenient service
- A dial for regulating temperature
- A timer. Often the completed drying time may occur during the night, and a timer turns the dehydrator off to prevent scorching.

Types of Dehydrators

There are two basic designs for dehydrators. One has horizontal air flow and the other has vertical air flow. In units with horizontal flow, the heating element and fan are located on the side of the unit. The major advantages of horizontal flow are: it reduces flavor mixture so several different foods can be dried at one time; all trays receive equal heat penetration; and juices or liquids do not drip down into the heating element. Vertical air flow dehydrators have the heating element and fan located at the base. If different foods are dried, flavors can mix and liquids can drip into the heating element.

Fruit Drying Procedures

Apples—Select mature, firm apples. Wash well. Pare, if desired, and core. Cut in rings or slices ⅛ to ¼ inch thick or cut in quarters or eighths. Soak in ascorbic acid, vinegar, or lemon juice for 10 minutes. Remove from solution and drain well. Arrange in single layer on trays, pit side up. Dry until soft, pliable, and leathery; there should be no moist area in center when cut.

Apricots—Select firm, fully ripe fruit. Wash well. Cut in half and remove pit. Do not peel. Soak in ascorbic acid, vinegar, or lemon juice for 10 minutes. Remove

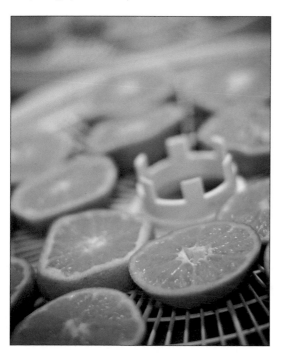

from solution and drain well. Arrange in single layer on trays, pit side up with cavity popped up to expose more flesh to the air. Dry until soft, pliable, and leathery; there should be no moist area in center when cut.

Bananas—Select firm, ripe fruit. Peel. Cut in ⅛-inch slices. Soak in ascorbic acid, vinegar, or lemon juice for 10 minutes. Remove and drain well. Arrange in single layer on trays. Dry until tough and leathery.

Berries—Select firm, ripe fruit. Wash well. Leave whole or cut in half. Dip in boiling water 30 seconds to crack skins. Arrange on drying trays not more than two berries deep. Dry until hard and berries rattle when shaken on trays.

Cherries—Select fully ripe fruit. Wash well. Remove stems and pits. Dip whole cherries in boiling water 30 seconds to crack skins. Arrange in single layer on trays. Dry until tough, leathery, and slightly sticky.

Citrus peel—Select thick-skinned oranges with no signs of mold or decay and no color added to skin. Scrub oranges well with brush under cool running water. Thinly peel outer 1/16 to ⅛ inch of the peel; avoid white bitter part. Soak in ascorbic acid, vinegar, or lemon juice for 10 minutes. Remove from solution and drain well. Arrange in single layers on trays. Dry at 130°F for 1 to 2 hours, then at 120°F until crisp.

Figs—Select fully ripe fruit. Wash or clean well with damp towel. Peel dark-skinned varieties if desired. Leave whole if small or partly dried on tree; cut large figs in halves or slices. If drying whole figs, crack skins by dipping in boiling water for 30 seconds. For cut figs, soak in ascorbic acid, vinegar, or lemon juice for 10 minutes. Remove and drain well. Arrange in single layers on trays. Dry until leathery and pliable.

Grapes and black currants—Select seedless varieties. Wash, sort, and remove stems. Cut in half or leave whole. If drying whole, crack skins by dipping in boiling water for 30 seconds. If halved, dip in ascorbic acid or other antimicrobial solution for 10 minutes. Remove and drain well. Dry until pliable and leathery with no moist center.

Melons—Select mature, firm fruits that are heavy for their size; cantaloupe dries better than watermelon. Scrub outer surface well with brush under cool running water. Remove outer skin, any fibrous tissue, and seeds. Cut into ¼- to ½-inch-thick slices. Soak in ascorbic acid, vinegar, or lemon juice for 10 minutes. Remove and drain well. Arrange in single layer on trays. Dry until leathery and pliable with no pockets of moisture.

Nectarines and peaches—Select ripe, firm fruit. Wash and peel. Cut in half and remove pit. Cut in quarters or slices if desired. Soak in ascorbic acid, vinegar, or lemon juice for 10 minutes. Remove and drain well. Arrange in single layer on trays, pit side up. Turn halves over when visible juice disappears. Dry until leathery and somewhat pliable.

Pears—Select ripe, firm fruit. Bartlett variety is recommended. Wash fruit well. Pare, if desired. Cut in half lengthwise and core. Cut in quarters, eighths, or slices ⅛ to ¼ inch thick. Soak in ascorbic acid, vinegar, or lemon juice for 10 minutes. Remove and drain. Arrange in single layer on trays, pit side up. Dry until springy and suede-like with no pockets of moisture.

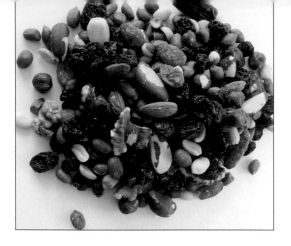

Plums and prunes—Wash well. Leave whole if small; cut large fruit into halves (pit removed) or slices. If left whole, crack skins in boiling water 1 to 2 minutes. If cut in half, dip in ascorbic acid or other antimicrobial solution for 10 minutes. Remove and drain. Arrange in single layer on trays, pit side up, cavity popped out. Dry until pliable and leathery; in whole prunes, pit should not slip when squeezed.

Fruit Leathers

Fruit leathers are a tasty and nutritious alternative to store-bought candies that are full of artificial sweeteners and preservatives. Blend the leftover fruit pulp from making jelly or use fresh, frozen, or drained canned fruit. Ripe or slightly overripe fruit works best.

Chances are the fruit leather will get eaten before it makes it into the cupboard, but it can keep up to one month at room temperature. For storage up to one year, place tightly wrapped rolls in the freezer.

Ingredients
2 cups fruit
2 tsp lemon juice or ⅛ tsp ascorbic acid (optional)
¼ to ½ cup sugar, corn syrup, or honey (optional)

Directions
1. Wash fresh fruit or berries in cool water. Remove peel, seeds, and stem.
2. Cut fruit into chunks. Use 2 cups of fruit for each 13 x 15-inch inch fruit leather. Purée fruit until smooth.
3. Add 2 teaspoons of lemon juice or ⅛ teaspoon ascorbic acid (375 mg) for each 2 cups light-colored fruit to prevent darkening.
4. Optional: To sweeten, add corn syrup, honey, or sugar. Corn syrup or honey is best for longer storage because these sweeteners prevent crystals. Sugar is fine for immediate use or short storage. Use ¼ to ½ cup sugar, corn syrup, or honey for each 2 cups of fruit. Avoid aspartame sweeteners as they may lose sweetness during drying.
5. Pour the leather. Fruit leathers can be poured into a single large sheet (13 x 15 inches) or into several smaller sizes. Spread purée evenly, about ⅛ inch thick, onto drying tray. Avoid pouring purée too close to the edge of the cookie sheet.
6. Dry the leather. Dry fruit leathers at 140°F. Leather dries from the outside edge toward the center.

Larger fruit leathers take longer to dry. Approximate drying times are 6 to 8 hours in a dehydrator, up to 18 hours in an oven, and 1 to 2 days in the sun. Test for dryness by touching center of leather; no indentation should be evident. While warm, peel from plastic and roll, allow to cool, and rewrap the roll in plastic. Cookie cutters can be used to cut out shapes that children will enjoy. Roll, and wrap in plastic.

Spices, Flavors, and Garnishes

To add interest to your fruit leathers, include spices, flavorings, or garnishes.

- **Spices to try**—Allspice, cinnamon, cloves, coriander, ginger, mace, mint, nutmeg, or pumpkin pie spice. Use sparingly; start with ⅛ teaspoon for each 2 cups of purée.
- **Flavorings to try**—Almond extract, lemon juice, lemon peel, lime juice, lime peel, orange extract, orange juice, orange peel, or vanilla extract. Use sparingly; try ⅛ to ¼ teaspoon for each 2 cups of purée.
- **Delicious additions to try**—Shredded coconut, chopped dates, other dried chopped fruits, granola, miniature marshmallows, chopped nuts, chopped raisins, poppy seeds, sesame seeds, or sunflower seeds.
- **Fillings to try**—Melted chocolate, softened cream cheese, cheese spreads, jam, preserves, marmalade, marshmallow cream, or peanut butter. Spread one or more of these on the leather after it is dried and then roll. Store in refrigerator.

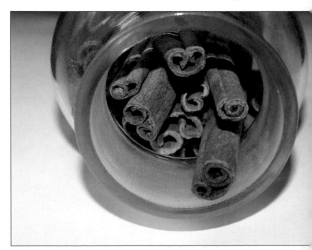

Vegetable Leathers

Pumpkin, mixed vegetables, and tomatoes make great leathers. Just purée cooked vegetables, strain, spread on a tray lined with plastic wrap, and dry. Spices can be added for flavoring.

Mixed-Vegetable Leather

2 cups cored, cut-up tomatoes
1 small onion, chopped
¼ cup chopped celery
Salt to taste
Combine all ingredients in a covered saucepan and cook over low heat 15 to 20 minutes. Purée or force through a sieve or colander. Return to saucepan and cook until thickened. Spread on a cookie sheet or tray lined with plastic wrap. Dry at 140°F.

Pumpkin Leather

2 cups canned pumpkin or 2 cups fresh pumpkin, cooked and puréed
½ cup honey
¼ tsp cinnamon
⅛ tsp nutmeg
⅛ tsp powdered cloves
Blend ingredients well. Spread on tray or cookie sheet lined with plastic wrap. Dry at 140°F.

Tomato Leather

Core ripe tomatoes and cut into quarters. Cook over low heat in a covered saucepan, 15 to 20 minutes. Purée or force through a sieve or colander and pour into electric fry pan or shallow pan. Add salt to taste and cook over low heat until thickened. Spread on a cookie sheet or tray lined with plastic wrap. Dry at 140°F.

Vine Drying

One method of drying outdoors is vine drying. To dry beans (navy, kidney, butter, great northern, lima, lentils, and soybeans) leave bean pods on the vine in the garden until the beans inside rattle. When the vines and pods are dry and shriveled, pick the beans and shell them. No pretreatment is necessary. If beans are still moist, the drying process is not complete and the beans will mold if not more thoroughly dried. If needed, drying can be completed in the sun, an oven, or a dehydrator.

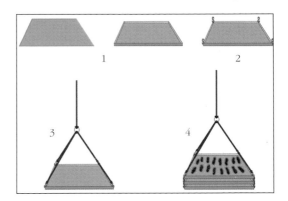

How to Make a Woodstove Food Dehydrator

1. Collect pliable wire mesh or screens (available at hardware stores) and use wire cutters to trim to squares 12 to 16 inches on each side. The trays should be of the same size and shape. Bend up the edges of each square to create a half-inch lip.
2. Attach one S hook from the hardware store or a large paperclip to each side of each square (four clips per tray) to attach the trays together.
3. Cut four equal lengths of chain or twine that will reach from the ceiling to the level of the top tray. Use a wire or metal loop to attach the four pieces together at the top and secure to a hook in the ceiling above the woodstove. Attach the chain or twine to the hooks on the top tray.
4. To use, fill trays with food to dry, starting with the top tray. Link trays together using the S hooks or strong paperclips. When the foods are dried, remove the entire stack and disassemble. Remove the dried food and store.

Herbs

Drying is the easiest method of preserving herbs. Simply expose the leaves, flowers, or seeds to warm, dry air. Leave the herbs in a well-ventilated area until the moisture evaporates. Sun drying is not recommended because the herbs can lose flavor and color.

The best time to harvest most herbs for drying is just before the flowers first open when they are in the bursting, bud stage. Gather the herbs in the early morning after the dew has evaporated to minimize wilting. Avoid bruising the leaves. They should not lie in the sun or unattended after harvesting. Rinse herbs in cool water and gently shake to remove excess moisture. Discard all bruised, soiled, or imperfect leaves and stems.

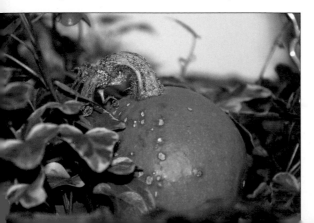

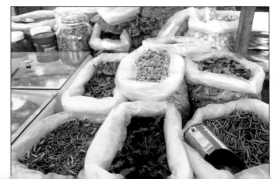

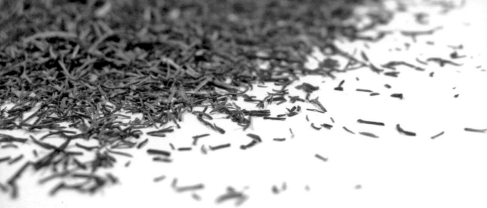

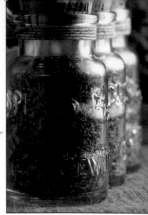

Dehydrator drying is another fast and easy way to dry high-quality herbs because temperature and air circulation can be controlled. Preheat dehydrator with the thermostat set to 95°F to 115°F. In areas with higher humidity, temperatures as high as 125°F may be needed. After rinsing under cool, running water and shaking to remove excess moisture, place the herbs in a single layer on dehydrator trays. Drying times may vary from one to four hours. Check periodically. Herbs are dry when they crumble, and stems break when bent. Check your dehydrator instruction booklet for specific details.

Less-tender herbs—The more sturdy herbs, such as rosemary, sage, thyme, summer savory, and parsley, are the easiest to dry without a dehydrator. Tie them into small bundles and hang them to air dry. Air drying outdoors is often possible; however, better color and flavor retention usually results from drying indoors.

Tender-leaf herbs—Basil, oregano, tarragon, lemon balm, and the mints have a high moisture content and will mold if not dried quickly. Try hanging the tender-leaf herbs or those with seeds inside paper bags to dry. Tear or punch holes in the sides of the bag. Suspend a small bunch (large amounts will mold) of herbs in a bag and close the top with a rubber band. Place where air currents will circulate through the bag. Any leaves and seeds that fall off will be caught in the bottom of the bag.

Another method, especially nice for mint, sage, or bay leaf, is to dry the leaves separately. In areas of high humidity, it will work better than air drying whole stems. Remove the best leaves from the stems. Lay the leaves on a paper towel, without allowing leaves to touch. Cover with another towel and layer of leaves. Five layers may

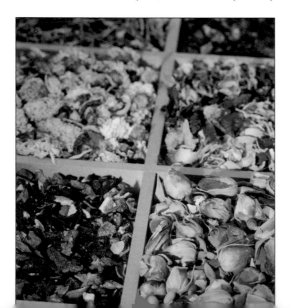

be dried at one time using this method. Dry in a very cool oven. The oven light of an electric range or the pilot light of a gas range furnishes enough heat for overnight drying. Leaves dry flat and retain a good color.

Microwave ovens are a fast way to dry herbs when only small quantities are to be prepared. Follow the directions that come with your microwave oven.

When the leaves are crispy, dry, and crumble easily between the fingers, they are ready to be packaged and stored. Dried leaves may be left whole and crumbled as used, or coarsely crumbled before storage. Husks can be removed from seeds by rubbing the seeds between the hands and blowing away the chaff. Place herbs in airtight containers and store in a cool, dry, dark area to protect color and fragrance.

Dried herbs are usually three to four times stronger than the fresh herbs. To substitute dried herbs in a recipe that calls for fresh herbs, use ¼ to ⅓ of the amount listed in the recipe.

Jerky

Jerky is great for hiking or camping because it supplies protein in a very lightweight form—not to mention the fact that it can be very tasty. A pound of meat or poultry weighs about four ounces after being made into jerky. In addition, because most of the moisture is removed, it can be stored for one to two months without refrigeration.

Jerky has been around since the ancient Egyptians began drying animal meat that was too big to eat all at once. Native Americans mixed ground dried meat with dried fruit or suet to make pemmican. *Biltong* is dried meat or game used in many African countries. The English word *jerky* came from the Spanish word *charque*, which means "dried, salted meat."

Drying is the world's oldest and most common method of food preservation. Enzymes require moisture in order to react with food. By removing the moisture, you prevent this biological action.

Jerky can be made from ground meat, which is often less expensive than strips of meat and allows you to combine different kinds of meat if desired. You can also make it into any shape you want! As with strips of meat, an internal temperature of 160°F is necessary to eliminate disease-causing bacteria such as *E. coli*, if present.

Food Safety

The USDA Meat and Poultry Hotline's current recommendation for making jerky safely is to heat meat to 160°F and poultry to 165°F before the dehydrating process.

This ensures that any bacteria present are destroyed by heat. If your food dehydrator doesn't heat up to 160°F, it's important to cook meat slightly in the oven or by steaming before drying. After heating, maintain a constant dehydrator temperature of 130°F to 140°F during the drying process.

According to the USDA, you should always:

- Wash hands thoroughly with soap and water before and after working with meat products.
- Use clean equipment and utensils.
- Keep meat and poultry refrigerated at 40°F or slightly below; use or freeze ground beef and poultry within two days, and whole red meats within three to five days.
- Defrost frozen meat in the refrigerator, not on the kitchen counter.
- Marinate meat in the refrigerator. Don't save marinade to re-use. Marinades are used to tenderize and flavor the jerky before dehydrating it.
- If your food dehydrator doesn't heat up to 160°F (or 165°F for poultry), steam or roast meat before dehydrating it.
- Dry meats in a food dehydrator that has an adjustable temperature dial and will maintain a temperature of at least 130°F to 140°F throughout the drying process.

Preparing the Meat

1. Partially freeze meat to make slicing easier. Slice meat across the grain ⅛ to ¼ inch thick. Trim and discard all fat, gristle, and membranes or connective tissue.
2. Marinate the meat in a combination of oil, salt, spices, vinegar, lemon juice, teriyaki, soy sauce, beer, or wine.

Marinated Jerky

¼ cup soy sauce
1 tbsp Worcestershire sauce
1 tsp brown sugar
¼ tsp black pepper
½ tsp fresh ginger, finely grated
1 tsp salt
1½ to 2 lbs of lean meat strips (beef, pork, or venison)

1. Combine all ingredients except the strips, and blend. Add meat, stir, cover, and refrigerate at least one hour.
2. If your food dehydrator doesn't heat up to 160°F, bring strips and marinade to a boil and cook for 5 minutes.

3. Drain meat in a colander and absorb extra moisture with clean, absorbent paper towels. Arrange strips in a single layer on dehydrator trays, or on cake racks placed on baking sheets for oven drying.
4. Place the racks in a dehydrator or oven preheated to 140°F, or 160°F if the meat wasn't precooked. Dry until a test piece cracks but does not break when it is bent (10 to 24 hours for samples not heated in marinade, 3 to 6 hours for preheated meat). Use a paper towel to pat off any excess oil from strips, and pack in sealed jars, plastic bags, or plastic containers.

Freezing Foods

Many foods preserve well in the freezer and can make preparing meals easy when you are short on time. If you make a big pot of soup, serve it for dinner, put a small container in the refrigerator for lunch the next day, and then stick the rest in the freezer. A few weeks later, you'll be ready to eat it again and it will only take a few minutes to thaw out and serve. Many fruits also freeze well and are perfect for use in smoothies and desserts, or served with yogurt for breakfast or dessert. Vegetables frozen shortly after harvesting keep many of the nutrients found in fresh vegetables and will taste delicious when cooked.

Containers for Freezing

The best packaging materials for freezing include rigid containers such as jars, bottles, or Tupperware, and freezer bags or aluminum foil. Sturdy containers with rigid sides are especially good for liquids such as soup or juice because they make the frozen contents much easier to get out. They are also generally reusable and make it easier to stack foods in the refrigerator. When using rigid containers, be sure to leave headspace so that the container won't explode when the contents expand with freezing. Covers for rigid containers should fit tightly. If they do not, reinforce the seal with freezer tape. Freezer tape is specially designed to stick at freezing temperatures. Freezer bags or aluminum foil are good for meats, breads and baked goods, or fruits and vegetables that don't contain much liquid. Be sure to remove as much air as possible from bags before closing.

Headspace to Allow Between Packed Food and Closure

Headspace is the amount of empty air left between the food and the lid. Headspace is necessary because foods expand when frozen.

Type of Pack	Container with Wide Opening		Container with Narrow Opening	
	Pint	Quart	Pint	Quart
Liquid pack*	½ inch	1 inch	3/4 inch	1½ inch
Dry pack**	½ inch	½ inch	½ inch	½ inch
Juices	½ inch	1 inch	1½ inch	1½ inch

*Fruit packed in juice, sugar syrup, or water; crushed or puréed fruit
**Fruit or vegetable packed without added sugar or liquid

Foods That Do Not Freeze Well

Food	Usual Use	Condition After Thawing
Cabbage*, celery, cress, cucumbers*, endive, lettuce, parsley, radishes	As raw salad	Limp, waterlogged; quickly develops oxidized color, aroma, and flavor
Irish potatoes, baked or boiled	In soups, salads, sauces or with butter	Soft, crumbly, waterlogged, mealy
Cooked macaroni, spaghetti, or rice	When frozen alone for later use	Mushy, tastes warmed over
Egg whites, cooked	In salads, creamed foods, sandwiches, sauces, gravy, or desserts	Soft, tough, rubbery, spongy
Meringue	In desserts	Soft, tough, rubbery, spongy
Icings made from egg whites	Cakes, cookies	Frothy, weeps
Cream or custard fillings	Pies, baked goods	Separates, watery, lumpy
Milk sauces	For casseroles or gravies	May curdle or separate
Sour cream	As topping, in salads	Separates, watery
Cheese or crumb toppings	On casseroles	Soggy
Mayonnaise or salad dressing	On sandwiches (not in salads)	Separates
Gelatin	In salads or desserts	Weeps
Fruit jelly	Sandwiches	May soak bread
Fried foods	All except French fried potatoes and onion rings	Lose crispness, become soggy

* Cucumbers and cabbage can be frozen as marinated products such as "freezer slaw" or "freezer pickles." These do not have the same texture as regular slaw or pickles.

Effect of Freezing on Spices and Seasonings

- Pepper, cloves, garlic, green pepper, imitation vanilla, and some herbs tend to get strong and bitter.
- Onion and paprika change flavor during freezing.
- Celery seasonings become stronger.
- Curry develops a musty off-flavor.
- Salt loses flavor and has the tendency to increase rancidity of any item containing fat.
- When using seasonings and spices, season lightly before freezing, and add additional seasonings when reheating or serving.

How to Freeze Vegetables

Because many vegetables contain enzymes that will cause them to lose color when frozen, you may want to blanche your vegetables before putting them in the

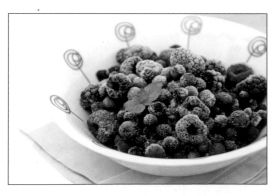

freezer. To do this, first wash the vegetables thoroughly, peel if desired, and chop them into bite-size pieces. Then pour them into boiling water for a couple of minutes (or cook longer for very dense vegetables, such as beets), drain, and immediately dunk the vegetables in ice water to stop them from cooking further. Use a paper towel or cloth to absorb excess water from the vegetables, and then pack in resealable airtight bags or plastic containers.

Blanching Times for Vegetables

Artichokes	3–6 minutes
Asparagus	2–3 minutes
Beans	2–3 minutes
Beets	30-40 minutes
Broccoli	3 minutes
Brussels sprouts	4–5 minutes
Cabbage	3–4 minutes
Carrots	2–5 minutes
Cauliflower	6 minutes
Celery	3 minutes
Corn (off the cob)	2–3 minutes
Eggplant	4 minutes
Okra	3–4 minutes
Peas	1–2 minutes
Peppers	2–3 minutes
Squash	2–3 minutes
Turnips or Parsnips	2 minutes

How to Freeze Fruits

Many fruits freeze easily and are perfect for use in baking, smoothies, or sauces. Wash, peel, and core fruit before freezing. To easily peel peaches, nectarines, or apricots, dip them in boiling water for 15 to 20 seconds to loosen the skins. Then chill and remove the skins and stones.

Berries should be frozen immediately after harvesting and can be frozen in a single layer on a paper towel--lined tray or cookie sheet to keep them from clumping together. Allow them to freeze until hard (about 3 hours) and then pour them into a resealable plastic bag for long-term storage.

Some fruits have a tendency to turn brown when frozen. To prevent this, you can add ascorbic acid (crush a vitamin C in a little water), citrus juice, plain sugar, or a sweet syrup (1 part sugar and 2 parts water) to the fruit before freezing. Apples, pears, and bananas are best frozen with ascorbic acid or citrus juice, while berries, peaches, nectarines, apricots, pineapple, melons, and berries are better frozen with a sugary syrup.

How to Freeze Meat

Be sure your meat is fresh before freezing. Trim off excess fats and remove bones, if desired. Separate the meat into portions that will be easy to use when preparing meals and wrap in foil or place in resealable plastic bags or plastic containers. Refer to the chart to determine how long your meat will last at best quality in your freezer.

Meat	Months
Bacon and sausage	1 to 2
Ham, hotdogs, and lunchmeats	1 to 2
Meat, uncooked roasts	4 to 12
Meat, uncooked steaks or chops	4 to 12
Meat, uncooked ground	3 to 4
Meat, cooked	2 to 3
Poultry, uncooked whole	12
Poultry, uncooked parts	9
Poultry, uncooked giblets	3 to 4
Poultry, cooked	4
Wild game, uncooked	8 to 12

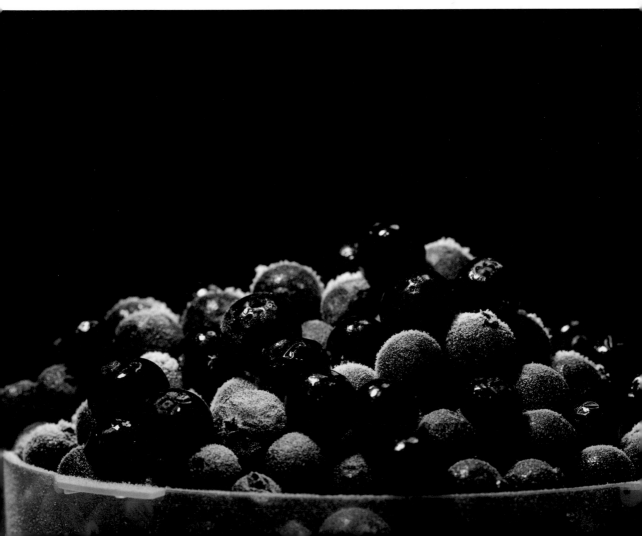

Edible Wild Plants and Mushrooms

Wild Vegetables, Fruits, and Nuts

Agave

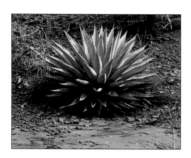

Description: Agave plants have large clusters of thick leaves that grow around one stalk. They grow close to the ground and only flower once before dying.

Location: Agave like dry, open areas and are found in the deserts of the American west.

Edible Parts and Preparing: Only agave flowers and buds are edible. Boil these before consuming. The juice can be collected from the flower stalk for drinking.

Other Uses: Most agave plants have thick needles on the tips of their leaves that can be used for sewing.

Asparagus

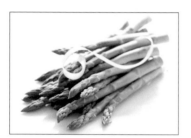

Description: When first growing, asparagus looks like a collection of green fingers. Once mature, the plant has fernlike foliage and red berries (which are toxic if eaten). The flowers are small and green and several species have sharp, thornlike projections.

Location: It can be found growing wild in fields and along fences. Asparagus is found in temperate areas in the United States.

Edible Parts and Preparing: It is best to eat the young stems, before any leaves grow. Steam or boil them for 10 to 15 minutes before consuming. The roots are a good source of starch, but don't eat any part of the plant raw, as it could cause nausea or diarrhea.

Beech

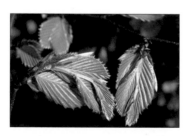

Description: Beech trees are large forest trees. They have smooth, light gray bark, very dark leaves, and clusters of prickly seedpods.

Location: Beech trees prefer to grow in moist, forested areas. These trees are found in the Temperate Zone in the eastern United States.

Edible Parts and Preparing: Eat mature beechnuts by breaking the thin shells with your fingers and removing the sweet, white kernel found inside. These nuts can also be used as a substitute for coffee by roasting them until the kernel turns hard and golden brown. Mash up the kernel and boil or steep in hot water.

Blackberry and Raspberry

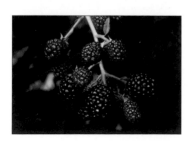

Description: These plants have prickly stems that grow upright and then arch back toward the ground. They have alternating leaves and grow red or black fruit.

Location: Blackberry and raspberry plants prefer to grow in wide, sunny areas near woods, lakes, and roads. They grow in temperate areas.

Edible Parts and Preparing: Both the fruits and peeled young shoots can be eaten. The leaves can be used to make tea.

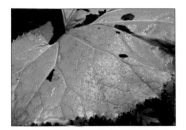

Burdock

Description: Burdock has wavy-edged, arrow-shaped leaves. Its flowers grow in burrlike clusters and are purple or pink. The roots are large and fleshy.

Location: This plant prefers to grow in open waste areas during the spring and summer. It can be found in the Temperate Zone in the north.

Edible Parts and Preparing: The tender leaves growing on the stalks can be eaten raw or cooked. The roots can be boiled or baked.

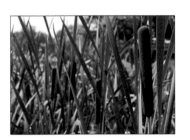

Cattail

Description: These plants are grasslike and have leaves shaped like straps. The male flowers grow above the female flowers; have abundant, bright yellow pollen; and die off quickly. The female flowers become the brown cattails.

Location: Cattails like to grow in full-sun areas near lakes, streams, rivers, and brackish water. They can be found all over the country.

Edible Parts and Preparing: The tender, young shoots can be eaten either raw or cooked. The rhizome (rootstalk) can be pounded and made into flour. When the cattail is immature, the female flower can be harvested, boiled, and eaten like corn on the cob.

Other Uses: The cottony seeds of the cattail plant are great for stuffing pillows. Burning dried cattails helps repel insects.

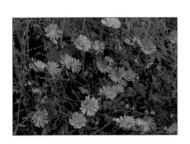

Chicory

Description: This is quite a tall plant, with clusters of leaves at the base of the stem and very few leaves on the stem itself. The flowers are sky blue in color and open only on sunny days. It produces a milky juice.

Location: Chicory grows in fields, waste areas, and alongside roads. It grows primarily as a weed all throughout the country.

Edible Parts and Preparing: The entire plant is edible. The young leaves can be eaten in a salad. The leaves and roots may also be boiled as you would regular vegetables. Roast the roots until they are dark brown, mash them up, and use them as a substitute for coffee.

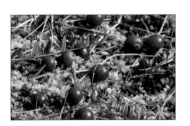

Cranberry

Description: The cranberry plant has tiny, alternating leaves. Its stems crawl along the ground and it produces red berry fruits.

Location: Cranberries only grow in open, sunny, wet areas. They thrive in the colder areas in the northern states.

Edible Parts and Preparing: The berries can be eaten raw, though they are best when cooked in a small amount of water, adding a little bit of sugar if desired.

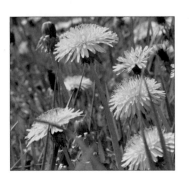

Dandelion

Description: These plants have jagged leaves and grow close to the ground. They have bright yellow flowers.

Location: Dandelions grow in almost any open, sunny space in the United States.

Edible Parts and Preparing: All parts of this plant are edible. The leaves can be eaten raw or cooked and the roots boiled. Roasted and ground roots can make a good substitute for coffee.

Other Uses: The white juice in the flower stem can be used as glue.

Elderberry

Description: This shrub has many stems containing opposite, compound leaves. Its flower is white, fragrant, and grows in large clusters. Its fruits are berry-shaped and are typically dark blue or black.

Location: Found in open, wet areas near rivers, ditches, and lakes, the elderberry grows mainly in the eastern states.

Edible Parts and Preparing: The flowers can be soaked in water for eight hours and then the liquid can be drunk. The fruit is also edible but don't eat any other parts of the plant—they are poisonous.

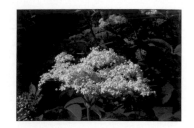

Hazelnut

Description: The nuts grow on bushes in very bristly husks.

Location: Hazelnut grows in dense thickets near streambeds and in open areas and can be found all over the United States.

Edible Parts and Preparing: In the autumn, the hazelnut ripens and can be cracked open and the kernel eaten. Eating dried nuts is also tasty.

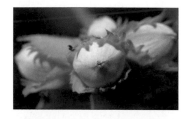

Juniper

Description: Also known as cedar, this shrub has very small, scaly leaves that are densely crowded on the branches. Berrylike cones on the plant are usually blue and are covered with a whitish wax.

Location: They grow in open, dry, sunny places throughout the country.

Edible Parts and Preparing: Both berries and twigs are edible. The berries can be consumed raw or the seeds may be roasted to make a substitute for coffee. Dried and crushed berries are good to season meat. Twigs can be made into tea.

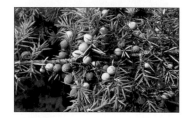

Lotus

Description: This plant has large, yellow flowers and leaves that float on or above the surface of the water. The lotus fruit has a distinct, flattened shape and possesses around 20 hard seeds.

Location: Found on fresh water in quiet areas, the lotus plant is native to North America.

Edible Parts and Preparing: All parts of the lotus plant are edible, raw or cooked. Bake or boil the fleshy parts that grow underwater and boil young leaves. The seeds are quite nutritious and can be eaten raw or they can be ground into flour.

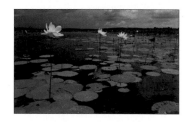

Marsh Marigold

Description: Marsh marigold has round, dark green leaves and a short stem. It also has bright yellow flowers.

Location: The plant can be found in bogs and lakes in the northeastern states.

Edible Parts and Preparing: All parts can be boiled and eaten. Do not consume any portion raw.

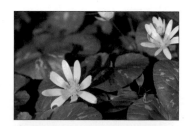

Mulberry

Description: The mulberry tree has alternate, lobed leaves with rough surfaces and blue or black seeded fruits.

Location: These trees are found in forested areas and near roadsides in temperate and tropical regions of the United States.

Edible Parts and Preparing: The fruit can be consumed either raw or cooked and it can also be dried. Make sure the fruit is ripe or it can cause hallucinations and extreme nausea.

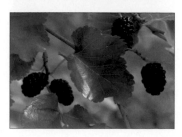

Nettle

Description: Nettle plants grow several feet high and have small flowers. The stems, leafstalks, and undersides of the leaves all contain fine, hairlike bristles that cause a stinging sensation on the skin.

Location: This plant grows in moist areas near streams or on the edges of forests. It can be found throughout the United States.

Edible Parts and Preparing: The young shoots and leaves are edible. To eat, boil the plant for 10 to 15 minutes.

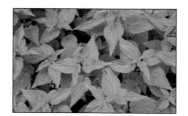

Oak

Description: These trees have alternating leaves and acorns. Red oaks have bristly leaves and smooth bark on the upper part of the tree and their acorns need two years to reach maturity. White oaks have leaves with no bristles and rough bark on the upper part of the tree. Their acorns only take one year to mature.

Location: Found in various locations and habitats throughout the country.

Edible Parts and Preparing: All parts of the tree are edible, but most are very bitter. Shell the acorns and soak them in water for one or two days to remove their tannic acid. Boil the acorns to eat or grind them into flour for baking.

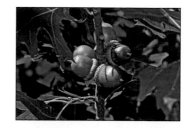

Palmetto Palm

Description: This is a tall tree with no branches and has a continual leaf base on the trunk. The leaves are large, simple, and lobed and it has dark blue or black fruits that contain a hard seed.

Location: This tree is found throughout the southeastern coast.

Edible Parts and Preparing: The palmetto palm fruit can be eaten raw. The seeds can also be ground into flour, and the heart of the palm is a nutritious source of food, but the top of the tree must be cut down in order to reach it.

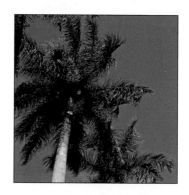

Persimmon

Description: The persimmon tree has alternating, elliptical leaves that are dark green in color, and inconspicuous flowers. It has orange fruits that are very sticky and contain many seeds.

Location: Growing on the margins of forests, it resides in the eastern part of the country.

Edible Parts and Preparing: The leaves provide a good source of vitamin C and can be dried and soaked in hot water to make tea. The fruit can be consumed either baked or raw and the seeds may be eaten once roasted.

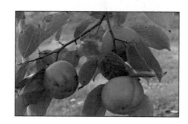

Pine

Description: Pine trees have needlelike leaves that are grouped into bundles of one to five needles. They have a very pungent, distinguishing odor.

Location: Pines grow best in sunny, open areas and are found all over the United States.

Edible Parts and Preparing: The seeds are completely edible and can be consumed either raw or cooked. Also, the young male cones can be boiled or baked and eaten. Peel the bark off of thin twigs and chew the juicy inner bark. The needles can be dried and brewed to make tea that's high in vitamin C.

Other Uses: Pine tree resin can be used to waterproof items. Collect the resin from the tree, put it in a container, heat it, and use it as glue or, when cool, rub it on items to waterproof them.

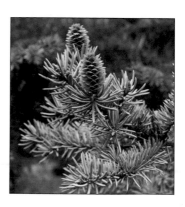

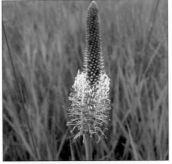

Plantain

Description: The broad-leafed plantain grows close to the ground and the flowers are situated on a spike that rises from the middle of the leaf cluster. The narrow-leaf species has leaves covered with hairs that form a rosette. The flowers are very small.

   Location: Plantains grow in lawns and along the side of the road in the northern Temperate Zone.

   Edible Parts and Preparing: Young, tender leaves can be eaten raw, and older leaves should be cooked before consumption. The seeds may also be eaten either raw or roasted. Tea can also be made by boiling 1 ounce of the plant leaves in a few cups of water.

Pokeweed

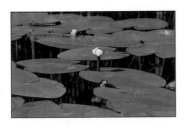

Description: A rather tall plant, pokeweed has elliptical leaves and produces many large clusters of purple fruits in the late spring.

   Location: Pokeweed grows in open and sunny areas in fields and along roadsides in the eastern United States.

   Edible Parts and Preparing: If cooked, the young leaves and stems are edible. Be sure to boil them twice and discard the water from the first boiling. The fruit is also edible if cooked. Never eat any part of this plant raw, as it is poisonous.

Prickly Pear Cactus

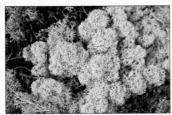

Description: This plant has flat, pad-like green stems and round, furry dots that contain sharp-pointed hairs.

   Location: Found in arid regions and in dry, sandy areas in wetter regions, it can be found throughout the United States.

   Edible Parts and Preparing: All parts of this plant are edible. To eat the fruit, peel it or crush it to make a juice. The seeds can be roasted and ground into flour.

Reindeer Moss

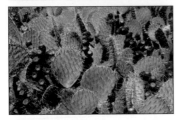

Description: This is a low plant that does not flower. However, it does produce bright red structures used for reproduction.

   Location: It grows in dry, open areas in much of the country.

   Edible Parts and Preparing: While having a crunchy, brittle texture, the whole plant can be eaten. To remove some of the bitterness, soak it in water and then dry and crush it, adding it to milk or other foods.

Sassafras

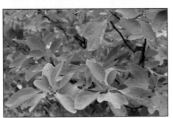

Description: This shrub has different leaves—some have one lobe, others two lobes, and others have none at all. The flowers are small and yellow and appear in the early spring. The plant has dark blue fruit.

   Location: Sassafras grows near roads and forests in sunny, open areas. It is common throughout the eastern states.

   Edible Parts and Preparing: The young twigs and leaves can be eaten either fresh or dried—add them to soups. Dig out the underground portion of the shrub, peel off the bark, and dry it. Boil it in water to make tea.

   Other Uses: Shredding the tender twigs will make a handy toothbrush.

Spatterdock

Description: The leaves of this plant are quite long and have a triangular notch at the base. Spatterdock has yellow flowers that become bottle-shaped fruits, which are green when ripe.

   Location: Found in fresh, shallow water throughout the country.

   Edible Parts and Preparing: All parts of the plant are edible and the fruits have brown seeds that can be roasted and ground into flour. The rootstock can be dug out of the mud, peeled, and boiled.

Strawberry

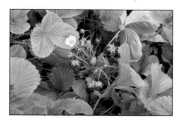

Description: This is a small plant with a three-leaved pattern. Small, white flowers appear in the springtime and the fruit is red and very fleshy.

   Location: These plants prefer sunny, open spaces, are commonly planted, and appear in the northern Temperate Zone.

   Edible Parts and Preparing: The fruit can be eaten raw, cooked, or dried. The plant leaves may also be eaten or dried to make tea.

Thistle

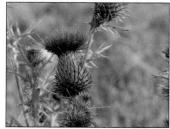

Description: This plant may grow very high and has long-pointed, prickly leaves.

   Location: Thistle grows in woods and fields all over the country.

   Edible Parts and Preparing: Peel the stalks, cut them into smaller sections, and boil them to consume. The root may be eaten raw or cooked.

Walnut

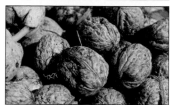

Description: Walnuts grow on large trees and have divided leaves. The walnut has a thick, outer husk that needs to be removed before getting to the hard, inner shell.

   Location: The black walnut tree is common in the eastern states.

   Edible Parts and Preparing: Nut kernels become ripe in the fall and the meat can be obtained by cracking the shell.

Water Lily

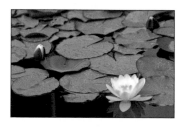

Description: With large, triangular leaves that float on water, these plants have fragrant flowers that are white or red. They also have thick rhizomes that grow in the mud.

   Location: Water lilies are found in many temperate areas.

   Edible Parts and Preparing: The flowers, seeds, and rhizomes can be eaten either raw or cooked. Peel the corky rind off of the rhizome and eat it raw or slice it thinly, dry it, and grind into flour. The seeds can also be made into flour after drying, parching, and grinding.

Wild Grapevine

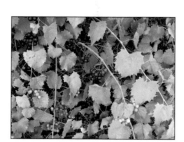

Description: This vine will climb on tendrils, and most of these plants produce deeply lobed leaves. The grapes grow in pyramidal bunches and are black-blue, amber, or white when ripe.

   Location: Climbing over other vegetation on the edges of forested areas, they can be found in the eastern and southwestern parts of the United States.

   Edible Parts and Preparing: Only the ripe grape can be eaten.

Wild Onion and Garlic

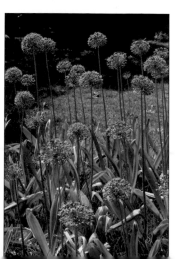

Description: These are recognized by their distinctive odors.

   Location: They are found in open areas that get lots of sun throughout temperate areas.

   Edible Parts and Preparing: The bulbs and young leaves are edible and can be consumed either raw or cooked.

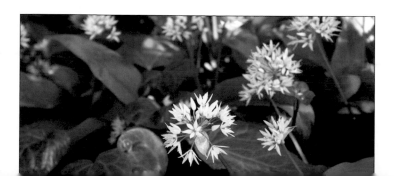

Wild Rose

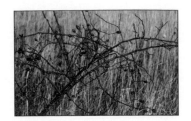

Description: This shrub has alternating leaves and sharp prickles. It has red, pink, or yellow flowers and fruit (rose hip) that remains on the shrub all year.

   Location: These shrubs occur in dry fields throughout the country.

   Edible Parts and Preparing: The flowers and buds are edible raw or boiled. Boil fresh, young leaves to make tea. The rose hips can be eaten once the flowers fall and they can be crushed once dried to make flour.

Violets

Violets can be candied and used to decorate cakes, cookies, or pastries. Pick the flowers with a tiny bit of stem, wash, and allow to dry thoroughly on a paper towel or a rack. Heat ½ cup water, 1 cup sugar, and ¼ teaspoon almond extract in a saucepan. Use tweezers to carefully dip each flower in the hot liquid. Set on wax paper and dust with sugar until every flower is thoroughly coated. If desired, snip off remaining stems with small scissors. Allow flowers to dry for a few hours in a warm, dry place.

Edible Wild Mushrooms

A walk through the woods will likely reveal several varieties of mushrooms, and chances are that some are the types that are edible. However, because some mushrooms are very poisonous, it is important never to try a mushroom of which you are unsure. Never eat a mushroom with gills, or, for that matter, any mushroom that you cannot positively identify as edible. Also, never eat mushrooms that appear wilted, damaged, or rotten.

   Here are some common edible mushrooms that you can easily identify and enjoy.

Chanterelles

These trumpet-shaped mushrooms have wavy edges and interconnected blunt-ridged gills under the caps. They are varied shades of yellow and have a fruity fragrance. They grow in summer and fall on the ground of hardwood forests. Because chanterelles tend to be tough, they are best when slowly sautéed or added to stews or soups.

   Notes: Beware of Jack O'Lantern mushrooms, which look and smell similarly to chanterelles. Jack O'Lanterns have sharp, knifelike gills instead of the blunt gills of chanterelles, and generally grow in large clusters at the base of trees or on decaying wood.

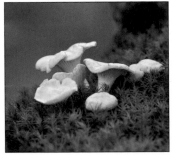
Chanterelles.

Coral Fungi

Corel fungi.

These fungi are aptly named for their bunches of upward-facing branching stems, which look strikingly like coral. They are whitish, tan, yellowish, or sometimes pinkish or purple. They may reach 8 inches in height. They grow in the summer and fall in shady, wooded areas.

   Notes: Avoid coral fungi that are bitter, have soft, gelatinous bases, or turn brown when you poke or squeeze them. These may have a laxative effect, though are not life-threatening.

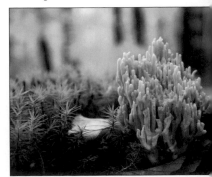

Morels

Morels are sometimes called sponge, pinecone, or honeycomb mushrooms because of the pattern of pits and ridges that appears on the caps. They can be anywhere from 2 to 12 inches tall. They may be yellow, brown, or black and grow in spring and early summer in wooded areas and on river bottoms. To cook, cut in half to check for insects, wash, and sauté, bake, or stew.

Notes: False morels can be poisonous and appear similar to morels because of their brainlike, irregularly shaped caps. However, they can be distinguished from true morels because false morel caps bulge inward instead of outward. The caps have lobes, folds, flaps, or wrinkles, but not pits and ridges like a true morel.

Puffballs

These round or pear-shaped mushrooms are often mistaken for golf balls or eggs. They are always whitish, tan, or gray and sometimes have a thick stem. Young puffballs tend to be white and older ones yellow or brown. Fully matured puffballs have dark spores scattered over the caps. Puffballs are generally found in late summer and fall on lawns, in the woods, or on old tree stumps. To eat, peel off the outer skin and eat raw or batter-fried.

Notes: Slice each puffball open before eating to be sure it is completely white inside. If there is any yellow, brown, or black, or **if there is a developing mushroom inside with a stalk, gills, and cap, do not eat!** Amanitas, which are very poisonous, can appear similar to puffballs when they are young. Do not eat if the mushroom gives off an unpleasant odor.

Shaggy Mane Mushrooms

This mushroom got its name from its cap, which is a white cylinder with shaggy, upturned, brownish scales. As the mushroom matures, the bottom outside circumference of the cap becomes black. Shaggy manes are generally 4 to 6 inches tall and grow in all the warm seasons in fields and on lawns.

Shaggy manes are tastiest eaten when young, but they're easiest to identify once the bottoms of the caps begin to turn black. They are delicious sautéed in butter or olive oil and lightly seasoned with salt, garlic, or nutmeg.

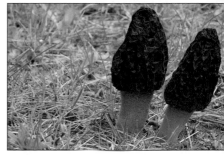

Morels

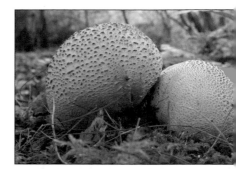

Puffballs

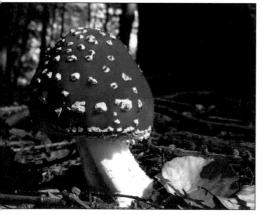

Poisonous amanita mushroom

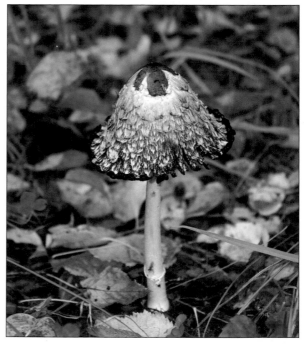

Shaggy mane mushroom

Make Your Own Foods

Make Your Own Butter

Making butter the old-fashioned way is incredibly simple and very gratifying. It's a great project to do with kids, too. All you need is a jar, a marble, some fresh cream, and about 20 minutes.

1. Start with about twice as much heavy whipping cream as you'll want butter. Pour it into the jar, drop in the marble, close the lid tightly, and start shaking.
2. Check the consistency of the cream every three to four minutes. The liquid will turn into whipped cream, and then eventually you'll see little clumps of butter forming in the jar. Keep shaking for another few minutes and then begin to strain out the liquid into another jar. This is buttermilk, which is great for use in making pancakes, waffles, biscuits, and muffins.
3. The butter is now ready, but it will store better if you wash and work it. Add ½ cup of ice-cold water and continue to shake for two or three minutes. Strain out the water and repeat. When the strained water is clear, mash the butter to extract the last of the water, and strain.
4. Scoop the butter into a ramekin, mold, or wax paper.

If desired, add salt or chopped fresh herbs to your butter just before storing or serving. Butter can also be made in a food processor or blender to speed up the processing time.

Make Your Own Yogurt

Yogurt is simple to make and is delicious on its own, as a dessert, in baked goods, or in place of sour cream. Yogurt is basically fermented milk. You can make it by adding the active cultures *Streptococcus thermophilus* and *Lactobacillus bulgaricus* to heated milk, which will produce lactic acid, creating yogurt's tart flavor and thick consistency.

Yogurt is thought to have originated many centuries ago among the nomadic tribes of Eastern Europe and Western Asia. Milk stored in animal skins would acidify and coagulate. The acid helped preserve the milk from further spoilage and from the growth of pathogens (disease-causing microorganisms).

Ingredients

Makes 4 to 5 cups of yogurt

- **1 quart milk** (cream, whole, low-fat, or skim)—In general the higher the milk fat level in the yogurt, the creamier and smoother it will taste. **Note:** If you use home-produced milk it *must* be pasteurized before preparing yogurt. See the center box for tips on pasteurizing milk.
- **Nonfat dry milk powder**—Use ⅓ cup powder when using whole or low-fat milk, or use ⅔ cup powder when using skim milk. The higher the milk solids, the firmer the yogurt will be. For even more firmness add gelatin (directions below).
- **Commercial, unflavored, cultured yogurt**—Use ¼ cup. Be sure the product label indicates that it contains a live culture. Also note the content of the culture. *L. bulgaricus* and *S. thermophilus* are

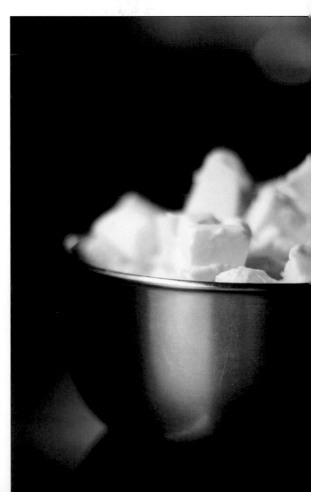

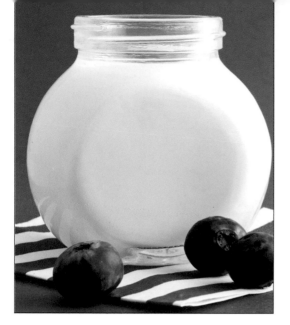

required in yogurt, but some manufacturers may add *L. acidophilus* or *B. bifidum*. The latter two are used for slight variations in flavor, but more commonly for health reasons attributed to these organisms. All culture variations will make a successful yogurt.

- **2 to 4 tablespoons sugar or honey (optional)**
- **1 teaspoon unflavored gelatin (optional)**— For a thick, firm yogurt, swell 1 teaspoon gelatin in a little milk for 5 minutes. Add this to the milk and nonfat dry milk mixture before cooking.

Supplies
- **Double boiler or regular saucepan**—1 to 2 quarts in capacity larger than the volume of yogurt you wish to make.
- **Cooking or jelly thermometer**—A thermometer that can clip to the side of the saucepan and remain in the milk works best. Accurate temperatures are critical for successful processing.
- **Mixing spoon**
- **Yogurt containers**—cups with lids or canning jars with lids.
- **Incubator**—a yogurt-maker, oven, heating pad, or warm spot in your kitchen. To use your oven, place yogurt containers into deep pans of 110°F water. Water should come at least halfway up the containers. Set oven temperature at lowest point to maintain water temperature at 110°F. Monitor temperature throughout incubation, making adjustments as necessary.

Processing
1. Combine ingredients and heat. Heating the milk is necessary to change the milk proteins so that they set together rather than form curds and whey. Do not substitute this heating step for pasteurization. Place cold, pasteurized milk in a double boiler and stir in nonfat, dry milk powder. Adding nonfat, dry milk to heated milk will cause some milk proteins to coagulate and form strings. Add sugar or honey if a sweeter, less tart yogurt is desired. Heat milk to 200°F, stirring gently and hold

for 10 minutes for thinner yogurt, or hold 20 minutes for thicker yogurt. Do not boil. Be careful and stir constantly to avoid scorching if not using a double boiler.

2. Cool and inoculate. Place the top of the double boiler in cold water to cool milk rapidly to 112°F to 115°F. Remove one cup of the warm milk and blend it with the yogurt starter culture. Add this to the rest of the warm milk. The temperature of the mixture should now be 110°F to 112°F.

3. Incubate. Pour immediately into clean, warm containers; cover and place in prepared incubator. Close the incubator and incubate about 4 to 7 hours at 110°F, ± 5°F. Yogurt should set firm when the proper acid level is achieved (pH 4.6). Incubating yogurt for several hours past the time after the yogurt has set will produce more acidity. This will result in a more tart or acidic flavor and eventually cause the whey to separate.

4. Refrigerate. Rapid cooling stops the development of acid. Yogurt will keep for about 10 to 21 days if held in the refrigerator at 40°F or lower.

Yogurt Types

Set yogurt: A solid set where the yogurt firms in a container and is not disturbed.

Stirred yogurt: Yogurt made in a large container then spooned or otherwise dispensed into secondary serving containers. The consistency of the "set" is broken and the texture is less firm than set yogurt. This is the most popular form of commercial yogurt.

Drinking yogurt: Stirred yogurt into which additional milk and flavors are mixed. Add fruit or fruit syrups to taste. Mix in milk to achieve the desired thickness. The shelf life of this product is four to 10 days, since the pH is raised by the addition of fresh milk. Some whey separation will occur and is natural. Commercial products recommend a thorough shaking before consumption.

Fruit yogurt: Fruit, fruit syrups, or pie filling can be added to the yogurt. Place them on top, on bottom, or stir them into the yogurt.

Troubleshooting

- If milk forms some clumps or strings during the heating step, some milk proteins may have jelled. Take the solids out with a slotted spoon or, in difficult cases, after cooking pour the milk mixture through a clean colander or cheesecloth before inoculation.

How to Pasteurize Raw Milk

If you are using fresh milk that hasn't been processed, you can pasteurize it yourself. Heat water in the bottom section of a double boiler and pour milk into the top section. Cover the milk and heat to 165°F while stirring constantly for uniform heating. Cool immediately by setting the top section of the double boiler in ice water or cold running water. Store milk in the refrigerator in clean containers until ready for making yogurt.

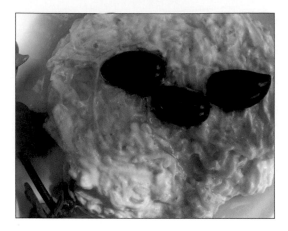

- When yogurt fails to coagulate properly, it's because the pH is not low enough. Milk proteins will coagulate when the pH has dropped to 4.6. This is done by the culture growing and producing acids. Adding culture to very hot milk (+115°F) can kill bacteria. Use a thermometer to carefully control temperature.
- If yogurt takes too long to make, it may be because the temperature is off. Too hot or too cold of an incubation temperature can slow down culture growth. Use a thermometer to carefully control temperature.
- If yogurt just isn't working, it may be because the starter culture was of poor quality. Use a fresh, recently purchased culture from the grocery store each time you make yogurt.
- If yogurt tastes or smells bad, it's likely because the starter culture is contaminated. Obtain new culture for the next batch.
- If yogurt has over-set or incubated too long, refrigerate yogurt immediately after a firm coagulum has formed.
- If yogurt tastes a little odd, it could be due to overheating or boiling of the milk. Use a thermometer to carefully control temperature.
- When whey collects on the surface of the yogurt, it's called syneresis. Some syneresis is natural. Excessive separation of whey, however, can be caused by incubating yogurt too long or by agitating the yogurt while it is setting.

Storing Your Yogurt

- Always pasteurize milk or use commercially pasteurized milk to make yogurt.
- Discard batches that fail to set properly, especially those due to culture errors.
- Yogurt generally has a 10- to 21-day shelf life when made and stored properly in the refrigerator below 40°F.
- Always use clean and sanitized equipment and containers to ensure a long shelf life for your yogurt. Clean equipment and containers in hot water with detergent, then rinse well. Allow to air dry.

Make Your Own Cheese

There are endless varieties of cheese you can make, but they all fall into two main categories: soft and hard. Soft cheeses (like cream cheese) are easier to make because they don't require a cheese press. The curds in hard cheeses (like cheddar) are pressed together to form a solid block or wheel, which requires more time and effort, but hard cheeses will keep longer than soft cheeses, and generally have a much stronger flavor.

Cheese is basically curdled milk and is made by adding an enzyme (typically rennet) to milk, allowing curds to form, heating the mixture, straining out the whey, and finally pressing the curds together. Cheeses such as *queso fresco* or *queso blanco* (traditionally eaten in Latin American countries) and *paneer* (traditionally eaten in India), are made with an acid such as vinegar or lemon juice instead of bacterial cultures or rennet.

You can use any kind of milk to make cheese, including cow's milk, goat's milk, sheep's milk, and even buffalo's milk (used for traditional mozzarella). For the richest flavor, try to get raw milk from a local farmer. If you don't know of one near you, visit realmilk.com/where.html for a listing of raw milk suppliers in your state. You can use homogenized milk, but it will produce weaker curds and a milder flavor. If your milk is pasteurized, you'll need to "ripen" it by heating it in a double boiler until it reaches 86°F and then adding 1 cup of unpasteurized, preservative-free, cultured buttermilk per gallon of milk and letting it stand 30 minutes to three hours (the longer you leave it, the sharper the flavor will be). If you cannot find unpasteurized buttermilk, diluting ⅛ teaspoon calcium chloride (available from online cheesemaker suppliers) in ¼ cup of water and adding it to your milk will create a similar effect.

Rennet (also called rennin or chymosin) is sold online at cheesemaking sites in tablet or liquid form. You may also be able to find Junket rennet tablets near the pudding and gelatin in your grocery store. One teaspoon of liquid rennet is the equivalent of one rennet tablet, which is enough to turn 5 gallons of milk into cheese (estimate four drops of liquid rennet per gallon of milk). Microbial rennet is a vegetarian alternative that is available for purchase online.

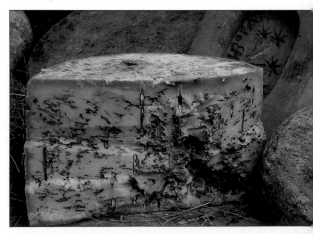

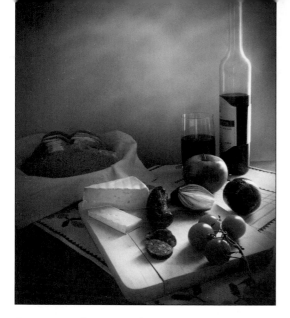

Preparation

It's important to keep your hands clean and all equipment sterile when making cheese.

1. Wash hands and all equipment with soapy detergent before and after use.
2. Rinse all equipment with clean water, removing all soapy residue.
3. Boil all cheesemaking equipment between uses.
4. For best-quality cheese, use new cheesecloth each time you make cheese. (Sterilize cheesecloth by first washing, then boiling.)
5. Squeaky clean is clean. If you can feel a residue on the equipment, it is not clean.

Yogurt Cheese

This soft cheese has a flavor similar to sour cream and a texture like cream cheese. A pint of yogurt will yield approximately ¼ pound of cheese. The yogurt cheese has a shelf life of approximately seven to 14 days when wrapped and placed in the refrigerator and kept at less than 40°F.

Ingredients
Plain, whole-milk yogurt

Directions

1. Line a large strainer or colander with cheesecloth.
2. Place the lined strainer over a bowl and pour in the yogurt. Do not use yogurt made with the addition of gelatin, as gelatin will inhibit whey separation.
3. Let yogurt drain overnight, covered with plastic wrap. Empty the whey from the bowl.
4. Fill a strong, plastic storage bag with some water, seal, and place over the cheese to weigh it down. Let the cheese stand another 8 hours and then enjoy!

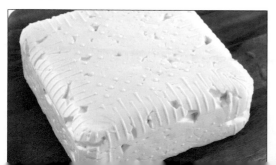

Queso Blanco

Queso blanco is a white, semi-hard cheese made without culture or rennet. It is eaten fresh and may be flavored with peppers, herbs, and spices. It is considered a "frying cheese," meaning it does not melt and may be deep-fried or grilled. *Queso blanco* is best eaten fresh, so try this small recipe the first time you make it. If it disappears quickly, next time double or triple the recipe. This recipe will yield about ½ cup of cheese.

Ingredients
2 cups milk
4 tsp white vinegar
Salt
Minced jalapeño, black pepper, chives, or other herbs to taste

Directions

1. Heat milk to 176°F for 20 minutes.
2. Add vinegar slowly to the hot milk until the whey is semi-clear and the curd particles begin to form stretchy clumps. Stir for 5 to 10 minutes. When it's ready, you should be able to stretch a piece of curd about ⅓ inch before it breaks.
3. Allow to cool, and strain off the whey by filtering through a cheesecloth-lined colander or a cloth bag.
4. Work in salt and spices to taste.
5. Press the curd in a mold or simply leave in a ball.
6. *Queso blanco* may keep for several weeks if stored in a refrigerator, but is best eaten fresh.

Ricotta Cheese

Making ricotta is very similar to making *queso blanco*, though it takes a bit longer. Start the cheese in the morning for use at dinner, or make a day ahead. Use it in lasagna, in desserts, or all on its own.

Ingredients
1 gallon milk
⅓ cup plus 1 tsp white vinegar
¼ tsp salt

Directions

1. Pour milk into a large pot, add salt, and heat slowly while stirring until the milk reaches 180°F.
2. Remove from heat and add vinegar. Stir for one minute as curds begin to form.
3. Cover and allow to sit undisturbed for two hours.
4. Pour mixture into a colander lined with cheesecloth, and allow to drain for two or more hours.
5. Store in a sealed container for up to a week.

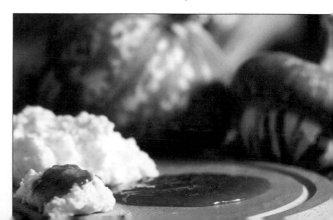

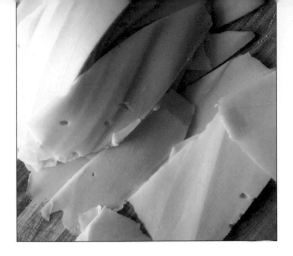

Mozzarella

This mild cheese will make your homemade pizza especially delicious. Or slice it and eat with fresh tomatoes and basil from the garden. Fresh cheese can be stored in saltwater but must be eaten within two days.

Ingredients

1 gallon 2 percent milk

¼ cup fresh, plain yogurt (see recipe on page 130)

One tablet rennet or 1 tsp liquid rennet dissolved in ½ cup tap water

Brine: use 2 pounds of salt per gallon of water

Directions

1. Heat milk to 90°F and add yogurt. Stir slowly for 15 minutes while keeping the temperature constant.
2. Add rennet mixture and stir for 3 to 5 minutes.
3. Cover, remove from heat, and allow to stand until coagulated, about 30 minutes.
4. Cut curd into ½-inch cubes. Allow to stand for 15 minutes with occasional stirring.
5. Return to heat and slowly increase temperature to 118°F over a period of 45 minutes. Hold this temperature for an additional 15 minutes.
6. Drain off the whey by transferring the mixture to a cheesecloth-lined colander. Use a spoon to press the liquid out of the curds. Transfer the mat of curd to a flat pan that can be kept warm in a low oven. Do not cut mat, but turn it over every 15 minutes for a 2-hour period. Mat should be tight when finished.
7. Cut the mat into long strips 1 to 2 inches wide and place in hot water (180°F). Using wooden spoons, tumble and stretch it under water until it becomes elastic, about 15 minutes.
8. Remove curd from hot water and shape it by hand into a ball or a loaf, kneading in the salt. Place cheese in cold water (40°F) for approximately 1 hour.
9. Store in a solution of 2 teaspoons salt to 1 cup water.

Cheddar Cheese

Cheddar is a New England and Wisconsin favorite. The longer you age it, the sharper the flavor will be. Try a slice with a wedge of homemade apple pie.

Ingredients

1 gallon milk

¼ cup buttermilk

1 tablet rennet, or 1 tsp liquid rennet

1½ tsp salt

Directions

1. Combine milk and buttermilk and allow the mixture to ripen overnight.
2. The next day, heat milk to 90°F in a double boiler and add rennet.
3. After about 45 minutes, cut curds into small cubes and let sit 15 minutes.
4. Heat very slowly to 100°F and cook for about an hour or until a cooled piece of curd will keep its shape when squeezed.
5. Drain curds and rinse out the double boiler.

6. Place a rack lined with cheesecloth inside the double boiler and spread the curds on the cloth. Cover and reheat at about 98°F for 30 to 40 minutes. The curds will become one solid mass.
7. Remove the curds, cut them into 1-inch wide strips, and return them to the pan. Turn the strips every 15 to 20 minutes for one hour.
8. Cut the strips into cubes and mix in salt.
9. Let the curds stand for 10 minutes, place them in cheesecloth, and press in a cheese press with 15 pounds for 10 minutes, then with 30 pounds for an hour.
10. Remove the cheese from the press, unwrap it, dip in warm water, and fill in any cracks.
11. Wrap again in cheesecloth and press with 40 pounds for 24 hours.
12. Remove from the press and let the cheese dry about five days in a cool, well-ventilated area, turning the cheese twice a day and wiping it with a clean cloth. When a hard skin has formed, rub with oil or seal with wax. You can eat the cheese after six weeks, but for the strongest flavor, allow cheese to age for six months or more.

Make Your Own Simple Cheese Press

1. Remove both ends of a large coffee can or thoroughly cleaned paint can, saving one end. Use an awl or a hammer and long nail to pierce the sides in several places, piercing from the inside out.
2. Place the can on a cooling rack inside a larger basin. Leave the bottom of the can in place.
3. Use a saw to cut a ¾-inch-thick circle of wood to create a "cheese follower." It should be small enough in diameter to fit easily in the can.
4. Place cheese curds in the can, and top with the cheese follower. Place several bricks wrapped in cloth or foil on top of the cheese follower to weigh down curds.
5. Once the cheese is fully pressed, remove the bricks and bottom of the can. Use the cheese follower to push the cheese out of the can.

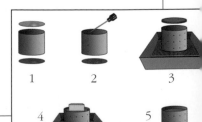

Make Your Own Ice Cream

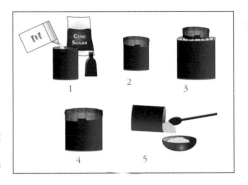

Supplies
1-pound coffee can
3-pound coffee can
Duct tape
1 cup salt

Ingredients
2 cups half and half
½ cup sugar
1 tsp vanilla Ice

Directions
1. Mix all the ingredients in the 1-pound coffee can. Cover the lid with duct tape to ensure it is tightly sealed.
2. Place the smaller can inside the larger can and fill the space between the two with ice and salt.
3. Cover the large can and seal with duct tape. Roll the can back and forth for 15 minutes. To reduce noise, place a towel on your working surface, or work on a rug.
4. Dump out ice and water. Stir contents of small can. Store ice cream in a glass or plastic container (if you leave it in the can it may take on a metallic flavor).

If desired, add cocoa powder, coffee granules, crushed peppermint sticks or other candy, or fruit.

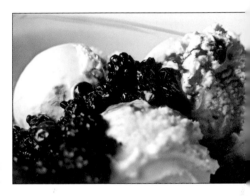

Brew Your Own Beer

Making your own brew is not difficult, but be sure to use water that is not heavily chlorinated or that has a strong mineral flavor. The sweetness of malt (from barley) and the bitterness of hops (the female flower of the hop vine) balance each other to create beer's rich flavor. The fermentation is caused by the yeast consuming the sugar, which produces carbon dioxide and alcohol.

Malt is barley that has begun to germinate, which creates enzymes necessary for converting starch to sugar. When you're first experimenting with brewing beer, use store-bought malt and hops, as they will have more predictable results. If you want to make your own malt, let the barley grains sprout. Once the shoots are the same length as the kernels, stop the growth by heating the barley to between 185°F and 230°F. At that point, the barley is malted and must be cracked and soaked in 150°F water for about six hours. Finally, strain the barley and use the liquid for your beer.

Supplies
10-gallon pail
Hydrometer
Siphon and clamp
12 2-liter bottles, sterilized

Ingredients
Water
40-oz can pre-hopped malt extract
6 to 7 cups white sugar or 8 to 9 cups
    corn sugar
1 tsp brewer's yeast
24 tsp white granulated sugar

Directions
1. Clean pail, hydrometer, and siphon with warm, soapy water and rinse thoroughly. Then sterilize by rinsing with a mix of 1 tablespoon household bleach and 1 gallon water. Rinse a final time with clean water.
2. Pour 2½ to 3 gallons cold water in the pail.
3. Bring 7½ quarts of water to a boil in a large pot. Add malt extract very slowly, stirring, and then simmer uncovered for 20 minutes.
4. Add sugar and stir until dissolved.
5. Dump the hot mixture into the pail containing the cold water, splashing it in to increase the oxygen in the liquid (yeast needs oxygen to do its job).
6. Add ice water until mixture is about 70°F (water that is too hot can kill the yeast).
7. Add the yeast and stir well.
8. Cover loosely (if the lid is too tight, the pail could explode) and allow to sit in a moderate to cool place (around 62°F to 68°F) for 6 to 10

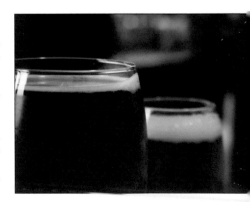

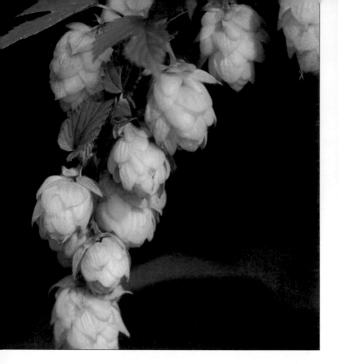

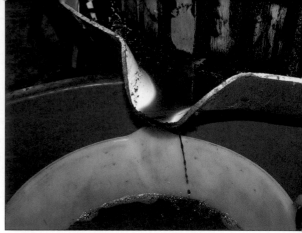

days. Don't open the pail, tip it, or shake it for at least 6 days.

9. Place the hydrometer in the beer and give it a spin to release air bubbles. The hydrometer should read about 1.008 for dark beers and 1.010 to 1.105 for light beers.

10. When the beer is ready, place the bucket on a bench or sturdy table and place the sterilized bottles on the floor below. Add about 2 teaspoons of white granulated sugar to each bottle to help carbonate the beer.

11. Use the siphon and clamp to siphon the beer into the bottles, screw on the lids, give the bottles a quick shake, and store the bottles in a warm, dark area for a few days, and then move into cool, dark area. Store at least three weeks before drinking.

Make Your Own Wine

Supplies
Colander or strainer
Large bowl or pot
1-gallon container with a secure lid
Spoon
Potato masher
Funnel

Ingredients
1 qt fruit
2 cups sugar
1 gallon water, divided
1 package active yeast

Directions
1. Thoroughly clean all your cooking utensils with warm, soapy water and rinse thoroughly. Then sterilize by rinsing with a mix of 1 tablespoon household bleach and 1 gallon water. Rinse a final time with clean water.

2. In a bowl, crush the fruit with a potato masher (or use a food processor) until smooth.

3. Dissolve the sugar in 1 cup of hot water. Allow to cool to room temperature and add to the fruit.

4. Dissolve the yeast in 2 cups of warm water and add to the fruit, along with the remaining water. Stir once every day for a week.

5. Strain through a colander into your 1-gallon container, close lid securely, and allow to rest in a cool, dark place for 6 weeks.

6. Strain the wine into your sterilized bottles (leaving one empty) and cork lightly. After three days, strain the wine from one bottle into the empty one, leaving about 1 inch headspace below the cork. Repeat until bottles are full.

7. Soak new corks in warm water for about 2 hours, rinse several times, place securely in bottles, and seal with paraffin.

Dandelion Wine

Ingredients
4 qts dandelion blossoms (use the full dandelion heads—not just the petals)
4 qts boiling water
2 oranges
2 lemons
4 lbs sugar
2 tbsp yeast

Directions
1. Wash dandelion blossoms and place them in a large pot. Pour 4 quarts of boiling water over them and let stand 24 hours.

2. Strain through cheesecloth and add grated rind and juice of two oranges and two lemons, four pounds of granulated sugar, and two tablespoonfuls yeast.

3. Let stand one week, then strain and fill bottles.

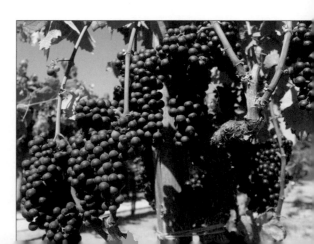

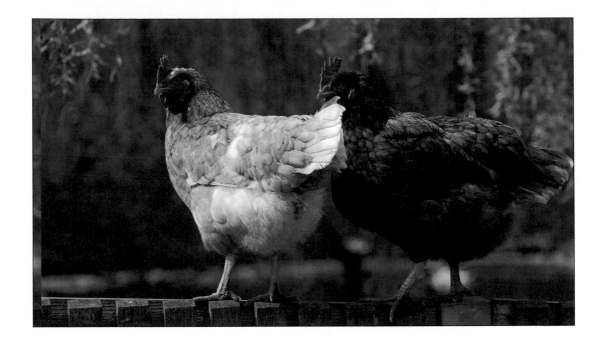

PART THREE   # The Backyard Farm

"The greatness of a nation and its moral progress can be judged by the way its animals are treated"

—*Mahatma Gandhi*

The prospect of raising farm animals in your backyard does not need to be overwhelming. If you're concerned about not having enough land, keep in mind that a few chickens can be raised on less than an eighth of an acre; you may be able to have a beehive on your rooftop; and a couple of goats or sheep will be perfectly content on a quarter of an acre. Worried about the cost? With chickens, the small amount you will invest in buying chicks will quickly pay itself back in fresh eggs or meat, and since chicken feed is very inexpensive, the upkeep costs are minimal. If you sheer your sheep or llamas, you can spin the wool and sell it at a local market or online to make a profit. However, if time is your concern, you should stop to think before purchasing animals or rescuing them from shelters. Any animal you bring onto your property deserves a portion of your time every day. You certainly don't have to spend every waking moment with your animals, but you will need to provide food, water, shelter, and a few other necessities. If you don't have the time for this on a regular basis, consider helping out at a local farm or shelter, or simply support other farmers by shopping at farmer's markets. If you do have the time to care properly for animals, very often you will find that they give you far more than you give them.

Chickens

Raising chickens in your yard will give you access to fresh eggs and meat, and because chickens are some of the easiest creatures to keep, even families in very urban areas are able to raise a few in a small backyard. Four or five chickens will supply your whole family with eggs on a regular basis.

Housing Your Chickens

You will need to have a structure for your chickens to live in to protect them from predators and inclement weather, and to allow the hens a safe place to lay their eggs. See "Poultry Houses" on page 175 to see several types of structures you can make for housing chickens and other poultry.

Placing your henhouse close enough to your own home will remind you to visit it frequently to feed the chickens and to gather eggs. It is best to establish the house and yard in dry soil, away from areas in your yard that are frequently damp or moist, as this is the perfect breeding ground for poultry diseases. The henhouse should be well-ventilated, warm, protected from the cold and rain, have a few windows that allow the sunlight to shine in (especially if you live in a colder climate), and have a sound roof.

The perches in your henhouse should not be more than 2½ feet above the floor, and you should place a smooth platform under the perches to catch the droppings so they can easily be cleaned. Nesting boxes should be kept in a darker part of the house and should have ample space around them.

The perches in your henhouse can be relatively narrow and shouldn't be more than a few feet from the floor.

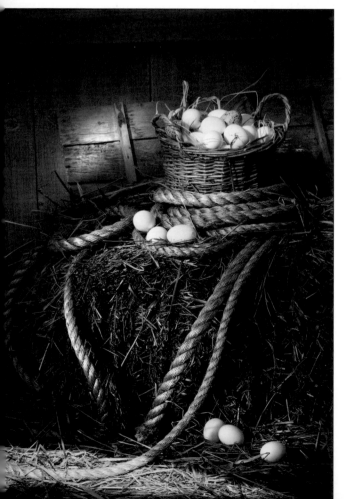

Selecting the Right Breed of Chicken

Take the time to select chickens that are well-suited for your needs. If you want chickens solely for their eggs, look for chickens that are good egg-layers. Mediterranean poultry are good for first-time chicken owners as they are easy to care for and only need the proper food to lay many eggs. If you are looking to slaughter and eat your chickens, you will want to have heavy-bodied fowl (Asiatic poultry) in order to get the most meat from them. If you are looking to have chickens that lay a good amount of eggs and that can also be used for meat, invest in the Wyandottes or Plymouth Rock breeds. These chickens are not incredibly bulky but they are good sources of both eggs and meat.

Wyandottes have seven distinct breeds: Silver, White, Buff, Golden, and Black are the most common. These breeds are hardy and they are very popular in the United States. They are compactly built and lay excellent dark brown eggs. They are good sitters and their meat is perfect for broiling or roasting.

Plymouth Rock chickens have three distinct breeds: Barred, White, and Buff. They are the most popular breeds in the United States and are hardy birds that grow to a medium size. These chickens are good for laying eggs, roost well, and also provide good meat.

Plymouth rock chickens are good all-around farm chickens with their docile dispositions, hardiness, tendency to be very productive egg-layers, and good meat.

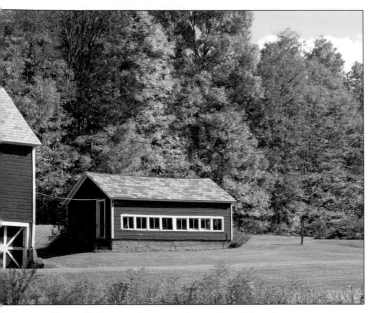

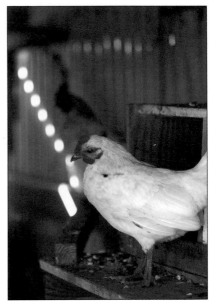

Building a chicken coop close to your house will make it easier to tend the chickens and gather eggs in inclement weather.

Feeding Your Chickens

Chickens, like most creatures, need a balanced diet of protein, carbohydrates, vitamins, fats, minerals, and water. Chickens with plenty of access to grassy areas will find most of what they need on their own. However, if you don't have the space to allow your chickens to roam free, commercial chicken feed is readily available in the form of mash, crumbles, pellets, or scratch. Or you can make your own feed out of a combination of grains, seeds, meat scraps or protein-rich legumes, and a gritty substance such as bone meal, limestone, oyster shell, or granite (to aid digestion, especially in winter). The correct ratio of food for a warm, secure chicken should be 1 part protein to 4 parts carbohydrates. Do not rely too heavily on corn as it can be too fattening for hens; combine corn with wheat or oats for the carbohydrate portion of the feed. Clover and other green foods are also beneficial to feed your chickens.

How much food your chickens need will depend on breed, age, the season, and how much room they have to exercise. Often it's easiest and best for the chickens to leave feed available at all times in several locations within the chickens' range. This will ensure that even the lowest chickens in the pecking order get the feed they need.

A simple movable chicken coop can be constructed out of two-by-fours and two wheels. The floor of the coop should have open slats so that the manure will fall onto the ground and fertilize the soil. An even simpler method is to construct a pen that sits directly on the ground, making sure that it has a roof to offer the chickens suitable shade. The pen can be moved once the area is well-fertilized.

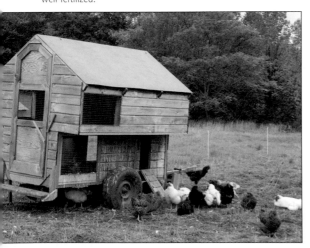

Wyandottes originated in the United States and were first bred in the 1870s. This one is a golden laced wyandott.

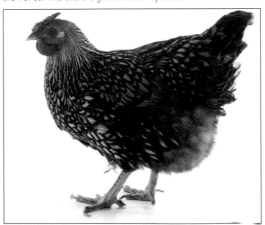

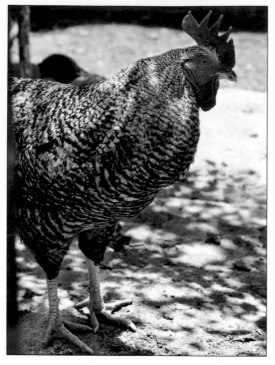

This one is a barred Plymouth rock chicken.

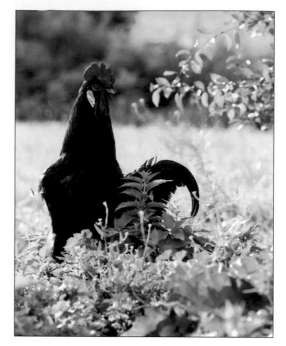

Chickens that are allowed to roam freely ("free-range" chickens) will be able to scavenge most of the food they need, as long as there is plenty of grass or other vegetation available.

Chicken Feed

4 parts corn (or more in cold months)
3 parts oat groats
2 parts wheat
2 parts alfalfa meal or chopped hay
1 part meat scraps, fish meal, or soybean meal
2 to 3 parts dried split peas, lentils, or soybean meal
2 to 3 parts bone meal, crushed oyster shell, granite grit, or limestone
½ part cod-liver oil

You may also wish to add sunflower seeds, hulled barley, millet, kamut, amaranth seeds, quinoa, sesame seeds, flax seeds, or kelp granules. If you find that your eggs are thin-shelled, try adding more calcium to the feed (in the form of limestone or oystershell). Store feed in a covered bucket, barrel, or other container that will not allow rodents to get into it. A plastic or galvanized bucket is good, as it will also keep mold-causing moisture out of the feed.

Hatching Chicks

If you are looking to increase the number of chickens you have, or if you plan to sell some chickens at the market, you may want your hens to lay eggs and hatch chicks. To hatch a chick, an egg must be incubated for a sufficient amount of time with the proper heat, moisture, and position. The period for incubation varies based on the species of chicken. The average incubation period is around 21 days for most common breeds.

If you are only housing a few chickens in your backyard, natural incubation is the easiest method with which to hatch chicks. Natural incubation is dependent upon the instinct of the mother hen and the breed of hen. Plymouth Rocks and Wyandottes are good hens to raise chicks. It is important to separate the setting hen from the other chickens while she is nesting and to also keep the hen clean and free from lice. The nest should also be kept clean, and the hens should be fed grain food, grit, and clean, fresh water.

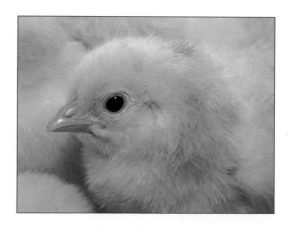

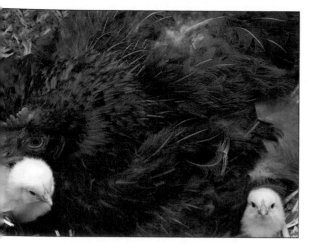

A nesting box should have plenty of clean hay or straw for the hen to rest in.

Bacteria Associated with Chicken Meat

- *Salmonella*—This is primarily found in the intestinal tract of poultry and can be found in raw meat and eggs.
- *Campylobacter jejuni*—This is one of the most common causes of diarrheal illness in humans and is spread by improper handling of raw chicken meat and not cooking the meat thoroughly.
- *Listeria monocytogenes*—This causes illness in humans and can be destroyed by keeping the meat refrigerated and by cooking it thoroughly.

It is important, when you are considering hatching chicks, to make sure your hens are healthy, have plenty of exercise, and are fed a balanced diet. They need materials on which to scratch and should not be infested with lice and other parasites. Free-range chickens, which eat primarily natural foods and get lots of exercise, lay more fertile eggs than do tightly confined hens. The eggs selected for hatching should not be more than 12 days old and they should be clean.

You'll need to construct a nesting box for the roosting hen and the incubated eggs. The box should be roomy and deep enough to retain the nesting material. Treat the box with a disinfectant before use to keep out lice, mice, and other creatures that could infect the hen or the eggs.

Make the nest of damp soil a few inches deep, placed in the bottom of the box, and then lay sweet hay or clean straw on top of that.

Place the nesting box in a quiet and secluded place away from the other chickens. If space permits, you can construct a smaller shed in which to house your nesting hen. A hen can generally sit on anywhere between 9 and 15 eggs. The hen should only be allowed to leave the nest to feed, drink water, and take a dust bath. When the hen does leave her box, check the eggs and dispose of any damaged ones. An older hen will generally be more careful and apt to roost than a younger female.

Once the chicks are hatched, they will need to stay warm and clean, get lots of exercise, and have access to food regularly. Make sure the feed is ground finely enough that the chicks can easily eat and digest it. They should also have clean, fresh water.

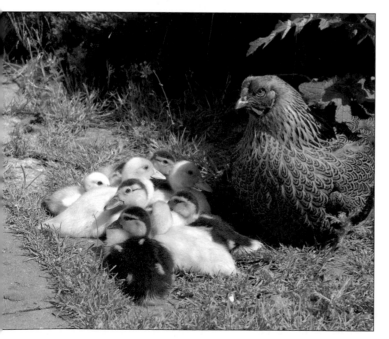

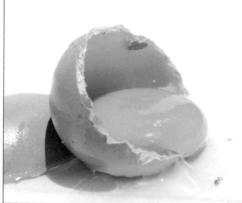

If an egg breaks, use it immediately or discard it. Once the egg is exposed to the air it spoils much more quickly

Storing Eggs

Eggs are among the most nutritious foods on earth and can be part of a healthy diet. Hens typically lay eggs every 25 hours, so you can be sure to have a fresh supply on a daily basis, in many cases. But eggs, like any other animal byproduct, need to be handled safely and carefully to avoid rotting and spreading disease. Here are a few tips on how to best preserve your farm-fresh eggs:

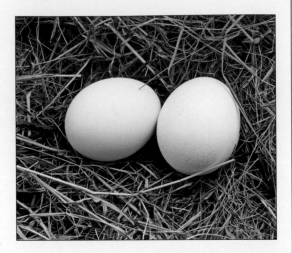

1. Make sure your eggs come from hens that have not been running with male roosters. Infertile eggs last longer than those that have been fertilized.
2. Keep the fresh eggs together.
3. Choose eggs that are perfectly clean.
4. Make sure not to crack the shells, as this will taint the taste and make the egg rot much more quickly.
5. Place your eggs directly in the refrigerator where they will keep for several weeks.

Wash fresh eggs and then refrigerate them immediately.

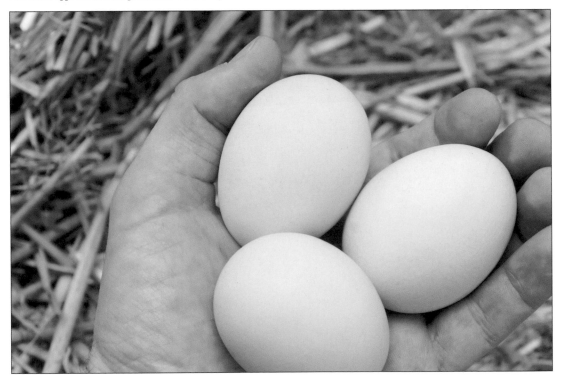

Ducks

Ducks tend to be somewhat more difficult than chicks to raise, but they do provide wonderful eggs and meat. Ducks tend to have pleasanter personalities than chickens and are often prolific layers. The eggs taste similar to chicken eggs, but are usually larger and have a slightly richer flavor. Ducks are happiest and healthiest when they have access to a pool or pond to paddle around in and when they have several other ducks to keep them company.

Breeds of Ducks

There are six common breeds of ducks: White Pekin, White Aylesbury, Colored Rouen, Black Cayuga, Colored Muscovy, and White Muscovy. Each breed is unique and has its own advantages and disadvantages.

1. White Pekin—The most popular breed of duck, these are also the easiest to raise. These ducks are hardy and do well in close confinement. They are timid and must be handled carefully. Their large frame gives them lots of meat, and they are also prolific layers.
2. White Aylesbury—This breed is similar to the Pekin but the plumage is much whiter and they are a bit heavier than the former. They are not as popular in the United States as the White Pekin duck.
3. Colored Rouens—These darkly plumed ducks are also quite popular and fatten easily for meat purposes.
4. Black Cayuga and Muscovy breeds—These are American breeds that are easily raised but are not as productive as the White Pekin.

Housing Ducks

You neither need a lot of space in which to raise ducks nor do you need water to raise them successfully, though they will be happier if you can provide at least a small pool of water for them to bathe and paddle around in. Housing for ducks is relatively simple. The houses do not have to be as warm or dry as for chickens but the ducks cannot be confined for as long periods as chickens

Ducks are social birds; they are happiest in groups.

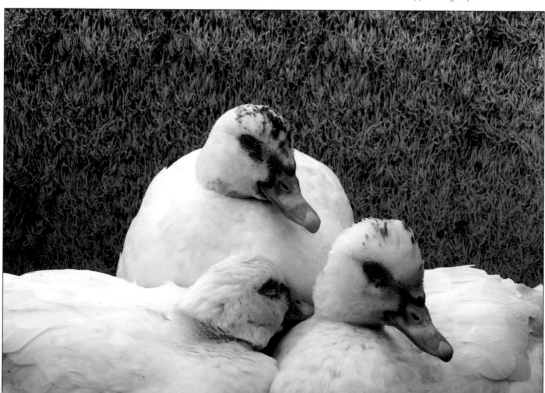

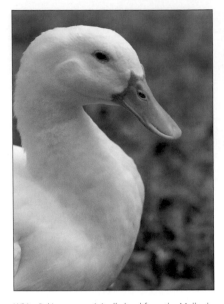

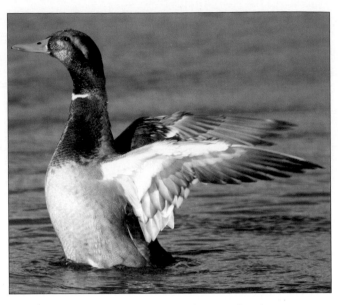

White Pekins were originally bred from the Mallard in China and came to the United States in 1873.

Ducks should have access to a lake, pond, or at least a small pool.

can. They need more exercise out-of-doors to be healthy and to produce more eggs. A house that is protected from dampness or excess rain water and that has straw or hay covering the floor is adequate for ducks. If you want to keep your ducks somewhat confined, a small fence about 2½ feet high will do the trick. Ducks don't require nesting boxes, as they lay their eggs on the floor of the house or in the yard around the house.

Feeding and Watering Ducks

Ducks require plenty of fresh water to drink, as they have to drink regularly while eating. Ducks eat both vegetable

According to Mrs. Beeton in her *Book of Household Management*, published in 1861, "[Aylesbury ducks'] snowy plumage and comfortable comportment make it a credit to the poultry-yard, while its broad and deep breast, and its ample back, convey the assurance that your satisfaction will not cease at its death."

and animal foods. If allowed to roam free and to find their own foodstuff, ducks will eat grasses, small fish, and water insects (if streams or ponds are provided).

Ducks need their food to be soft and mushy in order for them to digest it. Ducklings should be fed equal parts corn meal, wheat bran, and flour for the first week of life. For the next fifty days or so, the ducklings should be fed that mixture in addition to a little grit or sand and some green foods (green rye, oats, clover) all mixed together. After this time, ducks should be fed on a mixture of two parts cornmeal, one part wheat bran, one part flour, some coarse sand, and green foods.

Hatching Ducklings

The natural process of incubation (hatching ducklings underneath a hen) is the preferred method of hatching ducklings. It is important to take good care of the setting hen. Feed her whole corn mixed with green food, grit,

A Black Cayuga (right) stands with two Saxony ducks.

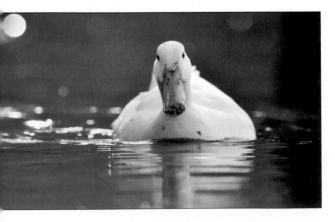

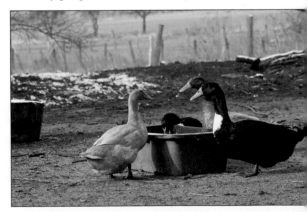

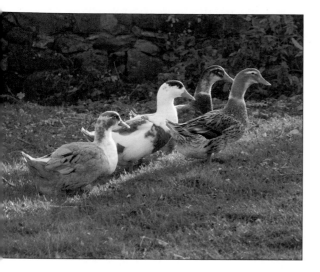

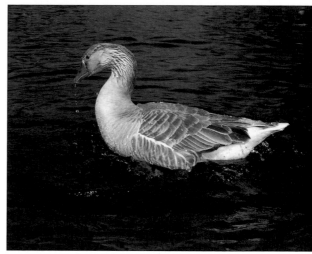

and fresh water. Placing the feed and water just in front of the nest for the first few days will encourage the hen to eat and drink without leaving the nest. Hens will typically lay their eggs on the ground, in straw or hay that is provided for them. Make sure to clean the houses and pens often so the laying ducks have clean areas in which to incubate their eggs.

Caring for Ducklings

Young ducklings are very susceptible to atmospheric changes. They must be kept warm and from getting chilled. The ducklings are most vulnerable during the first three weeks of life; after that time, they are more

likely to thrive to adulthood. Construct brooders for the young ducklings and keep them very warm by hanging strips of cloth over the door cracks. After three weeks in the warm brooder, move the ducklings to a cold brooder as they can now withstand fluctuating temperatures.

Common Diseases

On a whole, ducks are not as prone to the typical poultry diseases, and many of the diseases they do contract can be prevented by making sure the ducks have a clean environment in which to live (by cleaning out their houses, providing fresh drinking water, and so on).

Two common ailments found in ducks are botulism and maggots. Botulism causes the duck's neck to go limp, making it difficult or even impossible for the duck to swallow. Maggots infest the ducks if they do not have any clean water in which to bathe, and are typically contracted in the hot summer months. Both of these conditions (as well as worms and mites) can be cured with the proper care, medications, and veterinary assistance.

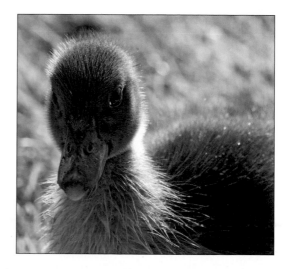

Turkeys

Turkeys are generally raised for their meat (especially for holiday roasts) though their eggs can also be eaten. Turkeys are incredibly easy to manage and raise as they primarily subsist on bugs, grasshoppers, and wasted grain that they find while wandering around the yard. They are, in a sense, self-sustaining foragers.

If you are looking to raise a turkey for Thanksgiving dinner, it is best to hatch the turkey chick in early spring, so that by November, it will be about 14 to 20 pounds.

Breeds of Turkeys

The largest breeds of turkeys found in the United States are the Bronze and Narragansett. Other breeds, though not as popular, include the White Holland, Black turkey, Slate turkey, and Bourbon Red.

Bronze breeds are most likely a cross between a wild North American turkey and domestic turkey, and they have beautiful rich plumage. This is the most common type of turkey to raise, as it is the largest, is very hardy, and is the most profitable. The White Holland and Bourbon Red, however, are said to be the most "domesticated" in their habits and are easier to keep in a smaller roaming area.

Housing Turkeys

Turkeys flourish when they can roost in the open. They thrive in the shelter of trees, though this can become problematic as they are more vulnerable to predators than if they are confined in a house. If you do build a house for them, it should be airy, roomy, and very clean.

It is important to allow turkeys freedom to roam; if you live in a more suburban or neighborhood area, raising turkeys may not be the best option

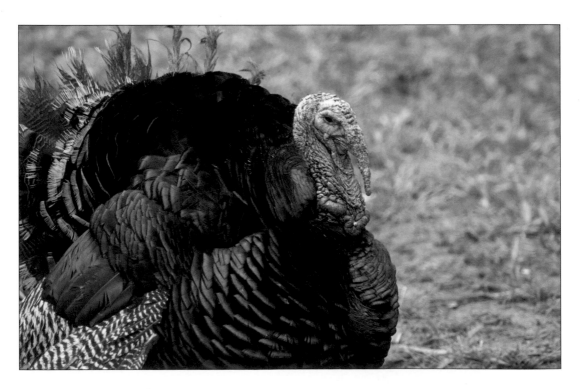

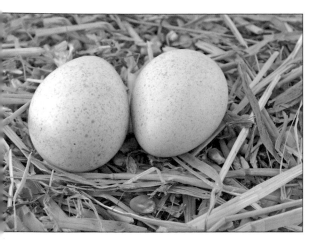

What Do Turkeys Eat?

Turkeys gain most of their sustenance from foraging, either in lawns or in pastures. They typically eat green vegetation, berries, weed seeds, waste grain, nuts, and various kinds of acorns. In the summer months, turkeys especially like to eat grasshoppers. Due to their love of eating insects that can damage crops and gardens, turkeys are quite useful in keeping your growing produce free from harmful insects and parasites.

Turkeys may be fed grain (similar to a mixture given to chickens) if they are going to be slaughtered, in order to make them larger.

for you, as your turkeys may wander into a neighboring yard, upsetting your neighbors. Turkeys need lots of exercise to be healthy and vigorous. When turkeys are confined for long periods of time, it is more difficult to regulate their feeding (turkeys are natural foragers and thrive best on natural foods), and they are more likely to contract disease than if they are allowed to range freely.

Hatching Turkey Chicks

Turkey hens lay eggs in the middle of March to the first of April. If you are looking to hatch and raise turkey chicks, it is vital to watch the hen closely for when she lays the eggs, and then gather them and keep the eggs warm until the weather is more stable. Turkey hens generally aim to hide their nests from predators. It is best, for the hen's sake, to provide her with a coop of some sort, which she can freely enter and leave. Or, if no coop is available, encourage the hen to lay her eggs in a nest close to your house (putting a large barrel on its side and heaping up brush near the house may entice the hen to nest there). This way, you can keep an eye on the eggs and hatchlings.

Hens are well-adapted to hatch all of the eggs that they lay. It takes 27 to 29 days for turkey eggs to hatch. While the hens are incubating the eggs, they should be given adequate food and water, placed close to their nest. Wheat and corn are the best food during the laying and incubation period.

Raising the Poults

Turkey chicks, also known as "poults," can be difficult to raise and require lots of care and attention for their first few weeks of life. In this sense, a turkey raiser must be "on call" to come to the aid of the hen and her poults at any time during the day for the first month or so. Many times, the hens can raise the poults well, but it is important that they receive enough food and warmth in the early weeks to allow them to grow healthy and strong. The poults should stay dry, as they become chilled

easily. If you are able, encouraging the poults and their mother into a coop until the poults are stronger will aid their growth to adulthood.

Poults should be fed soft and easily digestible foods. Stale bread, dipped in milk and then dried until it crumbles, is an excellent source of food for the young turkeys.

Diseases

Turkeys are hardy birds but they are susceptible to a few debilitating or fatal diseases. It is a fact that the mortality rate among young turkeys, even if they are given all the care and exercise and food needed, is relatively high (usually due to environmental and predatory factors).

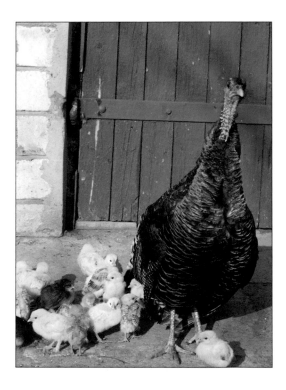

The most common disease in turkeys is blackhead. Blackhead typically infects young turkeys between 6 weeks and 4 months old. This disease will turn the head darker colored or even black and the bird will become very weak, will stop eating, and will have an insatiable thirst. Blackhead is usually fatal.

Another disease that turkeys occasionally contract is roup. Roup generally occurs when a turkey has been exposed to extreme dampness or cold drafts for long periods of time. Roup causes the turkey's head to swell around the eyes and is highly contagious to other turkeys. Nutritional roup is caused by a vitamin A deficiency, which can be alleviated by adding vitamin A to the turkey's drinking water. It is best to consult a veterinarian if your turkey seems to have this disease.

Slaughtering Poultry

If you are raising your own poultry, you may decide that you'd like to use them for consumption as well. Slaughtering your own poultry enables you to know exactly what is in the meat you and your family are consuming, and to ensure that the poultry is kept humanely before being slaughtered. Here are some guidelines for slaughtering poultry:

1. To prepare a fowl for slaughter, make sure the bird is secured well so it is unable to move (either hanging down from a pole or laid on a block that is used for chopping wood).
2. Killing the fowl can be done in two ways: one way is to hang the bird upside down and to cut the jugular vein with a sharp knife. It is a good idea to have a funnel or vessel available to collect the draining blood so it does not make a mess and can be disposed of easily. The other option is to place the bird's head on a chopping block and then, in one clean movement, chop its head off at the middle of the neck. Then, hang the bird upside down and let the blood drain as described earlier.
3. Once the bird has been thoroughly drained of blood, you can begin to pluck it. Have a pot of hot water (around 140 degrees Fahrenheit) ready, into which to dip the bird. Holding the bird by the feet, dip it into the pot of hot water and leave it for about 45 seconds—you do not want the bird to begin to cook! Then, remove the bird from the pot and begin plucking immediately. The feathers should come off fairly easily, but this process takes time, so be patient. Discard the feathers.
4. Once the bird has been completely rid of feathers, slip back the skin from the neck and cut the neck off close to the base of the body. Remove the crop, trachea, and esophagus from the bird by loosening them and pulling them out through the hole created by chopping off the neck. Cut off the vent to release the main entrails (being careful not to puncture the intestines or bacteria could be released into the meat) and make a horizontal slit about an inch above it so you can insert two fingers. Remove the entrails, liver (carefully cutting off the gallbladder), gizzard, and heart from the bird and set the last three aside if you want to eat them later or make them into stuffing. If you are going to save the heart, slip off the membrane enclosing it and cut off the veins and arteries. Make sure to clean out the gizzard as well if you will be using it later.
5. Wash the bird thoroughly, inside and out, and wipe it dry.
6. Cut off the feet below the joints and then carefully pull out the tendons from the drumsticks.
7. Once the carcass is thoroughly dry and clean, store it in the refrigerator if it will be used that same day or the next. If you want to save the bird for later use, place it in a moisture-proof bag and set it in the freezer (along with any innards that you may have saved).
8. Make sure you clean and disinfect any surface you were working on to avoid the spread of bacteria and other diseases.

Beekeeping

Beekeeping (also known as apiculture) is one of the oldest human industries. For thousands of years, honey has been considered a highly desirable food. Beekeeping is a science and can be a very profitable occupation it is also a wonderful hobby for many people in the United States. Keeping bees can be done almost anywhere—on a farm, in a rural or suburban area, and even in urban areas (even on rooftops!). Anywhere there are sufficient flowers from which to collect nectar, bees can thrive.

Apiculture relies heavily on the natural resources of a particular location and the knowledge of the beekeeper in order to be successful. Collecting and selling honey at your local farmers' market or just to family and friends can supply you with some extra cash if you are looking to make a profit from your apiary.

Why Raise Bees?

Bees are essential in the pollination and fertilization of many fruit and seed crops. If you have a garden with many flowers or fruit plants, having bees nearby will only help your garden flourish and grow year after year. Furthermore, nothing is more satisfying than extracting your own honey for everyday use.

How to Avoid Getting Stung

Though it takes some skill, you can learn how to avoid being stung by the bees you keep. Here are some ways you can keep your bee stings to a minimum:

1. Keep gentle bees. Having bees that, by sheer nature, are not as aggressive will reduce the number of stings you are likely to receive. Carniolan bees are one of the gentlest species, and so are the Caucasian bees introduced from Russia.

2. Obtain a good "smoker" and use it whenever you'll be handling your bees. Pumping smoke of any kind into and around the beehive will render your bees less aggressive and less likely to sting you.

3. Purchase and wear a veil. This should be made out of black bobbinet and worn over your face. Also, rubber gloves help protect your hands from stings.

4. Use a "bee escape." This device is fitted into a slot made in a board the same size as the top of the hive. Slip the board into the hive before you open it to extract the honey, and it allows the worker bees to slip below it but not to return back up. So, by placing the "bee escape" into the hive the day before you want to gain access to the combs and honey, you will most likely trap all the bees under the board and leave you free to work with the honeycombs without fear of stings.

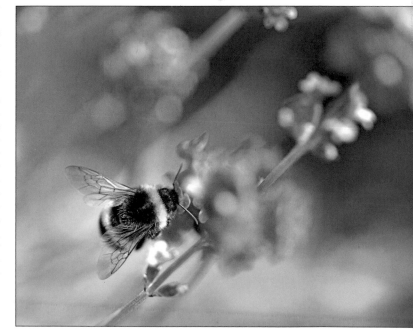

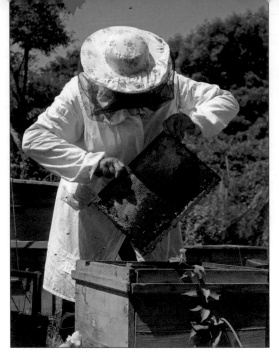

Wearing a hat and veil will help to prevent stings on your face and head.

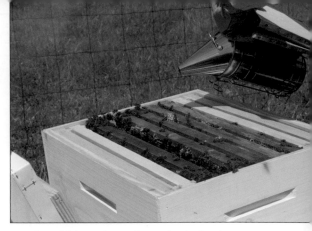

A smoker will help to relax your bees and make them less agressive.

What Type of Hive Should I Build?

Most beekeepers would agree that the best hives have suspended, movable frames where the bees make the honeycombs, which are easy to lift out. These frames, called Langstroth frames, are the most popular kind of frame used by apiculturists in the United States.

Whether you build your own beehive or purchase one, it should be built strongly and should contain accurate bee spaces and a close-fitting, rainproof roof. If you are looking to have honeycombs, you must have a hive that permits the insertion of up to eight combs.

Where Should the Hive Be Situated?

Hives and their stands should be placed in an enclosure where the bees will not be disturbed by other animals or humans and where it will be generally quiet. Hives should be placed on their own stands at least 3 feet from each other. Do not allow weeds to grow near the hives and keep the hives away from walls and fences. You, as the beekeeper, want to be able to easily access your hive without fear of obstacles.

Swarming

Swarming is simply the migration of honeybees to a new hive and is led by the queen bee. During swarming season (the warm summer days), a beekeeper must remain very alert. If you see swarming above the hive, take great care and act calmly and quietly. You want to get the swarm into your hive, but this will be tricky. It they land on a nearby branch or in a basket, simply approach and then "pour" them into the hive. Keep in mind that bees will more likely inhabit a cool, shaded hive than one that is baking in the hot summer sun.

Sometimes it is beneficial to try to prevent swarming, such as if you already have completely full hives Frequently removing the new honey from the hive before swarming begins will deter the bees from swarming. Shading the hives on warm days will also help keep the bees from swarming.

Bee Pastures

Bees will fly a great distance to gather food but you should try to contain them, as well as possible, to an area within 2 miles of the beehive. Make sure they have access to many honey-producing plants that you can grow in your garden. Alfalfa, asparagus, buckwheat, chestnut, clover, catnip, mustard, raspberry, roses, and sunflowers are some of the best honey-producing plants and trees. Also make sure that your bees always have access to pure, clean water.

Preparing Your Bees for Winter

If you live in a colder region of the United States, keeping your bees alive throughout the winter months is difficult. If your queen bee happens to die in the fall, before

Frame from a healthy beehive.

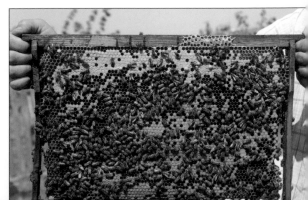

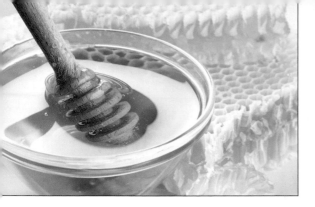

Raw honey is an anti-bacterial, anti-viral, and anti-fungal substance—besides being delicious.

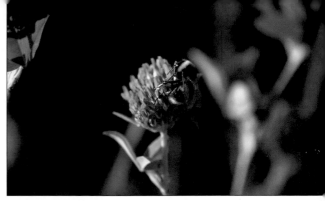

Bees thrive on sweet flowers, such as clover.

a young queen can be reared, your whole colony will die throughout the winter. However, the queen's death can be avoided by taking simple precautions and giving careful attention to your hive come autumn.

Colonies are usually lost in the winter months due to insufficient winter food storages, faulty hive construction, lack of protection from the cold and dampness, not enough or too much ventilation, or too many older bees and not enough young ones.

If you live in a region that gets a few weeks of severe weather, you may want to move your colony indoors, or at least to an area that is protected from the outside elements. But the essential components of having a colony survive through the winter season are to have a good queen; a fair ratio of healthy, young, and old bees; and a plentiful supply of food. The hive needs to retain a liberal supply of ripened honey and a thick syrup made from white cane sugar (you should feed this to your bees early enough so they have time to take the syrup and seal it over before winter).

To make this syrup, dissolve 3 pounds of granulated sugar in 1 quart of boiling water and add 1 pound of pure extracted honey to this. If you live in an extremely cold area, you may need up to 30 pounds of this syrup, depending on how many bees and hives you have. You can either use a top feeder or a frame feeder, which fits inside the hive in the place of a frame. Fill the frame with the syrup and place sticks or grass in it to keep the bees from drowning.

Extracting Honey

To obtain the extracted honey, you'll need to keep the honeycombs in one area of the hive or packed one above the other. Before removing the filled combs, you should allow the bees ample time to ripen and cap the honey. To uncap the comb cells, simply use a sharp knife (apiary suppliers sell knives specifically for this purpose). Then put the combs in a machine called a honey extractor to extract the honey. The honey extractor whips the honey out of the cells and allows you to replace the fairly undamaged comb into the hive to be repaired and refilled.

The extracted honey runs into open buckets or vats and is left, covered with a tea towel or larger cloth, to stand for a week. It should be in a warm, dry room where no ants can reach it. Skim the honey each day until it is perfectly clear. Then you can put it into cans, jars, or bottles for selling or for your own personal use.

Making Beeswax

Beeswax from the honeycomb can be used for making candles, can be added to lotions or lip balm, and can even be used in baking. Rendering wax in boiling water is especially simple when you only have a small apiary.

Collect the combs, break them into chunks, roll them into balls if you like, and put them in a muslin bag. Put the bag with the beeswax into a large stockpot and bring the water to a slow boil, making sure the bag doesn't rest on the bottom of the pot and burn. The muslin will act as a strainer for the wax. Use clean, sterilized tongs to occasionally squeeze the bag. After the wax is boiled out of the bag, remove the pot from the heat and allow it to cool. Then, remove the wax from the top of the water and then re-melt it in another pot on very low heat, so it doesn't burn.

Pour the melted wax into molds lined with wax paper or plastic wrap and then cool it before using it to make other items or selling it at your local farmers' market.

Extra Beekeeping Tips

General Tips

1. Clip the old queen's wings and go through the hives every 10 days to destroy queen cells to prevent swarming.
2. Always act and move calmly and quietly when handling bees.

Bees live off of the honey stored in the combs. In winter months they need a supply of ripe honey and benefit from extra sugary syrup.

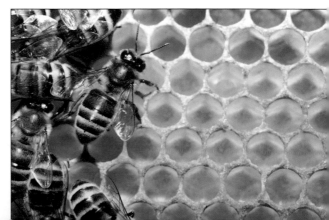

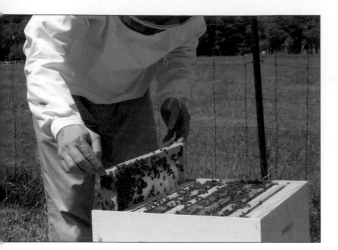

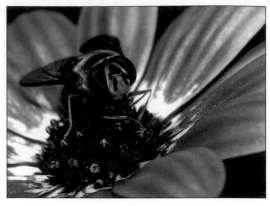

A beekeeper carefully removes frames from the hive.

3. Keep the hives cool and shaded. Bees won't enter a hot hive.

When Opening the Hive

1. Have a smoker ready to use if you desire.
2. Do not stand in front of the hive while the bees are entering and exiting.
3. Do not drop any tools into the hive while it's open.
4. Do not run if you become frightened.

5. If you are attacked, move away slowly and smoke the bees off yourself as you retreat.
6. Apply ammonia or a paste of baking soda and water immediately to any bee sting to relieve the pain. You can also scrape the area of the bee sting with your fingernail or the dull edge of a knife immediately after the sting.

When Feeding Your Bees

1. Keep a close watch over your bees during the entire season, to see if they are feeding well or not.
2. Feed the bees during the evening.

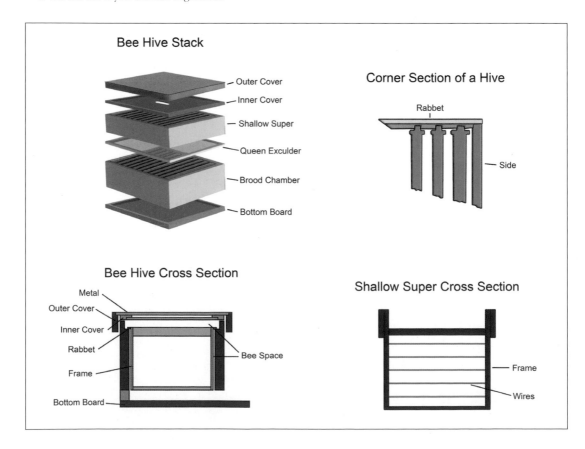

Bee Hive Stack

- Outer Cover
- Inner Cover
- Shallow Super
- Queen Exculder
- Brood Chamber
- Bottom Board

Corner Section of a Hive

Rabbet

- Side

Bee Hive Cross Section

Metal
Outer Cover
Inner Cover
Rabbet
Frame
Bottom Board

- Bee Space

Shallow Super Cross Section

- Frame
- Wires

3. Make sure the bees have ample water near their hive, especially in the spring.

Making a Beehive

The most important parts of constructing a beehive are to make it simple and sturdy. Just a plain box with a few frames and a couple of other loose parts will make a successful beehive that will be easy to use and manipulate. It is crucial that your beehive be well-adapted to the nature of bees and also the climate in which you live. Framed hives usually suffice for the beginning beekeeper. Below is a diagram of a simple beehive that you can easily construct for your backyard beekeeping purposes.

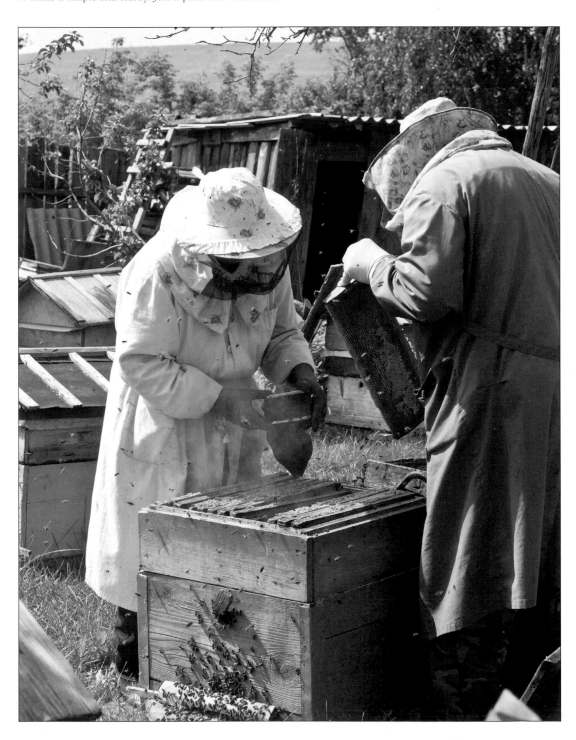

Goats

Goats provide us with milk and wool and thrive in arid, semitropical, and mountainous environments. In the more temperate regions of the world, goats are raised as supplementary animals, providing milk and cheese for families and acting as natural weed killers.

Breeds of Goats

There are many different types of goats. Some breeds are quite small (weighing roughly 20 pounds) and some are very large (weighing up to 250 pounds). Depending on the breed, goats may have horns that are corkscrew in shape, though many domestic goats are dehorned early on to lessen any potential injuries to humans or other goats. The hair of goats can also differ—various breeds have short hair, long hair, curly hair, silky hair, or coarse hair. Goats come in a variety of colors (solid black, white, brown, or spotted).

Feeding Goats

Goats can sustain themselves on bushes, trees, shrubs, woody plants, weeds, briars, and herbs. Pasture is the lowest-cost feed available for goats, and allowing goats to graze in the summer months is a wonderful and economic way to keep goats, even if your yard is small. Goats thrive best when eating alfalfa or a mixture of clover and timothy. If you have a lawn and a few goats, you don't need a lawn mower if you plant these types of plants for your goats to eat. The one drawback to this is that your goats (depending on how many you own) may quickly deplete these natural resources, which can cause weed growth and erosion. Supplementing pasture feed with other food-stuff, such as greenchop, root crops, and wet brewery grains will ensure that your yard does not become overgrazed and that your goats remain well-fed and healthy. It is also beneficial to supply your goats with unlimited access to hay while they are grazing. Make sure that your goats have easy access to shaded areas and fresh water, and offer a-salt-and mineral mix on occasion.

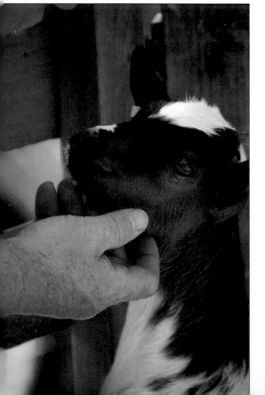

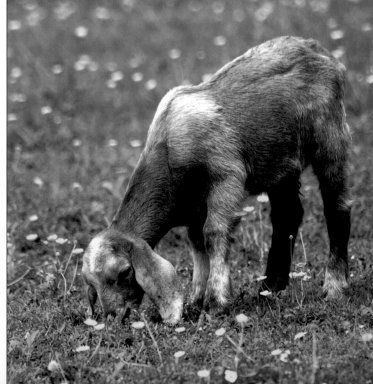

Six Major U.S. Goat Breeds

Alpine—Originally from Switzerland, these goats may have horns, are short haired, and are usually white and black in color. They are also good producers of milk.

Alpine goat

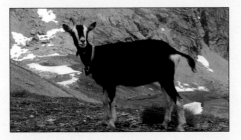

Anglo-Nubian—A cross between native English goats and Indian and Nubian breeds, these goats have droopy ears, spiral horns, and short hair. They are quite tall and do best in warmer climates. They do not produce as much milk, though it is much higher in fat than other goats'. They are the most popular breed of goat in the United States.

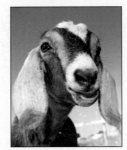

Anglo-Nubian goat

LaMancha—A cross between Spanish Murciana and Swiss and Nubian breeds, these goats are extremely adaptable, have straight noses, short hair, may have horns, and do not have external ears. They are not as good milk producers as the Saanen and Toggenburg breeds, and their milk fat content is much higher.

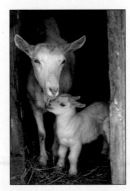

La Mancha goats

Pygmy—Originally from Africa and the Caribbean, these dwarfed goats thrive in hotter climates. For their size, they are relatively good producers of milk.

Pygmy goat

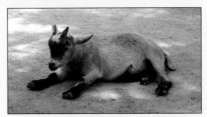

Saanen—Originally from Switzerland, these goats are completely white, have short hair, and sometimes have horns. Goats of this breed are wonderful milk producers.

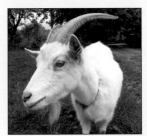

Saanen goat

Toggenburg—Originally from Switzerland, these goats are brown with white facial, ear, and leg stripes; have straight noses; may have horns; and have short hair. This breed is very popular in the United States. These goats are good milk producers in the summer and winter seasons and survive well in both temperate and tropical climates.

Toggenburg goat

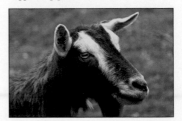

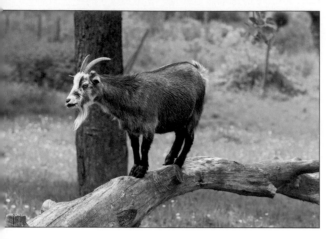

Goats enjoy having objects to climb on.

Dry forage is another good source of feed for your goats. It is relatively inexpensive to grow or buy and consists of good quality legume hay (alfalfa or clover). Legume hay is high in protein and has many essential minerals beneficial to your goats. To make sure your forages are highly nutritious, be sure that there are many leaves that provide protein and minerals and that the forage had an early cutting date, which will allow for easier digestion of the nutrients. If your forage is green in color, it most likely contains more vitamin A, which is good for promoting goat health.

Goat Milk

Goat milk is a wonderful substitute for those who are unable to tolerate cow's milk, or for the elderly, babies, and those suffering from stomach ulcers. Milk from goats is also high in vitamin A and niacin but does not have the same amount of vitamins B6, B12, and C as cow's milk.

Lactating goats do need to be fed the best quality legume hay or green forage possible, as well as grain. Give the grain to the doe at a rate that equals ½ pound grain for every pound of milk she produces.

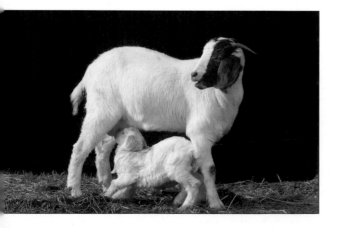

Common Diseases Affecting Goats

Goats tend to get more internal parasites than other herd animals. Some goats develop infectious arthritis, pneumonia, coccidiosis, scabies, liver fluke disease, and mastitis. It is advisable that you establish a relationship with a good veterinarian who specializes in small farm animals to periodically check your goats for various diseases.

Milking a Goat

Milking a goat takes some practice and patience, especially when you first begin. However, once you establish a routine and rhythm to the milking, the whole process should run relatively smoothly. The main thing to remember is to keep calm and never pull on the teat, as this will hurt the goat and she might upset the milk bucket. The goat will pick up on any anxiousness or nervousness on your part and it could affect how cooperative she is during the milking.

Supplies
- A grain bucket and grain for feeding the goat while milking is taking place
- Milking stand
- Metal bucket to collect the milk
- A stool to sit on (optional)
- A warm, sterilized wipe or cloth that has been boiled in water
- Teat dip solution (2 tbsp bleach, 1 quart water, one drop normal dish detergent mixed together)

Directions
1. Ready your milking stand by filling the grain bucket with enough grain to last throughout the entire milking. Then retrieve the goat, separating her from any other goats to avoid distractions and unsuccessful milking. Place the goat's head through the head hold of the milking stand so she can eat the grain and then close the lever so she cannot remove her head.
2. With the warm, sterilized wipe or cloth, clean the udder and teats to remove any dirt, manure, or bacteria that may be present. Then, place the metal bucket on the stand below the udder.
3. Wrap your thumb and forefinger around the base of one teat. This will help trap the milk in the teat so it can be squirted out. Then, starting with your middle finger, squeeze the three remaining fingers in one single, smooth motion to squirt the milk into the bucket. Be sure to keep a tight grip on the base of the teat so the milk stays there until extracted. Remember: The first squirt of milk from either teat should not be put into the bucket as it may contain dirt or bacteria that you don't want contaminating the milk.
4. Release the grip on the teat and allow it to refill with milk. While this is happening, you can repeat

this process on the other teat and alternate between teats to speed up the milking process.

6. When the teats begin to look empty (they will be somewhat flat in appearance), massage the udder just a little bit to see if any more milk remains. If so, squeeze it out in the same manner as above until you cannot extract much more.

7. Remove the milk bucket from the stand and then, with your teat dip mixture in a disposable cup, dip each teat into the solution and allow to air dry. This will keep bacteria and infection from going into the teat and udder.

8. Remove the goat from the milk stand and return her to the pen.

Making Cheese from Goat Milk

Most varieties of cheese that can be made from cow's milk can also be successfully made using goats' milk. Goats' milk cheese can easily be made at home. To make the cheese, however, at least one gallon of goat milk should be available. Make sure that all of your equipment is washed and sterilized (using heat is fine) before using it.

Cottage Cheese

1. Collect surplus milk that is free of strong odors. Cool it to around 40°F and keep it at that temperature until it is used.

2. Skim off any cream. Use the skim milk for cheese and the cream for cheese dressing.

3. If you wish to pasteurize your milk (which will allow it to hold better as a cheese) collect all the milk to be processed into a flat-bottomed, straight-sided pan and heat to 145°F on low heat. Hold it at this temperature for about 30 minutes and then cool to around 80°F. Use a dairy thermometer to measure the milk's temperature. Then, inoculate the cheese milk with a desirable lactic acid–fermenting bacterial culture (you can use commercial buttermilk for the initial source). Add about 7 ounces to 1 gallon of cheese milk, stir well, and let it sit undisturbed for about 10 to 16 hours, until a firm curd is formed.

4. When the curd is firm enough, cut the curd into uniform cubes no larger than ½ inch using a knife or spatula.

5. Allow the curd to sit undisturbed for a couple of minutes and then warm it slowly, stirring carefully, at a temperature no greater than 135°F. The curd should eventually become firm and free from whey.

6. When the curd is firm, remove from the heat and stop stirring. Siphon off the excess whey from the top of the pot. The curd should settle to the bottom of the container. If the curd is floating, bacteria that produces gas has been released and a new batch must be made.

7. Replace the whey with cold water, washing the curd and then draining the water. Wash again with ice-cold water to chill the curd. This will keep the flavor fresh.

8. Using a draining board, drain the excess water from the curd. Now your curd is complete.

9. To make the curd into a cottage cheese consistency, separate the curd as much as possible and mix with a milk or cream mixture containing salt to taste.

Domiati Cheese

This type of cheese is made throughout the Mediterranean region. It is eaten fresh or aged two to three months before consumption.

1. Cool a gallon of fresh, quality milk to around 105°F, adding 8 ounces of salt to the milk. Stir the salt until it is completely dissolved.

2. Pasteurize the milk as described in step 3 of the cottage cheese recipe.

3. This type of cheese is coagulated by adding a protease enzyme (rennet). This enzyme may be purchased at a local drug store, health food store, or a cheese maker in your area. Dissolve the concentrate in water, add it to the cheese milk, and stir for a few minutes. Use 1 milliliter of diluted rennet liquid in 40 milliliters of water for every 2½ gallons of cheese milk.

4. Set the milk at around 105°F. When the enzyme is completely dispersed in the cheese milk, allow the mix to sit undisturbed until it forms a firm curd.

5. When the desired firmness is reached, cut the curd into very small cubes. Allow for some whey separation. After 10 to 20 minutes, remove and reserve about ⅓ the volume of salted whey.

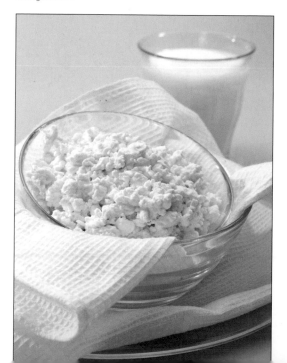

Cottage cheese

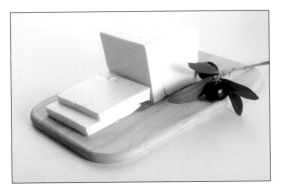

Damiati cheese

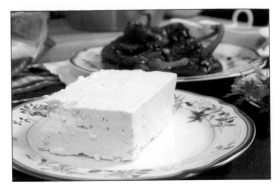

Feta cheese

6. Put the curd and remaining whey into cloth-lined molds (the best are rectangular stainless steel containers with perforated sides and bottom) with a cover. The molds should be between 7 and 10 inches in height. Fill the molds with the curd, fold the cloth over the top, allow the whey to drain, and discard the whey.

7. Once the curd is firm enough, apply added weight for 10 to 18 hours until it is as moist as you want.

8. Once the pressing is complete and the cheese is formed into a block, remove the molds and cut the blocks into 4-inch-thick pieces. Place the pieces in plastic containers with airtight seals. Fill the

containers with reserved salted whey from step 5, covering the cheese by about an inch.

9. Place these containers at a temperature between 60°F and 65°F to cure for 1 to 4 months.

Feta Cheese

This type of cheese is very popular to make from goats' milk. The same process is used as the Domiati cheese except that salt is not added to the milk before coagulation. Feta cheese is aged in a brine solution after the cubes have been salted in a brine solution for at least 24 hours.

Angora Goats

Angora goats may be the most efficient fiber producers in the world. The hair of these goats is made into mohair: a long, lustrous hair that is woven into fine garments. Angora goats are native to Turkey and were imported to the United States in the mid-1800s. Now, the United States is one of the two biggest produces of mohair on earth.

Angora goats are typically relaxed and docile. They are delicate creatures, easily strained by their year-round fleeces. Angora goats need extra attention and are more high-maintenance than other breeds of goat. While these goats can adapt to many temperate climates, they do particularly well in the arid environment of the southwestern states.

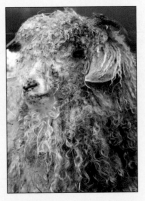

Angora goats can be sheared twice yearly, before breeding and before birthing. The hair of the goat will grow about ¾ inch per month and it should be sheared once it reaches 4 to 6 inches in length. During the shearing process, the goat is usually lying down on a clean floor with its legs tied. When the fleece is gathered (it should be sheared in one full piece), it should be bundled into a burlap bag and should be free of contaminants. Mark your name on the bag and make sure there is only one fleece per bag. For more thorough rules and regulations about selling mohair through the government's direct-payment program, contact the USDA Agricultural Stabilization and Conservation Service online or in one of their many offices.

Shearing can be accomplished with the use of a special goat comb, which leaves ¼ inch of stubble on the goat. It is important to keep the fleeces clean and to avoid injuring the animal. The shearing seasons are in the spring and fall. After a goat has been sheared, it will be more sensitive to changes in the weather for up to six weeks. Make sure you have proper warming huts for these goats in the winter and adequate shelter from rain and inclement weather.

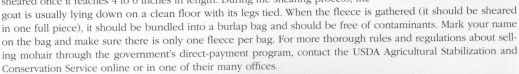

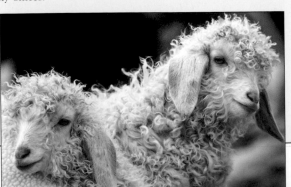

Sheep

Sheep were possibly the first domesticated animals and are now found all over the world on farms and smaller plots of land. Almost all the breeds of sheep that are found in the United States have been brought here from Great Britain. Raising sheep is relatively easy, as they only need pasture to eat, shelter from bad weather, and protection from predators. Sheep's wool can be used to make yarn or other articles of clothing and their milk can be made into various types of cheeses and yogurt, though this is not normally done in the United States.

Sheep are naturally shy creatures and are extremely docile. If they are treated well, they will learn to be affectionate with their owner. If a sheep is comfortable with its owner, it will be much easier to manage and to corral into its pen if it's allowed to graze freely. Start with only one or two sheep; they are not difficult to manage but do require a lot of attention.

Breeds of Sheep

There are many different breeds of sheep—some are used exclusively for their meat and others for their wool. Six quality wool-producing breeds are as follows:

1. Cotswold Sheep—This breed is very docile and hardy and thrives well in pastures. It produces around 14 pounds of fleece per year, making it a very profitable breed for anyone wanting to sell wool.
2. Leicester sheep—This is a hardy, docile breed of sheep that is a very good grazer. This breed has 6-inch-long, coarse wool that is desirable for knitting. It is a very popular breed in the United States.
3. Merino sheep—Introduced to the United States in the early twentieth century, this small- to medium-sized sheep has lots of rolls and folds of fine white wool and produces a fleece anywhere between 10 and 20 pounds. It is considered a fine-wool specialist, and though its fleece appears dark in color, the wool is actually white or buff. It is a wonderful foraging sheep, is hardy, and has a gentle disposition, but is not a very good milk producer.
4. Oxford Down sheep—A more recent breed, these dark-faced sheep have hardy constitutions and good fleece.
5. Shropshire sheep—This breed has longer, more open, and coarser fleece than other breeds. It is quite popular in the United States, especially in areas that are more moist and damp, as they seem to be better in these climates than other breeds of sheep.
6. Southdown sheep—One of the oldest breeds of sheep, these sheep are popular for their good quality wool and are deemed the standard of excellence for many sheep owners. Docile, hardy, and good grazing on pastures, their coarse and light-colored wool is used to make flannel.

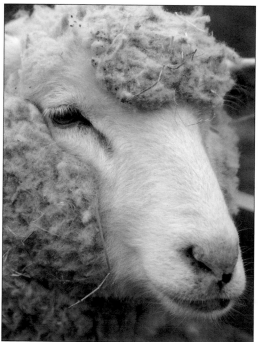

Housing Sheep

Sheep do not require much shelter—only a small shed that is open on one side (preferably to the south so it can stay warmer in the winter months) and is roughly 6 to 8 feet high. The shelter should be ventilated well to reduce any unpleasant smells and to keep the sheep cool in the summer. Feeding racks or mangers should be placed inside of the shed to hold the feed for the sheep. If you live in a

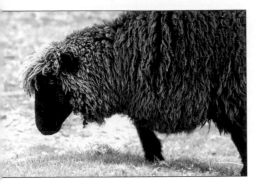

Cotswold sheep

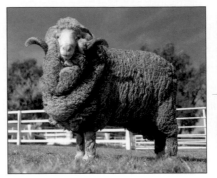

Merino sheep

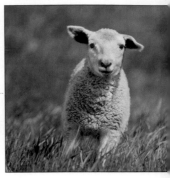

Southdown sheep

colder region of the country, building a sturdier, warmer shed for the sheep to live in during the winter is recommended.

Straw should be used for the sheep's bedding and should be changed daily to make sure the sheep do not become ill from an unclean shelter. Especially for the winter months, a dry pen should be erected for the sheep to exercise in. The fences should be strong enough to keep out predators that may enter your yard and to keep the sheep from escaping.

What Do Sheep Eat?

Sheep generally eat grass and are wonderful grazers. They utilize rough and scanty pasturage better than other grazing animals and, due to this, they can actually be quite beneficial in cleaning up a yard that is overgrown with undesirable herbage. Allowing sheep to graze in your yard or in a small pasture field will provide them with sufficient food in the summer months. Sheep also eat a variety of weeds, briars, and shrubs. Fresh water should always be available for the sheep.

Especially during the winter months, when grass is scarce, sheep should be fed hay (alfalfa, legume, or clover hay) and small quantities of grain. Corn is also a good winter food for the sheep (it can also be mixed with wheat bran), and straw, salt, and roots can also be occasionally added to their diet. Good food during the winter season will help the sheep grow a healthier and thicker wool coat.

Shearing Sheep

Sheep are generally sheared in the spring or early summer before the weather gets too warm. To do your own shearing, invest in a quality hand shearer and a scale on which to weigh the fleece. An experienced shearer should be able to take the entire wool off in one piece.

You may want to wash the wool a few days to a week before shearing the sheep. To do so, corral the sheep into a pen on a warm spring day (make sure there isn't a cold breeze blowing and that there is a lot of sunshine so the sheep does not become chilled). Douse the sheep in warm water, scrub the wool, and rinse. Repeat this a few times until most of the dirt and debris is out of the wool. Diffuse some natural oil throughout the wool to make it softer and ready for shearing.

Leicester sheep   Shropshire sheep

Oxford down sheep

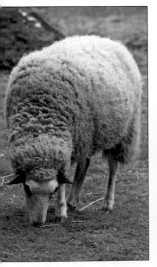

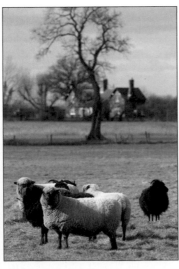

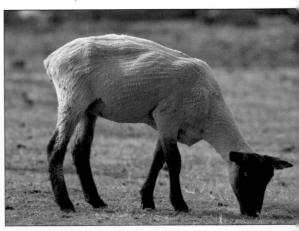

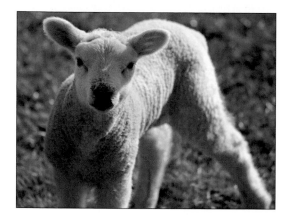

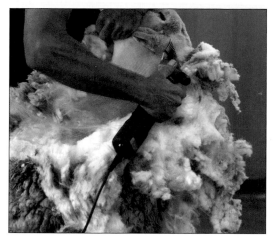

Sheer your sheep in the spring or early summer, before the weather gets hot.

The sheep should be completely dry before shearing and you should choose a warm—but not overly hot—day. If you are a beginner at shearing sheep, try to find an experienced sheep owner to show you how to properly hold and shear a sheep. This way, you won't cause undue harm to the sheep's skin and will get the best fleece possible. When you are hand-shearing a sheep, remember to keep the skin pulled taut on the part where you are shearing to decrease the potential of cutting the skin.

Once the wool is sheared, tag it and roll it up by itself, and then bind it with twine. Be sure not to fold it or bind it too tightly. Separate and remove any dirty or soiled parts of the fleece before binding, as these parts will not be able to be carded and used.

Carding and Spinning Wool

To make the sheared wool into yarn you will need only a few tools: a spinning wheel or drop spindle and wool-cards. Wool-cards are rectangular pieces of thin board that have many wire teeth attached to them (they look like coarse brushes that are sometimes used for dogs'

Wod-cards are used to soften and clean the wod fibers.

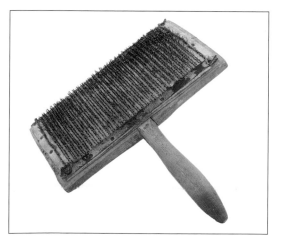

hair). To begin, you must clean the wool fleece of any debris, feltings, or other imperfections before carding it; otherwise your yarn will not spin correctly. Also wash it to remove any additional sand or dirt embedded in the wool and then allow it to dry completely. Then, all you need is to gather your supplies and follow these simple instructions:

Carding Wool

1. Grease the wool with rape oil or olive oil, just enough to work into the fibers.
2. Take one wool-card in your left hand, rest it on your knee, gather a tuft of wool from the fleece, and place it onto the wool-card so it is caught between the wired teeth of the card.

Spinning on a traditional spinning wheel

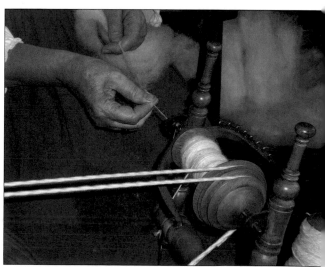

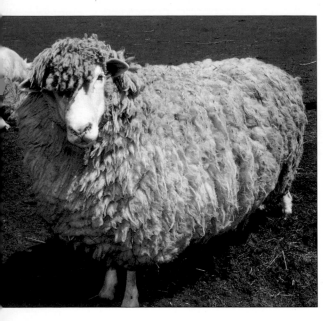

3. Take the second wool-card in your right hand and bring it gently across the other card several times, making a brushing movement toward your body.
4. When the fibers are all brushed in the same direction and the wool is soft and fluffy to the touch, remove the wool by rolling it into a small, fleecy ball (roughly a foot or more in length and only 2 inches in width) and put it in a bag until it is used for spinning.

Note: Carded wool can also be used for felting, in which case no spinning is needed. To felt a small blanket, place large amounts of carded wool on either side of a burlap sack. Using felting needles, weave the wool into the burlap until it is tightly held by the jute or hemp fabrics of the burlap.

Spinning Wool

1. Take one long roll of carded wool and wind the fibers around the spindle.
2. Move the wheel gently and hold the spindle to allow the wool to "draw," or start to pull together into a single thread.
3. Keep moving the wheel and allow the yarn to wind around the spindle or a separate spool, if you have a more complex spinning wheel.
4. Keep adding rolls of carded wool to the spindle until you have the desired amount of yarn.

Note: If you are unable to obtain a spinning wheel of any kind, you can spin your carded wool by hand, although this will not produce the same tightness in your yarn as regular spinning. All you need to do is take the carded wool, hold it with one hand, and pull and twist the fibers into one, continuous piece. Winding the end of the yarn around a stick, spindle, or spool and securing it in place at the end will help keep your fibers tight and your yarn twisted.

If you want your yarn to be different colors, try dying it with natural berry juices or with special wool dyes found in arts and crafts stores.

Milking Sheep

Sheep's milk is not typically used in the United States for drinking, making cheese, or other familiar dairy products. Sheep do not typically produce milk year-round, as cows do, so milk will only be produced if you bred your sheep and had a lamb produced. If you do have a sheep that has given birth and the lamb has been sold or taken away, it is important to know how to milk her so her udders do not become caked. Some ewes will still have an abundance of milk even after their lambs have been weaned and this excess milk should be removed to keep the ewe healthy and her udder free from infection.

To milk an ewe, bring her rear up to a fence so she cannot step backwards and, placing two knees against her shoulders to prevent her from moving forward, reach under with both hands and squeeze the milk into a bucket. When the udder is still soft but the ewe has been partly milked out, set her loose and then milk her again a few days later. If there is still milk to be had, wait another three days and then milk her again. By milking the ewes in this manner, you can prevent their udders from becoming infected and the milk from spoiling.

Diseases

The main diseases to which sheep are susceptible are foot rot and scabs. These are contagious and both require proper treatment. Sheep may also acquire stomach worms if they eat hay that has gotten too damp or has been lying on the floor of their shelter. As always, it is best to establish a relationship with a veterinarian who is familiar with caring for sheep and have your flock regularly checked for any parasites or diseases that may arise.

Llamas

Llamas make excellent pets and are a great source of wooly fiber (their wool can be spun into yarn). Llamas are being kept more and more by people in the United States as companion animals, sources of fiber, pack and light plow animals, therapy animals for the elderly, "guards" for other backyard animals, and good educational tools for children. Llamas have an even temperament and are very intelligent. Their intelligence and gentle nature make them easy to train, and their hardiness allows them to thrive well in both cold and warmer climates (although they can have heat stress in extremely hot and humid parts of the country).

Before you decide to purchase a llama or two for your yard, check your state requirements regarding livestock. In some places, your property must also be zoned for livestock.

Llamas come in many different colors and sizes. The average adult llama is between 5½ and 6 feet tall and weighs between 250 and 450 pounds. Llamas, being herd animals, like the company of other llamas, so it is advisable that you raise a pair to keep each other company. If you only want to care for one llama, then it would be best to also have a sheep, goat, or other animal that can be penned with the llama for camaraderie. Although llamas can be led well on a harness and lead, never tie one up as it could potentially break its own neck trying to break free.

Llamas tend to make their own communal dung heap in a particular part of their pen. This is quite convenient for cleanup and allows you to collect the manure, compost it, and use it as a fertilizer for your garden.

Feeding Llamas

Llamas can subsist fairly well on grass, hay (an adult male will eat about one bale per week), shrubs, and trees, much like sheep and goats. If they are not receiving enough nutrients, they may be fed a mixture of rolled corn, oats, and barley, especially during the winter season when grazing is not necessarily available. Make sure not to overfeed your llamas, though, or they will become overweight and constipated. You can occasionally give cornstalks to your llamas as an added source of fiber, and you may add mineral supplements to the feed mixture or hay if you want. Salt blocks are also acceptable to have in your llama pen, and a constant supply of fresh water is necessary. Nursing female llamas should receive a grain mixture until the cria (baby) is weaned.

Be sure to keep feed and hay off the ground. This will help ward off parasites that establish themselves in the feed and are then ingested by the llamas.

Housing Your Llamas

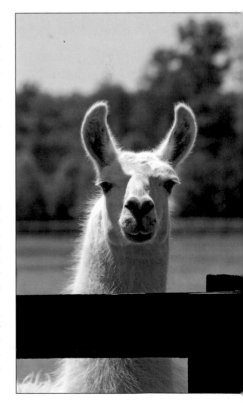

Llamas may be sheltered in a small stable or even a converted garage. There should be enough room to store feed and hay, and the shelter should be able to be closed off during wet, windy, and cold weather. Llamas prefer light, open spaces in which to live, so make sure your shed or shelter has large doors and/or big windows. The feeders for the hay and grain mixture should be raised above the ground. Adding a place where a llama can be safely restrained for toenail clippings and vet checkups will help facilitate these processes but is not absolutely necessary.

The llamas should be able to enter and exit the shelter easily and it is a good idea to build a fence or pen around the shelter so they do not wander off. A fence about four feet tall should be enough to keep your llamas safe and enclosed. If you happen to have both a male and female llama, it is necessary to have separate enclosures for them to stave off unwanted pregnancies.

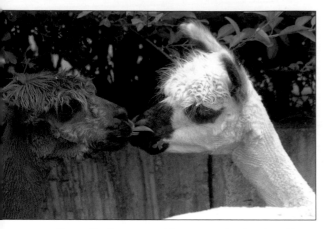

Alpacas, like llamas, are social creatures and are happiest with other alpacas.

Toenail Trimming

Llamas need their toenails to be trimmed so they do not twist and fold under the toe, making it difficult for the llama to move around. Laying gravel in the area where your llamas frequently walk will help to keep the toenails naturally trimmed, but if you need to cut them, be careful not to cut too deeply or you may cause the tip of the toe to bleed and this could lead to an infection in the toe. Use shears designed for this purpose to cut the nails. Use one hand to hold the llama's "ankle" just above where the foot bends. Hold the clippers in your other hand, cutting away from the foot toward the tip of the nail. The nail's are easiest to clip in the early morning or after a rain, since the wetness of the ground will soften them.

Shearing

It is important to groom and shear your llama, especially during hot weather. Brushing the llama's coat to remove

Llamas enjoy hay, but keep it off the ground to help prevent your llamas from ingesting parasites.

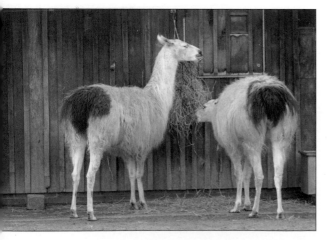

dirt and keep it from matting will not only make your llamas look clean and healthy but it will also improve the quality of their coats. If you want to save the fibers for spinning into yarn, it is best to brush, comb, and use a hair dryer to remove any dust and debris from the llama's coat before you begin shearing.

Shearing is not necessarily difficult, but if you are a first-time llama owner, you should ask another llama farmer to teach you how to properly shear your llama. To shear your llama, you can purchase battery-operated shears to remove the fibers for sale or use. Different llamas will respond in different ways to shearing. Try holding the llama with a halter and lead in a smaller area to begin the shearing process. Do not completely remove the llama from any other llamas you have, though, as their presence will help calm the llama you are shearing. It is best to have another person with you to aid in the shearing (to hold the llama, give it treats, and offer any other help). When shearing a llama, don't shear all the way down to the skin. Allowing a thin coating of hair to cover the llama's body will help protect it from the sun and from being scratched when it rolls in the dirt.

Start by shearing a flat top the length of the llama's back. Next, taking the shears in one hand, move them in a downward position to remove the coat. Shear a strip the length of the neck from the chin to the front legs about 3 inches wide to help cool the llama. Shearing can take a long time, so it may be necessary for both you and the llama to take a break. Take the llama for a quiet walk and allow it to go to the bathroom so it will not become antsy during the rest of the shearing process.

Collect the sheared fibers in a container and make sure you are working on a clean floor so you can collect any excess fibers and use them for spinning. Do not store the fiber in a plastic bag, as moisture can easily accumulate, ruining the fiber and making it unusable for spinning.

Caring for the Cria

Baby llamas require some additional care in their first few days of life. It is important for the cria to receive the

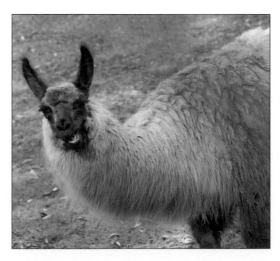

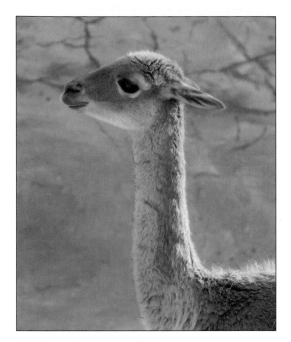

Baby llamas and alpacas are called "Crias."

colostrum milk from their mothers, but you may need to aid in this process. Approach the mother llama and pull gently on each teat to remove the waxy plugs covering the milk holes. Sometimes, you may need to guide the cria into position under its mother for it start nursing.

Weigh the cria often (at least for the first month) to see that it's gaining weight and growing strong and healthy. A bathroom scale, hanging scale, or larger grain scale can be used for this.

If the cria seems to need extra nourishment, goat or cow milk can be substituted during times when the mother llama cannot produce enough milk for the cria. Feed this additional milk to the cria in small doses, several times a day, from a milking bottle.

Diseases

Llamas are prone to getting worms and should be checked often to make sure they do not have any of these parasites. There is special worming paste that can be mixed in with their food to prevent worms from infecting them. You should also establish a relationship with a good veterinarian who knows about caring for llamas and can determine if there are any other vaccinations necessary in order to keep your llamas healthy. Other diseases and pests that can affect llamas are tuberculosis, tetanus, ticks, mites, and lice.

Using Llama Fibers

Llama fiber is unique from other animal fibers, such as sheep's wool. It does not contain any lanolin (an oil found in sheep's wool); thus, it is hypoallergenic and not as greasy. How often you can shear your llama will depend on the variety of llama, its health, and environmental conditions. Typically, though, every year llamas grow a fleece that is 4 to 6 inches long and that weighs between 3 and 7 pounds. Llama fiber can be used like any other animal fiber or wool, making it the perfect substitute for all of your fabric and spinning needs.

Llama fiber is made up of two parts: the undercoat (which provides warmth for the llama) and the guard hair (which protects the llama from rain and snow). The undercoat is the most desirable part to use due to its soft, downy texture, while the coarser guard hair is usually discarded.

Gathering llama hair is easy. To harvest the fiber, you must shear the llama. However, the steps involved in shearing when you are gathering the fiber are slightly different than when you are simply shearing to keep the llama cooler in the summer months. To shear a llama for fiber collection:

1. Clean the llama by blowing and brushing until the coat is free from dirt and debris.
2. Wash the llama. Be sure to rinse out all of the soap from the hair and let the llama air-dry.
3. You can use scissors or commercial clippers to shear the llama. Start at the top of the back, behind the head and neck and work backwards. If using clippers, shear with long sweeping motions, not short jerky ones. If using scissors, always point them downward. Leave about an inch of wool on the llama for protection against the sun and insect bites. You can shear just the area around the back and belly (in front of the hind legs and behind the front legs) if your main purpose is to offer the llama relief from the heat. Or you can shear the entire llama—from just below the head, down to the tail—to get the most wool. Once the shearing is complete, skirt the fleece by removing any little pieces or belly hair from the shorn fleece.

The fiber can be hand-processed or sent to a mill (though sending the fibers to a mill is much more expensive and is not necessary if you have only one or two llamas). Processing the fiber by hand is definitely more cost-effective but you will initially need to invest in some

Llama fiber can be dyed and spun to be used for knitting.

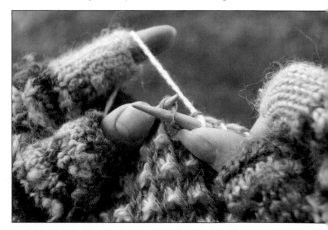

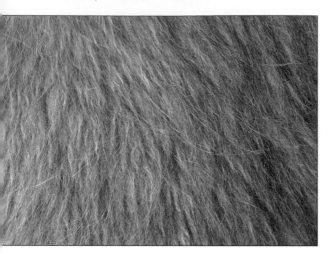

Llamas should be washed and allowed to air dry before shearing.

equipment (such as a spinning wheel, drop spindle, or felting needle).

To process the fiber by hand:

1. Pick out any remaining debris and unwanted (coarse) fibers.
2. Card the fiber. This helps to separate the fiber and will make spinning much easier. To card the fiber, put a bit of fiber on one end of the cards (standard wool-cards do the trick nicely) and gently brush it until it separates. This will produce a rolag (log) of fiber.
3. Once the fiber is carded, you can use it in a few different ways:

   a. Wet felting: To wet felt, lay the fiber out in a design between 2 pieces of material and soak it in hot, soapy water. Then, agitate the fiber by rubbing or rolling it. This will cause it to stick together. Rinse the fiber in cold water. When it dries, you will have produced a strong piece of felt that can be used in many crafting projects.

   b. Needle felting: For this type of manipulation, you will need a felting needle (available at your local arts and crafts or fabric store). Lay out a piece of any material you want over a pillow or Styrofoam piece. Place the fiber on top of the material in any design of your choosing. Push the needle through the fiber and the bottom material and then gently draw it back out. Continue this process until the fiber stays on the material of its own accord. This is a great way to make table runners or hanging cloths using your llama fiber.

   c. Spinning: Spinning is a great way to turn your llama fiber into yarn. Spinning can be accomplished by using either a spinning wheel or drop spindle, and a piece of fiber that is either in a batt, rolag, or roving. A spinning wheel, while larger and more expensive, will easily help you to turn the fiber into yarn. A drop spindle is convenient because it is smaller and easier to transport, and if you have time and patience, it will do just as good a job as the spinning wheel. To make yarn, twist two or more pieces of spun wool together.

   d. Other uses: carded wool can also be used to weave, knit, or crochet.

If you become very comfortable using llama fiber to make clothing or other craft items, you may want to try to sell these crafts (or your llama fiber directly) to consumers. Fiber crafts may be particularly successful if sold at local craft markets or even at farmers' markets alongside your garden produce.

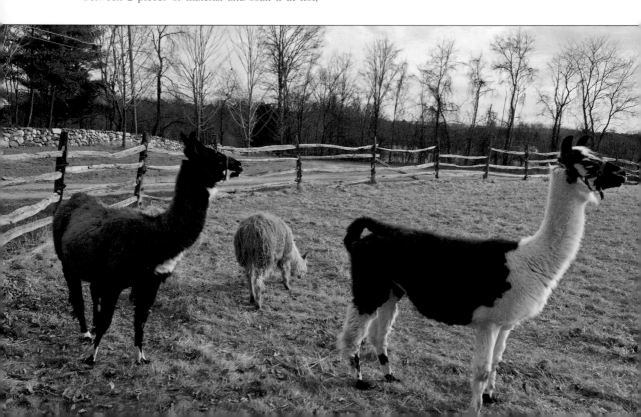

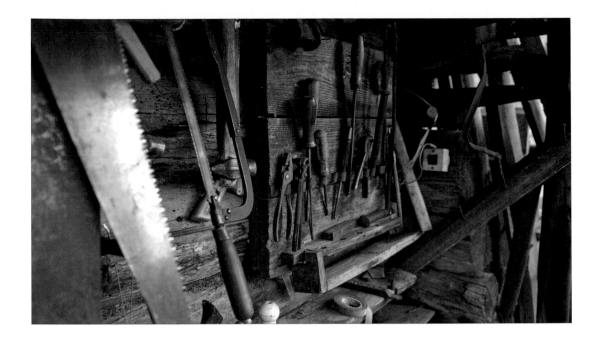

PART FOUR

Simple Structures for Your Land

"Regard it as just as desirable to build a chicken house as to build a cathedral."

—*Frank Lloyd Wright*

"Develop an infallible technique and then place yourself at the mercy of inspiration."

—*Lao-Tzu*

Even if you only have a small plot of land, it may be helpful to have a modest potting shed near your garden or a workshop where you can keep your tools. If you'll be raising animals, you'll need shelter for them—even a dog deserves a house it can call its own. Some of the projects in this chapter offer step-by-step instructions that will guide you through the entire building process. Others are meant to offer guidelines for a structure, which you can then alter to meet your own wants and needs. If you are new to woodworking, you may want to start off with one of the simpler projects, such as a birdhouse, and then progress to more complex structures as you build confidence. Follow the directions closely, measure materials carefully, and cross-reference with similar plans found online or in other books when needed. If you're an experienced builder, use the directions and illustrations here as inspiration to create your own unique masterpieces. Whatever your skill level, as with everything, try to enjoy the process as much as the end result.

Doghouses

Dog houses and kennels are easy to construct and are especially useful if you have dogs that primarily live out of doors. A dog kennel needs to protect the dog from harsh winds and heavy rains and should be spacious enough for the dog to move around in comfortably. Doghouses should be located near to your own house, so you can have easy access to your pet, and should be situated on a side of your house that creates a natural barrier from the wind and weather. Dogs should not be left outside overnight in very cold weather, even with access to a doghouse. Below are a couple of doghouses and kennels that can be easily constructed for your outdoor pet.

Standard Dog Kennel

This kennel is constructed to be warm and windproof, to direct the rain away from the base by creating large roof overhangs, and to be easily cleaned.

Materials
- Matched boards for the sides, ends, and bottom (standard measurements for the kennel are 30 inches long, 20 inches wide, and 30 inches tall)
- Weather boards for the roof
- Strip of sheet metal
- Wooden beading

Directions
1. Make the ends first by nailing lengths of matching boards across uprights of 2 x 1-inch batten *(f)*. At the top, halve the battens into the two roof pieces. Set the two outer uprights, X X, in about ¾ inch from the edges to allow the sides to be flush with the outside of the ends. Place these four uprights on the inside.
2. It is advisable to cut out the door—using a pad-saw for the semicircular top—before nailing on Y Y, which should be a little nearer to one another than are the rough edges of the door. Two short verticals on the outside, also projecting beyond the edges, prevent the dog injuring his coat on them. Pieces Z Z give the door a neat finish.

The dog house is wider and has the door set off to one side, which allows for even more protection from the elements.

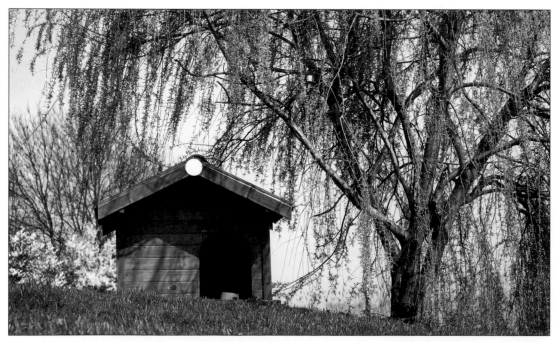

3. The battens may be omitted from the back end of the kennel, but they ultimately help strengthen the structure and so are advisable to include.

4. When the ends are finished, the horizontal boards for the sides are nailed on to each end (b). Begin at the bottom, arranging the lowest board with its tongue pointing upwards and add the upper boards one by one. The direction in which the tongue points is an important detail—if the boards are put on the wrong way, water will leak more easily into the kennel, rotting the boards and making your dog wet.

5. Battens (d) and (e) are nailed inside along the sides of the kennel and a third is nailed across the back, at a distance above the bottom edge equal to the thickness of the bottom boards and of the battens (b) and (c), to which they are attached. At each end a 2 x 2-inch deal, (f), is screwed to (b) and (c) to raise the bottom clear off the ground.

6. The roof weather boards must be long enough to project at least 6 inches beyond the door end, to prevent rain from coming through the entrance. The eaves overhang 3 inches and are supported, as shown in (a), by three brackets cut out of hard wood. Begin laying on the boards, starting at the eaves and finishing at the ridge, which is closed with a 6-inch strip of sheet metal placed on top of a wooden beading.

7. Stain all the exterior surfaces, including the bottom, and fill in the cracks with caulking to keep the water from seeping through.

The inside part of the kennel should be exposed to the sun occasionally by being turned on its end, and the bottom should be cleaned often.

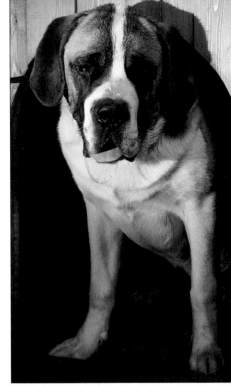

Modify the dog kennel plans here to fit your dog if it is a larger breed.

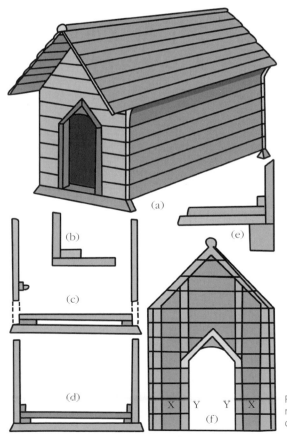

(a)

(b)

(c)

(d)

(e)

(f)

X Y   Y X

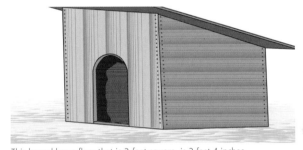

This kennel has a floor that is 2 feet square, is 3 feet 4 inches high in front, and the roof has an overhang of 8 inches.

Refer to this illustration when making the dog kennel. The kennel raised off the ground is shown by (c); (d) illustrates the parts in contact; (e) is a vertical section of the back end.

Birdhouses

If you are looking to attract birds to your yard during the spring, summer, and fall months, in particular, it is important to have shelter for the birds. Birdhouses do not need to be very elaborate and they should be rather inconspicuous so birds can easily come and go without attracting predators to their house and nest. All that is really required of a birdhouse is a good hiding place, with an opening just large enough for the bird to fit through, and a strong roof that keeps out the rain.

Birdhouses can be made from a variety of materials—even an old hat tacked to the side of a shed with a hole cut in the top can suffice for a birdhouse. Other usable materials include tin cans, barrels, flowerpots, wooden buckets, and small boxes (preferably wooden or metal).

Most standard birdhouses are made of wood pieces nailed together to look like a miniature house. If you are looking to have many birds nesting in your yard, you may want to build a few birdhouses during the winter so they can be ready for springtime, when birds are beginning to nest. To attract a particular kind of bird to your birdhouse, you must make the size of the hole appropriate for the type of bird. For wrens, make the hole about 1 inch; for bluebirds and tree-swallows, the hole should be 1½ inches; for martins, it should be 2½ inches. Below are a few examples of birdhouses you can easily make to attract beautiful birds to your yard.

Be creative with your birdhouse designs, experimenting with different shapes and materials.

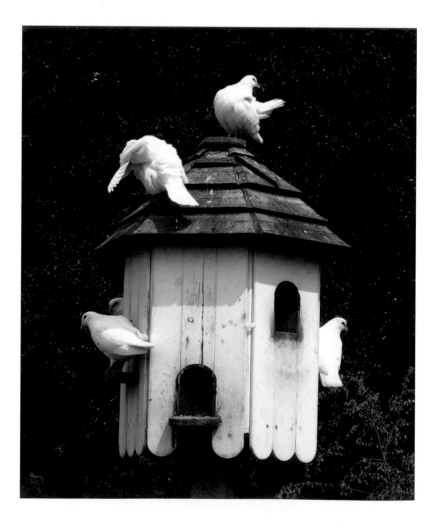

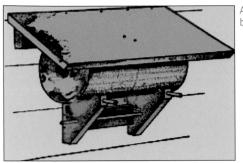

A bird ark birdhouse

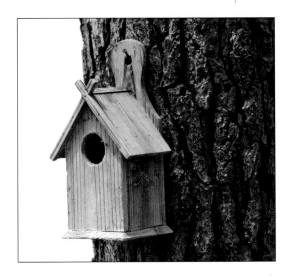

Bird Ark Birdhouse

This birdhouse is constructed of three tin cans joined together. Both ends of the center can are removed, but the bottom is left on both end cans. To make the bird ark, simply:

1. Cut a hole into the side of the center can and another through the bottom of each can. Do not remove the pieces of tin but bend them out to serve as perches.
2. Cut the roof boards of the correct size to project over the ends and sides about 1 inch, nail them together, and then fasten them in place by nailing the boards to the connecting blocks between the cans.
3. Fasten the ark between the blocks on a platform or board and then mount the platform on post supports and brace it with brackets, as seen in the picture above. Attach several sticks for perches.

Log Cabin Birdhouse

This birdhouse can be made out of any sized box. Nail pieces together to form the roof, and then thatch the roofing itself to blend into the surrounding environment. The more sloped the roof, the easier the rain can fall off

and not penetrate into the house. This house is slightly more elaborate in the sense that the support pole passes through the house to form a "chimney." The windows can be cut out and fake doors painted on for aesthetic purposes. Small branches should be cut to the proper lengths, split, and then nailed all over the exterior of the house to produce a sort of "log cabin" look—this also helps the birdhouse to better blend into the surrounding trees and foliage in your yard.

Temple Birdhouse

This is a small birdhouse, perfect for wrens. This birdhouse hangs from a tree branch.

Materials
- Large tin can
- Wooden board about 7 inches square
- Carpet or upholstery tacks
- Earthen flowerpot
- Small cork to plug up the flowerpot hole
- Eye screw
- Short stick
- Wire
- Small nails

Cross section of a log cabin birdhouse

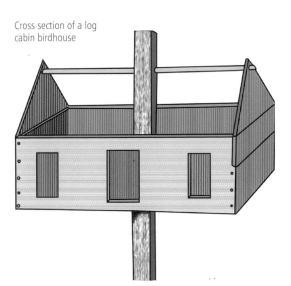

Temple birdhouse

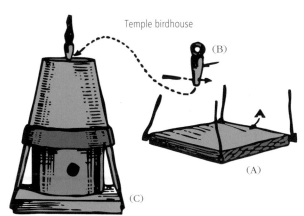

(A)

(B)

(C)

Directions

1. Mark the doorway on the side of the can and cut the opening with a can opener.
2. Fasten the can to the square baseboard (A) by driving large carpet tacks through the bottom of the can into the board.
3. Invert the flowerpot to make the roof. Plug up the drain hole to make the house waterproof (use a cork or other means of stopping up the hole) (B).
4. Screw the eye screw into the top of the plug to attach the suspending wire. Drill a small hole through the lower end of the plug so that a short nail can be pushed through after the plug has been inserted to keep it from coming out.
5. Fasten the flowerpot over the can with wire, passing the loop of wire entirely around the pot and then running short wires from this wire down to small nails driven into the four corners of the base, (C).
6. Now the bird temple can be painted and hung on a tree.

Birdhouses for Specific Bird Species

Species	Floor of cavity (inches)	Depth of cavity (inches)	Entrance above floor (inches)	Diam. of entrance (inches)	Height above ground (feet)
Bluebird	5 x 5	8	6	1½	5 to 10
Robin	6 x 8	8	(a)	(a)	6 to 15
Chickadee	4 x 4	8 to 10	8	1⅛	6 to 15
Tufted titmouse	4 x 4	8 to 10	8	1¼	6 to 15
White-breasted nuthatch	4 x 4	8 to 10	8	1¼	12 to 20
House wren	4 x 4	6 to 8	1 to 6	⅞	6 to 10
Bewick wren	4 x 4	6 to 8	1 to 6	⅞	6 to 10
Carolina wren	4 x 4	6 to 8	1 to 6	1⅛	6 to 10
Dipper	6 x 6	6	1	3	1 to 3
Violet-green swallow	5 x 5	6	1 to 6	1½	10 to 15
Tree swallow	5 x 5	6	1 to 6	1½	10 to 15
Barn swallow	6 x 6	6	(a)	(a)	8 to 12
Martin	6 x 6	6	1	2½	15 to 20
Song sparrow	6 x 6	6	(b)	(b)	1 to 3
House finch	6 x 6	6	4	2	8 to 12
Phoebe	6 x 6	6	(a)	(a)	8 to 12
Crested flycatcher	6 x 6	8 to 10	8	2	8 to 20
Flicker	7 x 7	16 to 18	16	2½	6 to 20
Red-headed woodpecker	6 x 6	12 to 15	12	2	12 to 20
Golden-fronted woodpecker	6 x 6	12 to 15	12	2	12 to 20
Hairy woodpecker	6 x 6	12 to 15	12	2	12 to 20
Downy woodpecker	4 x 4	8 to 10	8	1¼	6 to 20
Screech owl	8 x 8	12 to 15	12	3	10 to 30
Sparrow hawk	8 x 8	12 to 15	12	3	10 to 30
Saw-whet owl	6 x 6	10 to 12	10	2½	12 to 20
Barn owl	10 x 18	15 to 18	4	6	12 to 18
Wood duck	10 x 18	10 to 15	3	6	4 to 20

(a) One or more sides open
(b) All sides open

Simple Stables

If you are raising larger livestock—sheep, goats, horses, or llamas, for example—you will need a small stable where they can go for protection during inclement weather and especially during the winter months in cooler regions. Building stables can be done relatively easily and inexpensively, and doing it yourself means that you can customize the design to fit your and your animals' needs.

Stables should be built on relatively flat ground that does not become excessively wet or flooded during heavy rains. Laying down a thick bed of gravel or sand below the stable floor will help keep surface water drained. Also consider the positioning of the stable; try to find an area that is protected from strong winds but also near your own home so you don't have to go too far to tend the animals during bad weather. Facing the stable toward the south or west will help keep a nice breeze flowing through your stable while protecting it from harsh northerly winds. A place to store feed and hay for your animals is also a worthwhile addition when planning and building a simple stable.

General Stable Construction

When building a stable for your livestock, make sure that the interior walls are weatherproof and free of dampness. To keep moisture out of the stable, the building should be situated on slightly higher ground than that surrounding it. This will keep the ground from getting too damp, and vapors will not be as likely to rise through the floor and foundation walls. If possible, it is best to make the stable floor out of concrete between 4 and 6 inches thick.

The stable walls should be built solid. Brick and stone are preferable to wood, but wooden stables also do an adequate job of providing shelter and are much more common in the United States, due to the availability of wood. If you decide to build your stable using bricks, building the walls one brick (9 inches) thick should be suitable. Internal walls should be built solid, and the foundation must be deep and wide enough to give the whole structure stability. If one side of your stable gets the brunt of driving rain or moisture, it is a good idea to cover it with an extra layer of cement or stucco, or hang shingles to protect the wall.

The Dutch door on this stable can keep animals enclosed while allowing fresh air to circulate.

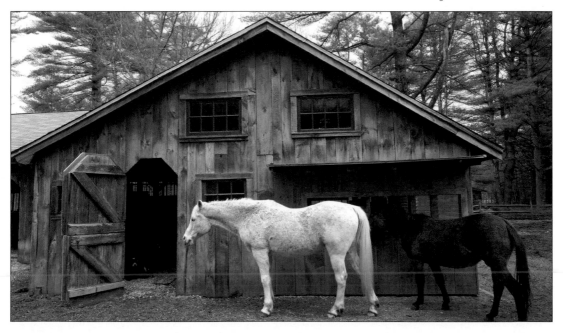

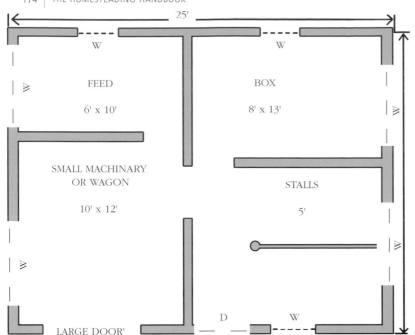

25'

W   W

FEED   BOX

6' x 10'   8' x 13'

SMALL MACHINARY
OR WAGON
                          STALLS
10' x 12'
                           5'

LARGE DOOR'   D   W

Plans for a small stable

The external angles of all of the doors and windows should be rounded. This can be done by using bull-nosed bricks. This way, horses and other livestock will not be injured by coming into contact with any sharp angles or ledges.

A Small Stable for Horses, Llamas, or Sheep

This simple stable is inexpensive to build and has plenty of room for two horses, llamas, or sheep, along with feed and tack. Hay and grain can be kept in the loft. Place the windows as high up as possible and hinge them at the bottom so they'll open inwardly to permit the air to pass over the animals without blowing directly on them. Make the stable door a "Dutch door"; that is, a door divided horizontally in the middle so that the upper half may be opened and the lower half remain closed.

A stable can be made out of a variety of materials, including brick and wood.

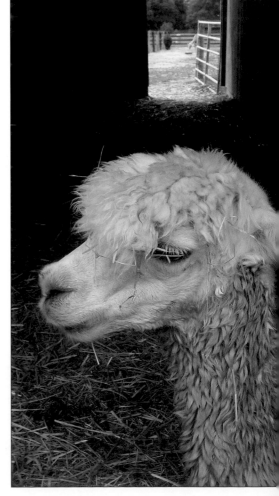

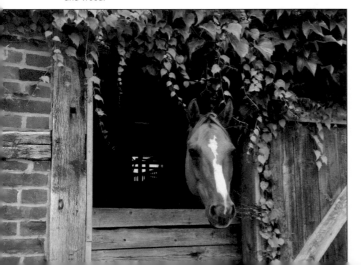

Poultry Houses

Poultry houses should be warm, dry, well-lighted, and ventilated shelters with convenient arrangements for roosts, feeding space, and nest boxes. In winter, if you're living in a cool climate, light and warmth are of the up most importance. Fowl will stop laying eggs and their health will suffer when confined in cold, wet, and dark conditions. Windows facing the south or southeast, large enough to admit the sun freely, should be provided and made to slide open to increase circulation during the summer.

Beyond these few requirements, houses for your poultry can be made in a variety of ways and are, generally, relatively easy to construct. Below are many different types of poultry houses that can be used to keep your fowl warm, dry, and healthy.

Simplest Poultry House

While poultry can survive in this type of cheaply and simply built coop, it is best used in warmer climates, where the winter months do not become incredibly cold and not much, if any, snow falls. Also, this type of coop is best suited for only one or two chickens or ducks.

Materials
*   Four pieces of 1 x 2-inch boards for the studs and rafters
*   Strong nails
*   Wire netting
*   Tarred paper

1. Take two of the boards and nail them together in a T shape. Repeat with the other two. Set these apart from each other about 2 feet 10 inches on the centers, and cover them with tightly drawn wire netting (cut to size).
2. Cover the wire netting with tarred paper, creating a barrier between the outside winds and weather and the fowl inside.

Young Poultry Coops

Chicks need extra warmth and protection from predators. This coop, if it houses small chicks, should not hold the other fowl, as they may bully or even harm the young chicks.

This pitched roof chicken coop consists of a pitched roof mounted on three boards, 6 feet high. This coop is 3 feet wide and 2 feet deep. Nail slats across the front to prevent the hen from getting out but to allow the chicks to enter and exit freely into a small fenced-in area surrounding the coop.

The coop pictured above is similar to the pitched roof chicken coop except that there is a canopy that keeps the rain out and shades the interior of the coop so it does not become too warm. This coop is 3 feet long, 2 feet wide, and 30 inches high at the front and 24 inches high in the back. The coop can be constructed from boards with matched edges and should be raised an inch or two above the ground to ensure the floor remains dry. Tack a piece of light canvas or muslin to the roof to serve as the awning.

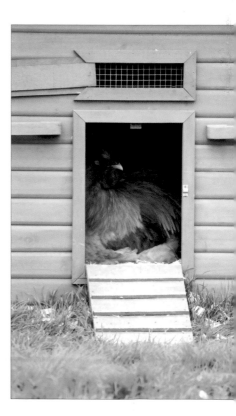

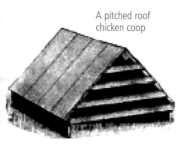

A pitched roof chicken coop

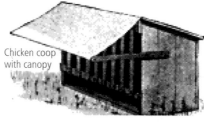

Chicken coop with canopy

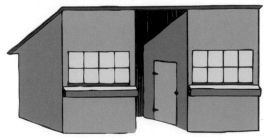

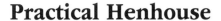

This henhouse has a scratching shed, which allows the chickens access to the open air while still being protected from the elements.

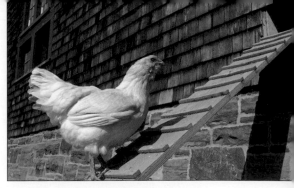

You can build a simple ramp to give your chickens easy access to the coop

Practical Henhouse

This simple and efficient henhouse has a shed roof and, as most poultry houses should, faces toward the south. This house can be up to 10 feet wide and as long as you need to accommodate your chickens.

A scratching shed is in the center of the building and has windows that let sunlight in. The sleeping quarters should be kept warm. An open, wire-enclosed front for the scratching shed should be included, too. The roosts should be made moveable and fresh bedding should be kept on the floor of the henhouse.

The roof of the henhouse should project out 1 foot over the south, east, and west sides. It should also be 5 inches higher than the siding, allowing for free ventilation. Two large windows will admit light and warmth into the henhouse. A laying box should extend the entire length of the room and must be divided into compartments and covered with a hinged lid. This allows the eggs to be gathered simply by raising the lid from the outside. Make sure the floor is cleaned weekly to keep out disease. The inside of the walls should be whitewashed often to keep out moisture and pests.

Two-Room Henhouse

This two-room henhouse has a south-facing front to allow ample sunlight and warmth into the house. It can be made as large as 10 x 12 feet and should be constructed of wood or timber planks. It is divided into two rooms by a partition made out of wire netting. This henhouse can serve two separate yards. A fence con-

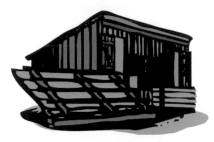

These pictures show how the perches can be moved to allow for easy cleaning

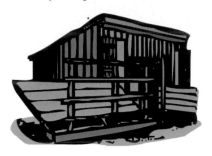

structed in the middle of the house yard should join the center of the front of the building (and at the back as well if you so desire). In this house, both hens and roosters can be kept and are easily separated while allowing each enough space and exercise.

The platform and perches should be constructed inside of each room. When the perches are in need of cleaning, they are raised up against the wall in the house, in a perpendicular position. To clean the trough, the perches and platform are raised perpendicular to the floor.

Duck Houses

Ducks, while they can survive rather well in any type of poultry house, are happiest when they have either a stream or pond in which to swim, bathe, and gather food. If you have a stream or pond on your property, situating a duck house nearby will help ensure that the duck eggs are safe and secure.

If you are raising a good number of ducks, your duck house should be about 30 feet long and 12 feet high. Doors should be situated in the front of the house and the house should have a few small windows that can be slid open to allow fresh air to circulate within the duck

A two-room henhouse with a south-facing front

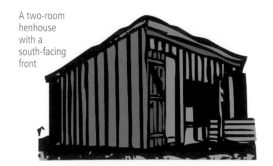

house. The rear of the house should hold the nests (boxes open at the front). A small door should be situated behind each nest so the eggs can be easily removed.

You can use a strip of wire netting to enclose a small, narrow yard in the front of the house. Do not use twine netting, however, as the ducks could get their heads twisted in it and strangle themselves.

Easy, Creative Coops

If you don't have much space in your yard and only have a few chickens to keep, very good coops can be made at a very small cost from items found around your house, yard, or at rummage sales:

1. Barrel Coop
   a. First, drive shingle nails through the hoops on both sides of each stave and clinch them down on the inside.
   b. Divide the barrel in half, if it is big enough, by cutting through the hoops and the bottom.
   c. Drive sticks into the ground to hold the coop in place, and drive a long stick at each side of the opened end just far enough from the coop to allow the front door to be slipped in and out.
   d. The night door can be made from the head of the barrel or any solid board, and the slatted door, used to confine the hen, can be made by nailing upright strips of lath to a cross-lath at top and bottom.
2. Box Coop
   a. Find a box that is roughly 2 to 2½ feet long, 16 inches deep, and 2 feet high and saw a hole, *d*, in one end.
   b. Strengthen the box with narrow strips of wood, *b, c*, on each side of the hole. This acts as a groove for the door, *a*, to slide in. By doing so, you will have a sliding door that opens and shuts easily.
   c. The front of the coop is enclosed with lath, or narrow strips, placed 2½ to 3 inches apart. The top should be covered with a good grade of roofing paper to make it completely waterproof.
3. Portable Coop—This type of coop will allow you to have a fresh yard for your chickens and other poultry to scrounge in and is easily transported to any place on your property.
   a. The coop is built of ordinary material on a base frame and with a V-shaped roof and side frames. The preferred length of the coop is about 2 feet and the yard should be around 3 to 4 feet.
   b. The ridge pole is extended, as shown at each end, to form a handle.
   c. If desired, the hen may be allowed to freely roam the yard or can be contained within the coop by slats, as is pictured in the drawing.

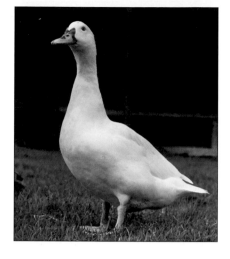

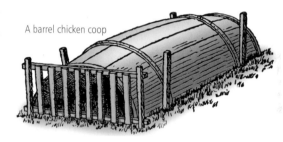
A barrel chicken coop

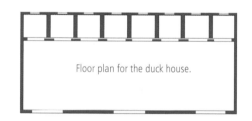
Floor plan for the duck house.

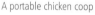
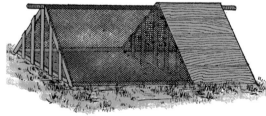
A portable chicken coop

A simple box coop

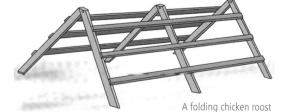
A folding chicken roost

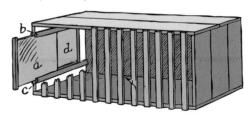

Poultry House Aids and Other Considerations

Folding Chicken Roost

This roost is made of 3-inch boards cut to any desired length that will fit within your poultry house. A small bolt fastens the upright pieces at their top ends and the horizontal pieces are fastened on with nails. This roost can be kept at any angle and may be quickly taken out of the house when it is time to clean. This sort of roost will accommodate more fowl in the same space than the flat kind.

Keeping Rats and Mice Out of the Poultry House

If you are building a permanent poultry house, you should try to make it as rodent-proof as possible. If rats and mice can easily enter your poultry house, they will not only steal eggs and spread diseases, but they could scare or even harm the fowl. Cheap and efficient walls can be made of small fieldstones in this way:

1. Dig trenches for the walls below the frost line.
2. Drive two rows of stakes into the trenches, one row at each side of the trench.
3. Set up boards in between the stakes. The boards will hold the stones and cement in place until the cement hardens. The top boards should have a straight upper edge and should be placed level to determine the top of the wall.
4. Place two or three layers of stone in the bottom of the trench, pour in thinly mixed cement, and pound it in. Repeat this until the desired height is reached.
5. The top of the wall should be smoothed off with a trowel and left until the cement completely hardens. The side boards can now be removed and the poultry house built.

Winter Care of Fowl

If chickens and other fowl are not kept warm in the winter, they will stop growing, cease laying eggs, and can become ill. There are several ways you can winterize chicken coops to ensure your birds' comfort and well-being.

Especially if you live in colder climates, having a house with hollow or double side walls will help keep your fowl warm during the winter season. Buildings with hollow side walls are warmer in the winter and are also cooler in the summer. They do not collect as much severe frost and result in less moisture seeping into the henhouse once the frost melts.

The outside walls of chicken coops can be plastered or lined with matched boards and the spaces between the boards filled with wood shavings, sawdust, or hay. The floor should be covered with several inches of dry sand, wood shavings, or straw, and the ventilating holes near the roof should be partly stopped up or shutters

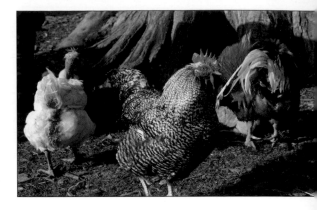

arranged to close most of them in very cold weather. You don't want to seal the place up completely, though. Nothing is more important to the health of fowl than pure air. Birds breathe with great rapidity and maintain a relatively high body temperature, so they need plenty of oxygen.

Constructing a solid, insulated roof for your poultry house for the winter is very important. A roof can be built either by sealing the inside with material to exclude draughts or by placing roof boards close together and covering them thoroughly with tarred paper before shingling. An ordinary shingled roof allows too much wind to come into the house and could cause your fowl to get frosted combs or wattles. If this happens, there will not be much, if any, egg production in the winter months.

Hanging curtains in front of the perches is also a great way to keep your fowl warm during the winter months. Make these curtains of burlap and hang them from the roof in such a way that the perches are enclosed in a little room. Make sure the curtains are long enough to touch the floor all around, and sew the edges of the burlap together, except at the corners. At night, the corners can be pinned together to keep the birds from leaving their sheltered perches. This pseudo-sleeping room allows air to move in without creating drafts and it also helps retain the birds' body heat. This maintains a comfortable temperature for the birds during cold, winter nights.

A drinking fountain for your chickens can be made with a can or bucket and a tray. Cut out one end of the can and poke holes along the edge as shown. Fill with water, cover with a shallow tray, and turn the whole thing over quickly. Chicks will be able to drink water easily without risk of drowning.

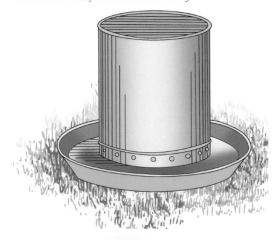

Fences, Gates, and Pens

Whether you are looking to add a lovely fence and gate around your garden plants or you have poultry or other livestock to keep in check, you may need to build a fence, gate, or animal pen. These structures can be attractive if well built and should be able to stand up to all kinds of weather and animals. Depending on your needs, here are some various fences, gates, and pens you can easily construct in your yard or on your property.

Fences

Fences are perfect for keeping animals or young children in a confined space or for drawing boundaries between yours and your neighbor's property lines—but check with your neighbors before you construct your fence to make sure they don't mind. Also call your local utility companies to make sure that you will not be digging up power or gas lines.

Wooden Fences

Wooden fences allow for good ventilation and an open, airy feel. They can provide protection for young shrubs and plants as well as keep animals and children safe within the yard or fenced-in space.

The most common type of wooden fence consists of horizontal rails nailed to posts or stakes that are placed vertically into the ground. These fences can be constructed with three or four horizontal rails that are made out of split wood, spruce, or pine wood planks. The posts are usually about 6 feet long and sharpened at the end that will be driven into the ground (to a depth of roughly 8 inches). These posts should be spaced about 6 feet apart.

In order to keep the pointed, earth-bound ends from rotting, dip them in melted pitch before inserting them into the ground. To do this, boil linseed oil and stir in pulverized coal until it reaches the consistency of paint. Brush a coat of this on the wooden post. Make sure the posts are completely dry before painting them. If properly done, this should keep moisture from seeping into the buried parts of the posts and will keep your fence upright for many, many years.

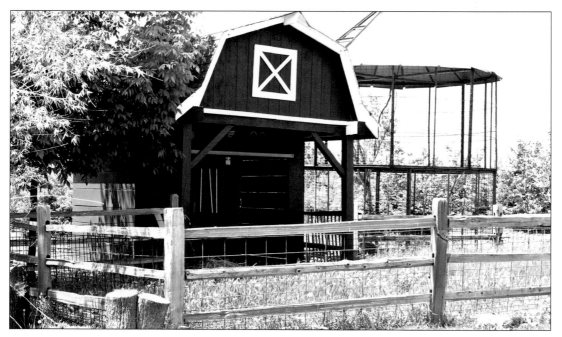

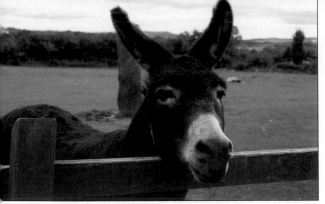

A simple wooden fence is enough to keep most animals in their pastures.

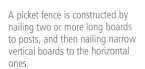

A hole borer lifts the soil from the hole without having to use spades. These borers can be used by hand or electric models can be purchased for the same purpose.

In order to drive the posts into the ground, you will need either a very good shovel or a heavy wooden mallet. For longer poles, use a post-hole borer. This saves lots of time and energy and will work with almost all types of soil.

To construct a basic wooden fence, you'll need:

Materials

- Post-hole diggers, a post-hole borer, or a shovel
- 4 x 4 wooden posts (wood that has been treated will last longer but is not necessary)
- 2 x 4 lumber (this too can be treated but does not need to be) or fence boards (which can be purchased at your local home and gardening center)
- Thick, long nails

Directions

1. Decide where the fence will be constructed and then lay a line of twine or string to mark out the border.
2. Decide how tall you want your fence to be. Take into consideration what the fence is being used for (if it's for larger animals, such as llamas, you may want a 6-foot-tall fence; if for decoration, a shorter fence may do the trick).
3. Dig holes for your end posts (in all four corners of your fence). Make sure the holes are deep enough to be able to support the end posts. Fill in dirt around the posts and pack in the soil very well.

You can nail wire mesh to the rails of a wooden fence for extra security or to allow vines or other climbing plants to grow up along the posts.

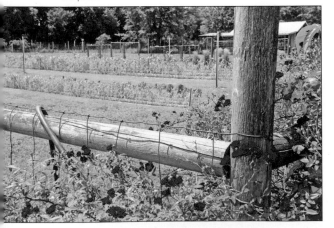

A picket fence is constructed by nailing two or more long boards to posts, and then nailing narrow vertical boards to the horizontal ones.

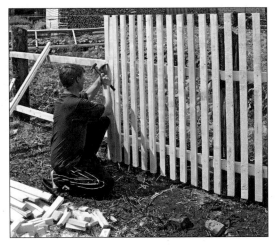

4. Start digging the remaining holes, trying to keep them in alignment with the end posts.
5. Insert the remaining posts into the holes, piling in the dirt and packing it down as before.
6. Nail on your fence boards, leaving a little space in between. Paint or stain the finished fence if you wish.

Note: If you want a privacy fence, you can nail thicker boards horizontally or vertically between each post, making sure the space in between is quite small.

Wire Fences

Wire fences are both portable and durable, making them convenient and economical to build. Wire fences usually have a longer staying power than wooden fences since they are less prone to deterioration or rot.

The most common type of wire fence is one that has wire lines strung between wooden posts. The wires are fastened to the posts by galvanized wire staples. The wooden posts should be spaced roughly 6 feet apart and should use five single wires.

A more substantial wire fence can be made with G-line wires. Each line consists of a three-ply strand. Instead of the wires being fastened to the post by staples, holes are bored through the posts and the lines

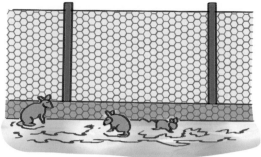

A wire netting fence

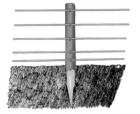

Drive your fence poles far enough into the ground that they stand firmly upright even when moderate pressure is applied to one side.

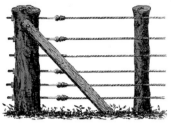

A G-line wire fence consists of three-ply strands of wire.

pass through. Straining eye bolts with nuts and washers are attached for tightening up the fence. This type of fence, however, is much more expensive to build and, unless you desire a fence that is incredibly strong, is probably not necessary.

[only one example below (and some pictures that have already been explained)]

Wire Netting Fence

Galvanized wire netting fences are used for enclosing root gardens and for poultry fences. The standard type of netting used when making this fence is 3-inch mesh netting that is 3 feet x 3 feet, and is rather inexpensive to buy.

A separate strip of 2-inch galvanized wire netting that is 6 inches wide can be laid flat on the ground on the side of the fence where the poultry are—this way they can not dig underneath, especially once grass and other natural materials hide the wire netting.

To dig in this type of fence, make a trench about 6 inches deep, drop the netting into it, and then fill the trench up with dirt, stones, or even concrete, depending on how permanent you want the fence to be.

Portable Fences

If you need a temporary fence or if you want to be able to easily move your livestock fence to new grazing areas on your property, you may want to consider one of these easily made moveable fences. Below are a few types of portable fences that can be tailored to your specific needs.

Convenient and Portable Fence

Often it is helpful to have a fence that can be quickly erected and disassembled. This fence is very cheap, strong, and convenient to use. It is built out of pine (any other wood can be substituted, but pine is typically lighter and easier to move), 1 x 6 inches for the bottom rail and 1 x 4 inches for the top rails. The braces that hold it upright are 2 x 4 inches and the base (cross piece) is 2 x 6 inches. The base is notched 2 inches and the bottom boards are notched with holes.

The base piece, which is more susceptible to rot, could be made out of a stronger wood, such as oak.

Make sure the panels aren't too long or they might warp out of shape. This fence can be put up very quickly and taken down again with ease if you want to move it to another part of your yard or get rid of it for a while.

Scotch Hurdle Fence

This moveable fence consists of two posts, each 2 x 3 inches and 4½ feet long. The lower ends are long and pointed—this allows them to easily enter the ground and prop up the fence. The brace and two diagonals are made of larch or fir wood. This fence is around 9 feet long and 4 feet high.

The Scotch Hurdle fence is easy to set up. The incline should be facing away from any livestock you might have contained inside of it. A stay should be placed between every two hurdles to keep them in position. One wooden peg should be fastened to one end of the hurdle and another peg driven through the other end and into the ground.

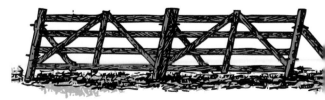

A portable fence

English Hurdle Portable Fence

This moveable fence is much lighter, cheaper, and more convenient than the Scotch hurdle fence. Usually made of split oak, this fence is tough and impenetrable. It consists of two upright end pieces that are joined by four or five mortised bars 7 to 9 feet long. These are strengthened by an upright bar in the middle and two

This Scotch hurdle fence is good for temporary use. If you live in a very windy area, however, this fence may not suit you well, as they do have a tendency to fall over in very strong gales.

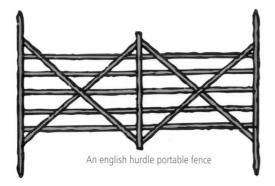

An english hurdle portable fence

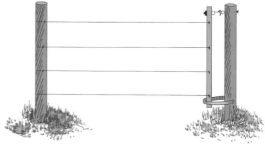

A basic wire gate can be constructed when you need an opening in your fence.

An easily opened gate

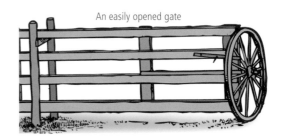

or more diagonals. The end pieces are long and pointed for setting into the ground. To set these into the earth, use an iron crowbar to avoid splitting the top of the wooden piece.

These fences are set erect and no stay is needed. The two adjoining ends of the fences are connected with a band that is passed over them.

Gates

Gates are a necessary part of any fence or pen and they can be situated in the fence wherever they can be easily accessed. If you have a field, your gate should be roughly 10 feet wide to allow small machinery through.

Most gates are made of either wood or iron (though iron is obviously much more expensive and more complicated to work with). Wooden gates will suffice for most of your homesteading needs. The following are a few simple gates that can be used for your garden, your backyard fences, and your pens housing livestock.

Inexpensive, Simple Gate

A light, useful, and durable gate can be made of sassafras poles (or other tall grass poles) and wire. Dig and place a strong post 4 feet in the ground in the middle of

Gates can be useful for entrances to a yard or walkway, as well as for animal pens or pastures.

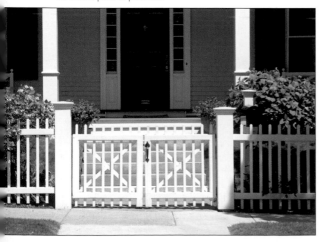

the gateway and balance the gate on it. The lower rail is made of two forked sassafras poles securely nailed together so they can be coiled back over the post.

Easily Opened Gate

To construct this simple gate, take an old wheel (possibly found at an antique store or rummage sale) and fasten it to make a gate that you will be opening frequently. The piece of board (C) drops between the spokes of the wheel and holds the gate either open or closed.

Simple Gate

This is a simple and appealing gate, especially for fences leading into pastures. The materials required to make this gate vary depending on what purpose the gate will serve.

For a paddock or pasture gate, make it out of seasoned boards, 1 x 6 inches and 12 to 14 feet long. The posts supporting the gate should be placed about 5 inches apart, the one on the inside being about 8 inches ahead of the other. These are joined together by cleats

A simple sliding gate can be made for any modern or wire fence.

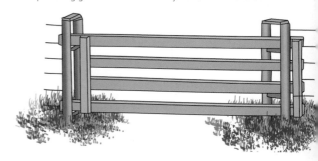

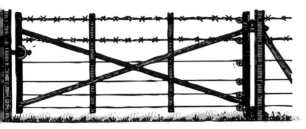

This wire gate is hung on ordinary iron posts. The heel of the gate, made of angle iron, is fitted with winding brackets for tightening the wire bars.

or rollers that support the gate and allow it to be pushed back and swing open. If rollers are not obtainable, cleats made of any hard wood are acceptable.

Pens

If you have built a simple stable to house your llamas, sheep, or other animals, it will be beneficial to build a small fence around it as an outdoor pen. A basic wooden fence or a simple wire fence will enclose most of your livestock in an area around the stable or shelter. If you have a llama or two, it is best to have at least a 4-foot

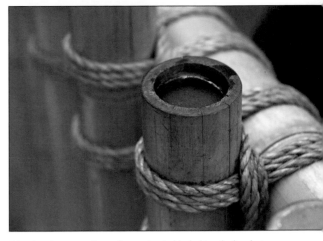

A bamboo fence or gate can be constructed by lashing the bamboo together with strong rope.

fence so they cannot escape. If you have ample space, having a pathway into a larger grazing field or pasture from your pen will allow your animals to come and go as they please. Or, if you want to keep them confined in the pen, a simple gate will suffice for when the animals need to be removed or relocated.

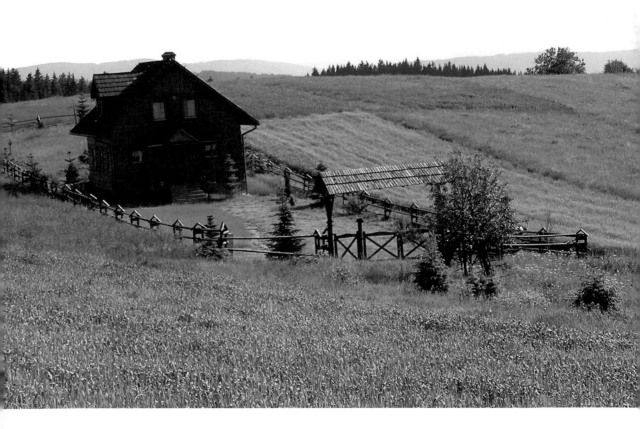

Basic Bridges

If you have a river or brook on your property, you may want to construct a simple bridge. Building these bridges can be quite easy, especially if you don't plan on transporting very heavy machinery or cars over them. Here are a few different ways to build basic bridges over streams, creeks, or other rather narrow waterways.

Footbridge

This natural-looking footbridge can be built between 8 feet and 12 feet long.

Excavate the banks of the stream or creek to allow for the building of a small, low rubble or stonewall. The sleepers will rest on this wall. The girders are formed of wooden spars (four are used in this plan). The girders should be between 8 and 10 inches in diameter. Lay the girders down and bolt them together in pairs with six ¾-inch-diameter coach bolts. Wedge the posts to fit mortises in the girders.

The posts and top rails should be roughly 4½ to 5½ inches in diameter and the intermediate rails 3 inches in diameter. Finally, join the rails to the posts.

The bridge should be anchored well if it's in a place where flooding is frequent, as you don't want your footbridge floating away in the stream. To do so, drive four short piles into the soil on the inside of the girders, near their ends. Fasten the girders to the piles with coach bolts. The pile tops are hidden by the ends of the floor battens.

Now, if you want to decorate your footbridge, you can use small twigs and nails to make patterns on your bridge.

Small Stream Bridge

If you have a small creek or stream on your property, you may want to construct a simple bridge for easy access to the other side. To build this bridge, you'll need lumber that is 6 inches wide and 2 inches thick, and additional lumber for the floor and four side braces.

Directions
1. Saw 11 pieces of wood the length required for the two sides.

Bridge can be fashioned in a range of shapes, styles, and sizes to meet your needs.

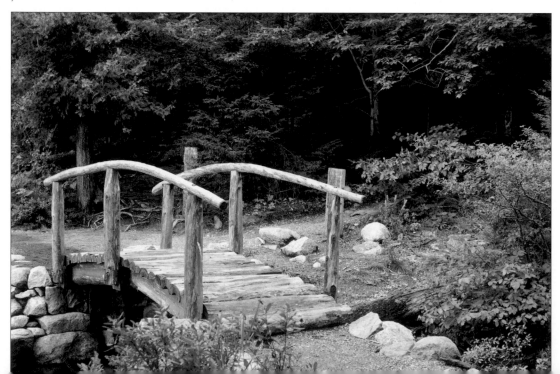

2. Bore bolt holes 1½ inches from each end. Use 5/8-inch bolts 8½ inches long for where four pieces come together, and use 6½-inch bolts where three pieces meet.

3. Bolt on the A-shaped supports and pieces for the approaches at one time, and then put on the side braces.

4. The sides of the bridge are made of triangles. The first triangle is made of pieces *a*, *b*, and *c*. The second triangle is made of pieces *b*, *d*, and *e*.

5. The piers for this bridge may be made of posts, stone, or even concrete, depending on how permanent you wish your small stream bridge to be.

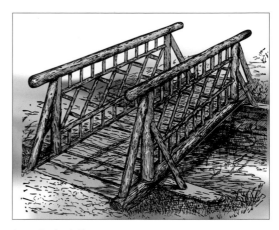

A wooden footbridge

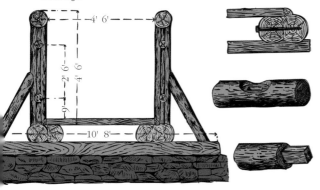

A cross section of the footbridge

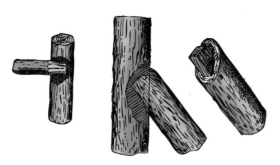

Join the rails of the footbridge to the posts as shown here.

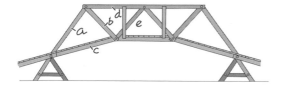

A bridge for a small stream

A Very Simple Bridge

Another very simple way of building a bridge across a creek or stream is to find a narrow part of the waterway and then find two logs that are longer than the creek is wide. These logs should be very sturdy (not rotted out) and thick. Place them across the creek, so they make a narrow beam over the water. Each log should have an extra foot at each end of the creek, so they can be securely walked upon with no danger of slipping into the creek bed. Place the logs roughly two feet apart.

If the water comes up close to the bottom of the logs, raise them so the bridge does not get washed away in heavy storms or during the course of the stream rising. To raise the bridge will require a bit more work, as each log will need to be set into another log on the edge of the streambed or even into stone to make it more permanent.

After you have the two base logs secured, find some sticks that are long enough (and relatively thick) to lay across the tops of the two logs. Or, if you have extra plywood or other boards, those can be used as well. Just make sure to place the sticks or boards fairly close to one another, leaving only little gaps between them. Then, once all the sticks have been laid down, secure these by tying twine or rope to them and the base logs.

If you'd like your bridge to last a little longer, you can pave it with clay or fine cement. Using a shovel, coat the bridge with the clay or cement until it's about 2 inches thick. Then shovel dirt onto the clay mixture, packing it down all over, and make the bridge as thick as you like. However, for just a simple bridge across a narrow stream or creek, the wooden sticks or boards will work just fine and won't require quite as much time and energy.

Tool Sheds and Workshops

Before building a tool shed, think about what you want to house in it. If you just need it for small tools, such as shovels, buckets, and a wheelbarrow, a smaller shed will be fine. However, if you plan to house your machinery there, such as a tractor, lawnmower, chainsaw, or rototiller, you'll need a larger shed and you may want to plan for a sliding garage door–style entrance. Will you want a workbench, space to pot plants, shelving, and drawers? Do you want electrical outlets for power tools and lights? Also consider location: It may be more convenient to have it close to your house, or you may prefer to have it nearer the garden. Below are a couple of examples of tool sheds that you can modify to meet your needs.

Medium-sized Tool Shed and Workshop

This shed is large enough to easily store your basic farm machinery. The shed is basically a giant umbrella with posts 30 feet apart in one direction and 12 or 16 feet apart in the other. There are no sides to this shed at all (though you could modify this if you want to store other tools here). If you park your main machinery (tractor, lawnmower, and so on) in the innermost part of the shed, you should still have an overhang of 10 feet. This shed would be most beneficial if it were 10 feet high—that way, most any kind of machine you want to house under it will fit well. Boarding up one, two, or three sides will help prevent snow from drifting in during the winter and rain from rusting your equipment. Making walls will also allow you to hang tools on the inside of the shed, such as clippers, weed whackers, or hoses.

The workshop housed above will hold a lot of smaller tools and is a good place to mend harnesses, make repairs, and store grain. The workshop gives about a 30-foot clearance space for the shed below. The entire building is built together using the following materials:

- 2 x 8-inch posts
- Three pieces of 2 x 12-inch wood materials (space these 2 inches apart)
- 2 x 10-inch box plates
- 6 x 6-inch bridge truss
- 2 x 4-inch or 2 x 6-inch beams for the rafters (depending on how much weight they must hold)

The floor of your shed should be either hard dirt or cement and the posts should be anchored firmly into the ground or on stone pillars. A shingle roof will ensure your smaller workshop tools are kept safe from the rain and snow.

Decide what you will want to store in your shed before you begin building so you know what size to make it.

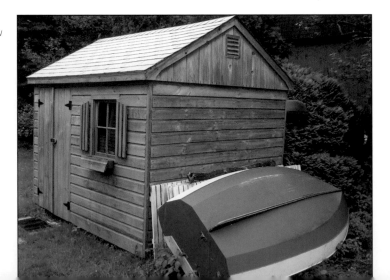

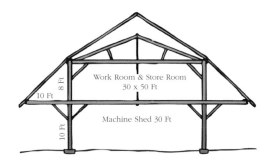

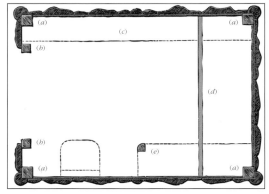

Plans for the inside of a rustic tool shed.

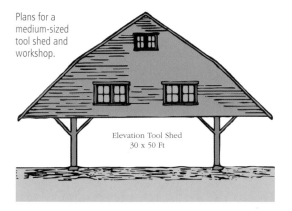

Plans for a medium-sized tool shed and workshop.

Small, Rustic Tool Shed

This small, rustic tool shed is made from "slabs" or "rough planks." If you are using trees from your own property to build the shed, you won't have to bother peeling the bark from the logs or cutting them as exactly. Slabs are cheap to buy (they can be found at saw mills and sometimes at home centers), and create an attractive, "woodsy" look. Although the boards are typically not uniform in size (some are wider than others), you can position them in such a way as to minimize the number of large cracks in your shed.

These boards may need to be straightened (especially the edges) with a saw or axe, and the interior of the tool shed should be lined with thin boards to cover up cracks and to keep out insects and animals.

When beginning construction on this type of shed, search for boards that lend themselves better to being end posts and those that are better suited for the walls. The corners of the four main posts (4 inches square) construct a building roughly 7 x 5 feet. Dig holes 2 feet into the ground and fit in the end posts.

On the tops of these posts, rest the wall plates—these should be 3 inches deep. These boards will be at the back and sides of the shed only. The sides will also need cross rails that are around 2 to 3 inches thick with ends flush to the corner posts. Nail the side and back boards to these cross boards to secure them.

Place two door posts in the front of the shed. They should stand 2 feet 8 inches apart and should be about

3 inches square. They should rise about 6 feet or so to attach to the rafters. Fill in the space between the door and corner posts with extra boards.

The roof for this tool shed can be thatched or made of boards and shingles, whichever you prefer. Make rafters and laths out of regular boards, arranging them about 1 foot apart, and the laths should be placed 6 inches apart for thatching. The shed can also be cheaply roofed with galvanized iron or tin roofing.

The door of the tool shed has the slabs nailed to it on the outside only, to make it aesthetically consistent. Attach hinges and the door should be ready. Inside the shed, sets of shelves may be hung in which tools and other items can be stored (c). A wheelbarrow can be stored upright at the back (d) and tools hung from hooks coming down from the rafters. Gardening tools and rakes can be stored on the right-hand side (e) and a chair can sit near the front of the door (f).

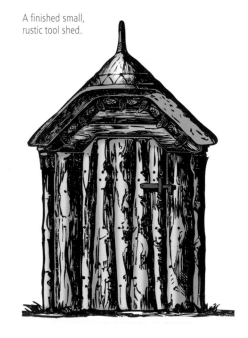

A finished small, rustic tool shed.

Smokehouses

If you are slaughtering your own poultry or other livestock, or if you just like the taste of smoked meat, try making your own smokehouse. Smokehouses help expose meats to the action of creosote and empyreumatic vapors resulting from the imperfect combustion of wood. The peculiar taste of smoked meat is from the creosote—this also helps preserve the meat. Other flavors are also imparted onto the meat by the choice of wood that is burned in the smokehouse, such as hickory.

To make a smokehouse you'll need a space (anything from the size of a barrel to a barn-sized area will work) that can be filled with smoke and closed up tightly. You'll also need a way to hang the meat that needs to be cured. In common smokehouses, a fire is made on a stone slab in the middle of the floor. In other instances, a pit is dug about a foot deep into the ground and the fire is built within it. Sometimes a stone slab covers the fire like a standard table. The possibilities are many, depending on your space and needs. Below are a few examples of smokehouses that can be built and used for smoking your own meats.

Standard Smokehouse

This smokehouse diffuses the rising smoke and prevents the direct heat of the fire from affecting the meats that are hung directly above it. In the picture, a section of the smokehouse is shown.

This standard smokehouse is 8 feet square and built of bricks—making it a somewhat permanent structure in your yard. If you want to make it out of wood, be sure to plaster is completely on the inside. The chimney, (c), has an 8-inch flue and the fireplace, (b), is outside, below the level of the floor. From this point, a flue, (f), is carried underneath the chimney into the middle of the floor where it opens up under a stone table, (e).

To kindle the fire, a valve is drawn to directly draft up through the chimney. The woodchips are thrown onto the fire and the valve is then placed so to direct the smoke into the brick smokehouse. There are openings, (g, g), in both the upper and lower parts of the chimney that are closed by valves (these

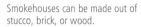
Smokehouses can be made out of stucco, brick, or wood.

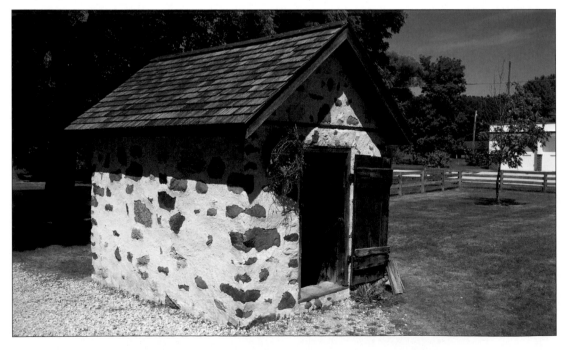

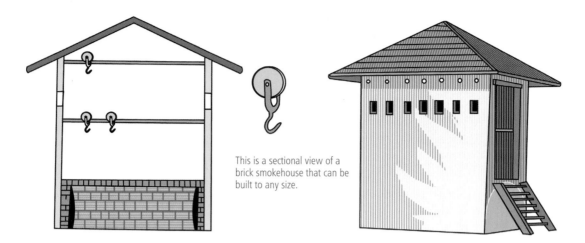

This is a sectional view of a brick smokehouse that can be built to any size.

can be manipulated from outside the smokehouse. The door of the smokehouse should be made to shut very tightly and, when building the smokehouse, be sure that there are not any cracks in the brick or mortar through which smoke can easily escape.

This type of smokehouse is nice because the smoke cools before it is pumped into the chamber and no ashes rise with the smoke. Meat may be kept in this smokehouse all year without tasting too smoky.

Another Brick Smokehouse

A smokehouse of this kind, built 7 x 9 feet, will be sufficient for private use. The bottom of this smokehouse has a brick arch with bricks left out sporadically. This is to allow the extraction of smoke from the house.

Located above the arch are two series of iron rods that have hooks with grooved wheels. You can find these at most local hardware stores. The open archway is for housing the fire and there is a door with steps leading up to it. A series of ventilating holes are situated above the lower bar and below the upper bar. These holes are meant to allow the smoke to escape from the house. By reinserting bricks into these holes, the smoke will stay mostly confined to the inside of the smokehouse.

The arch confines the fire and ashes, preventing any meat that might fall from being ruined or burned. The arch is made over a wooden frame of a few pieces of regular wood board, cut into an oval arch shape. Strips of wood are then nailed to this. When the brickwork is dry, the center is knocked out and removed. A small door can be fashioned to close up the arch when the fire is being kilned.

The drawing shows a common smokehouse that is built on a brick wall and over a brick arch. There are a number of holes left in it for smoke to escape. The ash pit is located beneath the arch, and there is also a door that opens to this pit. To reach the meat room door, use a sturdy ladder.

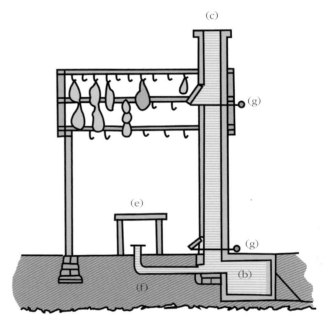

Interior view of a standard smokehouse

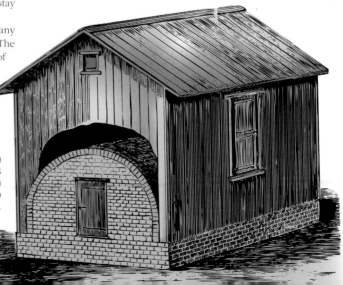

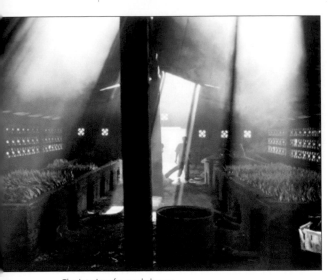

The interior of a smokehouse

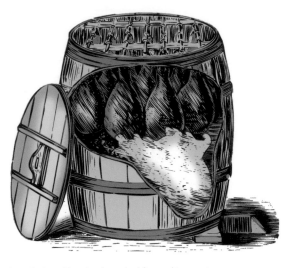

A smoke barrel is a simple method for smoking meats.

Simple Way to Smoke Meats

If you don't want to commit to building a permanent smokehouse in your yard but you would like to smoke meats occasionally, you can used a large cask or barrel as a smokehouse substitute.

To make the barrel into an effective smokehouse, just follow these steps:

1. Dig a small pit and place a flat stone or a brick across it. This is where the edge of the cask will rest.
2. Making sure that half of the pit is beneath the barrel and half is outside, remove the head and bottom of the barrel (or cut a hole into the bottom slightly larger than the portion of the pit beneath it).
3. Remove the top of the barrel and then hang the meat on cross-sticks. Rest these cross-sticks on crossbars that are made to fit into holes bored into the sides of the barrel, close to the top.
4. Put the lid on top of the barrel and cover it with a sack to confine the smoke inside.
5. Put coals into the pit outside of the cask, and then feed the fire with damp corncobs or a fine brush.
6. Cover the pit with a flat stone that will help regulate the fire and can be removed when more fuel is needed.

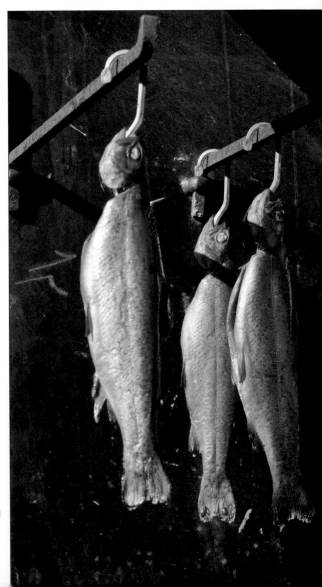

Fish that are hung and ready to be smoked

Root Cellars

While most modern houses have basements or crawl spaces in which to keep fresh vegetables and preserves cool and dry, you may want to construct an additional root cellar if you'll be storing significant amounts of these items. A root cellar should be located near to your home and should be dry, well ventilated, and frost proof. Creating your own root cellar is not terribly expensive and will give your yard and property a true back-to-basics feel.

Root Cellar

If you have a hilly area in your yard, this is the perfect place to make a root cellar. To construct the root cellar, follow these simple steps:

1. Make an excavation in the side of the hill, determining how large you'd like your root cellar to be.
2. In the excavation, erect a sturdy frame of timber and planks, or even of logs. Put up planks to stand as side walls, and build a strong roof over the frame.
3. Throw the excavated earth over the structure until it is completely covered by at least 2 feet of soil.
4. On the exposed end, make a door that is large enough for you to enter without ducking. Or, if you like, you can make a sort of "manhole" through which you can enter—this will actually protect your root cellar from the frost much better than a full-sized door.

If the soil in the hill is composed of stiff clay, you may not even need to construct any side walls, and the roof can be fitted directly into the clay. Then build up the front of the cellar with planks, bricks, or stone, and create a door.

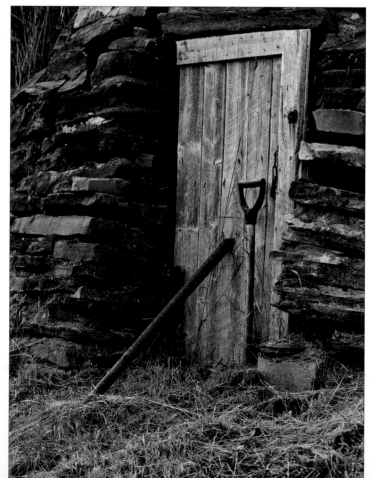

A root cellar can be built into the side of a hill using stone, bricks, or wood.

Root House

If you do not have a large hill on your property and would still like to construct a root cellar, find a knoll or other dry place and remove the soil over a space that is slightly larger than the size of the cellar (or root house if the structure is not built into a hill) and about 2 feet deep. To construct this root house:

1. Select poles or logs of two different sizes. The wider ones should be shorter than the other two.
2. Cut the ends of the logs very flat so they will fit closely together and make a very tight pen-like structure.
3. Cut two logs in each layer long enough to pass through and fit into the outer pen. This will help fasten the two walls together.
4. Build the doorway up with short logs passing from one layer of poles to the other. These serve as supports to the ends of the wall poles.
5. Fill in the space between these two walls with soil. It is important that these are filled in fully (sod may also be used to pack in spaces between the logs) to protect the inside storage items from frost and to keep the whole structure cool. Pack up the soil as you construct the walls so you can more easily compact it as you build up.
6. When the walls are about 5 or 6 feet on one side and 2 or 3 feet on the other, put the roof on. The roof is made of poles placed close together, secured to the logs, and covered with sod, then 18 inches of soil. It is then finished off with sod once again.

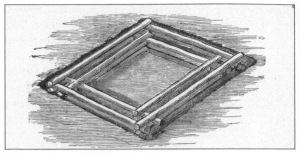

The base of the root house.

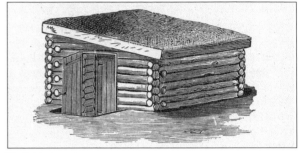

The finished root house.

Root cellars or houses are great for keeping vegetables like potatoes or carrots and for apples, which can keep for months in cool, dry storage.

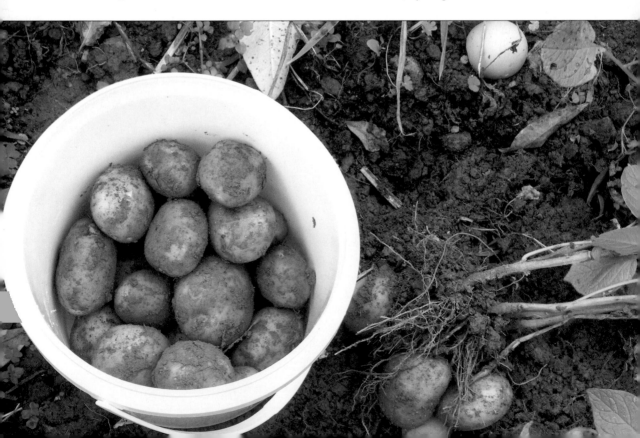

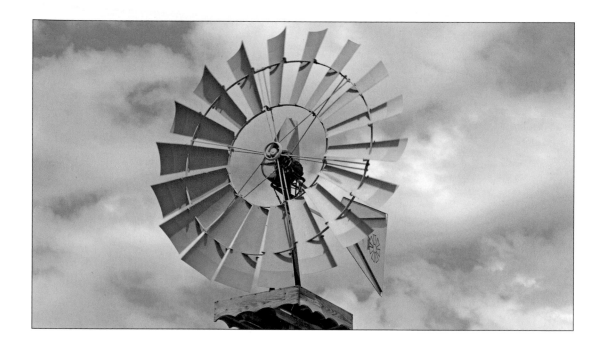

PART FIVE   Energy

With the extreme fluctuation in oil prices and ever-growing concerns about the state of our environment, it's no wonder that more and more people are turning to the natural elements for power. Sun, wind, water, and earth have provided for the basic needs of humanity since the beginning of time and it only makes sense to learn how to work with them more efficiently. The term "self-sufficiency," as it is commonly used, is something of a misnomer. We will never be able to meet all of our own needs alone. We don't create the natural world that supplies us with the light, heat, and other resources that we depend on. But we can learn how to make good use of those gifts. In these pages you will find both simple and advanced projects to do so, from fashioning and using solar cookers to building and installing wind turbines to utilizing geothermal systems. There's a lot here, but it's only a sampling of the methods available for harnessing natural energy. Look online or visit your library for more ideas, plans, and tips; you'll also find an extensive list of resources in the back of this book. Remember that the simplest and perhaps most effective way to be energy-efficient is to use less of it. The simple things, like turning off a light when you're not in the room—or even using candlelight in the evenings—can make a big difference. The more you understand about the process of turning the natural elements into usable energy, the more you'll appreciate the value of electricity and want to conserve it in any way you can.

Solar Energy

Solar energy is, in its simplest form, the sun's rays that reach the earth (also known as solar radiation). When you step outside on a hot, sunny summer day, you can feel the power of the sun's heat and light. Solar energy can be harnessed to do a variety of things in your home. These include:

- Heating your home through passive solar design or through active solar heating systems
- Generating electricity
- Heating water in your home
- Heating swimming pool water
- Lighting your home both inside and out
- Drying your clothes via a clothesline strung outside in direct sunlight

Solar energy can also be converted into thermal (heat) energy and used to heat water for use in homes, buildings, or swimming pools and also to heat spaces inside homes, greenhouses, and other buildings.

Photovoltaic energy is the conversion of sunlight directly into electricity. A photovoltaic cell, known as a solar or PV cell, is the technology used to convert solar energy into electrical power. A PV cell is a non-mechanical device made from silicon alloys. PV systems are often used in remote locations that are not connected to an electric grid. These systems are also used to power watches, calculators, and lighted road signs.

Solar Thermal Energy

Solar thermal (heat) energy is used most often for heating swimming pools, heating water to be used in homes, and heating specific spaces in buildings. Solar space heating systems are either passive or active.

Passive Solar Space Heating

Passive space heating is what happens in a car on a sunny summer day—the car gets hot inside. In buildings, air is circulated past a solar heat surface and through the building by convection—less dense, warm air tends to rise while the denser, cooler air moves downward. No mechanical equipment is needed for passive solar heating.

PV System Components.

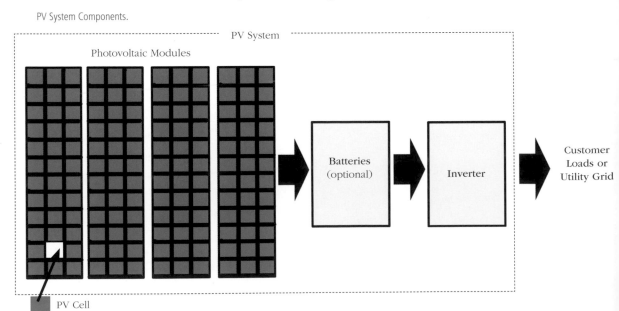

Advantages of Solar Energy

* It's free.
* Its supplies are unlimited.
* Solar heating systems reduce the amount of air pollution and greenhouse gases that result from using fossil fuels (oil, propane, and natural gas) for heating or generating electricity in your home.
* Solar heating systems reduce heating and fuel bills in the winter.
* It is most cost-effective when used for the entire year.

Disadvantages of Solar Energy

* The amount of sunlight that arrives at the earth's surface is not constant and depends on location, time of day and year, and weather conditions.
* A large surface area is required to collect the sun's energy at a useful rate.

Passive solar space heating takes advantage of the warmth from the sun through design features, such as large, south-facing windows and materials in the floors and/or walls that absorb warmth during the day and release it at night when the heat is needed most. Sunspaces and greenhouses are good examples of passive systems for solar space heating.

Passive solar systems usually have one of these designs:
1. Direct gain—This is the simplest system. It stores and slowly releases heat energy collected from the sun shining directly into the building and warming up the materials (tile or concrete). It is important to make sure the space does not become overheated.
2. Indirect gain—This is similar to direct gain in that it uses materials to hold, store, and release heat. This material is generally located between the sun and the living space, usually in the wall.
3. Isolated gain—This collects solar energy separately from the primary living area (a sunroom attached to a house can collect warmer air that flows through the rest of the house).

Active Solar Space Heating

Active heating systems require a collector to absorb the solar radiation. Fans or pumps are used to circulate the heated air or the heat-absorbing fluid. These systems often include some type of energy storage system.

There are two basic types of active solar heating systems. These are categorized based on the type of fluid (liquid or air) that is heated in the energy collectors. The collector is the device in which the fluid is heated by the sun. Liquid-based systems heat water or an antifreeze solution in a hydronic collector. Air-based systems heat air in an air collector. Both of these systems collect and absorb solar radiation, transferring solar heat to the

interior space or to a storage system, where the heat is then distributed. If the system cannot provide adequate heating, an auxiliary or backup system provides additional heat.

Liquid systems are used more often when storage is included and are well suited for radiant heating systems, boilers with hot water radiators, and absorption heat pumps and coolers. Both liquid and air systems can adequately supplement forced air systems.

Active solar space heating systems are comprised of collectors that absorb solar radiation combined with electric fans or pumps to distribute the solar heat. These systems also have an energy-storage system that provides heat when the sun is not shining.

Another type of active solar space heating system, the medium temperature solar collector, is generally used for solar space heating. These systems operate in much the same way as indirect solar water heating systems but have a larger collector area, larger storage units, and much more complex control systems. They are usually configured to provide solar water heating and can provide between 30 and 70 percent of residential heating requirements. All active solar space heating systems require more sophisticated design, installation, and maintenance techniques than passive systems.

Passive Solar Water Heaters

Passive solar water heaters rely on gravity and on water's natural tendency to circulate as it is heated. Since these heaters contain no electrical components, passive systems are more reliable, easier to maintain, and work longer than active systems. Two popular types of passive systems are:
1. Integral-collector storage systems—These consist of one or more storage tanks that are placed in an insulated box with a glazed side facing the sun. The solar collectors are best suited for areas where temperatures do not often fall below freezing. They work well in households with significant

A combination of an indirect water heater and a highly efficient boiler can provide a very inexpensive method of water heating.

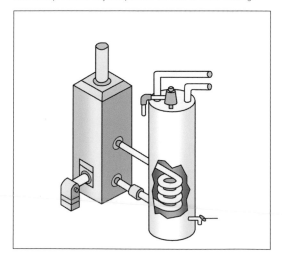

daytime and evening hot-water needs but they do not work as efficiently in households with only morning hot-water draws as they lose most of the collected energy overnight.

2. Thermospyhon systems—These are an economical and reliable choice particularly in newer homes. These systems rely on natural convection of warm water rising to circulate the water through the collectors and into the tank. As water in the collector heats, it becomes lighter and rises to the tank above it and the cooler water flows down the pipes to the bottom of the collector. In freeze-prone climates, indirect thermosyphons (using glycol fluid in the collector loop) can be installed only if the piping is protected.

Active Solar Water Heaters

Active solar water heaters rely on electric pumps and controllers to circulate the water (or other heat-transfer fluids). Two types of active solar water heating systems are:

1. Direct circulation systems—These use pumps to circulate pressurized potable water directly through the collectors. These systems are most appropriate for areas that do not have long freezes or hard/acidic water.

2. Indirect circulation systems—These pumps heat transfer fluids through the collectors. These heat exchangers then transfer the heat from the fluid to potable water. Some of these indirect circulation systems have overheat protectors so the collector and glycol fluid do not become superheated.

Common indirect systems include antifreeze, in which the heat transfer fluid is usually a glycol-water mixture, and drainback, in which pumps circulate the water through the collectors and then the water in the collector loop drains back into a reservoir tank when the pump stops.

Installing a Passive Solar Space Heater

A passive solar space heater works when the sun shines through the solar panels to heat the air inside a box. As the air heats up in the box, it rises and moves into the house. Cool air moves into the box and out of the house—in this way, the house is heated without the use of a mechanized heating system. Using a passive solar heater works best if you have a house that faces south and has both basement and first floor windows on that side of the house. If your house meets these requirements (and there aren't too many obstructions that would impede the sun from shining on the heater), then you can begin construction.

The passive solar space heater is made up of a floor and two triangular end walls, all of which can be made simply out of plywood. In between the open space, insulation can be placed. A lid can also be added to cover the heater in the summer.

To build such a solar space heater, first decide where on the southern wall your collector will be located. If you can place the heater in between windows, that is the best option. You may need to cut through the wall

A passive solar space heater.

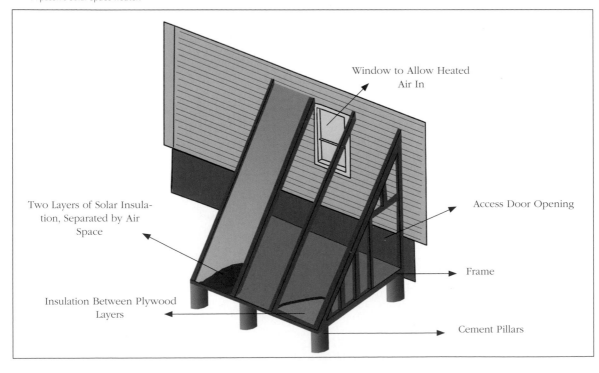

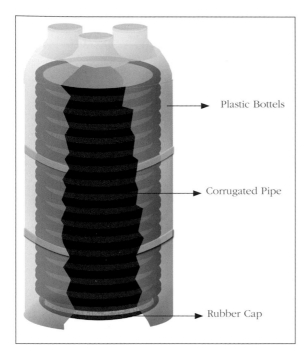

Plastic Bottles

Corrugated Pipe

Rubber Cap

A solar water heater

perfect for camping trips or other smaller water heating uses. Find the supplies online or at a hardware store.

Supplies

- Corrugated, high density polyethylene draining tube (4 inches is preferred)
- An EPDM rubber cap with clamp (available at hardware stores or online)
- Polyethylene terephthalate bottles (3-liter are preferred—soda bottles are fine)

To construct the water heater, simply stretch the EPDM rubber cap over one end of the draining tube and make certain the clamp is tight. Cut the ends off the bottles and fit them over the other end of the drainage pipe. This will serve as the glazing to heat the water. Each bottle should be able to fit tightly over the other bottle if you cut a small hole in the bottom of each. Fill the tube with water, place it in the sun, and allow the water inside the bottles and drainage tube to heat up. Once it's warm (around 120°F is the maximum it will heat the water), it can be used to wash dishes or clothes, or for a small bath.

Heating a Room Using Collectors

Air collectors can be installed on a roof or an exterior, south-facing wall to facilitate the heating of one or more rooms in a house. Factory-built collectors can be used but you can also make and install your own air collector, though note that this is not always cost-efficient.

The air collector should have an airtight and insulated metal frame and a black metal plate. This will absorb the heat through the glazing on the front. The sun's rays heat the plate, which then heats the air in the collector. A fan or blower can pull the air from the room through to the collector and blow it into the room.

Room Air Heating with Collectors

Air collectors can be installed on a roof or an exterior (south facing) wall for heating one or more rooms. Although factory-built collectors for on-site installation

Solar collectors on a roof

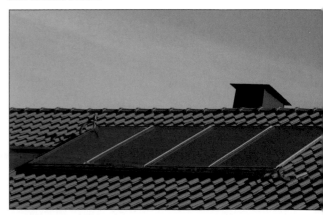

near a window to allow for the proper ventilation but if you don't want to do this, you can also purchase a detachable plywood "chimney" to move the heated air into the house. Next, find the studs that will support the fiberglass panel and find a panel that will be of the appropriate size.

Next, make the base for your solar heating system. The base can be made of 3/8-inch plywood board. Nail the board to a 2 x 4 and level it. Next, add insulation (the kind found on rolls is best), nailing it to the plywood. Then, nail the whole board to the side of the house. Make sloping supports out of 2 x 4s. Make sure the end wall studding is nailed in, and then attach the outside panel to it.

Under the shingles, install flashing or something else that will keep water out of the top of the solar heater. Then, install the fiberglass panels, making sure the edges are caulked so no water can come in. Enclose the edges of the fiberglass with small strips of plywood. Then, install the outer fiberglass panel so that it is flush with the top surface and caulk it. To finish up, paint the inside of the plywood surfaces black to absorb the heat. The inside of the cover panel should be painted white to reflect the light.

Building Your Own Solar Water Heater

This very simple and basic solar water heater is a low-pressure system and so should not be combined with your home plumbing system. This type of heater is

Roof Area Needed in Square Feet (shown in Bold Type)

PV module efficiency (¼)	PV capacity rating (watts)							
	100	250	500	1,000	2,000	4,000	10,000	100,000
4	30	75	150	300	600	1,200	3,000	30,000
8	15	38	75	150	300	600	1,500	15,000
12	10	25	50	100	200	400	1,000	10,000
16	8	20	40	80	160	320	800	8,000

*Although the efficiency (percent of sunlight converted to electricity) varies with the different types of PV modules available today, higher-efficiency modules typically cost more. So, a less-efficient system is not necessarily less cost-effective

are available, do-it-yourselfers may choose to build and install their own air collectors. A simple window air heat collector can be made for a few hundred dollars. Simple window box collector fans will fit in a window opening. These fans can be active or passive. A passive collector fan allows air to enter the bottom of the collector, rise as it heats, and enter the room. A damper keeps the room air from flowing back into the panel on overcast or cloudy days. Window box systems only provide a small amount of heat as the collectors are quite small.

Solar Collectors

Solar collectors are an essential part of active solar heating systems. These collectors harness the sun's energy and transform it into heat. Then, the heat is transferred to water, solar fluid, or air. Solar collectors can be one of two types:

1. Nonconcentrating collectors—These have a collector area that is the same size as the absorption area. The most common type is flat-plate collectors and these are used when temperatures below 200°F are sufficient for space heating.
2. Concentrating collectors—The area of these collectors gathering the solar radiation is much greater than the absorber area.

Solar thermal energy can be used for solar water heating systems, solar pool heaters, and solar space heating systems. There are many types of solar collectors, such as flat plate collectors, evacuated tube collectors, and integral collector storage systems.

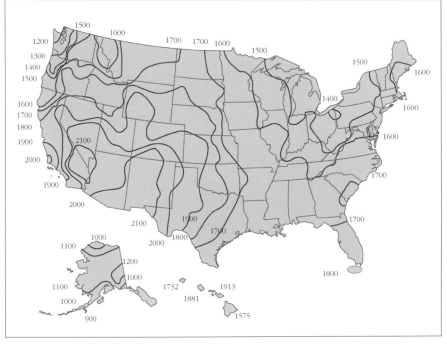

Calculating Electricity Bill Savings for a Net-Metered PV System

First determine the system's size in kilowatts (kW). A reasonable range is 1 to 5 kW. This value is the "kW of PV" input in the equations. Next, based on your geographic location, select the energy production factor from the map below for the kWh/kW-year input for the equations.

Energy from the PV system = (kW of PV) x (kWh/kW-year) = kWh/year. (Divide this number by twelve if you want to determine your monthly energy reduction.)

Energy bills savings = (kWh/year) x (Residential Rate)/100 = $/year saved. (Residential Rate in this above equation should be in dollars per kWh; for example, a rate of 10 cents per kWh is input as $0.10/kWh.)

For example, a 2-kW system in Denver, CO, at a residential energy rate of $0.07/kWh will save about $266 per year (1,900 kWh/kW-year x $0.07/kWh x 2kW = $266/year).

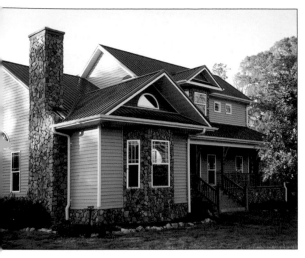

Including plenty of energy-efficient windows in your home will allow sunlight to warm your rooms naturally.

Another Form of Solar Heating: Daylighting

Solar collector panels are not the only way in which the sun's heat can be harnessed for energy purposes. Daylighting uses windows and skylights to bring sunlight into your home. Using energy-efficient windows, as well as carefully thought-out lighting design, reduces the need for artificial lighting during the daytime. These windows also cut down on heating and cooling problems.

The effectiveness of daylighting in your home will depend on your climate and the design of your house. The sizes and locations of window and skylights should be based on the way in which the sun hits your home and not on the outward aesthetics of your house. Facing windows toward the south is most advantageous for daylighting and for moderating seasonal temperatures.

A simple solar oven

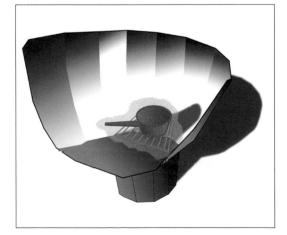

Placing windows that face toward the south will allow more sunlight into your home during the winter months. North-facing windows are also useful for daylighting as they allow a relatively even, natural light into a room, produce little glare, and capture no undesirable summer heat.

Make Your Own Solar Cooking Oven

This type of simple, portable solar oven is perfect for camping trips or if you want to do an outdoor barbeque with additional cooked foods in the summer. This homemade solar oven can reach around 350°F when placed in direct sunlight.

Supplies
- A reflective car sunshade or any sturdy but flexible material (such as cardboard) covered with tin foil and cut to the notched shape of a car sunshade
- Velcro
- A bucket
- A cooking pot
- A wire grill
- A baking bag

Directions
1. Place the car sunshade on the ground. Cut the Velcro into three separate pieces and stick on half of each piece onto the edge near the notch. Then, test the shade to see if the Velcro pieces, when brought together, form a funnel. Place the funnel atop the bucket.
2. Place the cooking pot on the wire grill. Put this all in the baking bag and put it inside the funnel. The rack should now be lying on top of the bucket. Now place the whole cooker in direct sunlight and angle the funnel in the direction of the sun. Adjust the angle as the sun moves.

Make Your Own Solar Panels

Making your own solar panels can be tricky and time-consuming, but with the right materials and lots of patience, you can certainly create an effective solar energy panel.

Supplies
- Pegboard
- Solar cells (quantity will be determined by how much power you want to get from your solar panel)
- Contact wire
- Wire cutters
- Solder
- Soldering iron
- Bolts with washers and wingnuts
- Plexiglass

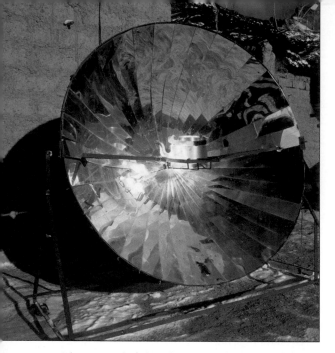

Solar ovens can be fashioned in a variety of ways. The goal is to have as much surface area as possible reflecting the sun toward your food.

- Aluminum framing
- Silicone caulking
- Screws

Directions

1. Apply silicone caulking in vertical strips between the rows of holes on the peg board. Place the solar cells face up along the caulking in straight rows, carefully aligning them so that the wires poke through the holes. The solar cells should completely cover the board.
2. Place a soft sheet or blanket on the ground or table (to prevent the cells from scratching) and care-

Refer to these illustrations while constructing your own solar panel.

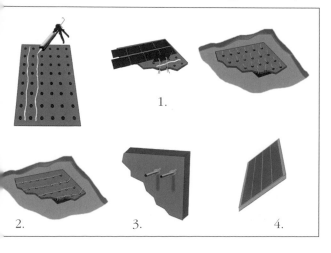

1.

2.   3.   4.

fully flip the baord so that it is face down. Solder together the wires coming out to create one thick wire stemming from each hole. Then use connecting wire or metal strips to connect the wires along horizontal lines. Be sure to connect all positive wires together and all negative wires together, without mixing the two.

3. Drill two holes in the back of your panel and attach a positive and negative bolt, washer, and wingnut. Solder the positive wires to the positive bolt and the negative wires to the negetaive bolt.
4. Build a watertight frame to size, using aluminum framing for the sides, plywood for the backing, and a plexiglass face to allow the sunlight to shine through. Seal all cracks and edges with silicone sealant.

Installing Your Heat Collector

If possible, install your own solar heat collector on the south side of your house (the side that receives the most sunlight during the day). It can be placed in a window to help minimize your heating costs during the winter months.

A solar heat collector can be made from heavy-duty foam insulation, window glass, sealant, aluminum foil, and heavy-duty tape. Paint the foam panel, or both sides of the aluminum sheets, black and then mount it on cubes that are cemented to the side of your house near a window. This will allow the air to come in on both sides of the heat collector.

All sides of the foam should be covered with aluminum foil and then adhered to the foam board. Then place and seal the glass panels over the foam, sealing it with the sealant and heavy-duty tape if needed. Another piece of foam can be utilized as a cover for the duct at night or

The more surface area you cover with solar panels, the more power you'll get. It's best to install your panels on the south side of your home.

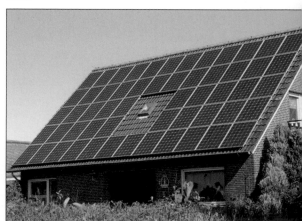

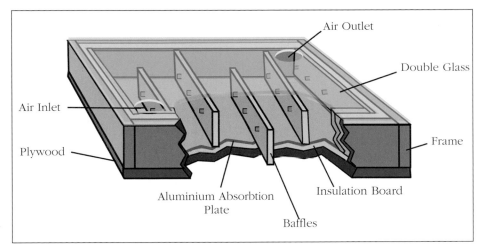

Air Outlet

Double Glass

Air Inlet

Plywood

Frame

Aluminium Absorbtion Plate

Insulation Board

Baffles

Alternate solar heating panel

during the warm, sunny summer months. Hinge this on with hinge brackets or clasps.

An Alternative Solar Heating Panel

This type of solar panel is quite different from the expensive, manufactured panels you can purchase and have installed on your roof or the side of your house. It is great for heating air but cannot produce electricity. You can either situate this heater in a south-facing window of your home or place it on the outside, southern wall or on the roof. Heating panels that are on the outside of a house generally create more heat and are much more effective in heating a room or area of your home.

To start, you will need to purchase glass or Plexiglas for your solar heating panel. Either one should be double-paned to keep out moisture. To build the frame for your solar heating panel, use 2 x 4s and create a square or rectangle that will fit your pane of glass. Nail

Solar panels can be placed in a field or other sunny area to collect energy, which is stored and then used as needed.

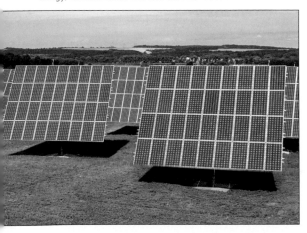

plywood to the back of the frame. Next, take a piece of insulation board and put it at the back of the panel. Heat absorption can be gained through aluminum flashing or copper. After this is inserted, screw down the window frame, if you are using one, and make sure it is caulked well to keep out any leaking water.

Add the interior boards that line the frame and the baffles to seal the top of the glass. Screw these interior boards to the sides of the panel to keep them secure. Then, cut out the air openings using a jigsaw. One circular opening should be in the lower left and the other in the upper right of your heating panel. Before hanging the panel up, you will need to determine where the studs are in the wall or where the roof rafters are located (if you are installing on your roof). It is also important that your openings do not fall on top of a stud or rafter as this will defeat their ability to direct airflow. Screw in

Regulations for Installing and Building Solar Heating Systems

Before you install a solar energy system, it is important to learn about the local building codes, zoning, and neighborhood covenants as they apply to these systems. You will most likely need to obtain a building permit to install a solar energy system onto an existing building. Common problems you may encounter as a homeowner in installing a solar energy system are: exceeding roof load, unacceptable heat exchangers, improper wiring, tampering with potable water supplies, obstructing property and yards, and placing the system too close to the street or lot lines. There are also local compliances that must be factored in before installing your system. Contact your local jurisdiction zoning and building enforcement divisions and any homeowner's, neighborhood, or community associations before building and installing any solar heating equipment.

boards along the studs or rafters, on which you will then mount the panel.

Once the panel is secured to the wall or roof, begin to install the air delivery system so the hot air can be circulated throughout your home. You may want to add a small fan (one used in a computer will be fine) to your heating panel so you can better circulate the air throughout the system, though this is not necessary to operate your heating panel effectively. If you do choose to use a fan, it must be able to fit inside the wall plate. You will need to drill a hole in your wall where the panel holes are situated on the outside. Cut the hole and add the connector to the ductwork, sliding it through the hole into the room, and seal off the edges of the hole.

Place the fan within the wall plate in the room, and place an electrical box near the fan to turn it on and off. If you aren't familiar with electrical work, you may want to ask an electrician to help you with connecting the electrical wiring. Next, mount the solar panel so it faces to the south, running a wire into the electrical box inside the room. This will save you money and energy while running your fan. Now turn on the fan and feel the warm air starting to blow through your room.

To finish your outside panel, simply paint the inside black to absorb more heat, add some weather stripping to seal the glass tightly, and screw the glass piece to the panel.

Solar Greenhouse

Greenhouses collect solar energy on sunny days and then store the heat for use in the evening and on days when it is overcast. A solar greenhouse can be situated as a free-standing structure (like a shed or larger enclosure) or in an underground hole.

For gardeners who want to grow small amounts of produce, passive solar greenhouses are a good option and help extend the growing season. Active systems take supplemental energy sources to move the solar heated air from its storage facility to other parts of the greenhouse. Solar greenhouses can utilize many of the same features and installation techniques as passive solar heating systems used in homes to stay heated.

While standard greenhouses also rely on the sun's rays to heat their interiors, solar greenhouses are different because they have special glazing that absorbs large amounts of heat during the winter months and also use

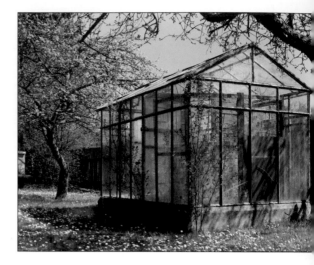

materials to store the heat. Solar greenhouses have a lot of insulation in areas with little sunlight to keep heat loss at a minimum.

Types of Solar Greenhouses

Two common types of solar greenhouses are the attached solar greenhouse and the freestanding solar greenhouse. Attached solar greenhouses are situated next to a house or shed and are typically lean-to structures. They are limited in the amount of produce they can grow and have passive solar heating systems.

Freestanding solar greenhouses are large structures that are best suited for producing a large variety and quantity of produce, flowers, and herbs. They can be constructed in the form of either a shed structure or a hoop house. In a shed greenhouse, the south wall is glazed to maximize the heating potential and the north wall is extremely well insulated. Hoop house greenhouses are rounded instead of shaped like an elongated shed. Solar energy is collected and stored in earth thermal storage and in water. These systems, while common,

Both flowers and vegetables can thrive in greenhouses.

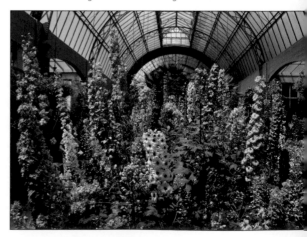

A solar greenhouse

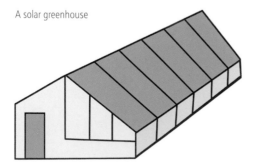

are not as effective in utilizing solar energy as the shed and lean-to structures.

Sites for Solar Greenhouses

The glazing portion of the solar greenhouse should ideally face directly south to gain the maximum exposure to the sun's heat. Situating the solar greenhouse on a slight slope facing upward will maximize the amount of solar energy it can absorb.

Materials Used in Solar Greenhouse Construction

For a solar greenhouse to be able to collect, circulate, and maintain the greatest amount of heat, it is important that it is constructed out of the proper materials. Glazing materials need to allow photosynthetic radiation to get through so it can reach the plants. Clear glass allows direct light into the greenhouse and so should be used as a glazing material. It is also imperative that when the glazing materials are mounted on the greenhouse, there are no cracks or holes that can allow for heat to escape. Thus, glazing material should have high heat efficiency and be made of resistant material to hold up in inclement weather and hail.

Solar greenhouses also need to be able to store the heat that is collected for use on cloudy days or at night. The easiest method for storing heat is to situate rocks, concrete, and/or water in the path of the sunlight that is entering the greenhouse. These materials will absorb the heat during the day and release it during the evening hours. Pools of water, rocks, and concrete slabs or small walls should be large enough to absorb and emit enough heat to last for the night or for a few cloudy days.

Phase-change materials may also be used to effectively store heat in your solar greenhouse. These materials consist of paraffin, fatty acids, and Glauber's salt. These materials store heat as they change into liquid and release it as they turn back into a solid form. They are kept in sealed tubes and many are needed to provide enough heat.

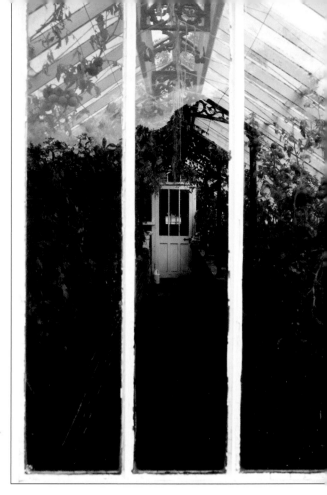

Greenhouses can be made in a range of shapes and sizes and can be attached to your home or separate from it.

All areas of the greenhouse that are not glazed need to be insulated to keep in the maximum amount of heat. Weather stripping is helpful in sealing doors and vents; foam insulation is helpful for walls. Place a polyethylene film between the insulation and the greenhouse walls to keep these materials dry—if they become too wet or saturated, they will be less effective and may start to mold. The floors of a solar greenhouse can also lose heat so they should be made out of brick or flagstone (with insulation foam underneath) to keep the heat in.

The solar greenhouse needs outdoor insulation as well, which can be attained by placing hay bales along the edges of the greenhouse, or the greenhouse can be situated slightly underground (a pit greenhouse). Of course, if a greenhouse is dug into the soil, it needs to be in an area that is above the water level to minimize leakage.

A solar greenhouse, like any other greenhouse, also needs proper ventilation for the warmer summer months. Vents in the sides of the greenhouse will help create air flow. Ridge vents in the roof will allow the hottest air to escape out of the top of the greenhouse as well. If a greenhouse needs more ventilation, a solar chimney can be hooked up to the passive solar collectors to release extra heat out into the air.

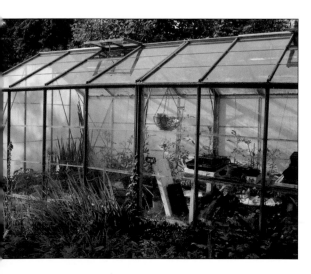

Wind Energy

Wind energy is created naturally by circulation patterns in the Earth's atmosphere driven by the heat from the sun. These winds are caused by the uneven heating of the atmosphere by the sun, the irregularities of the earth's surface, and the rotation of the earth. Wind patterns are modified by the earth's terrain, bodies of water, and vegetation. Since the earth's surface is made of very different types of land and water, it absorbs the sun's heat at different rates. During the day, the air above the land heats up very quickly. The warm air over the land expands and rises and the heavier, cooler air rushes in to take its place, creating winds. At night, the winds are reversed as the air cools rapidly over land. This air flow is used for many purposes: sailing, flying kites, and generating electricity.

Small Wind Electric Systems

Small wind electric systems are one of the most cost-effective, home-based renewable energy systems. These systems are nonpolluting and are fairly easy to set up. A small wind electric system can effectively:

- Lower your electricity bills by 50 to 90 percent
- Help you avoid high costs of having utility power lines extended to a remote location
- Help uninterruptible power supplies ride through extended utility outages

How Do Small Wind Electric Systems Work?

When the wind spins a wind turbine's blades, a rotor captures the kinetic energy of the wind, converting it into rotary motion to drive the generator. Most turbines have automatic overspeed-governing systems to keep the rotor from spinning out of control on very windy days.

A small wind system can be connected to an electric distribution system (grid-connected) or it can stand alone (off-grid). To capture and convert

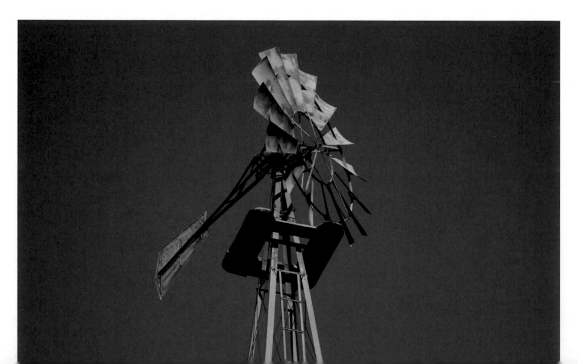

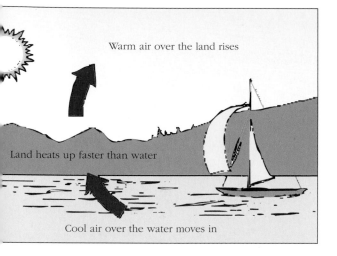

Warm air over the land rises

Land heats up faster than water

Cool air over the water moves in

A Brief History of Wind Energy

People have been harnessing energy from the wind since ancient times. Wind was used to sail ships and windmills were build to help grind wheat, corn, and other grains. Windmills were also used to pump water and to cut wood at sawmills in the formative years of the American colonies. Even into the early twentieth century, windmills were being used to generate electricity in rural parts of America. The windmill again gained national attention in the early 1980s when wind energy was finally considered a renewable energy source. It continues to be a growing industry throughout the United States.

the wind's kinetic energy into electricity, a home wind energy system must generally be comprised of the following:

1. A wind turbine—This consists of blades attached to a rotor, a generator/alternator mounted on a frame, and a tail
2. A tower
3. Balance-of-system components—i.e., controllers, inverters, and/or batteries

A wind-electric turbine generator, more commonly known as a "wind turbine," converts kinetic energy in the wind into mechanical power. This power can be used directly for specific tasks, like grinding grains or pumping water. A generator can also convert this mechanical power into a high-value, highly flexible and useful form of energy—electricity.

Wind turbines make electricity by working in the opposite way as a fan. Instead of using electricity to make wind, as a fan does, turbines use wind to make electricity. The wind turns the blades, spinning a shaft that connects to a generator, which makes electricity.

The basic parts of a small wind electric system

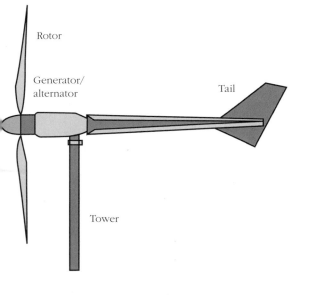

Rotor

Generator/
alternator

Tail

Tower

Installing a Small Electric Wind System

Small wind electric systems, with the proper installation and maintenance, can last over 20 years. Before installing your system, first find the best site, determine the appropriate size of your wind turbine, decide whether you want a grid-connected or stand-alone system, and find out about your local zoning, permitting, and neighborhood covenant requirements.

Many people decide to install these systems on their own (though the manufacturer and/or dealer should also be able to help you install the small wind electric system). However, before you attempt to install the wind turbine, make sure you can answer these do-it-yourself questions:

1. Can I pour a proper cement foundation?
2. Do I have access to a lift, ladder, or another way to erect the tower safely?
3. Do I know the difference between alternating current (AC) and direct current (DC) wiring?
4. Do I know enough about electricity to safely wire my turbine?
5. Do I know how to safely handle and install batteries?

If the answer to any of these questions is "No," then you should have someone help you install the system (contact the manufacturer or your state energy office).

Evaluating a Potential Site for Your Small Wind Turbine

The site on which you choose to install your system should meet the following criteria:
• Your property has a good wind resource—good annual wind speeds and a prevailing direction for the wind.

Inside a Wind Turbine

Parts of a wind turbine:

• Anemometer: measures the wind speed and transmits wind speed data to the controller.
• Blades: most turbines have either two or three blades and the wind blows over the blades, causing the blades to lift and rotate.
• Brake: a disc brake, applied mechanically, electrically, or hydraulically, and stops the rotor in emergencies.
• Controller: starts up the machine at wind speeds of about 8 to 16 mph and shuts off the machine at about 55 mph wind speeds. Turbines do not operate at wind speeds above 55 mph because they may be damaged.
• Gear box: gears connect the low-speed shaft to the high-speed shaft and increase the rotational speeds from about 30 to 60 rotations per minute (rpm) to about 1000 to 1800 rpm—the rotational speed required by most generators to produce electricity. The gear box is a costly and heavy part of the wind turbine.
• Generator: usually an off-the-shelf induction generator that produces 60-cycle AC electricity.
• High-speed shaft: drives the generator.
• Low-speed shaft: turned by the rotor at about 30 to 60 rpm.
• Nacelle: sits atop the tower and contains the gear box, low- and high-speed shafts, generator, controller, and brake. Some nacelles are large enough for a helicopter to land on.
• Pitch: Turns the blades out of the wind to control the rotor speed and keep the rotor from turning in winds that are too high or too low to produce electricity.
• Rotor: the blades and hub.
• Tower: made from tubular steel, concrete, or steel lattice. Since wind speed increases with height, taller towers enable turbines to capture more energy and generate more electricity.
• Wind direction: an "upwind" turbine operates facing into the wind while other turbines are designed to face "downwind" or away from the wind.
• Wind vane: measures wind direction and communicates with the yaw drive to orient the turbine properly with respect to the wind.
• Yaw drive: used to keep the rotor facing into the wind as the wind direction changes (not required for downwind turbines).
• Yaw motor: powers the yaw drive.

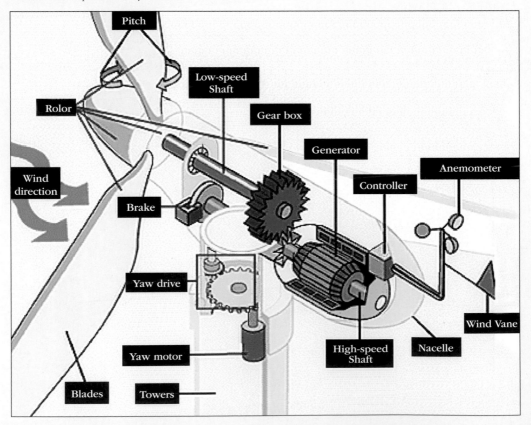

- Your home is located on at least one acre of land in a rural area.
- Your local zoning codes and covenants do not prohibit construction of a wind turbine.
- Your average electricity bill is $150 per month or more.

If you live in an area that has complex terrain, be careful when selecting an installation site. If you place your wind turbine on the top of a hill or on an exceptionally windy side, you will have more access to prevailing winds than in a gully or on the sheltered side of a hill. Additionally, it is important to consider any existing obstacles—trees, houses, sheds—that may be in the way of the wind's path. You should also plan for future obstructions, such as new buildings or landscaping. Your turbine needs to be positioned upwind of any buildings and trees, and it needs to be 30 feet above anything within 300 feet of its site.

When determining the suitability of your site for a small electric wind system, estimate your site's wind resource. Wind resource can vary significantly over an area of just a few miles because of local terrain's influence on wind flow. Use the following methods to help estimate your wind resource before installing your small electric wind system:

1. Consult a wind resource map. This is used to estimate the wind resource in your area. You can find a specific map for your state at the U.S. Department of Energy's Wind Powering America Program Web site. A general U.S. map is shown in the figure.
2. Obtain wind speed data. The easiest way to quantify the wind resource in your area is by obtaining the average wind speed information from a local airport. Airport wind data are typically measured 20 to 33 feet above ground. Average wind speeds increase with height and may be as much as 15 to 25 percent greater at a usual wind turbine hub (80 feet high) than those measured at airports.
3. Watch vegetation flagging. Flagging is the effect of strong winds on an area of vegetation. For example, if a group of trees on flat ground is leaning significantly in one direction, chances are they've become that way due to strong winds.
4. Use a measurement system. Direct monitoring using a measurement system at a certain site provides the best picture of the available wind resource. These are very expensive, however, and so may not be practical to use.
5. Obtain data from a local small wind system—if there is a small wind turbine near your area, you may be able to obtain information on the annual output of the system, as well as wind speed data.

Wind Power Classification

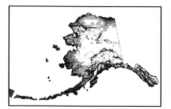

Wind power Class	Resource Potential	Wind Power Density at 50 m W/m2	Wind Speeda at 50m m/s	Wind Speeda at 50 m mph
3	Fair	300–400	6.4–7.0	14.3–15.7
4	Good	400–500	7.0–7.5	15.7–16.8
5	Excellent	500–600	7.5–8.0	16.8–17.9
6	Outstanding	600–800	8.0–8.8	17.9–19.7
7	Superb	800–1600	8.8–11.1	19.7–24.8

[a]Wind speeds are based on a Welbull k value of 2.0

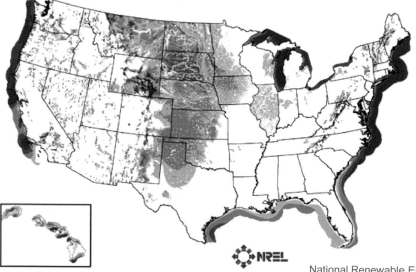

National Renewable Energy Laboratory
Innovation for Our Energy Future

Small Wind Turbines Used for Homes

Single, small, stand-alone turbines that are sized below 100 kilowatts are used for homes, telecommunication dishes, and water pumping. Used in residential applications, these small wind turbines can range from 400 watts to 20 kilowatts. In addition to being used for generating electricity and pumping water, they can be used for charging batteries. Most U.S. manufacturers rate their small wind turbines by the amount of power they can safely produce at wind speeds between 24 and 36 mph.

An average home uses about 9,400 kilowatt-hours of electricity per year. Thus, a wind turbine rated in the 5- to 15-kilowatt range would make a significant contribution to this energy demand. Before deciding on a wind turbine you should:

1. Establish an energy budget. Try to reduce the electricity use in your home so you will only need a small turbine.
2. Determine an appropriate height for the wind turbine's tower so it will generate the maximum amount of energy.
3. Remember that a small home-sized wind machine has rotors that are between 8 and 25 feet in diameter and stand around 30 feet tall. If your property does not have enough space to accommodate this, you may not be able to have a powerful enough turbine to help significantly reduce your energy costs.

Windmill blades can vary in shape but should always be angled to catch the most wind.

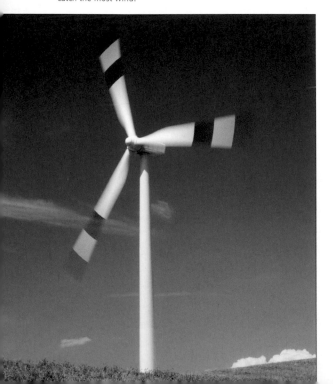

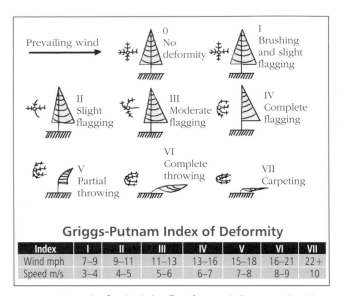

Griggs-Putnam Index of Deformity

Index	I	II	III	IV	V	VI	VII
Wind mph	7–9	9–11	11–13	13–16	15–18	16–21	22+
Speed m/s	3–4	4–5	5–6	6–7	7–8	8–9	10

Vegetation flagging is the effect of strong winds on vegetation. It's a good indicator of how strong the winds are in that area.

Maintaining Your Small Wind Turbine

In order to keep your turbine running smoothly and efficiently, do an annual check of the following:
- Check and tighten bolts and electrical connections as necessary.
- Check machines for corrosion.
- Check the guy wires for proper tension.
- Check for and replace any worn leading-edge tape on the turbine blades.
- Replace the turbine blades and/or bearings after 10 years.

Types of Wind Turbines

Modern wind turbines fall into two basic categories: horizontal-axis varieties and vertical-axis designs.

Horizontal-axis Wind Turbines

Most wind machines used today fall into this category. Horizontal-axis wind machines have blades like an airplane propeller. A standard horizontal wind machine stands about 20 stories tall and has three blades spanning 200 feet across. These are the machines most readily found in large fields and on wind farms.

The majority of small wind turbines made today are of the horizontal-axis style. They have two or three blades made of composite material, such as fiberglass. The turbine's frame is a structure to which the rotor, generator, and tail are all attached. The diameter of the rotor will determine the amount of energy the turbine will produce. The tail helps keep the turbine facing into the

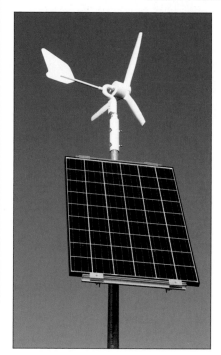

Stand-Alone and Small Hybrid Systems

Wind power can also be used in off-grid systems. These are called stand-alone systems because they are not connected to an electric distribution grid. In these systems, small wind turbines can be used in combination with other components, such as small solar electric systems, to create a hybrid power system. Hybrid power systems provide reliable off-grid power for homes (and even for entire communities in certain instances) that are far from local utility lines.

A hybrid electric system may be a practical system for you if:

- You live in an area with average annual wind speed of at least nine mph.
- A grid connection is not available or can only be made through a very costly extension.
- You would like to become independent from your energy utility company.
- You would like to generate clean power.

Small hybrid systems that combine wind and solar technologies offer several advantages over either single system. In many parts of the United States, wind speeds are low in the summer when the sun shines the brightest and for the longest hours. Conversely, the wind is stronger in the winter when less sunlight is available. These hybrid systems, therefore, are more likely to produce power when you need it.

If there are times when neither the wind nor the solar systems are producing energy, most hybrid systems will then provide power through batteries or an engine generator powered by diesel fuel (which can also recharge the batteries if they run low).

⩘ A solar and wind hybrid energy system

Hybrid power » systems combine multiple sources to deliver non-intermittent electric power.

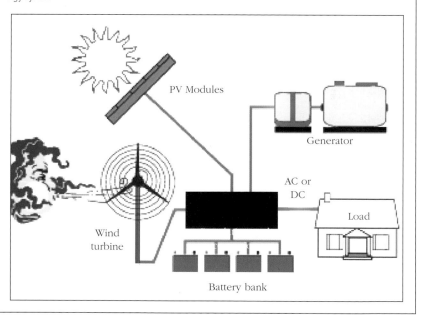

PV Modules

Generator

AC or DC

Load

Wind turbine

Battery bank

wind. Mounted on a tower, the wind turbine has better access to stronger winds.

These machines also require balance-of-system components. These parts are required for water pumping systems and other residential uses of your wind turbine. These also vary based on the type of system you are using: either a grid-connected, stand-alone, or hybrid.

For example, if you have a residential grid-connected wind turbine system, your balance-of-systems parts will include:

- A controller
- Storage batteries
- A power conditioning unit (inverter)
- Wiring

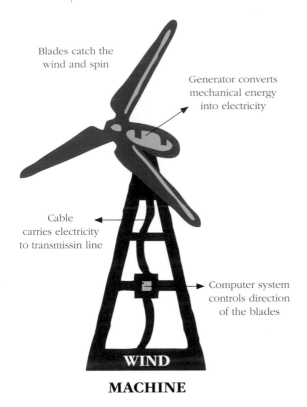

Blades catch the wind and spin

Generator converts mechanical energy into electricity

Cable carries electricity to transmissin line

Computer system controls direction of the blades

WIND MACHINE

A horizontal-axis wind turbine

A hybrid wind and solar energy system

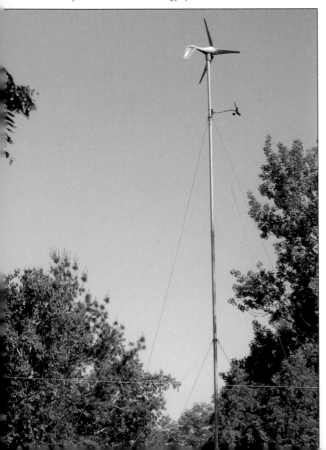

- Electrical disconnect switch
- Grounding system
- Foundation for the tower

Vertical-axis Wind Turbines

These machines have blades that go from top to bottom. The most common type looks like a giant two-bladed egg beater. Vertical-axis wind machines are generally 100 feet tall and 50 feet wide. Though these wind turbines have the potential to produce a great deal of energy, they make up only a small percentage of the wind machines that are in use currently due to the cost and effort required to set them up. In addition, they produce a great deal of noise, can be unsightly, hurt the bird population, and require large roads and heavy-duty equipment to get them up and running.

Grid-Connected Small Wind Electric Systems

Small wind energy systems can be connected to the electricity distribution system to become "grid-connected systems." These wind turbines can help reduce your consumption of utility-supplied electricity for appliances, electric heat, and lighting. The utility will make up the difference for any energy that your turbine cannot make. Any excess electricity that is produced by the system, and cannot be used by the household, can often be sent or sold to the utility. One drawback to this system, however, is that during power outages, the wind turbine is required to shut down for safety reasons.

Grid-connected systems are only practical if:

- You live in an area with average annual wind speeds of at least 10 mph.
- Utility-supplied electricity is expensive in your area.
- The utility's requirements for connecting your system to its grid are not exceedingly expensive.
- There are good incentives for the sale of excess electricity.

Mounting Your Small Wind Electric System on a Tower

Since wind speeds increase with height, it is essential that your small wind turbine be mounted on a tower. The higher the tower, the more power the wind system will be able to produce. To determine the best height for your tower, you will need to know the estimated annual energy output and the size of your turbine.

There are two types of towers: self-supporting (free-standing) and guyed. Most home wind power systems use a guyed tower as it is the least expensive. Guyed towers consist of these parts:

- Lattice sections

A grid-connected small wind electric system

- Pipe
- Tubing (depending on the design)
- Supporting guy wires

These towers are easier to install but they do require lots of space—the radius of the tower must be ½ to ¾ of the tower height.

Tilt-down towers, while more expensive, offer an easy way to maintain smaller, lightweight turbines that are less than 10 kilowatts. These towers can be lowered to the ground during severe weather or unusually high winds.

Generally, it is a good idea to install a small wind turbine on a tower with the bottom of the rotor blades around 30 feet above any obstacle that is within 300 feet from the tower.

Windmills

Windmills are used for pumping water, milling, and operating light machinery all around the world. They are constructed in a variety of shapes and some are quite picturesque. When set up properly, windmills cost nothing to operate and if the wheel is made well, it will last for many years without need for major repairs. To make a windmill requires a good understanding of carpentry and workmanship but it is not incredibly difficult or expensive to do.

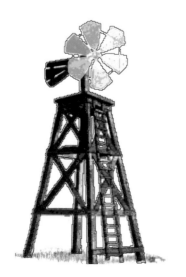

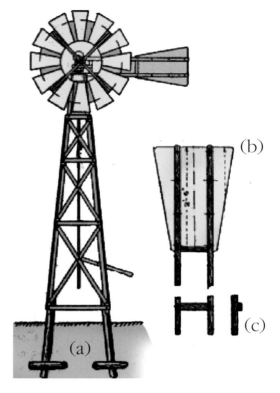

Details of the windmill. Figure (a) shows a general view with the tail turned to "off" position. Figure (b) shows details of the tail, and (c) shows a cross-piece of the tail.

Constructing a Windmill

Windmills can be of all sizes, though the larger the windmill, the more power it can generate. This windmill and tower can be easily constructed out of wood, an old wheel, and a few iron fittings you may be able to find at a hardware store or home center. Constructing the windmill in sections is the easiest way to create this structure. Simply follow these directions to make your own energy-producing windmill:

The Tower

1. The tower is the first part to be built and should be constructed out of four spruce sticks that are 16 feet long and 4 inches square, in a configuration that measures 30 inches square at the top and 72 inches square at the base.
2. The deck should be 36 inches square and should project 2 inches over the top rails.
3. The rails and cross braces can be spruce or pine strips and should measure 4 inches wide and 7/8 inch thick. Attach these to the corner posts with steel-wire nails.
4. Embed the corner posts 2 feet into the ground, leaving 14 feet above the surface. The rail at the bottom, which is attached to the four posts, should measure 3 feet above the ground. Midway between

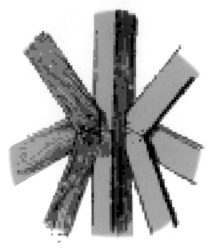

Beveled cross braces fit snugly against the corners.

this and the top rail of the deck, run a middle rail around the post. Make sure that where your wheel will be attached, this point rises at least 2 feet above any obstructions (buildings, trees, etc.) so it can have access to the blowing wind.

5. The cross braces should be beveled at the ends so they fit snugly against the corner.
6. The posts, rails, and braces should be planed so they present a nice appearance at the end of the building. A ladder can also be constructed at one side of the tower to allow easy access to the mill.
7. Nail a board across two of the rails halfway up the tower. Secure the lower end of a trunk tightly here

if you are constructing a pumping mill. However, if a wooden mill is what you are after, you can use an old wheel from a wagon and six blades of wood.

The Turntable

1. The turntable holds the wheel and tail. It should be built of 2½ x 2-inch timber and 2-inch galvanized wrought iron "water" tube and flanges.
2. The upper flange supports the timber framing. It should be countersunk, using a half-round file, and screwed tightly onto the tube as far as possible. The end of the tube should project just slightly beyond the face of the flange so that it can be riveted over to fill the countersink.
3. Bolt the two loose flanges to the framework of the tower. Use them with 2-inch pipe with the thread filed away so they may slide freely onto the tube. The upper loose flange should form a footstep bearing and the lower flange a guide for the turntable.
4. Now mount the turntable on the ball bearing to make sure the mill head can turn freely. Screw on two back nuts to guard against any possibility of the turntable being lifted out of place by a strong wind.

The Head

1. This is the part that will carry the wheel spindle.
2. Notch the joints and secure them with 2-inch bolts.
3. The upright, which carries a bolt or pin for the spur-wheel to revolve upon, is kept in place in the front and at the sides by a piece of hoop iron.

The windmill turntable (d, e, and f) holds the wheel and tail. The flange (detailed drawings g and h) forms a support for the timber framing.

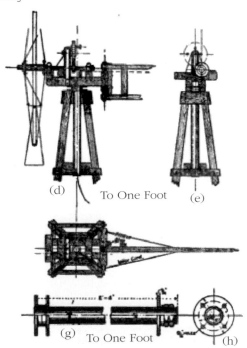

(d)   To One Foot   (e)

(g) To One Foot   (h)

Details of the wheel shaft frame (i, j); front and side views, (k, l); axle of wheel (m); attachment of inner end of vane to inner ring of frame (n); vane on rings (o); attachment of vane to outer brackets by bracket (p).

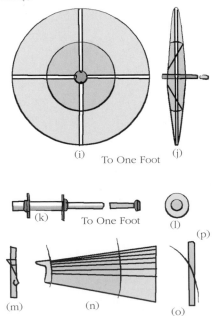

(i)   To One Foot   (j)

(k)   To One Foot   (l)

(p)

(m)   (n)   (o)

4. The tail vane swivel is a piece of 5-inch bore tube with back nuts and washers. Pass an iron bolt or other piece of iron through this, screw it to each end, and fit it with four nuts and washers.

The Wheel Shaft

1. Use wrought-iron tubing and flanges to create the wheel shaft. The bore of the tube is at least 5 inches, and the outside diameter should be roughly 1½ inches. Both the tube and the fittings should be of good quality and a thick gauge (steam quality is preferred).
2. If lathe is available, lightly skim it over the tubing. However, if it's not, a careful filing will do just as well to smooth down the edges.
3. Screw the tube higher up on one end to receive the flanges forming the hub. Screw these on and secure them on one side with back nuts and on the other with a distance piece made out of a 1½-inch bore tube. Fit a cap to close the open front end of the tube.
4. Grease two plummer blocks with some form of lubrication. These will be the bearings for the shaft.
5. A pinion is needed of at least 2½ inches in diameter at the pitch circle. Bore it to fit the wheel shaft. A spur wheel of 7 inches in diameter should follow that (gear wheels from a lawn mower can be used if available).

The Wheel

1. The wheel should be at least 5 feet in diameter to produce a good amount of energy. The framing consists of an inner and outer ring and four double arms with cross stays and diagonals (a regular wooden wheel will be sufficient, or you can find one made of galvanized steel).
2. Cut each spoke at an angle on one side so that the blades will have the necessary pitch to make the wind turn them.
3. The blades should be 18 inches long, 12 inches wide at the outer ends, and 6 inches wide next to the hub. Each blade should be only ¾ inch thick. Attach them to the spokes with simple screws.
4. If you desire, you can string a wire between the outer end of each blade to the end of the next spoke. This will help steady the blades.

The Tail

1. Run a fine saw cut up about 2 feet 6 inches from the outer end to receive the vane (optional).
2. Pass a cord over two pulleys and down the turntable tube. It is necessary to attach the end of the cord to a short cylinder of hard wood or metal (about 2 to 3 inches in diameter). This revolves with the turntable but can be slid up or down.

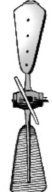

Each spoke should be cut at an angle so that the blades will have the pitch to make the wind turn them.

Total Lift	Gallons per Hour	Bore of Pump	Approximate Stroke
26 ft	100	2 in.	3½ in.
60 ft	50	2 in.	1½ in.
100 ft	25	1½ in.	1½ in.

3. If you plan on using a pump, it is important to cut a hole through the axis of the cylinder to fit the pump rod.
4. Cut a groove in the circumference of the cylinder, and bend two pieces of iron into shape and place them into the grooves. Now take the cords from the two bolts, untying the straps. Join these two cords to another cord, which acts as a reel or lever at the base of the tower. In this way, the position of the tail can be regulated from a stationary point.

Adding Pumps to Your Windmill

If you want to use this windmill to pump water, then you may need to do some experimenting with different lengths of pump stroke. Below is a table indicating what should be expected from the pump, and also providing the size of the single-action pump suitable for a given lift (using a ratio of 1 to 3).

Make sure that your pump is not too large; otherwise, it may not start in a light wind or breeze.

The pump is driven by a pin screwed into the side of the spur wheel and is secured with a lock nut. Drill and tap three or four holes at different distances from the center of the wheel so the length of the stroke can be adjusted. If the spokes on the wheel are too thin for drilling, you can use a clamp with a projecting pin instead.

A pump rod—a continuous wooden rod about 1 inch square and thicker at the top end—can be used in connecting the bottom end (by bolting) to the "bow" supplied with the pump. Intermediate joints, if needed, can be fashioned with 1 x ½-inch fish plates roughly 6 inches long. If the pump is no more than 12 feet below the crank pin, one guide will be adequate. The pump rod must be able to revolve with the head and will be need to be thickened up in a circular section where it passes through the guide. Make the guide in two halves and screw or bolt it to a bar running across the tower.

Final Touches

When construction is finished, paint all of the woodwork any color that complements your yard or property and, if desired, lacquer it to protect the wood from rain and snow. A windmill of this size will create at least a one quarter horsepower in a 15 mph wind.

Building a Small Wind Motor

This small wind motor can easily be made to generate energy for small machines, tool shed lightbulbs, and other small mechanics. The foundation for this wind-

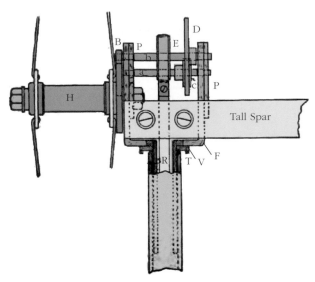

Details of small wind motor

wheel can be made out of the front wheel of an old bicycle with the front spindle and cones completely intact.

Attach eight to 12 vanes of stout sheet tin to the rim. These sheets should be around 8 inches long and 4 to 6 inches wide and should lie at a 30-degree angle to the plane of the rim. The vanes will be much more efficient if they are curved in a circular arc about the same radius as the wheel. The concave side should be positioned to face toward the wind.

On the back of each vane, rivet a rib of strip iron ½ inch thick. This strip should project about ½ inch beyond the tip and 1½ inches at the other end. There, twist and bend it to make a bracket and then bolt the vane to the center line of the rim.

The illustration above shows a side view of the motor with its gearing and supports. *A* is the rim and part of the spokes of a toothed wheel that are attached at several points to the spokes of the bicycle wheel. It is loosely fixed and adjusted until it runs well when the wheel is moved. It should not wobble. *A* drives a smaller cog, *B*,

mounted on the same spindle, *a*. This spindle revolves around two plates, *PP*, screwed to *F*. *C* drives a large cog, *D*, and an eccentric, *E*, which moves the eccentric rod, *R*, up and down. This works the small pump at the foot of the mast that supports the windmill. *E* can be quickly made out of a thick disc with two larger discs soldered to it. *R* is a piece of stout brass strip bent around *E* and closed with a screw.

When all of the vanes are in position, connect the tips of the ribs and vanes together with rings of stout wire and solder them on at all the contact points. Screw one of the spindle nuts tightly against its cone. The other end of the spindle should pass through one arm of the stirrup (*F*) made out of ½-inch iron 1½ inches wide. This is then secured by a washer and nut on the inside. The stirrup and circular plate (*V*) are bored to accommodate the end of the iron pipe (*T*).

Close off the top of the hole (*F*) and heat the top of the pipe to expand it to fit into the chamber. Clean these parts well and weld them together. It is important that the *T* is square with the stirrup. Then, cut the pipe off 9 inches below *V*. Solder a small ring to the underside of *V* to prevent moisture from working its way along *T* and ruining your motor.

The tail spar is a wooden bar 1½ x 2½ inches wide and 40 inches long. It is notched to fit the stirrup and tapered off toward the tail. A sheet of sturdy iron, 15 x 12 inches, is then fitted into the saw cut. Two bolts clip the wings of the forked end tightly against the sides of the stirrup. The tail should be able to balance the wheel on the vertical pivot to avoid stressing the joint at the top of *T*.

A wind-wheel this size will spin quite effectively in a blustery wind but will probably only generate enough energy to power a small pump. This will do nicely to fill a watering can for your garden or for powering other light machinery.

A Pumping Windmill

A pumping windmill can help you pump water from a well or other underground reservoir into a suction-pump. This windmill has a simple wheel with spokes

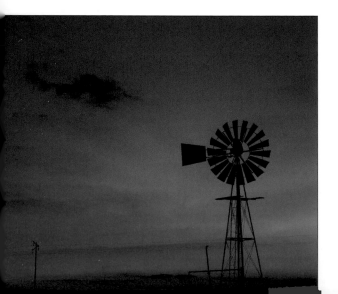

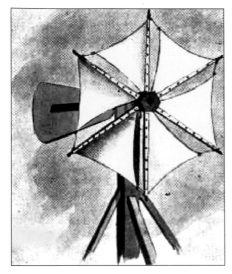

A pumping windmill

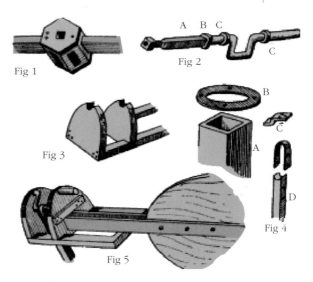

Windmill pump details

and sails. It consists of a hub, six spokes, a fan tail, and a trunk or pole for attaching the wheel.

The hub is a hexagon 6 x 6 inches. One spoke can be driven into a hole made on either side (Figure 1). The spokes should be 3 feet long, 3 x 1½ inches at the hub end, and 1 x 1½ inches on the outer end. The spokes are driven into the holes in the hub and pinned to hold them in place.

The hub should be made of hard wood and the holes may be cut with a mortise chisel and mallet. Make sure the holes are spaced evenly so the spokes will light up properly.

Attach triangular pieces of twilled muslin sheeting to the face of each spoke. The loose corner of each can be attached to the next spoke end with a piece of string. This creates an outlet between the leech and the spoke of each space between the spoke so that the wind can pass through. This, in effect, makes the wheel turn.

The wheel should be held in place at the top of the supporting post by a shaft passing through the hub and bolted to the front of the wheel with a nut. Figure 2 is a good example of what this should look like. The shaft should be about 1 inch square where it passes through the hub. At the front end, it should be tightened with a nut and washer. The square part, A, where the end of the hub will be, should be welded at B to hold the hub in the proper place. About an inch beyond the square shoulder, another one, C, should be welded to the shaft. This helps balance the wheel.

Now a crank can be formed, 2 inches wide and 3 inches out from the shaft. Another collar, C, C, should be welded onto the crank and then, beyond this point, the shaft should stick out about 6 inches.

The total length of the shaft is 15 inches, and the whole device can be painted. To attach the fan tail, a head made out of two blocks of wood should be

What would happen if we used more wind energy?

According to the American Wind Energy Association, if we increase our nation's wind energy capacity to 20 percent by 2030, it would have the following effects:

- *Reduce Greenhouse Gas Emission:* A cumulative total of 7,600 million tons of CO_2 would be avoided by 2030, and more than 15,000 million tons of CO_2 would be avoided by 2050.
- *Conserve Water:* Reduce cumulative water consumption in the electric sector by 8 percent or 4 trillion gallons from 2007 through 2030.
- *Lower Natural Gas Prices:* Significantly reduce natural gas demand and reduce natural gas prices by 12 percent, saving consumers approximately $130 billion.
- *Expand Manufacturing:* To produce enough turbines and components for the 20 percent wind scenario, the industry would require more than 30,000 direct manufacturing jobs across the nation (assuming that 30 to 80 percent of major turbine components would be manufactured domestically by 2030).
- *Generate Local Revenues:* Lease payments for wind turbines would generate well over $600 million for landowners in rural areas and generate additional local tax revenues exceeding $1.5 billion annually by 2030. From 2007 through 2030, cumulative economic activity would exceed $1 trillion or more than $440 billion in net present value terms.

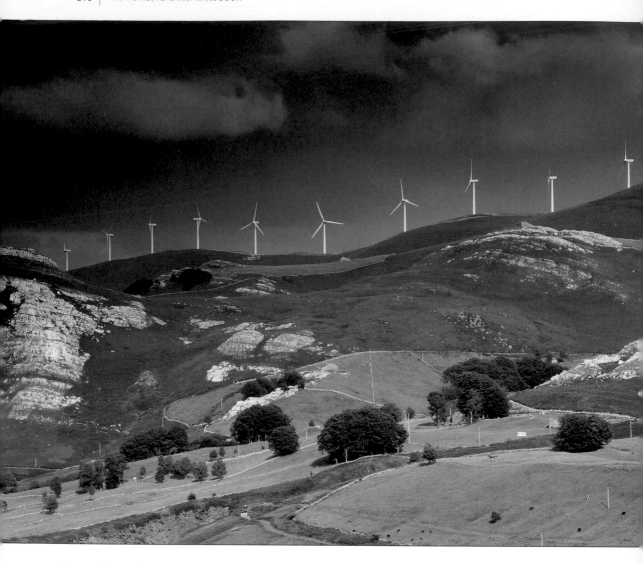

The use of large scale windmills is often controversial. They can provide a significant amount of clean energy, but they also clutter ridgelines, produce a lot of noise, and hurt the bird population.

attached and fastened 5 inches apart on the lower rails (Fig. 3). The upper ends of the blocks should be cut so as to allow the shaft to enter them. The collars, *C* and *C*, *C*, are placed at the inside of the blocks. To hold the shaft in place, small iron straps can be screwed tightly over the top of each block.

This head rests on the top of a hollow square post through which the rod passes, connecting the crank with the piston-rod of the pump (Fig. 4 A). A flat iron collar, *B*, should be screwed tightly at the top. To keep the head properly secured, four iron cleats (Fig. 4 C) should be screwed tightly under the corners of the head to help grip the projecting edge of the collar. This will hold the head rigid while allowing it to move about with the force of the wind.

Apply a little bit of grease or Vaseline to the top of the collar so the head will move easily. The top of the connecting rod should be attached to the crank and bolted to the top of the hard wood rod (Fig. 4 D).

The tail, which is 33 inches long and 24 inches wide at the end, is made of boards that are ¾ inch thick. The tail should be attached to the head (Fig. 5).

To place the windmill over a pump, build a platform that is braced with pieces of wood (see the illustration). Wires can also be run from the upper part of the trunk down to pegs driven into the ground. This will add additional support and steadiness to the upright shaft.

To start the wheel, snap the ends of the sheets to the spoke ends. To stop the wheel, unsnap the ends and furl the sails around the spokes, tying them securely with a piece of yarn or a cotton cord.

Hydropower

Water is constantly moving through a vast global cycle, evaporating from lakes and oceans, forming clouds, precipitating, and then flowing back into the ocean. The energy of this water cycle, which is mainly driven by the sun, can be tapped to produce electricity or to power machines—a process called hydropower. Hydropower uses water as a type of fuel that is neither reduced nor used up in the process. Since the water cycle is endless and will constantly recharge the system, hydropower is considered a renewable energy.

Hydropower (also known as hydroelectric power) is made when flowing water is captured and turned into electricity. There are many types of hydroelectric facilities that are all powered by the kinetic energy derived from flowing water as it moves downstream. Generators and turbines convert this energy into electricity. This is then fed into the electrical grid for use in homes, businesses, and other industries.

Types of Hydropower Plants

There are three types of hydropower plants:

1. Impoundment—Impoundment facilities are the most common type of hydroelectric power plants. This facility, typically a large hydropower system, uses a dam to store river water in a reservoir. Water that is released from the reservoir flows through a turbine, spinning it. This activates a generator to produce electricity. The water may be released either to meet the changing electricity needs or to maintain a constant reservoir level.

2. Diversion—A diversion facility, sometimes referred to as a run-of-river facility, channels a portion of a river through a canal or penstock. This does not always require the use of a dam.

3. Pumped storage—A pumped storage facility stores energy by pumping water from a lower reservoir to an upper reservoir when electricity demands are low. During times when electrical demands are high, water is then released back into the lower reservoir to generate electricity.

Some hydropower plants use dams and others do not. Many dams were originally built for other purposes and then hydropower was added at a later date. In the United States, only 2,400 of the 80,000 dams produce power—the rest are used for recreation, farm ponds, flood control, water supply, and irrigation.

Size of Hydropower Plants

Hydropower plants range in size from small and micro systems, which are operated for individual needs or to sell the power to utilities, to larger projects that produce electricity for utilities, supplying many consumers with electricity.

Micro hydropower plants have a capacity of up to 100 kilowatts. Small hydropower plants have a capacity between

≋ Water's never ending cycle

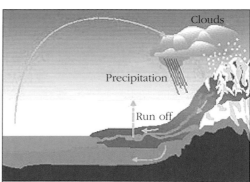

A Brief History of Hydropower

Humans have been using water to help them perform work for thousands of years. Water wheels have been employed for grinding grains into flour, to saw wood, and to power textile mills. The technology to use running water to create hydroelectricity has been around for over a hundred years. The modern hydropower turbine was created in the middle of the eighteenth century and developed into direct current technology. Today, an alternating current is in use and came about when the electric generator was combined with the turbine. The first hydroelectric plant in the United States was built in Appleton, Wisconsin in 1882.

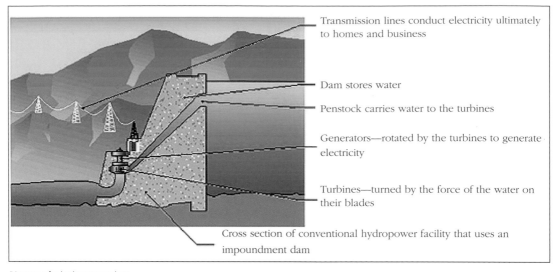

Transmission lines conduct electricity ultimately to homes and business

Dam stores water

Penstock carries water to the turbines

Generators—rotated by the turbines to generate electricity

Turbines—turned by the force of the water on their blades

Cross section of conventional hydropower facility that uses an impoundment dam

Diagram of a hydropower plant

100 kilowatts and 30 megawatts. Large hydropower plants have a capacity of more than 30 megawatts. The small and micro systems can produce enough electricity for a home, farm, or even a small village.

Hydropower Turbines

There are two main types of hydropower turbines: impulse and reaction. The type of turbine selected for a project is based on the height of the standing water (the "head") and the flow (volume) of the water at a particular site. It is also determined by how deep the turbine must be set, its efficiency, and its cost.

A micro hydropower plant.

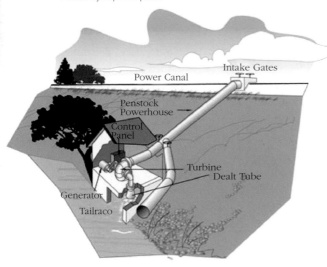

Impulse Turbine

An impulse turbine typically uses the velocity of water to move the runner and discharges to atmospheric pres-

Advantages of Hydropower

- It is fueled by water, making it a clean energy source.
- It does not pollute the air since it does not burn any fossil fuels.
- It is a domestic energy source.
- It relies on the water cycle and is a renewable energy source.
- It is usually available as needed.
- The water flow can be controlled through the turbine to produce energy on demand.
- The plants provide reservoirs for recreation (fishing, swimming, boating), water supply, and food control.

Disadvantages of Hydropower

- It can negatively impact fish populations by hampering fish migration upstream past dams, though there are ways to allow for passage both up- and downstream.
- It can impact the quality and flow of water, causing low dissolved oxygen levels that can negatively impact the riverbank habitats.
- The plants can be impacted by drought, and if they are not receiving adequate water, they cannot produce electricity.
- The plants compete for land use and can cause humans, plants, and animals to lose their natural habitat.

sure. The water stream then hits each bucket on the runner. The water flows out of the bottom of the turbine after hitting the runner. These turbines are suitable for high head, low flow applications.

Reaction Turbine

A reaction turbine generates power by the combined action of pressure and moving water. The runner is placed in the water stream, which flows over the blades instead of striking each one separately. These turbines are used for sites with lower head and higher flows.

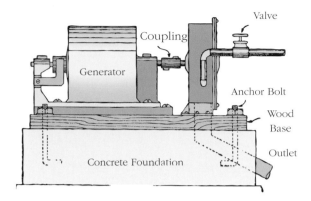

Diagram of a hydroelectric motor

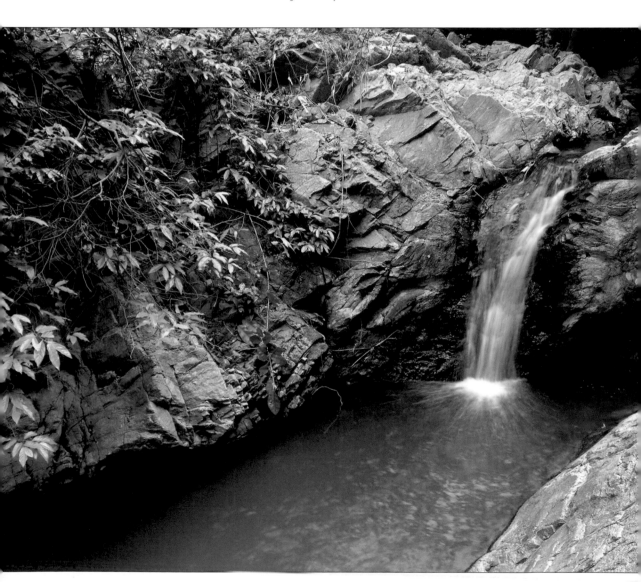

Even a small waterfall can provide a lot of power.

Geothermal Energy

Geothermal energy (the heat from the Earth) is accessible as an alternative source of heat and power. Geothermal energy can be accessed by drilling water or steam wells using a process much like drilling for oil. This resource is enormous but is sadly underused as an energy source. When it is employed, though, it proves to be clean (emitting little or no greenhouse gases), reliable, economical, and domestically found (geothermal energy can be harnessed from almost anywhere and thus makes countries less dependent on foreign oil).

Wells a mile or more deep can be drilled into underground reservoirs to tap steam and very hot water. This can then be brought to the surface and used in a variety of ways—such as to drive turbines and electricity generators. In the United States, most geothermal reservoirs are located in the western states, in Alaska, and in Hawaii. People in more than 120 locations in the United States are using geothermal energy for space and district heating.

Geothermal resources can range from shallow ground water to hot water found in rocks several miles below the surface of the earth. It can even be harnessed, in some cases, from magma (hot molten rock near the earth's core). Geothermal reservoirs of low to moderate temperature (roughly 68 to 302°F) can be used to heat homes, office, and greenhouses. Curiously, the dehydration of onions and garlic comprises the largest industrial use of geothermal energy in the United States.

Three Main Uses of Geothermal Energy

Some types of geothermal energy usage draw from the earth's temperatures closer to the surface and others require, as noted above, drilling miles into the earth. The three main uses of geothermal energy are:

1. Direct Use and District Heating Systems—These use hot water from springs and reservoirs near the earth's surface.
2. Electricity Generation—Typically found in power plants, this type of energy requires high-temperature water and steam (generally between 300 and 700°F). Geothermal power plants are built where reservoirs are positioned only a mile or two from the earth's surface.
3. Geothermal Heat Pumps—These use stable ground or water temperatures near the earth's surface to control building temperatures above the ground.

A geothermal power plant in action

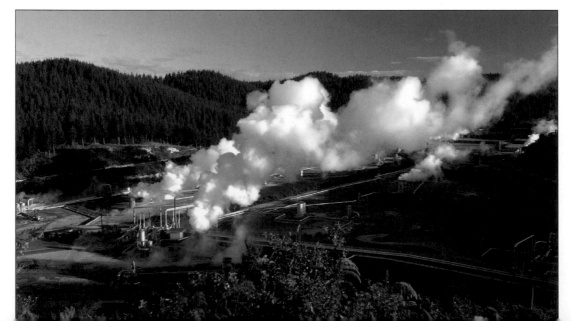

Additional Resources

The U.S. Department of Energy, in conjunction with the Geo-Heat Center, conducts research, provides technical support, and distributes information on a wide range of geothermal direct-use applications. Some information that is provided revolves around greenhouse informational packages, cost comparisons of heat pumps, low temperature resource assessments, cost analysis for homeowners, and information directed to aquaculture developers.

The greenhouse informational package provides information for people who are looking to develop geothermal greenhouses. This package includes crop market prices for vegetables and flowers, operating costs, heating system specifications, greenhouse heating equipment selection spreadsheets, and vendor information.

Groundwater heat pumps have also been identified as offering substantial savings over other types of pump systems. Informational packets about heat pump systems are provided to answer frequently asked questions concerning the application and usage of geothermal heat pumps.

The Geo-Heat Center examined the costs associated with the installation of district heating systems in single-family residential sectors. They discovered that cost-saving areas included installation in unpaved areas, using non-insulated return lines, and installation in areas that are unencumbered by existing buried utility lines.

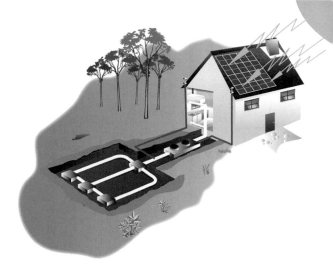

You can combine solar and geothermal energy to produce more consistent power in your home.

Besides bathing, the most common direct use of geothermal energy is for heating buildings. This is through district heating systems—these types of systems provide heat for roughly 95 percent of the buildings in Reykjavik, Iceland. District heating systems pipe hot water near the earth's surface directly into buildings in order to provide adequate heat.

Direct use of geothermal resources is a proven, economic, and clean energy option. Geothermal heat can be piped directly into facilities and used to heat buildings, grow greenhouse plants, heat water for fish farming, and even pasteurize milk. Some northern U.S. cities pipe hot water under roads and sidewalks to melt the snow.

Direct Use Geothermal Energy

Since ancient times, people have been directly using hot water as a source of energy. The Chinese, Native Americans, and Romans used hot mineral springs for bathing, cooking, and heating purposes. Currently, a number of hot springs are still used for bathing and many people believe these hot, mineral-rich waters possess natural healing powers.

Geothermal Heat Pumps

Even though temperatures above the surface of the earth change daily and seasonally, in general, temperatures in the top 10 feet of the Earth's surface stay fairly constant

A horizontal closed-loop heat pump system

A geothermal power plant

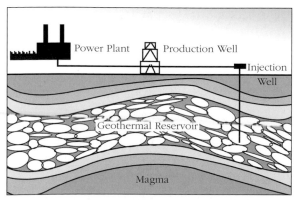

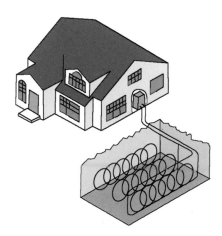

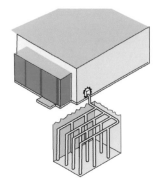

A vertical closed-loop heat pump system

at around 50 to 60°F. This means that, in most places, soil temperatures are typically warmer than air temperatures in the winter and cooler in the summer. Geothermal heat pumps (GHPs) use this constant temperature to heat and cool buildings. These pumps transfer heat from the ground (or underground water sources) into buildings during the winter and do the reverse process in the summer months.

Geothermal heat pumps, according to the U.S. Environmental Protection Agency (EPA), are the most energy-efficient, environmentally clean, and cost-effective systems for maintaining a consistent temperature control. These pumps are becoming more popular, even though most homes still use furnaces and air conditioners. Sometimes referred to as earth-coupled, ground-source, or water-source heat pumps, GHPs use the constant temperature of the earth as the exchange medium (using ground heat exchangers) instead of the outdoor air temperature. In this way, the system can be quite efficient on cold winter nights in comparison to air-source heat pumps.

Geothermal heat pumps can heat, cool, and, in some cases, even supply hot water to a house. These pumps are relatively quiet, long-lasting, need little to no maintenance, and do not rely on outside temperatures to function effectively. While geothermal systems are initially more expensive to install, these costs are quickly returned in energy savings in about five to 10 years. Systems have a life-span of roughly 25 years for inside components and more than 50 years for ground loop systems. Each year, about 50,000 geothermal heat pumps are installed in the United States.

Types of Geothermal Heat Pump Systems

There are four basic types of ground loop heat pump systems: horizontal, vertical, pond/lake, and open-loop systems. The first three are closed-loop systems while the fourth is, as its name suggests, open-loop. The type of system used is generally determined based on the climate, soil conditions, land availability, and local installation costs of the site for the pump. All four types of geothermal heat pump systems can be used for both residential and commercial building applications.

Horizontal Heat Pump System

This closed-loop installation is extremely cost-effective for residential heat pumps and is well suited for new construction where adequate land is available for the system. Horizontal heat pump systems need 4-foot trenches to be installed. These systems are typically laid out using two pipes—one buried 6 feet and the other buried 4 feet below the ground—or by placing two pipes side by side at 5 feet underground in a 2-foot-wide trench.

Vertical Heat Pump System

Schools and larger commercial buildings use vertical heat pump systems because they require less land to be effectively used. These systems are best used where the soil is too shallow for trenching. They also minimize any disturbance to established landscaping. To install a vertical system, holes that are roughly 4 inches in diameter are drilled about 20 feet apart and 100 to 400 feet deep. Two pipes are inserted into these holes and are connected at the bottom with a U-bend, forming a loop. The vertical loops are then connected with a horizontal pipe, placed in the trenches, and connected to the heat pump in the building.

Pond/Lake Heat Pump System

Another closed-loop system is the pond/lake heat pump system. If a site has enough water—usually in the form of a pond or even a lake—this system may be the most cost-effective. This heat pump system works by running a supply line pipe underground from a building to the water source. The piping is coiled into circles no less than 8 feet under the surface—this prevents the water in the pipes from freezing. The coils should be placed only in a water source that meets the minimum volume, depth, and quality criteria.

Open-Loop Heat Pump System

An open-loop system uses well or surface body water as the heat exchange fluid that will circulate directly through the geothermal heat pump system. Once this water has circulated through the system, it is returned to the ground through a recharge well or as surface discharge. The system is really only practical where there is a sufficient supply of clean water. Local codes and regulations for proper groundwater discharge must also be met in order for the heat pump system to be utilized.

Selecting and Installing a Geothermal Heat Pump System in Your Home

The heating efficiency of commercial ground-source and water-source heat pumps is indicated by their coefficient of performance (COP)—the ratio of heat provided in Btu per Btu of energy input. The cooling efficiency is measured by the energy efficiency ratio (EER)—the ratio of heat removed to the electricity required (in watts) to run the unit. Many geothermal heat pump systems are approved by the U.S. Department of Energy as being energy efficient products and so, if you are thinking of

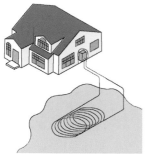
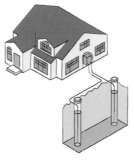

A closed-loop pond/lake heat pump system

An open-loop heat pump system

purchasing and installing this type of system, you may want to check to see if there is any special financing or incentives for purchasing energy efficient systems.

Evaluating Your Site

Before installing a geothermal heat pump, consider the site that will house the system. The presence of hot geothermal fluid containing low mineral and gas content, shallow aquifers for producing the fluid, space availability on your property, proximity to existing transmission lines, and availability of make-up water for evaporative cooling are all factors that will determine if your site is good for geothermal electric development. As a rule of thumb, geothermal fluid temperature should be no less than 300°F.

In the western United States, Alaska, and Hawaii, hydrothermal resources (reservoirs of steam or hot water) are more readily available than the rest of the country. However, this does not mean that geothermal heat cannot be used throughout the country. Shallow ground temperatures are relatively constant throughout the United States and this means that energy can be tapped almost anywhere in the country by using geothermal heat pumps and direct-use systems.

To determine the best type of ground loop systems for your site, you must assess the geological, hydrological, and spatial characteristics of your land in order to choose the best, most effective heat pump system to heat and cool your home:

1. Geology—This includes the soil and rock composition and properties on your site. These can affect the transfer rates of heat in your particular system. If you have soil with good heat transfer properties, your system will require less piping to obtain a good amount of heat from the soil. Furthermore, the amount of soil that is available also contributes to which system you will choose. For example, areas that have hard rock or shallow soil will most likely benefit from a vertical heat pump system instead of a system requiring large and deep trenches, such as the horizontal heat pump system.

2. Hydrology—This refers to the availability of ground or surface water, which will affect the type of system to be installed. Factors such as depth, volume, and water quality will help determine if surface water bodies can be used as a source of water for an open-loop heat pump system or if they would work best with

a pond/lake system. Before installing an open-loop system, however, it is best to determine your site's hydrology so potential problems (such as aquifer depletion or groundwater contamination) can be avoided.

3. Available land—The acreage and layout of your land, as well as your landscaping and the location of underground utilities, also play an important part in the type of heat pump system you choose. If you are building a new home, horizontal ground loops are an economical system to install. If you have an existing home and want to convert your heat and cooling to geothermal energy, vertical heat pump systems are best to minimize the disturbance to your existing landscaping and yard.

Installing the Heat Pumps

Geothermal heat pump systems are somewhat difficult to install on your own—though it can certainly be done. Make sure, before you begin any digging, to contact your local utility company to make sure you will not be digging into gas pipes or electrical wires.

The ground heat exchanger in a geothermal heat pump system is made up of closed- or open-loop pipe—depending on which type of system you've determined is best suited for your site. Since most systems employed are closed-loop systems, high density polyethylene pipe is used and buried horizontally at 4 to 6 feet deep or vertically at 100 to 400 feet deep. These pipes are filled with an environmentally friendly antifreeze/water solution that acts as a heat exchanger. You can find this at your local home store or contact a contractor to see where it is distributed. This solution works in the winter by extracting heat from the earth and carrying it into the building. In the summertime, the system reverses, taking heat from the building and depositing it into the ground.

Air delivery ductwork will distribute the hot or cold air throughout the house's ductwork like traditional, conventional systems. An air handler—a box that contains the indoor coil and fan—should be installed to move the house air through the heat pump system. The air handler contains a large blower and a filter, just like standard air conditioning units.

A vertical closed-loop system

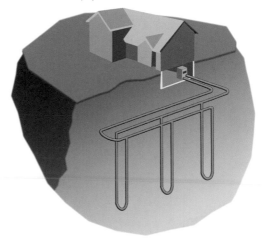

Cost-Efficiency of Geothermal Heat Pump Systems

By installing and using a geothermal heat pump system, you will save on the costs of operating and maintaining your heating and cooling system. While these systems are generally a bit pricier to install, they prove to be more efficient and thus save you money on a monthly and yearly basis. Especially in the colder winter months, geothermal heat pump systems can reduce your heating costs by about half. Annual energy savings by using a geothermal heat pump system range from 30 to 60 percent.

Benefits of Using Geothermal Energy

*   It is clean energy. Geothermal energy does not require the burning of fossil fuels (coal, gas, or oil) in order to produce energy.
*   Geothermal fields produce only about ⅙th of the carbon dioxide that natural gas-fueled power plants do. They also produce little to no sulfur-bearing gases, which reduces the amount of acid rain.
*   It is available at any time of day, all year round.
*   Geothermal power is homegrown, which reduces dependence on foreign oil.
*   It is a renewable source of energy. Geothermal energy derives its source from an almost unlimited amount of heat generated by the earth. And even if energy is limited in an area, the volume taken out can be reinjected, making it a sustainable source of energy.
*   Geothermal heat pump systems use 25 to 50 percent less electricity than conventional heating and cooling systems. They reduce energy consumption and emissions between 44 and 72 percent and improve humidity control by maintaining about 50 percent relative humidity indoors (GHPs are very effective for humid parts of the country).
*   Heat pump systems can be "zoned" to allow different parts of your home to be heated and cooled to different temperatures without much added cost or extra space required.
*   Geothermal heat pump systems are durable and reliable. Underground piping can last for 25 to 50 years and the heat pumps tend to last at least 20 years.
*   Heat pump systems reduce noise pollution since they have no outside condensing unit (like air conditioners).

Alternate "Geothermal" Cooling System

True geothermal energy systems can be very expensive to install and you may not be able to use one in your home at this time. However, here is a fun alternative way to use the concepts of geothermal systems to keep your house cooler in the summer and your air conditioning bills lower. All you need are a basement, small window fan, and dehumidifier.

Your basement is a wonderful example of how the top layers of earth tend to remain at a stable temperature throughout the year. In the winter, your basement may feel somewhat warm; in the summer, it's nice and refreshingly cool. This is due to the temperature of the soil permeating through the basement walls. And this cool basement air can be used to effectively reduce the temperature in your home by up to five degrees during the summer months. Here are the steps to your alternative "geothermal" cooling system:

1. Run the dehumidifier in your basement during the night, bringing the humidity down to about 60 percent.
2. Keep your blinds and curtains closed in the sunniest rooms in your home.
3. In the morning, when the temperature inside the house reaches about 77°F, open a small window in your basement, just a crack, and open one of the upstairs windows, placing a small fan in it and directing the room air out of the window.
4. With all other windows and outside doors closed, the fan will suck the cool basement air through your home and out the open window. Doing this for about an hour will bring down the temperature inside your home, buying you a couple of hours of reprieve before switching on the AC.

The hot springs at Yellowstone are a natural example of geothermal heating.

Composting Toilets

Toilets come in three common varieties: siphon-jet flush valve toilets (common in most homes), pressurized tank toilets, and gravity flow. These toilets, generally speaking, use up large amounts of water and the waste is flushed into a sewer system and then dumped in a variety of locations. Composting toilets require little to no water, which provides a solution to sanitation and environmental problems in areas that are rural, without sewers, and in the suburbs throughout the world. Although composting toilets are rare in private homes—they are generally found in park facilities and small highway rest stops—these waterless toilets can be utilized by the regular homeowner.

It is astonishing that Americans flush about 4.8 billion gallons of water down toilets every day, according to the U.S. Environmental Protection Agency. Just replacing all existing U.S. toilets with 1.6-gallon-per-flush, ultra-low-flow (ULF) models would save about 5,500 gallons of water per person per year! So, if you are unable to install a composting toilet in your home or on your property, you may choose to install ULF models in your home to help conserve water usage.

The Basics of the Composting Toilet

Composting (or biological) toilet systems contain and process excrement, toilet paper, carbon additive, and, at times, food wastes. These systems rely on unsaturated conditions where aerobic bacteria break down waste—unlike septic systems—much like a compost heap for your gardening necessities. The resulting soil-like material—humus—must be buried or removed. It's a good idea to check state and local regulations regarding proper handling methods.

In many parts of the country, public health officials are realizing that there is a definite need for environmentally sound human waste treatment and recycling methods, and compost toilets are an easy way to work toward these needs. Because they don't require any water to be used, composting toilets are ideal for remote areas and places that have high water tables, shallow soil, and rough terrain. These systems save water and allow for valuable plant nutrients to be recycled in the process.

Composting toilets are being used more regularly in parks around the world.

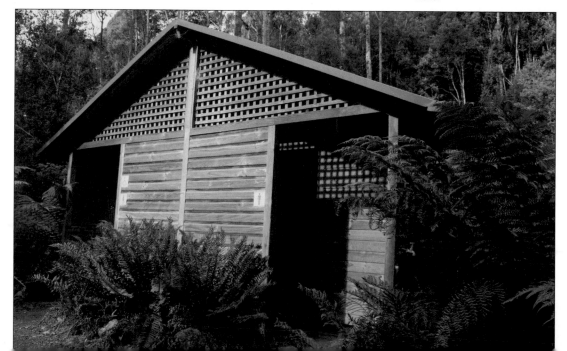

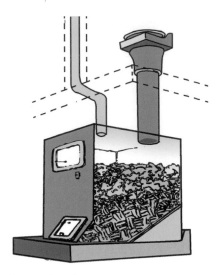

A composting toilet

There are a few key components for establishing a composting toilet:
- Composting reactor that is connected to a micro-flush toilet
- Screened air inlet and exhaust system to remove odors and heat, plus CO_2 and other decomposition byproducts
- Mechanism to provide proper ventilation that will help aerobic organisms in the compost heap
- Process controls
- Access door for the removal of the end product

It is important that the composting toilet separates the solid from the liquid waste and produces a humus-like material with less than 200 MPN per gram of fecal coliform. The compost chamber can be solar or electrically heated to maintain the right temperature for year-round use and bacterial decomposition.

Main Objective of the Composting Toilet

These systems are designed to contain, immobilize, and destroy pathogens. This reduces the risk of human infection and ensures that the toilets do not pollute the environment. If done correctly, the composted material should be able to be handled with little to no risk of harming the individual working with it.

A composting toilet consists of a well-ventilated container that breeds a good environment for unsaturated, moist human excrement that can be decomposed under sanitary conditions. A composting toilet can be large or small, depending on the space and its use. Organic matter is transformed into a humus-like product through the natural breaking down from bacteria and fungi. Most systems like this use the process of continuous composting, which includes a single chamber where the excrement is added to the top and the end product is taken from the bottom.

Advantages of Using a Composting Toilet

Composting toilets can be used practically anywhere a flush toilet can be. They are most likely to be used in homes in rural areas, seasonal cabins, recreation areas, and other places where flush toilets are either unnecessary or impractical. They are more cost-effective than establishing a central sewage system and there is no water wasted. These systems—since they aren't using copious amounts of water—also reduce the quantity of wastewater that is disposed of on a daily basis. These toilets can also be used to recycle and compost food wastes, thus reducing the amount of household garbage that is dumped every day. Finally, these toilet systems are beneficial to the environment as they divert nutrient and pathogen-containing effluent from the soil, surface water, and the groundwater.

Disadvantages of Using a Composting Toilet

Composting toilets are a big responsibility; the owner of a composting toilet must be committed to maintaining the system. Removing the compost can be unpleasant if the toilet is not properly set up and they could end up having odor issues.

Successful Management of the Composting Toilet

Composting toilets do not require highly trained people to deal with the sewage as it is relatively harmless to handle. But it is important to maintain your composting toilet so it can be effective and safe. Some composting toilets may need organic bulking agents added

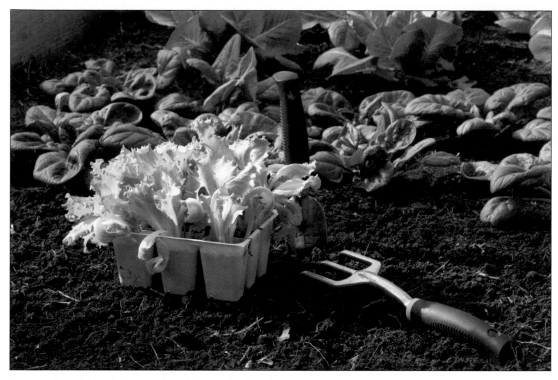

Compost will enrich the soil in your garden to help grow healthier plants.

to aid the composting process. Adding grass clippings, sawdust, and leaves to your composting toilet reservoir will help aid the process. The end product should be removed every three months for smaller systems and, if composted correctly, should not smell and should not be toxic to humans or animals. Be sure to dispose of the waste materials in accordance with your particular state and local regulations.

Making Your Own Composting Toilet

Building your own composting toilet can be quite inexpensive and takes only a short amount of time to assemble. In order to construct a composting toilet, you will need the following materials:

- Two or three 5-gallon buckets with lids
- A standard toilet seat (a used one will work just fine) with lid
- ¾ x 3 x 18-inch plywood sheets
- Boards to be cut and used for the sides of the toilet box and for the legs
- Two hinges
- Screws
- Saw and measuring tape
- Bag of sawdust, to be used for soaking up excess moisture in the compositing bucket

To begin, cut a hole in one of the pieces of plywood so that it fits the size of the bucket. Then, attach the pieces of plywood together using the hinges. Build a box with the boards and then screw in the solid piece of plywood to the box, allowing for the part with the hole to remain on the top. Attach legs to the box, allowing the bucket to lift just slightly above the hole cut in the top piece of plywood. Then, attach the toilet seat to the plywood top, making sure that it fits securely over the rim of the bucket. Finally, stain or paint the entire composting toilet so it will last longer and match the décor of your bathroom.

Before using your homemade composting toilet, sprinkle 1 to 2 inches of sawdust into the bottom of the bucket. This will help absorb extra moisture and will also add a necessary carbon element that is useful in composting. Sprinkle sawdust into the toilet after each use to facilitate the composting process and to minimize odors. When the first bucket is full, remove and cover (allowing the composting process to continue), insert another bucket, and continue use. When both buckets are full, remove them to your composting pile in your yard. Make a small indent in the center of your composting pile and dump the new compost into the depression, laying old compost and other organic materials on top of the new addition. If used properly, your composting toilet will be odorless and your compost will be rich and ready for use in your garden.

Greywater

Greywater is just wastewater. Greywater, however, does not include toilet wastewater, which is known as blackwater. These two different kinds of water should not be mixed together for basic health reasons. The main differences between greywater and blackwater are:

- Greywater contains less nitrogen than blackwater (and about half of the nitrogen that is found in greywater is organic nitrogen that can be filtered out and used by plants).
- Greywater contains fewer pathogens than blackwater and thus is not as likely to spread organisms that could be potentially harmful to humans.
- Greywater decomposes faster than blackwater and is less likely to cause water pollution because of this factor.

Greywater is not necessarily sewage to begin with, but if left untreated for a couple of days, it will become like blackwater and thus will be unusable. Therefore, it is important to know how best to treat and manage greywater so it can be successfully and safely reused.

What is Greywater?

Simply speaking, greywater is wash water—bath, dish, and laundry water that is free from toilet waste and garbage disposal remnants. Greywater, when it is managed properly, can be quite useful for growing things in your garden or yard. Greywater, in effect, is an excellent source of nutrients for plants when used properly.

Greywater Irrigation Systems

The practice of irrigating with greywater is common in areas where the water supply is short. To have effective greywater irrigation that successfully utilizes the nutrients in the greywater, it is important to take precautions before using it in irrigation.

Planning a greywater system requires either an assumption that the system is right for you and your family or an understanding that the system is needed for the house independent of who lives in it.

To assess whether your household could benefit from a greywater system, it is important to take inventory of all the sources of greywater in the house. Look at how many gallons of water you use, per person, per day, when doing the laundry, running the dishwasher, and taking a bath or shower, and then add up these numbers. Remember that the typical washing machine uses 30 gallons of water per cycle, a dishwasher uses between 3 and 5 gallons per cycle, and simply washing your hands and brushing your teeth daily wastes about 1 to 5 gallons of water per day. If you are able to recycle and reuse all of that wasted water, you can effectively reduce the amount of water consumption your family has every day and every year.

Once you've decided to use your greywater, it is important to check with your local authorities to see if there are any state or local regulations for greywater usage in your area. Once you have the go-ahead to proceed, you can begin reusing your greywater to the benefit of your garden and household.

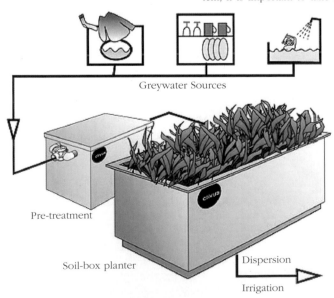

The pretreatment of greywater

Greywater Sources

Pre-treatment

Soil-box planter

Dispersion

Irrigation

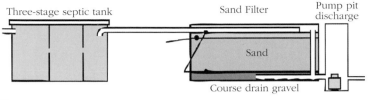

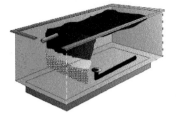

Greywater pretreatment

A planter soil box

Aerobic Pretreatment

This type of greywater treatment is suitable for shower, hand-washing, and laundry water. Aerobic pretreatment is a stretch filter technique that removes large particles and fibers to protect the pipes from clogging and transfers the greywater into a biologically active, aerobic soil-zone environment. Here microorganisms can survive and flourish. Stretch filters retain fibers and large particles and allow the rest of the materials to travel to the next processing stage. The filter is good for sinks and showers at public water facilities.

Anaerobic to Aerobic Pretreatment

If you have food waste entering the water system from dishwashers and kitchen sinks, this is the better option for treating your greywater. This system should have a three-stage septic tank to separate the sludge and grease from the water. This waste can then be removed easily. The outgoing water will be anaerobic and will need a sand filter to restore the aerobic conditions to the greywater. The final treatment leads the purified water to be treated in a planter bed. The system, while not inexpensive, is quite effective and is simple to maintain. A plan for this system can be seen above.

Planter Soil Box

Since 1975, soil boxes have been used to purify greywater. When using a soil box, however, it is vital that the planter bed be well drained to prevent water-logged zones from forming. Therefore, the bottom of the soil box should contain a layer of polyethylene pea gravel to provide for effective drainage. A layer of plastic mosquito netting should be placed over the gravel to prevent the layer of coarse sand from falling through. Atop the coarse sand should be a layer of concrete-mix sand and the top 2 feet should consist of humus-rich topsoil. Clay soils should not be used in soil boxes as they do not effectively allow water to pass through and drain.

Piping can usually be found in 5-foot sections.

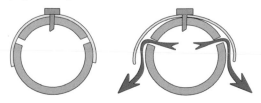

Pressure infiltration pipes should be designed to allow for the even distribution of water in both level and uneven terrain. These pipes are easy to clean and should be placed on the soil surface after planting. Then, they should be covered by a 2- to 4-inch layer of wood chip mulch. The pressure infiltration pipes consist of two concentric pipes that expand slightly due to the water pressure when the system is turned on. This causes the water to run out along the slot at the bottom of the soil box. When the water pressure is turned off, this causes the sleeve to close and prevents worms, insects, and roots from entering and clogging the pipe.

Gravity/Pressure Leaching Chambers

Leaching chambers can be successful in loading and receiving 2.4 gallons per square foot per day of greywater from a three-bedroom home. Using half of a PVC pipe that is 6 inches in diameter, this leaching chamber can be placed within a trench on a 1- to 2-inch mesh plastic netting to prevent the walls from sinking into the soil. No pre-filtration is used in these chambers. All that is required is a dosing pump chamber to pump every eight hours. The trench should have a minimum surface area of about 100 square feet—this will allow for a loading rate of around 2 to 2½ gallons per square foot per day for an average-sized home.

Gravity and Automatic Switch

The illustration below shows an example of an automatic switch system from a shallow leach chamber to one that is below the frost line—an important feature of

A leaching chamber

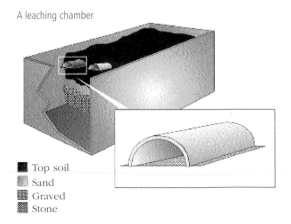

■ Top soil
░ Sand
▓ Graved
▓ Stone

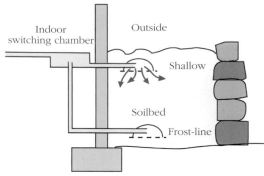

An automatic switch system

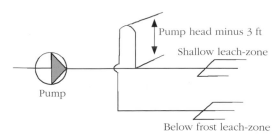

About 3 feet of water is a good margin for this automatic switch system.

any greywater system in the northern United States. If a shallow trench freezes and becomes clogged with ice, the water will back up and spill over into the pipe to the deeper, below-the-frost-line trench. It is worth noting that greywater is typically warmer than combined sewage and that the shallow leach zones that are operating in your system tend to stay freer of ice for longer periods of time than in places with combined waste water.

Automatic switching using pump pressure is different than gravity pressure switching. In an automatic switch system, a loop must be arranged indoors where the pressure needed for the shallow infiltration is normally lower than the pressure required to force the water up to the top of the loop. The top of the loop must, then, be no higher than the shut-off head of the pump. About 3 feet of water is a good margin for this system. The system can also be designed to be switched manually by the opening and closing of the valves that feed the different zones and levels of the greywater box.

An active cooling/passive heating greywater-irrigated greenhouse

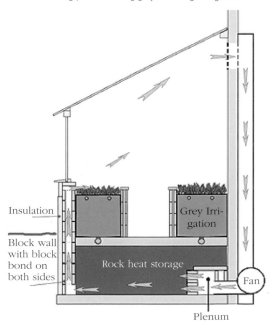

Options for Using Greywater in Cold Weather

Throughout New England, there are several greywater-irrigated greenhouses that feature a combination of automatically irrigated and fertilized growing beds that provide effective greywater treatment. Since these greenhouses are found in colder, northern states, it is important that these soil beds be deeper to store heat from both the sun and the greywater.

The greenhouse shown here provides enough salad greens for a family of four to six people throughout the long, cold northeastern winters. Growing broccoli, spinach, lettuce, mustard greens, and sorrel in these colder-climate greywater systems can be quite effective and profitable. To facilitate better distribution of greywater in the soil bed, a pipe-loop system can also be simply constructed to feed the bed from both sides.

Outdoor Planters

There are many variations of outdoor raised soil beds that are effective in replacing the soil needed for successful leach field treatment of greywater. Houses on ledges or in very sandy soils can be fitted with masonry soil boxes that serve to build up the site's soil profile. Such a strategy has been used in mounds or evapo-transpiration beds (a name derived from the assumption that all of the water will evaporate to the atmosphere even in wet and cold climates).

In parts of the country where construction density makes it very difficult to build a large mound or to locate planters for treating a significant volume of greywater, two adjacent neighbors can agree to build property dividers and plant hedges in their leaching area. This alternative combines privacy, landscaping aesthetics, and good environmental protection. Greywater gardens offer the added benefit of being able to garden at a higher elevation and in a raised garden bed.

Outdoor planters will have a less effective treatment during the winter seasons and during deep freezes. Yet,

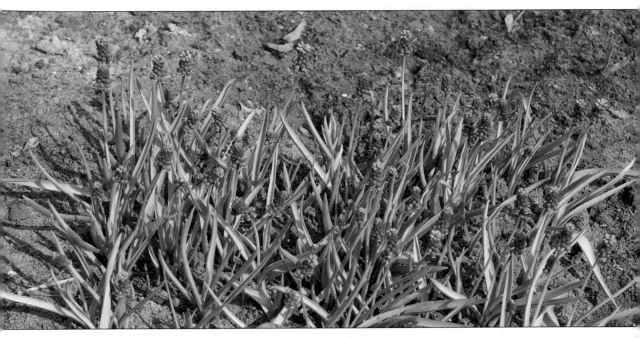

Greywater is especially useful in areas that are very dry.

when relatively warm greywater is injected into the soil, increased biological activity as well as warming of the soil tends to keep the injection area unfrozen for longer periods of time than the surrounding area. Raised beds or planters can also be ideal for compost bins in the fall. The decomposing leaves and grasses act as an insulator as well as a composting fuel source that further insures that the soil beneath does not go into a deep freeze.

Shallow Subsoil Irrigation

This type of irrigation (2 to 6 inches below the soil level) is preferable to surface irrigation when these factors are in play:
- The water used is "grey" (neither clean nor free of salts)
- The irrigation system is located in a high evaporation locale with water shortages
- It is desired to produce leaf or garden waste compost quickly
- Selective irrigation is needed (for a flower border, shrub, bush, tree, etc.)
- You want to automatically irrigate a drained planter indoors or outdoors

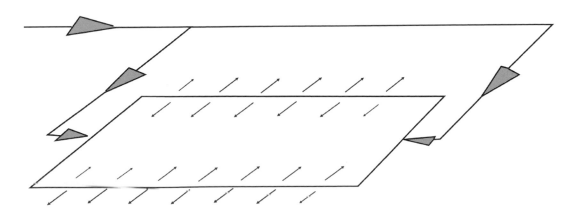

An injector pipe fork in the soil bed. Use 1-inch piping and drill ¼-inch holes on each side. Cover with canvas and a layer of soil to hide the pipe arrangement.

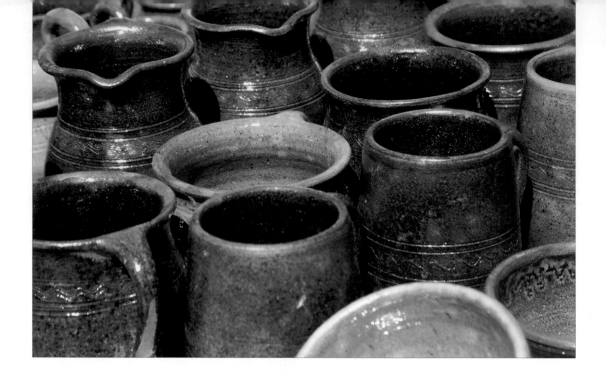

PART SIX

Crafts

Many people think of arts and crafts as something involving markers and construction paper that the kids do at summer camp. Certainly, the creativity that children express with scissors, tape, colored pencils, or clay is at the heart of crafting, but there's more to it than that. Most craft projects done for pleasure now were once done out of necessity—making candles, soaps, or baskets, for example—and many are still useful today. Beyond that, making things with your hands can be soothing, stimulating, or even enlightening, depending on the project and your frame of mind. Many people find knitting especially relaxing, and potters often discover within their art philosophical principles of intentionality, change, flexibility, and acceptance. In addition, crafting can become a lucrative and fulfilling business; handmade items are sought-after gifts and can be sold for significantly more than their factory-produced counterparts. In these pages you'll find an introduction to several diverse forms of crafting, from making soap and candles to pottery and even tying knots. Use the directions, descriptions, and images as a jumping-off point for your own creative endeavors, altering the projects as you're inspired in order to create one-of-a-kind pieces to use, give away, or sell . . . or just because they're fun to do.

Handmade Candles

Before the days of electricity, candles were a necessity in every home. Now they are enjoyed primarily for the unique way that they create ambience, or, for candles made with essential oils, for their aromatic properties. Turning off the lights for a few hours and enjoying the evening by candlelight can save money on your electric bill, too, and is a pleasant reminder of days gone by.

When making candles out of hot wax, it's a good idea to keep some baking soda nearby. If wax lights on fire, it reacts similarly to a grease fire, which is only aggravated by water. Douse a wax fire with baking soda, and it will extinguish quickly. Rather than pouring leftover wax down the drain (which will clog your drain and is bad for the environment), dump it into a jar and set it aside. If you continue to make candles, eventually your leftovers will become a unique layered jar candle.

Rolled Beeswax Candle

This is the simplest type of candle you can make and one that is great to do with children. Beeswax candles are cheap, eco-friendly, non-allergenic, drip-less, and non-toxic, and they burn cleanly and beautifully. And you can make a beeswax candle in about 20 minutes! So, if you are pressed for time and want to make a nice homemade gift—or you'd just like to have sweet-smelling candles in your home—making beeswax candles is the way to go.

Materials
Sheets of beeswax, any color you want (you can find this at your local arts and crafts store or even from a beekeeper or at a farmers' market)

Wick (you can purchase candle wicks at your local arts and crafts store)

Supplies
Scissors (to cut the wick and excess beeswax)

Hair dryer (optional)

Directions
1. Take one sheet of beeswax and fold it in half. Cut along the folded edge so you have two separate pieces.
2. Cut your wick to be about 2 inches longer than the length of the beeswax sheet.

Beeswax candles are easy to make, non-allergenic, and dripless.

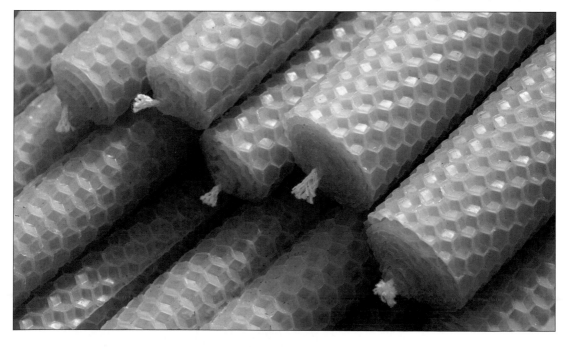

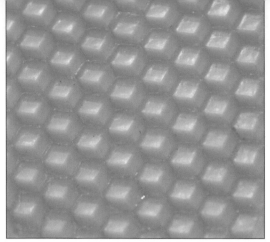

Purchase beeswax in sheets from crafts stores or gather them from your own hives.

3. Lay the wick on the edge of the beeswax sheet, closest to you. Make sure the wick hangs off of each end of the sheet.

4. Start rolling the beeswax over the wick, making sure it is tucked tightly around the wick. The tighter you begin rolling the beeswax, the more sturdy your candle will be and the better it will burn.

5. Carefully roll up the wick in the beeswax (as you would roll modeling clay). Stop about 2 inches from the other side and make sure the ends are smooth and straight. Apply slight pressure as you roll to keep the wax tightly bound.

6. When you reach the end, you must seal off your candle. To do so, start in the middle of the edge and gently press it into the candle, letting your body heat melt the wax into the rolled candle.

7. Trim the wick on the bottom (you may also want to cut the bottom slightly so it will stand up straight) and then cut the wick to about ½ inch at the top.

Note: If you are having trouble using the beeswax and want to facilitate the adhering process, you can use a hair dryer to soften the wax and to help you roll it. Start at the end with the wick and, moving the hair dryer over the wax, heat it up. Keep rolling until you reach a section that is not as warm, heat that up, and continue all the way to the end.

Taper Candles

Taper candles are perfect for candlesticks, and they can be made in a variety of sizes and colors.

Materials

Wick (be sure to find a spool of wick that is made specifically for taper candles)

Wax (paraffin is ideal for making taper candles)

Candle fragrances and dyes (optional)

Supplies

Pencil or chopstick (to wind the wick around to facilitate dipping and drying)

Weight (such as a fishing lure, bolt, or washer)

Dipping container (this should be tall and skinny. You can find these containers at your local arts and crafts store, or you can substitute a spaghetti pot)

Stove

Large pot for boiling water

Small trivet or rack

Newspaper (to prevent spills)

Glass or candle thermometer

Drying rack

Directions

1. Cut the wick to the desired length of your candle, leaving about 5 additional inches that will be tied onto the pencil or chopstick for dipping and drying purposes. It's also a good idea to put a weight on the dipping end of the wick (a fishing lure, bolt, or heavy metal washer) to help with the first few dips into the wax.

2. Ready your dipping container. Put the wax (preferably in smaller chunks to speed up the melting process) into the container and set aside.

3. In a large pot, start to boil water. Before putting the dipping container full of wax into the larger pot, place a small trivet, rack, or other elevating device into the bottom of the larger pot. This will keep the dipping container from touching the bottom of the larger pot and will prevent the wax from burning and possibly combusting.

4. Put the dipping container into the pot and start to melt the wax, keeping a thermometer in the wax at all times. The wax should be heated and melted between 150°F and 165°F. Stir frequently to keep the chunks of paraffin from burning and to ensure all the wax is thoroughly melted. (If you want to add fragrance or dye, do so when the wax is completely melted and stir until the additives are dissolved.)

5. Once your wax is completely melted, it's time to start the dipping process. Removing the container from the stove, take your wick that's tied onto a stick and dip it into the wax, leaving it there for a few minutes. Continue to lower the wick in and out of the dipping container, and by the eighth or ninth dip, cut off the weight from the bottom of the wick—the candle should be heavy enough now to dip well on its own.

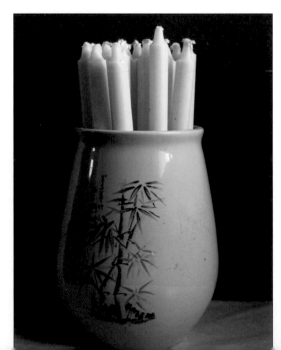

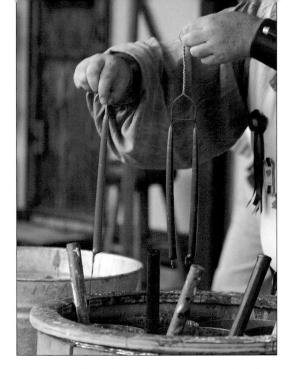

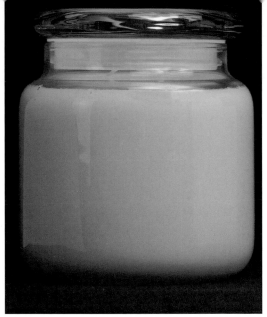

6. To speed up the cooling process—and to help the wax continue to adhere and build up on the wick—blow on the hot wax each time you lift the candle out of the dipping pot.

7. When the candle is at the desired length and thickness, you may want to lay it down on a very smooth surface (such as a countertop) and gently roll it into shape.

8. On a drying rack (which can be made from a box long enough so the candles do not touch the bottom or from another device), carefully hang your taper candle to dry for a good 24 hours.

9. Once the candle is completely hardened, trim the wick to just above the wax.

Jarred Soy Candles

Soy candles are environmentally friendly and easy candles to make. You can find most of the ingredients and materials needed to make soy candles at your local arts and crafts store—or even in your own kitchen!

Materials

1 lb soy wax (either in bars or flakes)
1 ounce essential oil (for fragrance)
Natural dye (try using dried and powdered beets for red, turmeric for yellow, or blueberries for blue)

Supplies

Stove
Pan to heat wax (a double boiler is best)
Spoon
Glass thermometer
Candle wick (you can find this at your local arts and crafts store)
Metal washers
Pencils or chopsticks
Heatproof cup to pour your melted wax into the jar(s)
Jar to hold the candle (jelly jars or other glass jars work well)

Directions

1. Put the wax in a pan or a double boiler and heat it slowly over medium heat. Heat the wax to 130°F to 140°F or until it's completely melted.

2. Remove the wax from the heat. Add the essential oil and dye (optional) and stir into the melted wax until completely dissolved.

3. Allow the wax to cool slightly, until it becomes cloudy.

4. While the wax is cooling, prepare your wick in the glass container. It is best to have a wick with a metal disk on the end—this will help stabilize it while the candle is hardening. If your wick does not already have a metal disk at the end, you can easily attach a thin metal washer to the end of the wick, tying a knot until the wick can no longer pass through the washer. Position the wick in the glass container and, using a pencil or chopstick, wrap the excess wick around the middle and then, laying the pencil or chopstick on the rim of the container, position the wick so it falls in the center.

5. Using a heat proof cup or the container from the double boiler, carefully pour the cloudy wax into the glass container, being careful not to disturb the wick from the center.

6. Allow the candle to dry for at least 24 hours before cutting off the excess wick and using.

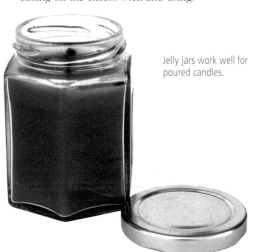

Jelly jars work well for poured candles.

Making Your Own Soap

Making your own soap can be a very rewarding process. It does, however, require a good amount of time, patience, and caution, because you'll be using some caustic and potentially dangerous ingredients—the main one being lye (sodium hydroxide). It is important, whenever you are making soap, that you are careful to avoid coming into direct contact with the lye. Wear goggles, rubber gloves, and long sleeves, and work in a well-ventilated area. Be sure, as well, that you never breathe in the fumes produced by the lye and water mixture.

Soap is made up of three main ingredients: water, lye, and fats or oils. While lard and tallow were once used exclusively for making soaps, it is perfectly acceptable to use a combination of pure oils for the "fat" needed to make soap. For these ingredients to become soap, they must go through a process called saponification, in which the mixture becomes completely blended and the chemical reactions between the lye and the oils, over time, turn the mixture into a hardened bar of usable soap.

Once you've become comfortable with the basic soap-making process, you can experiment with adding different colored dyes, essential oils, and other ingredients to make a personalized and interesting bar of soap—perfect for your own use or for giving as a gift.

Basic Recipe for Cold-Pressed Soap

Ingredients
6.9 ounces lye (sodium hydroxide)
2 cups distilled water, cold (from the refrigerator is the best)
2 cups canola oil
2 cups coconut oil
2 cups palm oil

Supplies
Goggles, gloves, and mask to wear while making the soap
Mold for the soap (a cake or bread loaf pan will work just fine; you can also find flexible plastic molds at your local arts and crafts store)
Plastic wrap or wax paper to line the molds
Glass bowl to mix the lye and water
Wooden spoon for mixing

You can pour your soap into molds, use stamps, or carve the finished bars to make them unique.

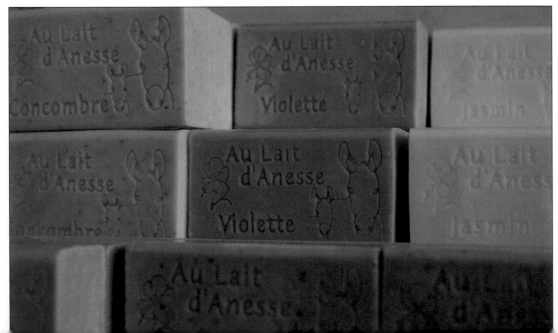

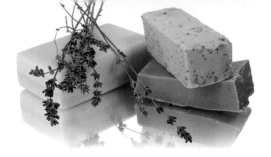

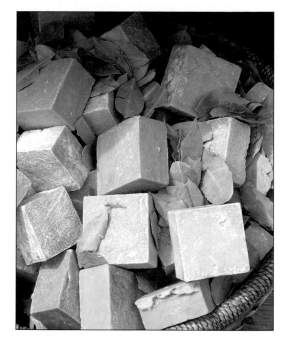

2 thermometers (one for the lye and water mixture and one for the oil mixture)

Stainless steel or cast iron pot for heating oils and mixing in lye mixture

Handheld stick blender (optional)

Directions

1. Put on the goggles and gloves and make sure you are working in a well-ventilated room.
2. Ready your mold(s) by lining with plastic wrap or wax paper. Set them aside.
3. Add the lye to the cold, distilled water in a glass bowl (never add the water to the lye) and stir continually for at least a minute, or until the lye is completely dissolved. Place one thermometer into the glass bowl and allow the mixture to cool to around 110°F (the chemical reaction of the lye mixing with the water will cause it to heat up quickly at first).
4. While the lye is cooling, combine the oils in a pot on medium heat and stir well until they are melted together. Place a thermometer into the pot and allow the mixture to cool to 110°F.
5. Carefully pour the lye mixture into the oil mixture (make sure you pour the lye solution in a small, steady stream), stirring continuously so that the lye and oils mix properly. Continue stirring, either by hand (which can take a very long time) or with a handheld stick blender, until the mixture traces (has the consistency of thin pudding). This may take anywhere from 30 to 60 minutes or more, so just be patient. It is well worth the time invested to make sure your mixture traces. If it doesn't trace all the way, it will not saponify correctly and your soap will be ruined.
6. Once your mixture has traced, pour carefully into the mold(s) and let sit for a few hours. Then, when the mixture is still soft but congealed enough not to melt back into itself, cut the soap with a table knife into bars. Let sit for a few days, then take the bars out of the mold(s) and place on brown paper (grocery bags are perfect) in a dark area. Allow the bars to cure for another 4 weeks or so before using.

If you want your soap to be colored, add special soap-coloring dyes (you can find these at the local arts and crafts store) after the mixture has traced, stirring them in. Or try making your own dyes using herbs, flowers, or spices.

To make a yummy-smelling bar of soap, add a few drops of your favorite essential oils (such as lavender, lemon, or rose) after the tracing of the mixture and stir in. You can also add aloe and vitamin E at this point to make your soap softer and more moisturizing.

To add texture and exfoliating properties to your soap, you can stir some oats into the traced mixture, along with some almond essential oil or a dab of honey. This will not only give your soap a nice, pumice-like quality but it will also smell wonderful. Try adding bits of lavender, rose petals, or citrus peel to your soap for variety.

To make soap in different shapes, pour your mixture into molds instead of making them into bars. For round soaps, you can take a few bars of soap you've just made, place them into a resealable plastic bag, and warm them by putting the bag into hot water (120°F) for 30 minutes. Then, cut the bars up and roll them into balls. These soaps should set in about an hour or so.

Natural Dyes for Soap or Candles

Light/Dark Brown	Cinnamon, ground cloves, allspice, nutmeg, coffee
Yellow	Turmeric, saffron, calendula petals
Green	Liquid chlrophyll, alfalfa, cucumber, sage, nettles
Red	Annatto extract, beets, grape-skin extract
Blue	Red cabbage
Purple	Alkanet root

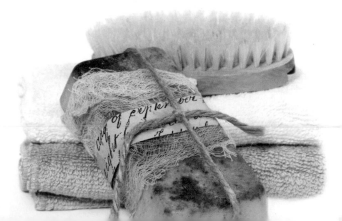

Pottery Basics

Pottery is enjoyable to make because of its flexibility and simplicity as a means of art expression, its utility, and its timelessness.

Clay is the basic ingredient for making pottery. Clay is decomposed rock containing water (both in liquid and chemical forms). Water in its liquid form can be separated from the clay by heating the mass to a boiling point—a process that restores the clay to its original condition once dried. The water in the clay that is found in chemical forms can also be removed by ignition—a process commonly referred to as "firing." After being fired, clay cannot be restored to any state of plasticity—this is what we term "pottery." Some clay requires greater heat in order to be fired, and these are known as "hard clays." These types of clay must be subjected to a "hard-firing" process. However, in the making of simple pottery, soft clay is generally used and is fired in an over-glaze (soft glaze) kiln.

Pottery clays can either be found in certain soils or bought from craft stores. If you have clay soil available on your property, the process of separating the clay from the other soil materials is simple. Put the earthen clay into a large bucket of water to wash the soil away. Any rocks or other heavy matter will sink to the bottom of the bucket. The milky fluid that remains—which is essentially water mixed with clay—may then be drawn off and allowed to settle in a separate container, the clear water eventually collecting on the top. Remove the excess water by using a siphon. Repeating of this process will refine the clay and make it ready for use.

You can also purchase clay at your local craft store. Usually, clay sold in these stores will be in a dry form (a grayish or yellowish powder), so you will need to prepare it before using it your pottery. To prepare it for use, you must mix the powder with water. If there are directions on your clay packet, then follow those closely to make your clay. In general, though, you can make your clay by mixing equal parts of clay powder and water in a bowl and allowing the mixture to soak for 10 to 12 hours. After it has soaked, knead the mixture thoroughly to disperse the water evenly throughout the clay and pop any air bubbles. Air bubbles, if left in the clay, could be detrimental to your pottery once kilned, because the bubbles would generate steam and possibly crack your creation. However, be careful not to knead your clay mixture too much,

A potter carefully forms a bowl which will eventually be glazed and fired in a kiln.

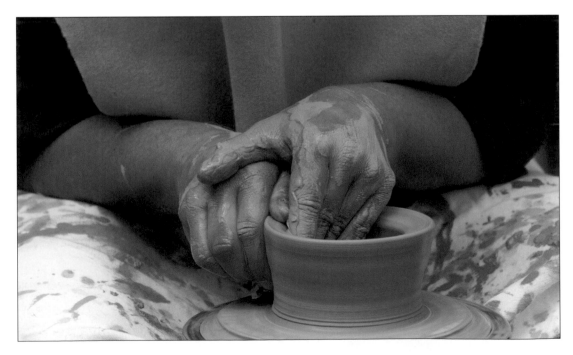

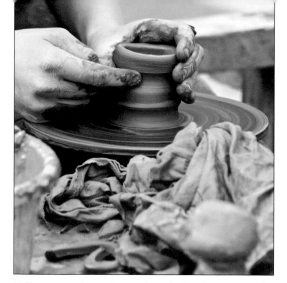

Making pottery takes patience and practice, but the process can be very enjoyable.

or you may increase the chance of air bubbles becoming trapped in the mixture.

If, after kneading, you find that the clay is too wet to work with (test the wetness of the clay on your hands and if it to slips around your palm very easily, it is probably too wet), the excess water can be removed by squeezing or blotting out with a dry towel or dry board.

The main tools needed for making pottery are simply your fingers. There are wooden tools that can be used for adding finer detail or decoration, but typically, all you really need are your own two hands. A loop tool (a piece of fine, curved wire) may also be used for scraping off excess clay where it is too thick. Another tool has ragged edges and this can be used to help regulate the contour of the pottery. Remember that homemade pottery will not always be symmetrical, and that is what makes it so special.

Sticks and other tools can be used to help you form and decorate your pottery.

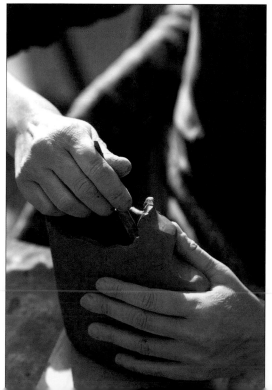

Basic Vase or Urn

Try making this simple vase or urn to get used to working with clay.

1. Take a lump of clay. The clay should be about the size of a small orange and should be elastic feeling. Then, begin to mold the base of your object—let's say it is either a bowl or a vase.

2. Continue molding your base. By now, you'll have a rather heavy and thick model, hollowed to look a little like a bird's nest. Now, using this base as support, start adding pieces of clay in a spiral shape. Press the clay together firmly with your fingers. Make sure that your model has a uniform thickness all around.

3. Continue molding your clay and making it grow. As you work with the clay, your hands will become more accustomed to its texture and the way it molds, and you will have less difficulty making it do what you want. As you start to elongate and lengthen the model, remember to keep the walls of the piece substantial and not too thin—it is easier to remove extra thickness than it is to add it.

4. Don't become frustrated if your first model fails. Even if you are being extra careful to make your bowl or vase sturdy, there is always the instance when a nearly complete vase will fall over. This usually happens when one side of the structure becomes too thin or the clay is too wet. To keep this from happening, it is sometimes helpful to keep one hand inside the structure and the other outside. If you are building a vase, you can extract one finger at a time as you reach closer and closer to the top of the model.

5. The clay should be moist throughout the entire molding process. If you need to stop molding for an extended period of time, cover the item with a moist cloth to keep it from drying out.

6. When your model has reached the size you want, you may turn it upside down and smooth and refine the contours of the object. You can also make the base much more detailed and shaped to a more pleasing design.

7. Allow your model to air dry.

Embellishing Your Clay Models

You may eventually want to make something that requires a handle or a spout, such as a cup or teapot. Adding handles and spouts can be tricky, but only if you don't remember some simple rules. Spouts can be modeled around a straw or any other material that is stiff enough to support the clay and light enough to burn out in the firing. In the designing of spouts and handles, it is still important to keep them solid and thick. Also, keeping them closer to the body of your model is more practical, as handles and spouts that are elongated

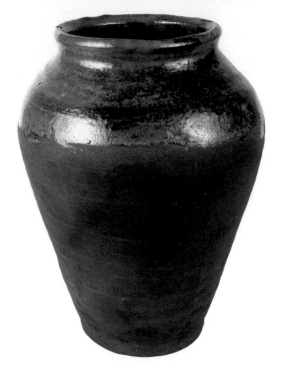

public). For schools that have pottery classes, over-glaze kilns may be installed there. It is important, whenever you are using a kiln, that you are with a skilled pottery maker who knows how to properly operate a kiln.

After the pottery has been colored and fired, a simple design may be made on the pottery by scraping off the surface color so as to expose the original or creamy-white tint of the clay.

Unglazed pottery may be worked with after firing by rubbing floor wax on the outer surface. This fills up the pores and gives a more uniform quality to the whole piece.

Pottery offers so many opportunities for personal experimentation and enjoyment; there are no set rules as to how to make a piece of pottery. Keep a journal about the different things you try while making pottery so you can remember what works best and what should be avoided in the future. Note the kind of clay you used and its consistency, the types of colors that have worked well, and the temperature and positioning within the kiln, if you use firing. Above all, enjoy making unique pieces of pottery!

are harder to keep firm and can also break off easily. Although more time-consuming and difficult to manage, handles and spouts can add a nice aesthetic to your finished pottery.

The simplest way to decorate your pottery is by making line incisions. Line incision designs are best made with wooden, finger-shaped tools. It is completely up to you as to how deep the lines are and into what pattern they are made.

Wheel-working and Firing Pottery

If you want to take your pottery-making one step further, you can experiment with using a potters' wheel and also glazing and firing your model to create beautiful pottery. Look online or at your local craft store for potters' wheels. Firing can leave your pottery looking two different ways, depending on whether you decide to leave the clay natural (so it maintains a dull and porous look) or to give it a color glaze.

Colored glazes come in the form of powder and are generally metallic oxides, such as iron oxides, cobalt oxide, chromium oxide, copper oxide, and copper carbonate. The colors these compounds become will vary depending on the atmosphere and temperature of the kiln. Glazes often come in the form of powder and need to be combined with water to be applied to the clay. Only apply glaze to dried pottery, because it won't adhere well to wet clay. Use a brush, sponge, or putty knife to apply the glaze. Your pottery is then ready to be fired.

There are various different kinds of kilns in which to fire your pottery. An over-glaze kiln is sufficient for all processes discussed here, and you can probably find a kiln in your surrounding area (check online and in your telephone book for places that have kilns open to the

Making Jars, Candlesticks, and Bowls

Making pottery at home is simple and easy, and is a great way for you to make personalized, unique gifts for family and friends. Clay can be purchased at local arts and crafts stores. Clay must always be kneaded before you model with it because it contains air that, if left in the clay, would form air bubbles in your pottery and spoil it. Work out this air by kneading it the same way that you knead bread. Also guard against making the clay too moist, because that causes the pottery to sag, and sagging, of course, spoils the shape.

To make your own pottery, you need modeling clay, a board on which you can work, a pie tin on which to build, a knife, a short stick (one side should be pointed), and a ruler.

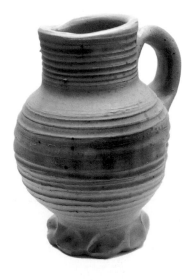

Keep spouts and handles thick so they will not crack or break off. Use a stick or dowel to create line incisions like these.

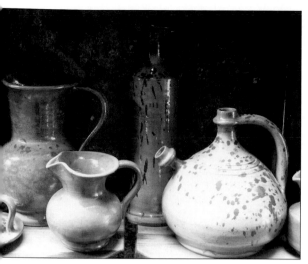

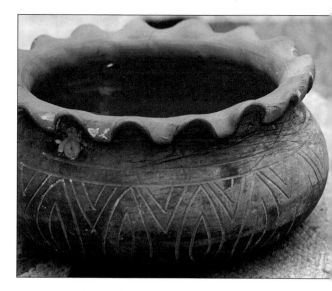

Using different glazes will give your pottery variances in odor and texture.

Jars

To start a jar, put a handful of clay on the board, pat it out with your hand until it is an inch thick, and smooth off the surface. Then, take a coffee cup, invert it upon the base, and, with your stick, trim the clay outside the rim.

To build up the walls, put a handful of clay on the board and use a knife to smooth it out into a long piece, ¼ inch thick. With the knife and a ruler, trim off one edge of the piece and cut a number of strips ¾ inch wide. Take one strip, stand it on top of the base, and rub its edge into the base on both sides of the strip. Take another strip and add it to the top of the first one, and continue building in this way, placing one strip on another, joining each to the one beneath it, and smoothing over the joints as you build. Keep doing this until the walls are as high as you want them to be. Remember to keep one hand inside the jar while you build, for extra support. Fill uneven places with bits of clay and smooth out rough spots with your fingers, having moistened your fingers with water first. When you are finished, you may also add decorations, or ornaments, to your jar.

Candlestick

Making a pottery candlestick requires a round base ½ inch thick and 4 inches in diameter. After preparing the base, put a lump of clay in the center, work it into the base, place another lump on top, work it into the piece, and continue in this way until the candlestick has been built as high as you want it. Then, force a candle into the moist clay, twisting it around until it has made a socket deep enough to place a candle into.

A cardboard "templet", with one edge trimmed to the proper shape, will make it easy to keep the walls of the candlestick symmetrical and the projecting cap on the top equal on all sides. Run the edge of the templet around the walls as you work, and it will show

you exactly where and how much to fill out, trim, and straighten the clay.

If you want to make a candlestick with a handle, make a base just as described earlier. Then cut strips of clay and build up the wall as if building a jar, leaving a center hole just large enough to hold a candle. When the desired height for the wall has been reached, cut a strip of clay ½ inch wide and ½ inch thick, and lay it around the top of the wall with a projection of ¼ inch over the wall. Smooth this piece on top, inside, and outside with your modeling stick and fingers. For the handle, prepare a strip 1 inch wide and ⅜ inch thick, and join one end to the top band and the other end to the base. Use a small lump of clay for filling around where you join the piece, and smooth off the piece on all sides.

When the candlestick is finished, run a round stick the same size as the candle down into the hole, and let it stay put until the clay is dry, to keep the candlestick straight.

Bowls

Bowls are quite easy to make. Starting with a base, lay strips of clay around the base, building upon each strip as you did when making a jar. Once the bowl reaches its desired height and width, allow it to dry.

Glazing and Firing

Most pottery that you buy is glazed and then fired in a pottery kiln, but firing is not necessary to make beautiful, sturdy pottery. The clay will dry hard enough, naturally, to keep its shape, and the only thing you must provide for is waterproofing (if the pottery will be holding liquids). To do this, you can take bathtub enamel and apply it to the inside (and outside, if desired) of the pottery to seal off any cracks and keep the item from leaking.

If you do want to try glazing and firing your own pottery, you will need a kiln. Below are instructions for making your own.

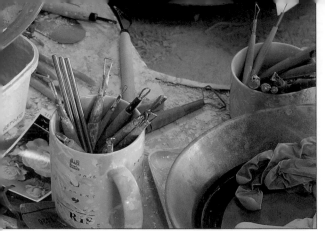

Pottery may be ornamented by scratching a design on it with the end of a modeling stick. You can do a simple, straight-line design by using a ruler to guide the stick in drawing the lines.

Sawdust Kiln

This small, homemade kiln can be used to bake and fire most small pottery projects. It will only get up to about 1200 degrees Fahrenheit, which is not hot enough to fire porcelain or stonewear. However, it will suffice for clay pinch pots and other decorative pieces.

You will need:

- Sawdust
- 20–30 red or orange bricks
- Chicken wire
- Sheet metal
- Newspaper and kindling

1. Choose a spot outdoors that is protected from strong winds. Clear away any dried branches or other flammables from the immediate area. A concrete patio or paved area makes an ideal base, but you can also place bricks or stones on the ground.
2. Stack bricks in a square shape, building each wall up at least four bricks high. Fill the kiln with sawdust.
3. Place the chicken wire on top of the bricks and add another layer or two of bricks. Carefully place your pottery n the center of the mesh, spacing the pieces at least ½ inch apart. Cover the pottery with sawdust.
4. Add another piece of chicken wire, add bricks and pottery, and cover with sawdust. Repeat until your kiln is the desired height.
5. Light the top layer of sawdust on fire, using kindling and newspaper if needed. Cover with the sheet metal, using another layer of bricks to hold it in place.
6. Once the kiln stops smoking, leave it alone until it completely cools down. Then carefully remove the sheet metal lid.

Permanent Homemade Pottery Kiln

As you continue to create pottery, you may find that you enjoy the art enough that you would like to continue this craft for years to come. In that case, and if you have enough space in your yard, you may think about constructing a permanent kiln for all of your pottery needs.

This kiln requires some intense construction, but having your own wood-burning pottery kiln will make firing your creations easier and more effective.

The essentials of this kiln are: a fire box, an oven, and a chimney. The kiln works by allowing the fire to pass up from the fire box through the oven floor, between the bricks (spaced about 1½ inches apart), and out through the chimney at the top of the oven.

The Construction of the Kiln

1. Begin by laying out a space for the foundation of the kiln. This should be on solid, dry ground. It is advisable to make an excavation a few inches below the surface and fill it in with cinders or broken brick. The place you choose for your kiln should also allow water to run off and not collect underneath.
2. Build the walls of the kiln three bricks deep on each of the sides and the back. Leave the front of the kiln open for the fire mouths.
3. Halfway between the two side walls, build a thin, central support, made of three courses of brick on the edge. This will leave a narrow ledge where the grates of the fire boxes can rest. Build the other edge of each grate into the side wall.

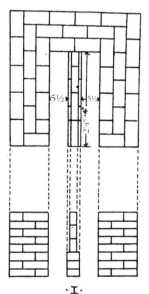

·I·

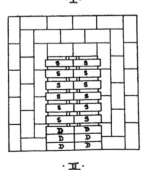

·II·

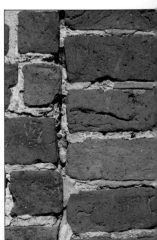

The top illustrations shows plan and front view of the kiln foundation up to the oven floor. The walls are three bricks thick on each side and the front is left open. The bottom illustration shows the bricks that rest on the side walls and on the central support. These should be made of fire bricks, since they'll be subjected to the most extreme heat.

The size of the kiln will be dependent on the amount of bricks you lay. Lay bricks endwise to make a stronger wall.

4 Make the mortar of common clay (or you can buy it if you desire). Mix the clay with water into a mortar. You can add some regular sand to give the mortar better working qualities, and this will also help prevent shrinkage.

5. Spread the mortar over the cinder foundation and start to lay the bricks. In building the walls and central support, make the joints between the bricks as tight and thin as possible. Tap the bricks into place so there will be no settling of the wall later on.

6. Build the walls and central support up to the point where the oven floor will be. To make the oven floor, arrange the bricks on their edges about 1½ inches apart from the front to the back of the kiln. These bricks should rest on the side walls and central support. Since this oven floor is going to be subjected to high heat, use fire bricks. Also be sure to project the bricks out in the front for the oven door to sit on.

7. Continue to build the side and back walls up nine more bricks. Then, you can start to taper the bricks into a chimney formation. Lay the next two levels of bricks (on the side walls only) in toward the center of the kiln about 1½ inches or so. The space between the walls at the top should not be more than 9 inches. Bridge the opening at the top across the front and back of the kiln, leaving an opening in the center just large enough for the chimney (about 8 or 9 inches square). You can do this by using large pieces of terra cotta flue lining (purchased at any hardware or home center store). The size of the flue lining should be about 2 feet x 8 inches x 6 inches.

8. Carefully cut lines in the flue lining from end to end, until the side falls away. Cut this in two and use the two halves for closing in the top of the kiln. Put these bricks in place with plenty of mortar and finish out the rest of the bricking over the walls with other pieces of flue lining, making them level.

9. Build two more levels of brick all around, leaving the chimney opening 9 inches by 9 inches.

10. Now build the chimney straight up with a single layer of bricks (or two bricks to each layer, if you desire). The inside diameter of the chimney should not be less than 7 inches by 7 inches. When complete, the chimney should be about 3 feet high.

11. You can also build the chimney 1 foot high and then let one brick on each side project into the chimney cavity about 2 inches. Then, fit ordinary stovepipe with a square end to rest on these projections inside the chimney. This is a lighter method than building brick all the way up.

12. Install grates to produce a better and cleared fire. You can find grates at your local hardware store or use old stove grates. Build these grates into the walls of the fire box and central support. Leave the front end of the oven open.

14. Place pottery in the oven. Brick up the front of the oven without any mortar and fill in the joints with wet sand.

15. The kiln will now need to be heated with wood. You should begin with a very simple fire lasting about an hour or two. This is extremely important, as the flame comes into contact with the raw clay, which, unless it is heated very gradually, could crack and split apart. After thoroughly warming the kiln, increase the heat more rapidly. After the firing is well underway (three or so hours later), close the doors of the fire boxes with pieces of sheet iron or bricks piled up in front. Only allow air in through the grates. Only remove the temporary doors to add fuel to the fire.

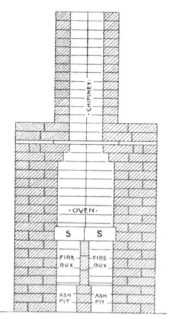

Cross section of the finished kiln. The space between the walls at the top should not be more than nine inches.

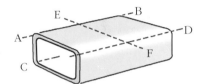

Cut lines in the flue lining from end to end at AB and CD. Then cut in two at EF and use the two halves for closing in the top of the kiln.

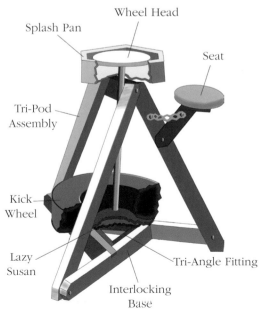

Knitting

The art of knitting was supposedly invented by the Spanish nobility as a means of relaxation for noble women in the country. The Scottish also claim to have developed knitting, and King Henry VII was the first to wear knitted stockings in England. Queen Elizabeth also wore knitted silk stockings made by Mistress Montegue.

Whenever and wherever knitting was first "discovered," it is useful, relaxing, and can be done while enjoying a good conversation with a friend.

Knitting Basics

Stitches

Knitting can be done in rows of plain or purl stitches or by incorporating a variety of stitches and knitting techniques in one project. However, the simpler stitches are better when first starting to knit. Just be sure not to pull the thread too tight or keep it too loose—as you continue to knit, you will learn the proper amount of tension to apply to your string so you create a perfect, knitted item.

Tools Needed for Knitting

1. **Gauge**—This measures the knitting needles. Most needles already have their gauge listed on them, but if your needles do not, you should find this measuring tool at your local arts and crafts store.
2. **Knitting needles**—These are made of steel, wood, or plastic and are used to knit your material together.
3. **Knitting shields**—Although these are not a necessary tool for knitting, you may find that you want these so the material does not slip off of your needle.
4. **Material to be knitted**—Beginners should use thicker yarn in their knitted items. When you have become more proficient in knitting, you can experiment with different types of threads and materials to create your various knitted items.

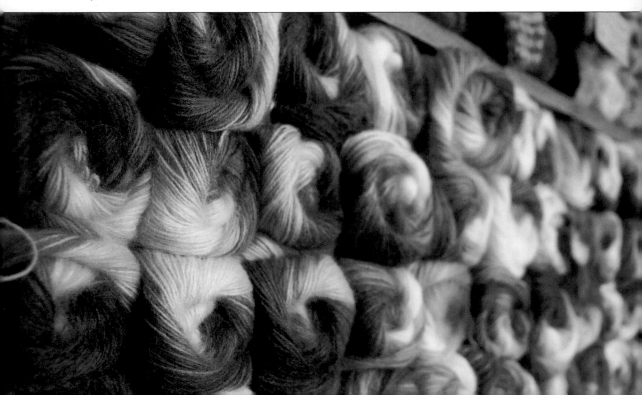

Knitting Terminology

To bring the thread forward—This means to pass the thread between the needles toward the knitter's body.

To cast off—You do this by knitting two stitches, passing the first over the second, and proceeding in this manner until the last stitch, which is secured by passing the thread through it.

To cast on the loops or stitches—Take the material in your right hand and twist it around the little finger, bringing it under the next two fingers, and passing it over the pointer finger. Then, take the end of the material in your left hand (holding the needle with your right), wrap it around the little finger, and then bring it over the thumb and around the second and third fingers. By doing so, you will have formed a loop. Now, bring the needle under the lower thread of the material and above the material that is over the right-hand pointer finger under the needle. The thread in the left hand should be pulled tightly, completing this step. You can repeat this process as many times as needed until you've cast the amount of stitches you want.

To cast over—This means to bring the material around the needle (bringing it forward).

To fasten on—This refers to fastening the end of the material when it's needed during the process of knitting. The best way to fasten on is to place the two ends in opposite directions and knit a few stitches with both.

Knitting stitch—In this stitch, the needle must be put through the cast-on stitch and the material should be turned over. This will be taken up and under the loop (or stitch) and then let off. This is also known as a plain stitch and will be continued until an entire round is complete.

A loop stitch—This is made by passing the thread before the needle.

Narrowing—This is to decrease the number of stitches by knitting two together, so you only form one loop.

Purl stitch—This is also known as a seam, ribbed, or turn stitch. It is formed by knitting with the material before the needle and instead of bringing the needle over the upper thread, the material is brought under it. This is the opposite of a knitting stitch.

Raising—This is to increase the number of stitches and is made by knitting one stitch in the usual way and then omitting to slip out the left-hand needle. Then, the material is passed forward, and a second stitch is formed by pulling the needle under the stitch. The material must be put back to its normal place when the extra stitch is completed.

To rib—To alternately knit plain and purled stitches (three plain then three purl, etc.).

A round—This is all of the stitches on two, three, or more needles.

A row—This refers to the stitches from one end of the needle to the other.

To seam—To knit a purl stitch every alternate row.

A slip stitch—This is made by passing the thread from one needle to another without knitting.

To turn—To change the type of stitch.

Welts—These are alternating plain and ribbed stitches and are used for anything that you don't want to twist or curl up.

How to Knit

1. To cast on, hold the two needles loosely in your hands. Pass a loop over the left-hand needle near the end of the yarn and hold the right-hand needle loosely. Put the right-hand needle into the loop, passing it from left to right and keeping the right-hand needle under the left needle. Pass the string over this needle—between it and the left-hand needle—and pull the loop up toward the right. Now, bring the right needle up and pass the stitch on it to the left needle by putting the left needle through the left side of the loop, keeping the right needle in the loop. It is ready to begin the next stitch. Repeat.

2. Knitting stitch: After you have made the correct number of stitches, hold the needle that has the stitches on it in your left hand and pass the right needle into the first stitch from left to right. Put the yarn around between the two needles, pull the loop through the other loop on the left needle, and slip that loop off the left needle. Repeat.

3. Purling stitch: Keep the yarn in the front of the work and put the right needle into a stitch from right to left, passing it upward through the front loop of the stitch. The right needle should be resting on the left. Pass the yarn around the front of the needle and bring it back between the two needles. Pull the right needle slightly back, so as to secure the loop on the right needle and then draw off the loop on the left needle. Repeat. Note: This is basically the knitting stitch, only backwards.

4. Slipping a stitch: This is done by passing a stitch from one needle to another without knitting it at the beginning of a row. This should always been done when using two needles at the beginning of each row, so the rows remain even.

5. Casting (binding) off: Knit two stitches, passing the first stitch over the second, and then knit a third stitch, passing the second over the third. Continue in this way until all the stitches are off the needle.

Two Simple Knitting Patterns

1. Patent Knitting, or Brioche Knitting

Cast on any number of stitches divisible by three.

Yarn forward, slip one, knit two together. Work every row in the same way.

2. Cane-work Pattern

Cast on any number of stitches divisible by four.

General Tip for Beginning Knitters

Hold the needles loosely in your hands and close to the points. To knit easily and quickly, your hands should neither move too much nor should you make large gestures with the needles.

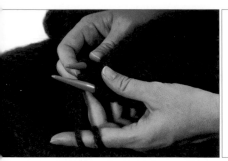
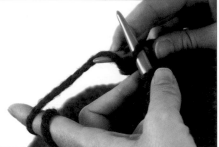
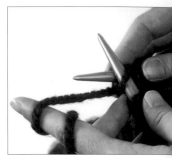

Hold the needles loosely in your hands with the loose yarn wrapped around your pointer finger.

Slip the right needle into the top loop on the left needle, keeping the left needle above the right needle. To do a purl stitch, the right needle would go on top of the right needle.

Wrap the loose strand of yarn over and behind the right needle. For a purl stitch, wrap the yarn behind first and then over the needle. Slip the loop off of the left needle to finish the stitch.

First Row: make one, knit one, make one, knit three. Repeat.

Second Row: purl.

Third Row: knit three, make one, slip one, knit two together, pass the slip-stitch over the two knitted together, make one. Repeat.

Fourth Row: purl.

Fifth Row: make one, slip one, knit two together, pass the slip-stitch over, make one, knit three. Repeat.

Sixth Row: purl.

Seventh Row: repeat the third row.

Eighth Row: purl.

Ninth Row: make one, slip one, knit two together, pass the slip-stitch over, make one, knit three. Repeat.

Tenth Row: purl.

Repeat from the third row until the item is complete.

Simple Scarf

Materials

Mid-weight or 4-ply yarn of any color (use at least one full bundle of yarn)

Knitting needles (size 8 to 10.5 are best for knitting scarves)

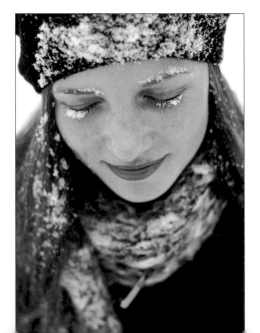

Alternating rows of knit and purl stitches.

Directions

1. Decide how wide you want your scarf to be (26 to 35 stitches are the standard width for a scarf).
2. First row: knit 26 to 36 stitches
3. Second row: knit 26 to 35 stitches (if you want something a little more challenging, purl this row instead)
4. Continue knitting (or knitting and purling alternately) until you reach the desired length (60 inches is a good length for a scarf).
5. At the end, cast (bind) off the stitches.

Hat

Materials

Yarn of a medium-heavy weight, any color of your choosing

Knitting needles (depending on the head size for the hat, use No. 6 or No. 8 needles)

Directions

1. Cast on 72 stitches.
2. First row: knit 72 stitches.
3. Second row: purl 72 stitches.

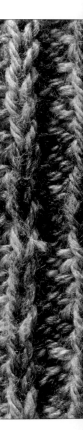

This hat shows the "knit one row, purl one row" pattern. You can also follow this pattern for six or eight rows and then switch to just knitting to give your hat a differentiated band around the bottom. If desired, use round needles (two knitting needles that are attached by a plastic or rubber cord) to avoid having to sew a seam at the end.

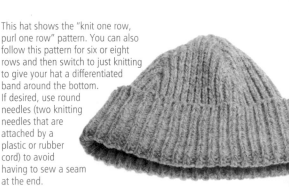

4. Continue in this fashion until your hat is about 9 inches tall.
5. To begin to cast (bind) off your hat, follow this pattern:
   a. Knit five stitches, knit two together, and continue to the end of the row.
   b. Purl the next row.
   c. Knit four stitches, knit two together, and continue to the end of the row.
   d. Purl the next row.
   e. Knit three stitches, knit two together, and continue to the end of the row.
   f. Purl the next row.
   g. Knit two stitches, knit two together, and continue to the end of the row.
   h. Purl the next row.
   i. Knit every two stitches together.
7. Take the excess yarn, pull it through the last stitches, and cut off so only about an inch and a half remains. Sew a seam, put the remaining yarn through the loops, and fold your hat inside out.

Fingerless Mittens

Fingerless mittens are wonderful to use if your hands are cold but you still need to have complete access to things, such as typing on a computer or making a meal. They make wonderful gifts for friends and family members.

Materials
150 yards of worsted-weight yarn or wool/yarn blend
Double-pointed knitting needles, No. 8

Directions
1. To make the cuff, cast on 28 stitches, making sure these stitches are even. Then, begin to knit in the round. Do not twist the stitches. Use the yarn tail to keep track of the round ends. Knit three rounds. Switching to the twisted rib pattern, knit one stitch through the back loop in order to twist it. Purl one, and repeat this pattern until the cuff measures roughly 2½ inches.
2. Using a stocking stitch, begin the hand and thumb portion of the mitten.
3. First row: knit one, purl one, make one (increase the stitch), knit one, make one, purl one, knit until the end of the round.
4. Second row: knit one, purl one, knit until you reach the next purl stitch in the row above, purl one, knit until the end of the round.
5. Third row: knit one, purl one, make one, knit until the next purl, make one, purl one, knit until the end of the round.
6. Repeat the second and third rows until you have nine stitches between the purls. The glove should now measure about 5½ inches from the edge of the cast-off point.
7. Place two purl and nine thumb gore stitches on a piece of scrap yarn. Cast off three stitches and knit four rounds of stocking stitch. Change to twisted rib stitch and make six rounds. Bind this off very loosely.

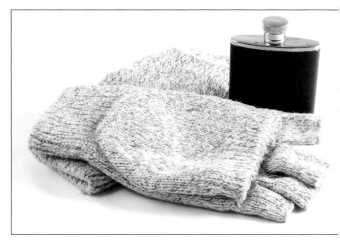

You can easily modify the pattern described here to include these individual finger openings and the finger "hood." Simply follow the steps to make the thumb hole (steps 8–10) for each of the additional finger openings. For the "hood," follow the directions for making a hat (only make it much smaller) and sew it onto the mitten above the knuckles.

8. To make the thumb, put 11 stitches on hold for the thumb onto an extra knitting needle. Pick up three stitches at the base of the thumb and make 14 stitches.
9. Knit one round of only 12 stitches.
10. Using the twisted rib stitch, make six more rounds and bind off loosely.
11. To finish up, weave in the yarn ends and, if necessary, sew closed any holes at the sides of the thumb base.

Knitted Square Blanket

Materials
Thick yarn, any color you like (if you want a multicolored blanket, feel free to use different- colored yarn for each individual square)
Knitting needles, No. 6

Directions
1. Begin by making smaller squares that will be sewn together to form a larger blanket.
2. Cast on any number of stitches divisible by three. For a square of 6 inches, you'll need 45 stitches.
3. First row: Slip one, knit two. Turn the yarn around the needle and bring it again in front. Then, slip one, knit two together. Purl the last two stitches.
4. Second row: Turn the yarn around the needle, bringing it to the front. Slip one, knit two together. Knit the last two stitches in the row.
5. Continue the pattern in step 4 (alternating purled and knitted last two stitches) until you reach the end and cast off your square.
6. Continue making as many squares as you want to get the desired size of your blanket.
7. When you have all your knitted squares, take a knitting needle and sew each square together.

Tying Knots

Knowing how to tie different types of knots is a useful skill to have, especially if you are involved in boating, rock climbing, fishing, or other outdoor activities.

Strong knots are typically those that are neat in appearance and are not bulky. If a knot is tied properly, it will almost never loosen and will still be easy to untie when necessary.

The best way to learn how to tie knots effectively is to sit down and practice with a piece of cord or rope. Practice, in this case, definitely makes tying knots much faster and easier. Listed below are a few common knots that are useful to know:

- **Bowline knot:** Fasten one end of the line to some object. After the loop is made, hold it in position with your left hand and pass the end of the line up through the loop, behind and over the line above, and through the loop once again. Pull it tightly and the knot is now complete.

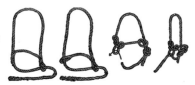

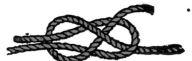

- **Clove hitch:** This knot is particularly useful if you need the length of the running end to be adjustable.

- **Halter:** If you need to create a halter to lead a horse or pony, try this knot.

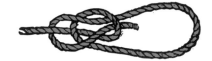

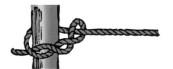

- **Sheepshank knot:** This is used for shortening ropes. Gather up the amount to be shortened and then make a half hitch around each of the bends.

- **Slip knot:** Slip knots are adjustable, so that you can tighten them around an object after they're tied.

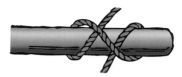

- **Timber hitch:** If you need to secure a rope to a tree, this is the knot to use. It is easy to untie, too.

Qualities of a Good Knot

1. It can be tied quickly.
2. It will hold tightly.
3. It can be untied easily.

- **Two half hitches:** Use this knot to secure a rope to a pole, boat mooring, washer, tire, or similar object.

Three Parts of a Rope

1. **The standing part:** this is the long, unused part of the rope.
2. **The bight:** this is the loop formed whenever the rope is turned back.
3. **The end:** this is the part used in leading.

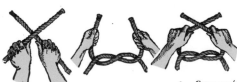

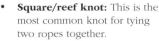

- **Square/reef knot:** This is the most common knot for tying two ropes together.

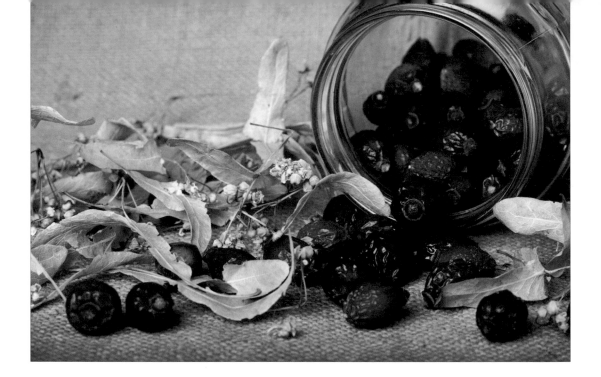

PART SEVEN Well-Being

"Health is a state of complete harmony of the body, mind, and spirit. When one is free from physical disabilities and mental distractions, the gates of the soul open."

—*B.K.S. Iyengar*

On some level, we all know what we need for optimum health. Our bodies are built to give us clues, from simple ones—if we're tired, we probably need rest—to ones that require a little more attention to discern, such as a headache or stomachache, which can stem from a wide range of issues. Many of us consistently ignore the clues, masking exhaustion with caffeine, or popping an aspirin every time a pain begins to surface without even considering the cause. Well-being begins with taking the time to listen to ourselves, being honest about what needs healing or improvement, and nurturing the desire to reach a healthier level of being. Once the desire for health is strong, you will find a myriad of channels for achieving it. This section offers suggestions for finding well-being through natural means, from herbal medicine to natural spa products. There are times when the best thing to do is to go straight to a doctor, whether a doctor of Western medicine, a homeopath, or another type of medical practitioner. But part of leading a self-sufficient life is learning to recognize and meet your own needs, even in the areas of health and safety. From there, you can begin to help those around you, too. So start paying attention to your physical, mental, and spiritual state, and find out what you can do to be the best version of who you already are.

Herbal Medicine

An herb is a plant or plant part used for its scent, flavor, or therapeutic properties. For centuries herbs have been used in various forms for their health benefits. Many are now sold as tablets, capsules, powders, teas, extracts, and fresh or dried plants. However, some have side effects and may interact with other drugs you are taking.

To use an herbal product as safely as possible:

* Consult your doctor first.
* Do not take a bigger dose than the label recommends.
* Take it under the guidance of a trained medical professional.
* Be especially cautious if you are pregnant or nursing.

Herbal supplements are sold in many forms: as fresh or dried products; liquid or solid extracts; and tablets, capsules, powders, and tea bags. For example, fresh ginger root is often found in the produce section of food stores; dried ginger root is sold packaged in tea bags, capsules, or tablets; and liquid preparations made from ginger root are also sold. A particular group of chemicals or a single chemical may be isolated from a botanical and sold as a dietary supplement, usually in tablet or capsule form. Common preparations include teas, decoctions, tinctures, and extracts:

A *tea*, also known as an *infusion*, is made by adding boiling water to fresh or dried botanicals and steeping them. The tea may be drunk either hot or cold.

Some roots, bark, and berries require more forceful treatment to extract their desired ingredients. They are simmered in boiling water for longer periods than teas, making a *decoction*, which also may be drunk hot or cold.

A *tincture* is made by soaking a botanical in a solution of alcohol and water. Tinctures are sold as liquids and are used for concentrating and preserving a botanical. They are made in different strengths that are expressed as botanical-to-extract ratios (i.e., ratios of the weight of the dried botanical to the volume or weight of the finished product).

An *extract* is made by soaking the botanical in a liquid that removes specific types of chemicals. The liquid can be used as is or evaporated to make a dry extract for use in capsules or tablets.

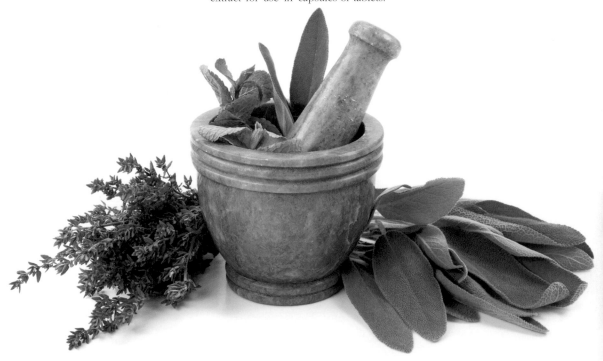

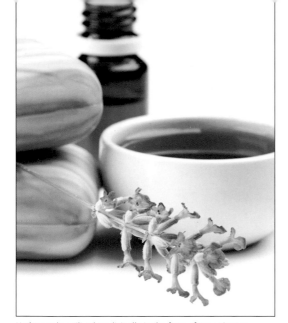

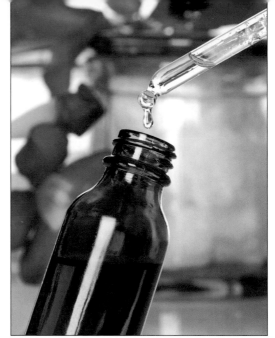

Herbs can be utilized medicinally in the form of teas, tincture, extracts, or as an addition to soaps, lotions, or salves.

Add several drops of your tincture to tea or juice to receive the healing benefits without the strong flavor.

Make Your Own Herbal Tincture

Tinctures help to concentrate and preserve the health benefits of your herbs. To use, mix 1 teaspoon of tincture with juice, tea, or water and drink no more than three times a day.

1. Pick the fresh herbs, removing any dirty, wilted, or damaged parts. Do not wash. Be sure you know whether it is the stems, leaves, roots, or flowers that have the health benefits, and use only those parts.
2. Coarsely chop the plant parts. Flowers can be left whole.
3. Clean and dry a small glass jar with an airtight lid and put the herbs inside. Fill the jar with 100-proof vodka or warm cider vinegar until plant parts are fully immersed. Screw the lid on securely and label the jar.
4. Store for 6 to 8 weeks, gently shaking a few times a week.
5. Strain out the herbs and store the liquid tincture in a clean, dry bottle. Be sure to label the jar with the ingredients, and date and store it in a safe place away from children's reach.

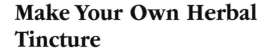

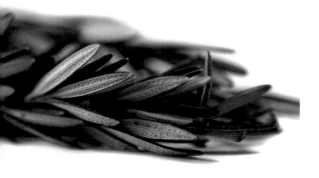

Common Herbal Remedies

Here is a list of common herbs that can be used to cure or alleviate the symptoms of conditions ranging from cancer to acne to the common cold. If you are taking any other medications or supplements, check with your doctor before trying any herbs. As with any medication, every body is unique and certain herbs can have adverse side effects for certain people, so pay attention to your body and cease taking any herbs that make you feel worse in any way. It's a good idea to try one herb at a time per condition and to keep a journal documenting what you take when and how you feel. This way you'll be able to tell more easily what effects the herbs are having.

Aloe Vera

Uses: The clear gel in aloe is used topically to treat osteoarthritis, burns, and sunburn. The green part can be made into a juice or dried and taken orally to treat a variety of conditions, such as diabetes, asthma, epilepsy, and osteoarthritis.

Cautions: Using aloe vera on surgical wounds may inhibit their healing. If taken orally, aloe vera can produce abdominal cramps and diarrhea, which can decrease the absorption of many drugs.

If you have diabetes and take glucose-lowering medication, you should be careful of taking aloe orally, as studies suggest that aloe may decrease blood glucose levels.

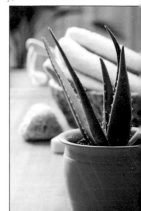

Aloe vera can be used topically to treat and soothe a variety of skin irritations.

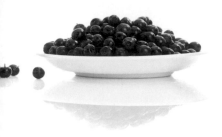

Bilberries are a close relative of blueberries and can be eaten whole or made into an extract.

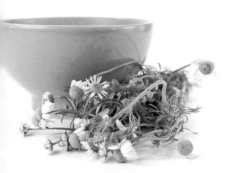

Chamomile flowers can be used to make a relaxing tea.

Echinacea is beautiful as well as useful medicinally. It grows well in moderately dry soil.

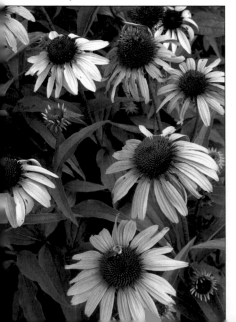

Astragalus

Uses: Astragalus was traditionally used in Chinese medicine in combination with other herbs to help boost the immune system. It is still used widely in China for chronic hepatitis and as an additional cancer therapy. Astragalus is commonly used to boost the immune system to help colds and upper respiratory infections and has also been used to fight heart disease. The astragalus plant root is used in soups, teas, extracts, and capsules and is generally used with other herbs, like ginseng, angelica, and licorice.

Cautions: Astragalus may interact with medications that suppress the immune system (such as those taken by cancer patients or organ transplant recipients).

Bilberry

Uses: Bilberry fruit is used to treat diarrhea, menstrual cramps, eye problems, varicose veins, and circulatory problems. The leaf of a bilberry is used to treat diabetes. It's claimed that bilberry fruit also helps improve night vision, but this is not clinically proven. The bilberry fruit can be eaten or made into an extract. Likewise, its leaves can be used in tea or made into an extract.

Cautions: Though bilberry fruit is considered safe, high doses of the leaf or leaf extract may have possible toxic side effects.

Chamomile

Uses: Chamomile has a calming effect and is often used to counteract sleeplessness and anxiety, as well as diarrhea and gastrointestinal conditions. Topically, chamomile is used in the treatment of skin conditions and for mouth ulcers (particularly due to cancer treatment). The chamomile plant has flowering tops, which are used to make teas, extracts, capsules, and tablets. It can also be applied as a skin cream or ointment or even be used as a mouth rinse.

Cautions: Some people have developed rare allergic reactions from eating or coming into contact with chamomile. These reactions include skin rashes, swelling of the throat, shortness of breath, and anaphylaxis. People allergic to related plants, such as daisies, ragweed, or marigolds, should be careful when coming into contact with chamomile.

Cranberry

Uses: Cranberry fruit and leaves are used in healing many conditions, including wounds, urinary disorders, diarrhea, diabetes, and stomach and liver problems. Cranberries are often used in treating urinary tract infections and stomach ulcers. They may also be useful in preventing dental plaque and in preventing *E.coli* bacteria from adhering to cells along the urinary tract wall. Cranberry fruit can be eaten straight; made into juice; or used in the form of extracts, tea, or tablets and taken as a dietary supplement.

Cautions: Drinking copious amounts of cranberry juice can cause an upset stomach and diarrhea.

Dandelion

Uses: Dandelions, throughout history, have been most commonly used to treat liver and kidney diseases and spleen problems. Dandelions are sometimes used in liver and kidney tonics, as a diuretic, and for simple digestive issues. The dandelion's leaves and roots (and sometimes the entire plant) are used in teas, capsules, and extracts. The leaves are used in salads or are cooked, and the flowers are used to make wine.

Cautions: While using dandelions is typically safe, there are a few instances of upset stomach and diarrhea caused by the plant, as well as allergic reactions. If your gallbladder is inflamed or infected, you should avoid using dandelion products.

Echinacea

Uses: Traditionally, echinacea has been used to boost the immune system to help prevent colds, flu, and various infections. Echinacea can also be used for wounds, acne, and boils. The roots and exposed plant are used, either fresh or dried, for teas, juice, extracts, or in preparations for external use.

Cautions: Echinacea, taken orally, generally does not cause any problems. Some people do have allergic reactions (rashes, increased asthma, anaphylaxis), but typically only gastrointestinal problems are experienced. If you are allergic to any plants in the daisy family, it may be best to steer clear of echinacea.

Evening Primrose Oil

Uses: Since the 1930s, evening primrose oil has been used to fight eczema and recently, it has been used for other inflammatory conditions. Evening primrose oil is also used in the treatment of breast pain during the menstrual cycle, symptoms of menopause, and premenstrual issues. It may also relieve pain associated with rheumatoid arthritis.

The oil is extracted from the evening primrose seeds. You'll find it in capsule form at many health food stores.

Cautions: There may be some mild side effects, such as gastrointestinal upset or headache.

Flaxseed and Flaxseed Oil

Uses: Flaxseed is typically used as a laxative and to alleviate hot flashes. Flaxseed oil is used for treating arthritis pain. Both herbs are used to fight high cholesterol and can be beneficial for those with heart disease. Flaxseed, in either its whole or crushed form, may be mixed with water or juice and ingested. It is also available as a powder. Flaxseed oil can be taken in either a liquid or capsule form.

Cautions: It is essential to take flaxseed with lots of water, or constipation could worsen. Further, flaxseed fiber may decrease the body's ability to absorb other oral medications and so should not be taken together.

Garlic

Uses: Garlic is typically used as a dietary supplement for those with high cholesterol, heart disease, and high blood pressure. It may help decrease the hardening of the arteries and is also used in the prevention of stomach and colon cancer. It is also used topically or orally to heal some infections, including ear infections. Garlic cloves may be eaten either raw or cooked, or they may be dried or powdered and used in capsules. Oil and other extracts can be obtained from garlic cloves.

Cautions: Some common side effects of garlic are breath and body odor, heartburn, upset stomach, and allergic reactions. Garlic can also thin blood and so should not be used before surgeries or dental work, especially if you have a bleeding disorder. It also has an adverse effect on drugs used to fight HIV.

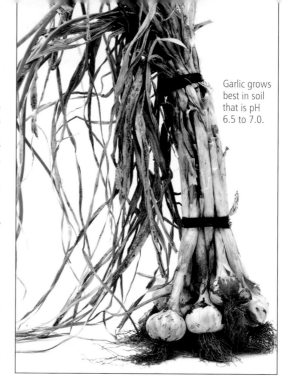

Garlic grows best in soil that is pH 6.5 to 7.0.

Ginger

Uses: Ginger is commonly used in Asian medicines to treat stomachaches, nausea, and diarrhea. Many U.S. dietary supplements containing ginger are used to help fight cold and flu and can be used to relieve post-surgery nausea or nausea related to pregnancy. It has also been used for arthritis and other joint and muscle pain. Ginger root can be found fresh or dried, in tablets, capsules, extracts, and teas.

Cautions: Side effects are rare but can include gas, bloating, heartburn, and, for some people, nausea.

Ginkgo

Uses: Traditionally, extract from ginkgo leaves has been used in the treatment of illnesses such as asthma, bronchitis, fatigue, and tinnitus. People use gingko leaf extract in the hopes that it will help improve their memory (especially in the treatment of Alzheimer's disease and dementia). It is also taken to treat sexual dysfunction, multiple sclerosis, and other health issues. Ginkgo leaf extracts are made into tablets, capsules, or teas. Sometimes the extracts can also be found in skin care products.

Cautions: Some common side effects are headache, nausea, gastrointestinal upset, diarrhea, dizziness, or skin irritations. Ginkgo may also increase bleeding risks, so those having surgery or with bleeding disorders should consult a doctor before using any ginkgo products. Uncooked ginkgo seeds are toxic and can cause seizures.

Ginkgo leaves can be made into an extract and ingested for a wide range of health benefits.

Ginseng (Asian)

Uses: Ginseng is used to help boost the immune system and contribute to the overall health of an individual. It has been used traditionally and currently for improving those who are recovering from illnesses, increasing stamina and mental and physical performance, treating erectile dysfunction and symptoms of menopause, and lowering blood glucose levels and blood pressure. In some studies, ginseng has been proven to lower blood glucose levels and boost immune systems. The ginseng root is dried and made into tablets, capsules, extracts, and teas. It can also be made into creams for external use.

Cautions: Limiting ginseng intake to three months at a time will most likely reduce any potential side effects. The most common side effects are headaches and sleep issues, along with some allergic reactions. If you have diabetes and are taking blood-sugar lowering medications, it is advisable not to use ginseng, as it too lowers blood sugar.

Grape Seed Extract

Uses: Grape seed extract is used for treating heart and blood vessel conditions, such as high blood pressure, high cholesterol, and low circulation. It is also used for those struggling with complications from diabetes, such as nerve and eye damage. Grape seed extract is also used in treating vision problems, reducing swelling after surgery, and cancer prevention. Extracted from grape seeds, it is readily available in tablets and capsules.

Cautions: Common side effects of prolonged grape seed oil use are headaches; dry, itchy scalp; dizziness; and nausea.

Green Tea

Uses: Green tea and its extracts have been used in preventing and treating breast, stomach, and skin cancers, as well as improving mental alertness, aiding weight loss, lowering cholesterol, and preventing the sun from damaging the skin. Green tea is typically brewed and drunk. Extracts can be taken in capsule form and sometimes green tea can be found in skin care products.

Cautions: While green tea is generally safe for most adults, there have been a few reports of liver problems occurring in those who take green tea extracts. Thus, these extracts should always be taken with food and should not be taken at all by those with liver disorders. Green tea also contains caffeine and can cause insomnia, anxiety, irritability, nausea, diarrhea, or frequent urination.

Lavender

Uses: Lavender, in the past, has been used as an antiseptic and to help with mental health issues. Now it is more commonly taken for anxiety, restlessness, insomnia, and depression, and can also be used to fight headaches, upset stomach, and hair loss.

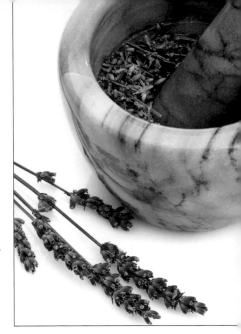

Lavender has a soothing, relaxing aroma. It can also be ingested in the form of tea or extracts, or even in baked goods.

Most commonly used in aromatherapy, lavender essential oil can also be diluted with other oils and rubbed on the skin. When dried, lavender flowers can be made into teas or liquid extracts and ingested.

Cautions: Lavender oil applied to the skin may cause some irritation and is poisonous if ingested. Lavender tea may cause headache, appetite change, and constipation. If used with sedatives, it may increase drowsiness.

Licorice Root

Uses: Traditionally, licorice root is used as a dietary supplement for the treatment of stomach ulcers, bronchitis, and sore throat. It is also used to help cure infections caused by viruses. When licorice root is peeled, it can be dried and made into powder. It is available in capsules, tablets, and extracts.

Cautions: If taken in large doses, licorice root can cause high blood pressure, water retention, and low potassium levels, leading to heart conditions. Taken with diuretics, it could cause the body's potassium levels to fall to dangerously low levels. If you have heart disease or high blood pressure, you should practice caution when taking licorice root. Large doses of licorice root may cause preterm labor in pregnant women.

Milk Thistle

Uses: Milk thistle is used as a protective measure for liver problems and in the treatment of liver cirrhosis, chronic hepatitis, and gallbladder diseases. It is also used to lower cholesterol, reduce insulin resistance in those with type 2 diabetes, and reduce the growth of cancerous cells in the breast, cervix, or prostate. Milk thistle seeds are used to make capsules, extracts, and strong teas.

Milk thistle grows in a wide range of soil types and will thrive in sunny or partly shady areas.

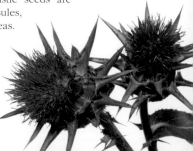

Cautions: Occasionally, milk thistle may cause diarrhea, upset stomach, or bloating. It may also cause allergic reactions, especially in those with allergies to the daisy family.

Mistletoe

Uses: For hundreds of years, mistletoe has been used to treat seizures and headaches. In Europe, mistletoe is used to treat cancer and to boost the immune system. The shoots and berries of mistletoe are used in oral extracts. In Europe, these extracts are prescription drugs, available only by injection.

Cautions: Eating raw and unprocessed mistletoe may cause vomiting, seizures, a slowing of the heart rate, and even death. American mistletoe cannot be used for medical purposes. Injected mistletoe extract can irritate the skin and produce low-grade fevers or flu-like symptoms. There is also a slight risk for severe allergic reactions that could cause breathing difficulty.

Peppermint Oil

Uses: Usually, peppermint oil is used to treat nausea, indigestion, and cold symptoms and it can also be used to allay headaches, muscle and nerve pain, and irritable bowel syndrome. Peppermint essential oil can be taken orally in small doses. It can also be diluted with other oils and applied to the skin.

Cautions: Common side effects include allergic reactions and heartburn, though peppermint oil is relatively safe in small doses.

Red Clover

Uses: Red clover has been used for treating cancer, whooping cough, asthma, and indigestion. It is also used to allay menopausal symptoms, breast pain, high cholesterol, osteoporosis, and enlarged prostate. The red clover flower is used in preparing extracts in tablets and capsules as well as teas.

Cautions: No serious side effects have been reported, though it is unclear if it is safe for use by pregnant women, women who are breastfeeding, or women with breast or other hormonal cancer. The estrogen in red clover may also increase a woman's chance of contracting cancer in the uterus.

Soy

Uses: Soy products are typically used for treating high cholesterol, menopausal symptoms, osteoporosis, problems with memory, breast and prostate cancer, and high blood pressure. Available in dietary supplements, soy can be found in tablet or capsule form. Soybeans may be cooked and eaten, or made into tofu, soy milk, and other foods.

Cautions: Using soy supplements or eating soy products can create minor stomach and bowel problems, and in rare cases, allergic reactions causing breathing difficulties and rashes. While there is no conclusive evidence linking soy with increased risk of breast cancer, women who have or are at risk of getting breast cancer should consult a doctor about using soy products.

St. John's Wort

Uses: St. John's wort has been used for hundreds of years to treat mental illness and nerve pain. It has also been used as a sedative; in malaria treatment; and as a balm for wounds, burns, and insect bites. It is commonly used to treat depression, anxiety, and sleep disorders. The flowers are used, in extract form, for tea and capsules.

Cautions: A possible side effect of using St. John's wort is increased light sensitivity. Other common side effects are anxiety, dry mouth, dizziness, gastrointestinal symptoms, fatigue, headache, and sexual dysfunction. St. John's wort also interacts with drugs and may interfere with the way the body breaks down those drugs. It may affect antidepressants, birth control pills, cyclosporine, digoxin, indinavir and other HIV drugs, irinotecan and other cancer drugs, and anticoagulants.

If you are taking antidepressants, be careful if also taking St. John's wort, as it may increase the likelihood of nausea, anxiety, headache, and confusion.

Turmeric

Uses: Traditionally used in Chinese medicine, turmeric was supposed to aid digestion and liver function and to relieve arthritis pain. It was also taken to regulate the menstrual cycle. Applied directly to the skin, it was used to treat eczema and wounds. Now, turmeric is used in the treatment of heartburn, stomach ulcers, and gallstones. Turmeric is also used to reduce inflammation and in the prevention and treatment of certain cancers.

The underground stems of the turmeric plant are dried and taken orally in capsules, teas, or liquid extracts. It can also be made into a paste to be used on the skin.

Cautions: Considered safe for most adults, long-term use of turmeric may cause indigestion. Those with gallbladder problems should avoid turmeric, however, as it may worsen the condition.

Make St. John's wort flowers into tea and drink to boost your mood and ease tension.

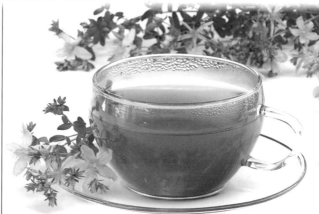

Valerian

Uses: For many years, valerian has been used for sleep disorders and to treat anxiety. Valerian has also been used to alleviate headaches, depression, irregular heart-beat, and trembling. The roots and underground stems of the valerian plant are usually made into supplements in capsule, tablet, or liquid extract form. It can also sometimes be made into teas.

Cautions: Valerian is typically safe to use for short periods of time (no more than six weeks) but there is no proof about its long-term effectiveness. Some common side effects of valerian use are headaches, dizziness, upset stomach, and grogginess the morning after use.

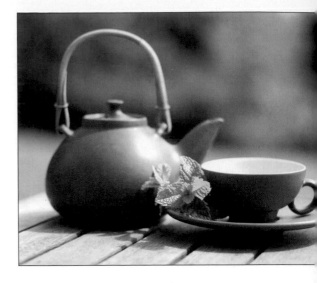

Homemade Herbal Teas

Herbal teas can be very tasty and deliver between 50 and 90 percent of the medicinal qualities of the herbs used. Teas you make yourself will be more potent and flavorful than those you can buy at the store, and much less expensive. Try experimenting with different herbal combinations, but be careful to avoid any plants you cannot confidently identify as edible, or any plants sprayed with pesticides. If using dried herbs, you can store your tea mixes in sealed containers for months. Be sure to label each container with the name of the tea.

Use 1 to 2 teaspoons of dried herbs per cup of hot water or 3 teaspoons of fresh herbs per pint of water. Steep the herbs for about 10 minutes and then strain. The following plants can all be safely used in teas:

Flowers

Alliums, bee balm, carnations, echinacea (roots and flowers), hibiscus, hollyhocks, honeysuckle (avoid the poisonous berries), lavender, marshmallow (use the roots), red clover, nasturtiums, roses (flowers or hips), violets.

Herbs

Basil, chamomile flowers, chives, dill, eucalyptus, ginger root, lemon balm, lemongrass, marjoram, mint, oregano, parsley, peppermint, linden leaves, mint, rosemary, sage, thyme, valerian root, verbena.

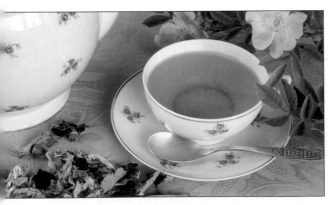

Bushes and Trees

Birch leaves, blackberry leaves, citrus blossoms, elderberry flowers, gardenia, pine needles, raspberry leaves.

Weeds

Chickweed, chicory, dandelions, goldenrod, stinging nettle.

Tea for the Common Cold

Combine the following herbs in any proportion you like. Boil for 10 minutes, strain, and add honey to taste.

Marshmallow root (eases body aches, reduces inflammation)

Peppermint (reduces congestion, eases headaches, soothes stomach)

Echinacea roots and flowers (boosts the immune system)

Thyme (reduces chest and nasal congestion, increases circulation)

Cinnamon (reduces inflammation and fights infection)

Rosehips, finely chopped (full of vitamin C, which boosts the immune system and energizes)

Ginger root, peeled and finely chopped (warms from the inside out)

Lavender, crushed (eases migraines)

Lemon peel, finely grated (full of vitamin C)

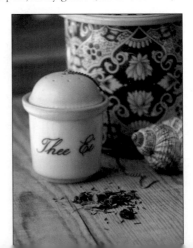

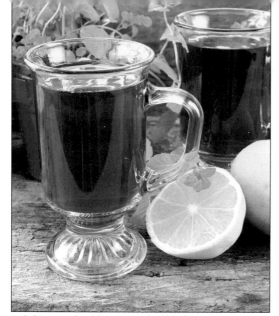

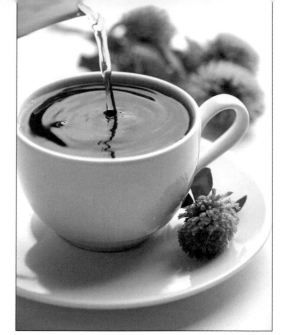

Herbal teas are also delicious served cold in the summer months.

Red clover blossoms promote estrogen and nourish the uterus.

Calming Tea

Combine the following calming herbs, using about ¼ as much valerian as the other herbs (valerian can be very potent). Boil for 10 minutes, strain, and add honey to taste.

Lemon balm leaves
Chamomile flowers
Valerian root, crushed
Ginger root, peeled and finely chopped

Fertility Tea

Drink one cup of fertility tea a day to help balance your hormones and to get nutrients that can aid in becoming pregnant. Combine the herbs in equal proportion, boil for 10 minutes, strain, and add honey to taste.

Red clover blossoms (nourishes the uterus, promotes estrogen, rich in magnesium and calcium)
Nettle leaves (rich in calcium, potassium, phosphorous, iron, and sulfur)

Red raspberry leaves (aids the fertilized egg in attaching to the uterine lining, rich in minerals, helps to tone muscles in the pelvic region)
Peppermint (aids in absorption of red raspberry leaf nutrients)

Cleansing Tea

The herbs in this tea will improve your digestion, help your body in its natural detoxification process, and give you more energy. Combine the herbs in any proportion (go easy on the cayenne), boil for 10 minutes, strain, and add honey if desired.

Peppermint leaves
Dandelion root
Whole allspice berries
Ginger root, peeled and finely chopped
Licorice root, crushed
Cayenne pepper

Natural Cosmetics

Homemade Lip Gloss

You only need a few ingredients to make your own lip gloss, though once you understand the basic recipe you can begin to experiment by adding different essential oils, aloes, and food products to create your own, unique type of gloss.

Homemade lip gloss containers can be any small glass jar or tin, or you can reuse an old lip gloss container (just make sure all the old gloss is out of the container). To sterilize the container, wash with soap and hot water, dunk the container in a jar of rubbing alcohol, rinse clean, and then allow the container to completely dry before pouring in your melted gloss. Allow the gloss mixture to cool completely before using (you can speed

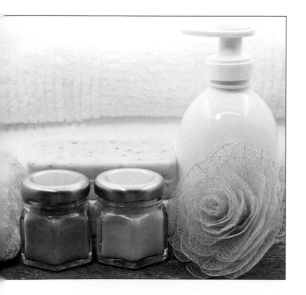

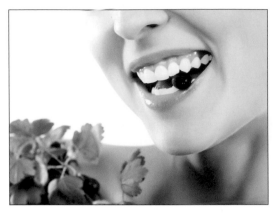

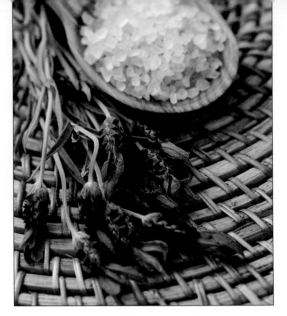

up this process by placing the container of gloss into the refrigerator for a few hours).

Honey Lip Gloss

Ingredients

1 tsp beeswax (you can find this at a craft store or at your local farmers' market)

½ tsp honey

2 tsp almond oil (optional)

Vitamin E oil from a capsule (optional)

Directions

1. Melt the beeswax and honey in a heat-proof jar in the microwave or use a double boiler method.
2. When the wax and honey are just melted, remove from the heat source and whisk in the almond oil and vitamin E oil, if you so desire. To remove the vitamin E oil from the capsule, simply prick the end of the capsule with a safety pin and squeeze it out.
3. Pour the mixture into the containers and allow to cool fully before using.

Note: If you want to add a citrus flavoring to this lip gloss, you can add a few drops of lemon or lime essential oil during the whisking stage.

"Make-up" Lip Balm

If you have leftover make-up (such as blush, lipstick, or shimmering eye shadow), don't let it go to waste. You can use it in this "recycled" lip balm.

Ingredients

Petroleum jelly

Blush, mineral eye shadow with shimmer, lipstick (only use one or two of these for your balm)

Essential oil for flavoring (optional)

Directions

1. Mix together the petroleum jelly and either the blush (add a little at a time until the desired color is attained), eye shadow, or the last remnants of any lipstick. Add essential oil and mix thoroughly.
2. Scoop the mixture into containers and put in the refrigerator to harden.

Note: You can also experiment by melting the jelly with some beeswax and then adding in the leftover makeup. The possibilities are endless.

Homemade Bath Products

Lavender Bath Salt

Pour several tablespoons of this into your bath as it fills for an extra-soothing, relaxing, and cleansing experience. You can also add powdered milk or finely ground old-fashioned oatmeal to make your skin especially soft. Toss in a few lavender buds if you have them.

Ingredients

2 cups coarse sea salt

½ cup Epsom salts

½ cup baking soda

4 to 6 drops lavender essential oil

Red and blue food coloring, if desired (use more red than blue to achieve a lavender color)

Mix all ingredients thoroughly and store in a glass jar or other airtight container.

Citrus scrub

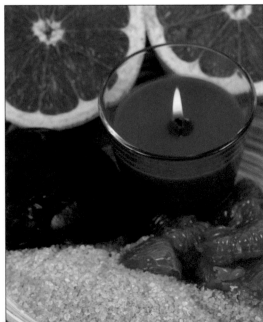

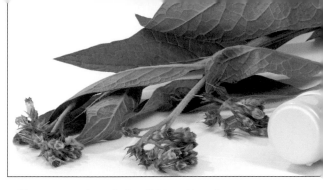

Citrus Scrub

Use this invigorating scrub to wake up your senses in the morning. The vitamin C in oranges serves as an astringent, making it especially good for oily skin.

Ingredients

½ orange or grapefruit

3 tbsp cornmeal

2 tbsp Epsom salts or coarse sea salt

Squeeze citrus juice and pulp into a bowl and add cornmeal and salts to form a paste. Rub gently over entire body and then rinse.

Healing Bath Soak

This bath soak will relax tired muscles, help to calm nerves, and leave skin soft and fragrant. You may also wish to add blackberry, raspberry, or violet leaves. Dried or fresh herbs can be used.

2 tbsp comfrey leaves

1 tbsp lavender

1 tbsp evening primrose flowers

1 tsp orange peel, thinly sliced or grated

2 tbsp oatmeal

Combine herbs and tie up in a small muslin or cheese-cloth sack. Leave under faucet as the tub fills with hot water. If desired, empty herbs into the bath water once the tub is full.

Rosemary Peppermint Foot Scrub

Use this foot rub to remove calluses, soften skin, and leave your feet feeling and smelling wonderful.

Ingredients

1 cup coarse sea salt

¼ cup sweet almond or olive oil

2 to 3 drops peppermint essential oil

1 to 2 drops rosemary essential oil

2 sprigs fresh rosemary, crushed, or ½ tsp dried rosemary

Combine all ingredients and massage into feet and ankles. Rinse with warm water and follow with a moisturizer.

Minty Cucumber Facial Mask

1 tbsp powdered milk

1 tsp plain yogurt (whole milk yogurt is best)

1 tsp honey

1 tsp fresh mint leaves

½ cucumber, peeled

Blend ingredients thoroughly, using a food processor or blender if available. Apply to face, avoiding eyes. Leave on for 10 to 15 minutes, then rinse.

After-Sun Comfrey Lotion

Comfrey root soothes skin and minimizes inflammation. Apply this lotion to sunburned skin for immediate relief and faster healing.

Ingredients

3 tbsp fresh comfrey root

1 cup water

1 tbsp beeswax, unrefined

¾ cup sweet almond oil or light cooking oil

¼ cup cocoa butter

4 vitamin E capsules

¼ cup aloe vera gel

1 tsp borax powder

12 to 16 drops essential oil (peppermint, lavender, or sandalwood are all good choices)

Directions

1. Place the comfrey root and water in a small pot and bring to a boil, simmering for about 30 minutes. Strain, retaining the water. Discard the root.
2. In a double boiler, combine beeswax, oil, and cocoa butter, stirring over low heat until melted. Remove from heat. Pierce the vitamin E capsules and add the oil from inside, stirring to combine.
3. In a separate saucepan, combine the comfrey water, aloe vera gel, and borax powder, stirring over low heat until the borax is fully dissolved. Allow to cool.
4. Once both mixtures are cooled to room temperature, pour the beeswax and oil mixture in a thin stream into the comfrey water mixture, whisking vigorously to combine (or use a food processor). Add the essential oils and continue mixing until thoroughly combined.
5. Cover and store in a cool, dark place.

Shampoo

Cleaning your hair can be as simple as making a baking soda and water paste, scrubbing it into your hair, and rinsing well. However, if you enjoy the feel of a sudsy, soapy, scented shampoo, try this recipe. You can substitute homemade soap flakes for the castile soap, if desired.

Ingredients

4 ounces liquid castile soap

3 tbsp fresh or dried herbs of your choice, boiled for 30 minutes in 2 cups water and strained

Pour the soap and herbal water into a jar, cover, and shake until well combined.

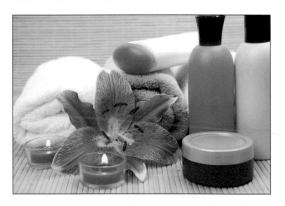

Hair Conditioner

This conditioner will add softness and volume to your hair. Avocado, bananas, and egg yolks are also great hair conditioners. Apply conditioner, allow to sit in hair a minimum of five minutes (longer for a deeper conditioning), and then rinse well. You may wish to shampoo a second time after using this conditioner.

Ingredients

1 cup olive oil
1 tsp lemon juice
1 tsp cider vinegar
2 tsp honey
6 to 10 drops essential oils, if desired

Whisk all ingredients together or blend in a food processor. Store in an airtight container.

Herbs for Your Hair

Herbs for dry hair	Burdock root, comfrey, elderflowers, lavender, marshmallow, parsley, sage, stinging nettle
Herbs for oily hair	Calendula, horsetail, lemon juice, lemon balm, mints, rosemary, witch hazel, yarrow
Herbs to combat dandruff	Burdock root, garlic, onion, parsley, rosemary, stinging nettle, thyme
Herbs for body and luster	Calendula, catnip, horsetail, licorice, lime flowers, nasturtium, parsley, rosemary, sage, stinging nettle, watercress
Herbs for shine	Horsetail, parsley, nettle, rosemary, sage, calendula
Herbs for hair growth	Aloe, arnica, birch, burdock, catmint, chamomile, horsetail, licorice, marigold, nettles, parsley, rosemary, sage, stinging nettle
Herbs for coloring	Brown: henna (reddish brown), walnut hulls, sage Blonde: calendula, chamomile, lemon, saffron, turmeric, rhubarb root

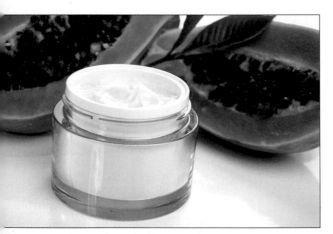

Papaya is ofen used in face creams for its anti-aging anti-acne properties.

Fruits and Vegetables for Your Skin

These fruits and vegetables can be applied directly to your face or blended together to make a mask. Leave on skin for 20 to 30 minutes and then rinse thoroughly with clean water.

Beneficial for Oily Skin	Beneficial for Normal Skin	Beneficial for Dry Skin
Lemons, grapes, limes, strawberries, grapefruits, apples	Peaches, papayas, tomatoes, apricots, bananas, persimmons, bell peppers, cucumbers, kiwi, pumpkins, watermelons	Carrots, iceberg lettuce, honeydew melons, avocados, cantaloupes

Tropical Face Cleanser

The vitamin C in kiwi has enzymatic and cleansing properties, and the apricot oil serves as a moisturizer. The ground almonds act as an exfoliant to remove dead skin cells. Yogurt has cleansing and moisturizing properties.

1 kiwi
¾ cup avocado, banana, apricot, peach, strawberry, or papaya (or some of each)
2 tbsp plain yogurt (whole milk is best)
1 tbsp apricot oil (almond oil also works well)
1 tbsp honey
1 tsp finely ground almonds

Purée all ingredients together. Massage into face and neck and rinse thoroughly with cool water. Store excess in refrigerator for one to two days.

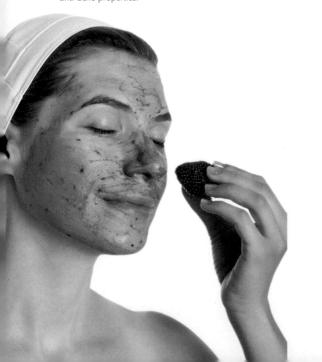

First Aid

It's impossible to predict when an accident will occur, but the more you educate yourself ahead of time, the better you'll be able to help should the need arise. The first step in an emergency situation should always be to call for help, but there are many things you can do to help the victim while you're waiting for assistance to arrive. The most important procedures are described in this section.

Drowning

1. As soon as the patient is in a safe place, loosen the clothing, if any.
2. Empty the lungs of water by laying the body breastdown and lifting it by the middle, with the head hanging down. Hold for a few seconds until the water drains out.
3. Turn the patient on his breast, face downward.
4. Give artificial respiration: Press the lower ribs down and forward toward the head, then release. Repeat about twelve times to the minute.
5. Apply warmth and friction to extremities, rubbing toward the heart.
6. Don't give up! Persons have been saved after hours of steady effort, and after being underwater for more than twenty minutes.
7. When natural breathing is reestablished, put the patient into a warm bed, with hot-water bottles, warm drinks, fresh air, and quiet.

Sunstroke

1. Move the patient to a cool place, or set up a structure around the patient to produce shade.
2. Loosen or remove any clothing around the neck and upper body.
3. Apply cold water or ice to the head and body, or wrap the patient in cold, damp cloths.
4. Encourage the patient to drink lots of water.

Burns and Scalds

1. Cover the burn with a thin paste of baking soda, starch, flour, petroleum jelly, olive oil, linseed oil, castor oil, cream, or cold cream.
2. Cover the burn first with the paste, then with a soft rag soaked in the paste.
3. Shock always accompanies severe burns, and must be treated.

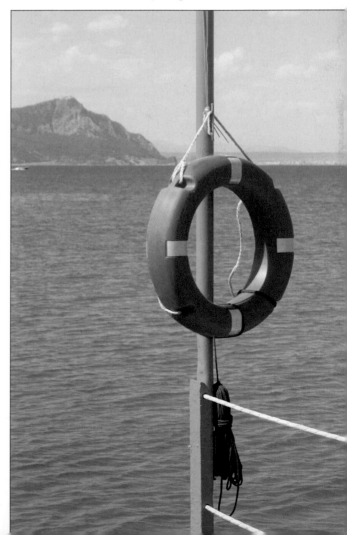

Keep a buoy nearby whenever spending time in or near the water.

A simple hand bandage can be made from any square cloth or handkerchief.

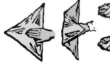

Shock or Nervous Collapse

A person suffering from shock has a pale face, cold skin, feeble breathing, and a rapid, feeble pulse, and will appear listless or half-dead.

1. Place the patient on his back with head low.
2. Give stimulants, such as hot tea or coffee.
3. Cover the patient with blankets.
4. Rub the limbs and place hot-water bottles around the body.

Cuts and Wounds

1. After making sure that no dirt or foreign substance is in the wound, apply a tight bandage to stop the bleeding.
2. Raise the wound above the heart to slow the bleeding.
3. If the blood comes out in spurts, it means an artery has been cut. For this, apply a tourniquet: Make a big knot in a handkerchief, tie it around the limb, with the knot just above the wound, and twist it until the flow is stopped.

Hemorrhage or Internal Bleeding

Internal bleeding usually comes from the lungs or stomach. If from the lungs, the blood is bright red and frothy, and is coughed up; if from the stomach, it is dark, and is vomited.

1. Help the patient to lie down, with head lower than body.
2. Encourage the patient to swallow small pieces of ice, and apply ice bags, snow, or cold water to the place where the bleeding is coming from.
3. Hot applications may be applied to the hands, arms, feet, and legs, but avoid stimulants, unless the patient is very weak.

How to Make a Tourniquet

The tourniquet is an appliance used to check severe bleeding. It consists of a bandage twisted more or less lightly around the affected part. The bandage—a cloth, strap, belt, necktie, neckerchief or towel—should be long enough to go around the arm or leg affected. It can then be twisted by inserting the hand, and the blood stopped.

If a stick is used, there is danger of twisting too tightly.

The tourniquet should not be used if bleeding can be stopped without it. When used it should be carefully loosened every 15 to 20 minutes to avoid permanent damage to tissues.

Fainting

Fainting is caused by a lack of blood supply to the brain and is cured by getting the heart to correct the lack.

1. Have the person lie down with the head lower than the body.
2. Loosen the clothing. Give fresh air. Rub the limbs. Use smelling salts.
3. Do not let the person get up until fully recovered.

Snake Bite

1. Put a tight cord or bandage around the limb between the wound and the heart. This should be loose enough to slip a finger under it.
2. Keep the wound lower than the heart. Try to keep the patient calm, as the faster the heart beats, the faster the venom will spread.
3. If you cannot get to a doctor quickly, suck the wound many times with your mouth or use a poison suction kit, if available.

Insect Stings

1. Wash with oil, weak ammonia, or very salty water, or paint with iodine.
2. A paste of baking soda and water also soothes stings.

Poison

1. First, get the victim away from the poison. If the poison is in solid form, such as pills, remove it from the victim's mouth using a clean cloth wrapped around your finger. Don't try this with infants because it could force the poison further down their throat.
2. If the poison is corrosive to the skin, remove the clothing from the affected area and flush with water for 30 minutes.
3. If the poison is in contact with the eyes, flush the victim's eyes for a minimum of 15 minutes with clean water.

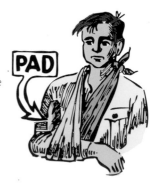

For elbow, arm, or wrist injuries, a simple sling can be made out of a piece of cloth or clothing.

How to Put Out Burning Clothing

1. If your clothing should catch fire, do not run for help, as this will fan the flames.
2. Lie down and roll up as tightly as possible in an overcoat, blanket, rug, or any woolen article—or lie down and roll over slowly, at the same time beating the fire with your hands. Smother the fire with a coat, blanket, or rug. Remember that woolen material is much less flammable than cotton.

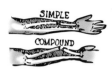

A compound fracture is one that breaks through the flesh.

Ice Rescue

1. Always have a rope nearby if you're working or playing on ice. This way, if someone falls through, you can tie one end to yourself and one to a tree or other secure anchor onshore before you attempt to rescue the person.
2. You could also throw one end to the victim if his head is above water.
3. Do not attempt to walk out to victim. Push out to him or crawl out on a long board or rail or tree trunk.
4. The person in the water should never try to crawl up on the broken ice, but should try merely to support himself and wait for help, if it is at hand.

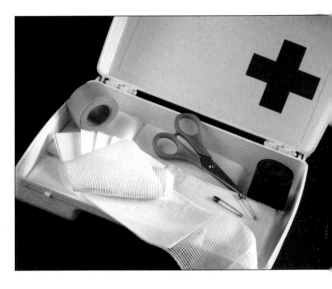

Broken Bone

A simple fracture is one in which the bone is broken but does not break the skin. In a compound fracture, the bone is broken and the skin and tissue are punctured or torn. A simple fracture may be converted into a compound fracture by careless handling, as a broken bone usually has sharp, saw-tooth edges, and just a little twist may push it through the skin.

1. Do not move the patient without supporting broken member by splints.
2. In a compound fracture, bleeding must be checked—by bandage over compress, if possible, or by tourniquet in extreme cases. Then splints may be applied.
3. Where skin is broken, infection is the great danger, so exercise care that compress or dressing is sterile and clean.

There are many ways to carry someone with an injury. If neck or spine injury is suspected, do not attempt to move the victim if you can get help to come to the victim instead. If the victim must be moved, the head and neck must first be carefully stabilized.

Dislocation

A dislocation is an injury where the head of a bone has slipped out of its socket at a joint.

1. Do not attempt to replace the joint. Even thumb and finger dislocations are more serious than usually realized.
2. Cover the joint with cloths wrung out in very hot or very cold water. For the shoulder—apply padding and make a sling for the arm.
3. Seek medical assistance.

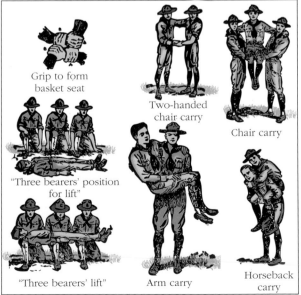

Grip to form basket seat

Two-handed chair carry

Chair carry

"Three bearers' position for lift"

"Three bearers' lift"

Arm carry

Horseback carry

First Aid Checklist

To administer effective first aid, it is important to maintain adequate supplies in each first aid kit. A first aid kit should include:

- Adhesive bandages: These are available in a large range of sizes for minor cuts, abrasions, and puncture wounds.
- Butterfly closures: These hold wound edges firmly together.
- Rolled gauze: These allow freedom of movement and are recommended for securing a wound dressing and/or pads. These are especially good for hard-to-bandage wounds.
- Nonstick sterile pads: These are soft, super-absorbent pads that provide a good environment for wound healing. These are recommended for bleeding and draining wounds, burns, or infections.
- First aid tapes: Various types of tapes should be included in each kit. These include adhesive, which is waterproof and extra strong for times when rigid strapping is needed; clear, which stretches with the body's movement and is good for visible wounds; cloth, recommended for most first aid taping needs, including taping heavy dressings (less irritating than adhesive); and paper, which is recommended for sensitive skin and is used for light and frequently changed dressings.
- Items that can also be included in each kit are tweezers, first aid cream, thermometer, an analgesic or equivalent, and an ice pack.

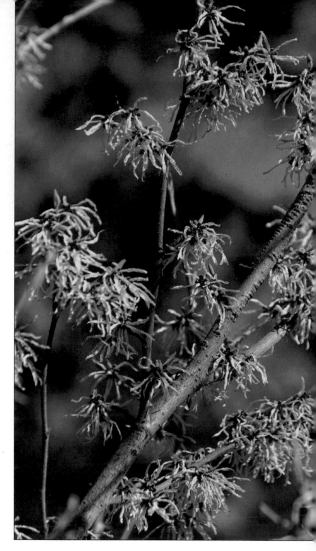

Witch hazel bark can be brewed and used to soothe irritated skin or eyes.

Nature's First Aid

Antiseptic or *wound-wash*: A handful of salt in a quart of hot water.

Balm for wounds: Balsam fir. The gum can be used as healing salve, usually spread on a piece of linen and laid over the wound for a dressing.

Cough remedy: Slippery elm or black cherry inner bark boiled, a pound to the gallon, boiled down to a pint, and given a teaspoonful every hour.

Linseed can be used the same way; add honey if desired. Or boil down the sap of the sweet birch tree and drink it on its own or mixed with the other remedies.

Diuretic: A decoction of the inner bark of elder is a powerful diuretic.

Inflammation of the eyes or skin: Wash with a strong tea made of the bark of witch hazel.

Lung balm: Infusion of black cherry bark and root is a powerful tonic for lungs and bowels. Good also as a skin wash for sores.

Poison ivy: Wash every hour or two with hot soapy water, then with hot salt water.